POPULAR MEDICINE
IN THIRTEENTH-CENTURY ENGLAND

POPULAR MEDICINE
IN THIRTEENTH-CENTURY ENGLAND

INTRODUCTION AND TEXTS

Tony Hunt

D. S. BREWER

First published 1990 by D. S. Brewer, Cambridge
Reprinted 1994

D. S. Brewer is an imprint of Boydell & Brewer Ltd
PO Box 9, Woodbridge, Suffolk IP12 3DF, UK
and of Boydell & Brewer Inc.
PO Box 41026, Rochester, NY 14604–4126, USA

ISBN 0 85991 290 6

British Library Cataloguing in Publication Data available
Popular medicine in thirteenth-century England
   1. England. Folk medicine. Remedies, 1200–1300
   I. Hunt, Tony
   615.8'82'0942
   ISBN 0–85991–290–6

Library of Congress Catalog Card Number 88–37097

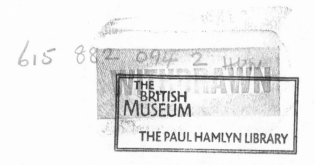
This publication is printed on acid-free paper

Printed in the United States of America

To the Memory of Stevie Hilton

Contents

Preface

As early as 1912, on the occasion of a meeting of the British Medical Association in Liverpool, Burroughs Wellcome & Co. were able to issue a beautifully illustrated historical sketch of early English medicine entitled 'Anglo-Saxon Leechcraft'[1] and since that time the subject has continued to attract expert scholarly attention.[2] The history of medieval English medicine in the post-Conquest period, however, has fared much less well.[3] Health services in the reigns of Henry I and Stephen have been described and applauded by E. J. Kealey,[4] who identifies 90 physicians and 113 hospitals in the period 1110–1154 and Lady Clay's study of English hospitals has been usefully reissued.[5] Unfortunately, R. S. Gottfried's *Doctors and Medicine in Medieval England 1340–1530* (Princeton, 1986) cannot be said to have rendered comparable service.[6] What has been totally lacking is a study of the thirteenth century when medical knowledge began to be disseminated in the vernacular. Whilst Rossell Hope Robbins opened our eyes to the vast storehouse of medical knowledge represented by unpublished and unstudied Middle English manuscripts,[7] no scholar has yet attended to the Anglo-Norman materials, some of which, of course, may have been sources of the Middle English writings. I have therefore set myself the task of rescuing Anglo-Norman medical texts from oblivion. In a later volume I shall edit a series of relatively learned treatises in which quite technical medical terminology is for the first time rendered in the vernacular. In the present volume, however, I have contented myself with presenting a conspectus of what I prefer to call popular medicine, using the term to indicate a non-theoretical medicine exclusively concerned with the therapeutic administration of naturally occurring *materia medica*. Some students of the subject may use the expressions ethnopharmacy, ethnomedicine or ethnoiatry, whilst others may cling to the rather traditional 'folk medicine'.[8] My principal purpose is to put into print for the first time a collection of primary materials which adequately represents the state of popular medicine in thirteenth-century England,[9] whether the texts be in Latin, French or English. A conspicuous omission here is a set of versified receipts known as the *Novele Cirurgerie*. Having drawn attention to it in an earlier publication,[10] I now refer the reader to a forthcoming edition of the work from Professors C. B. Hieatt and R. F. Jones rather than duplicate their work here. The printing of reliable texts based on sound philological principles is an essential condition for any future assessment of the debt of medieval popular medicine to Roman medicine and the *antidotaria* and *receptaria* of the early Middle Ages. I have written a short history of the medical receipt simply to set the stage for such an assessment. My analysis of the medical receipts printed in the present volume makes it clear that we are dealing essentially with lists of *materia medica*.

A significant proportion of the renewed interest in the early history of medicine is, in fact, concerned with pharmacognosy and the general study of *materia medica*. Whilst the debt of medieval medicine to the authorities of Antiquity has been well documented in this respect,[11] it is becoming clear that its relation to popular medicine in other ages and other places is of prime importance.[12] There is a fascinating continuity to be observed from the ancients' debt to popular medicine to widespread practices in those parts of today's world which have not been cured to death by the pharmaceutical industry.[13] Ironically, the latter's debt to popular medical knowledge should not be underestimated. Again and again we see how modern therapeutic discoveries can be related to earlier practices. J. M. Riddle has remarked, for example, that A. P. Dustin's report in 1938 on the antimitotic properties of colchicine drawn from the autumn crocus (*Colchicum autumnale* L.) corresponds to a suggestion found in Dioscorides.[14] It is hardly possible to consult an issue of the *Journal of Ethnopharmacology* or the quarterly *Current Research in Medicinal and Aromatic Plants*, published by the Central Institute of Medicinal and Aromatic Plants, Lucknow, without noting correspondences between modern research discoveries, popular practices in the modern world, and the records of ancient and medieval medicine.[15] It is not surprising that Alexander Nelson wrote in his handbook *Medical Botany* 'Even today it is not wise to dismiss out of hand "traditional remedies" as useless and "country cures" as without foundation'.[16] Thus both technical literature and popular medical practices have been drawn on for nominations for screening in connection with a catalogue of potential plant anti-tumour agents.[17] The potential relevance of previously exploited medicinal plants[18] to the treatment of a whole range of recalcitrant medical conditions makes the careful recording of medieval medical receipts a far from merely antiquarian task. For this reason I have appended glossaries of the *materia medica* to each collection of receipts that I have printed below. For practical reasons I have suggested the most likely identification for each medicinal plant but the full range of possibilities can be discovered by consulting my *Plant Names of Medieval England* (Cambridge, 1989).[19] The empirical tradition of medieval medicine[20] is important not only to screening programmes set up in modern drug research, but also, in consequence, to the whole issue of conservation. Sir Peter Scott wrote 'There still remains today a vast number of plant species whose potential is unknown. Maybe they will never have more than aesthetic value to mankind. But who knows where, for example, the next anti-cancer agent may be found'.[21] At the time of writing doctors at Nottingham University Hospital have conducted trials which strongly suggest the efficacy of feverfew in the treatment of migraine. At Kew Professor Vernon Heywood, Director of the Plants Programme for the International Union for the Conservation of Nature, has been a tireless campaigner for conservation, arguing that 'No one on earth can say that there is one single plant we could afford to lose'. With almost eighty percent of the world's population still dependent on popular medicine[22] and the increasing challenges to the pharmaceutical companies to find new cures, it is clear that the estimated loss of thousands of plant species through the projected thinning out of the world's rain forests over the next half century would represent a drastic step backwards in terms of world health care. The present study therefore seeks to record as accurately as possible the *materia medica* of the thirteenth century on the basis of previously unstudied documents which provide a wealth of lexical material which has not entered the standard dictionaries. With so little comparable material yet in print,[23] it would be premature to embark on any extended source study, though this will be an important task in the future. From the linguistic point of view the evidence of the following pages confirms the view of the inseparability of Latin, French and English in the thirteenth century when they did not function as discrete units but mingled in a process of reciprocal support whereby deficiencies, for example of terminology, in one were remedied by another in an attempt to overcome the disadvantages produced by the lack of a consistent or systematic teaching programme.[24]

The writing of this study has been immeasurably facilitated by the ever helpful staff of the Wellcome Historical Medical Library, London, where it is always a pleasure to work. For much stimulus and encouragement I am greatly indebted to Professor Linda Voigts who has taken every opportunity to share her knowledge with me and to put me in touch with other workers in the field. To the Committee on Research in Arts and Divinity in the University of St Andrews I am immensely grateful for a generous grant towards the costs of publication. My greatest benefactor, however, has been the British Academy, which through its award of a Research Readership (1986–88) has enabled me to work in an area which I otherwise could not even have approached and has already engendered further projects. The encouragement offered by such an award has been of incalculable value at a time when greater political faith has been placed in Britain's supermarkets than in its universities. Finally, to my friends in London I am grateful for much help and encouragement and, particularly, to Diana Harrison for her long-standing hospitality.

Chapter One

INTRODUCTION

History of the Medical Receipt

The medical receipt has a long and unusually stable history.[1] From Ancient China and India, the Sumerians, Assyrians, Babylonians and Egyptians, its fortunes can be traced by a continuous evolution in the West which takes in Hippocratic medicine, the schools of Rome and Alexandria, the renovation of Greek medical texts by the translators of early medieval Islam, the transfer of such materials to the celebrated schools of Toledo and Salerno, and the gradual absorption of a vast residue of medical prescriptions by the monastic schools of Western Europe. All this attests to an extraordinary continuity of copying over several thousand years. As W. R. Dawson remarks,

> When a drug really possesses the virtues attributed to it, and is an effective remedy for disease, its survival into modern times is quite natural, but the fact that many quite fantastic remedies have been carried on almost to our own days, is definite proof of the slavish copying from the works of one writer to another in a continuous line that originated many centuries ago on the banks of the Nile.[2]

Equally striking is the receipt's continuity of form. Its characteristic structure is already discernible in Babylonian medicine where the scheme *indication – preparation – application* was early established, and a comparable stability in its linguistic features gave rise to set formulae constituting a model which was followed by the writers of the *Corpus Hippocraticum*, albeit with some degree of flexibility.[3] The use of linguistic formulae remained a characteristic feature of the receipt, the nature of the formulae naturally varying according to the language employed.[4]

In contrast to such striking consistency in form and phraseology there are important differences of medical outlook which helped to shape the development of the receipt. The Babylonian conception of illness rested on metaphysical, even irrational, beliefs including the notion that illness is punishment for sins. In Greek therapeutic writings illness is not given metaphysical interpretation, but is closely related to the conduct, circumstances and constitution of the patient. Further, illness is seen as a dynamic process with its own pattern or progression of changes which may be carefully charted, and not as a state which arrives and departs with unforeseeable suddenness. Dietary control therefore becomes an essential part of medical treatment.[5] Inevitably, however, the evolution of the medical receipt displays a mixture of aetiological notions and for many centuries in the Christian era mingles charms and magic with pharmaceutical preparations.

The foundations of Western medicine were immovably laid by the 'Father of Medicine', Hippocrates, and the rationalist philosopher of Pergamon, Galen. The *Corpus Hippocraticum*[6] is a disparate collection of some 65 works mostly dating from the period 450–350 BC, all but a few of them anonymous, and many of them teeming with problems which involve fundamental historical questions such as the influence exerted by the schools of Cos and Cnidos.[7] Whilst the Corpus is significant for establishing the dignity and rigour of medical practice[8] and for combating the irrational, the incompetent and the false,[9] its pragmatic emphasis on studying the course of the disease, on control of diet, and on the administration of a restricted number of drugs (substantially those of its Eastern predecessors) would suggest that there is relatively little to be gleaned on the subject of receipts and *materia medica*. Yet a recent investigation[10] proposes that there are 3000 references to plants and vegetable products, covering approximately 230 different vegetable substances, including, in order of frequency, wine, honey, oil, vinegar, myrrh, hellebore, hydromel, cumin etc. They are largely concentrated in the treatises on gynaecology.[11] In its understanding of how drugs work Hippocratic pharmacology marks a considerable advance on Aristotelian drug theory and elaborates a clear explanation based on *krasis* of humours, elements and qualities. But there is more than *krasis* theory and pharmaceuticals. Parts of the *Corpus* display considerable familiarity with herbal medicine and ancient lore concerning herbs, minerals and animal products. Much of what was of value in the old receipts was clearly retained. The influence of the *Corpus Hippocraticum* was, of course, largely indirect, the early Latin translations being mostly limited to a few treatises dealing with practical matters of diagnosis and cure.[12] The Middle Ages produced its own *Corpus Hippocraticum*,[13] but it is difficult to ascertain exactly how its texts were used and whether they received much study independently of Galen's commentaries and of the influence of Rhazes in his *Liber Almansoris*.[14]

Between Hippocrates and Galen there exists a sort of 'silence des siècles' – six centuries! Most of what we can safely recover from this interval survives as excerpts in Galen himself.[15] These excerpts from his predecessors are predominantly medical receipts.[16] At the beginning of *De compositione medicamentorum secundum locos* Galen promises to emulate his predecessors in following the order of the parts of the body, starting with the head and working down to the toes – the *a capite ad calcem* technique continued throughout the Middle Ages. The full form of the receipt is composed of four parts; rubric (προγραφή), indication (ἐπαγγελία), composition (σύνθεσις) and preparation (σκευασία). The *rubric* is the most variable in extent: the medicament may be described in terms of its type, its effect, the human organ it is destined for, or the rubric may include supplementary information on a person with whom it is connected, perhaps a successful promoter of the cure or a patient who has been effectively treated with it. In the medieval receipts the rubric is usually much simplified. The *indication* lists the complaints and disorders for which the receipt is deemed efficacious. The *composition* enumerates the ingredients and their proportions and quantities. Dawson had already remarked in his study of Egyption medicine that 'The quantities of each drug are meticulously specified in the prescriptions, minute fractional notation being employed, and from this may be inferred that considerable care was used in dispensing'.[17] This is a feature which disappears almost completely from the medieval vernacular receipts and leads to the contrary inference. Dawson also remarked that the ingredients might vary in number from 3 or 4 to 37, with 'a preference for rare and bizarre elements'.[18] The medieval receipts, whilst being infinitely variable in the number of their ingredients, do not display the taste for the bizarre or exotic which is sometimes imagined. Finally, the *preparation* provides instructions for producing the medicament and for its administration. Also found in Galen, but less commonly, is a short-form receipt which lacks both detail and precision and exhibits no consistent structure. It usually lists a small number of ingredients, without quantities, and the συμμετρία is missing. Such receipts are frequently found under 'indications'. Galen's works also provide much useful information on antidotes and theriacs.[19] The *materia medica* treated by him is estimated at approximately 473 vegetable products.[20] Galen's reception in medieval Europe is in need of detailed study.[21] We know that a major avenue of access was formed by the Greek-Arabic translations in Salerno and Toledo which were rapidly accepted in university medicine. For the study of medical receipts the most important writings are *De compositione medicamentorum secundum locos, De compositione medicamentorum secundum genera* and *De antidotis*. Galen was a fiercely honest controversialist and his rationalist ideas, though embodied in a tiresomely prolix style, dominated medicine until the Renaissance. Heavily dependent on the theory of humours and never less than reverential towards Hippocrates, he added to the number of drugs in use, generally following the theory of 'contraria contrariis', and sometimes indulging in extremely complicated pharmaceutical preparations.

A fundamental influence on the medieval medical receipt was the popular tradition bequeathed by Roman medicine. At first heavily impregnated with magic and superstition, the practice of medicine in Rome was for long left to foreigners until, after the third century BC, under Greek influence, medicine grew in prestige and medical writings were produced.[22] Whilst an idea of the Roman pharmacopeia is best obtained from the exhaustive treatment of *materia medica* in Dioscorides and Pliny (see below pp.5f.), the tradition of receipt collections is attested by a series of writers who were exploited throughout the Middle Ages and modern knowledge of whom is largely due to the editions prepared by Valentin Rose, which are gradually being replaced by the work of recent scholars. At the head of the tradition stands Aulus Cornelius Celsus (c. 25 BC – c. 50 AD) who reproduces much of the teaching of the Alexandrian school.[23] Book 5 of his *De medicina* deals with maladies affecting the whole body that are combated by *medicamenta* rather than general rules of regimen (*victus*) and Book 6 with disorders affecting specific parts of the body, beginning with the head. In these books the receipts are embedded in lengthy descriptions of the various disorders and of their treatment.

A more influential text was the *Compositiones* (c. 43–48 AD) of Scribonius Largus (fl. c.14–54 AD) which contains 271 receipts involving 242 plants and vegetable products.[24] They are ordered by indications, that is under the illnesses for which they are efficacious. The simpler preparations are described first, then the more complex ones. Scribonius was probably a Greek freedman and military doctor and he seems to have been familiar, even if not directly, with the work of Nicander of Colophon (2nd C. BC), especially the *Alexipharmaca*.[25] Like Nicander, Scribonius divides his receipts into symptomatology and therapy. As in the case of his debt to Celsus, it is most likely that he had access to a common source. Indeed, his most recent editor, Sconocchia, explains many of the similarities in his writings with other authors by suggesting the existence of a 'medico-cultural koiné' in the second half of the first century.[26] In his turn Scribonius influenced Galen, Marcellus Empiricus, Cassius Felix, the *Medicina Plinii* and a number of *antidotaria*.

Similar in arrangement to Scribonius's work and equally redolent of the practices of magic and folklore (including amulets and incantations) is the *Liber Medicinalis* of Quintus Serenus Sammonicus about whom almost nothing is surely known.[27] The *Liber* may, in fact, date from any point between the end of the second century and the first half of the fourth. It is a collection of versified medical receipts comprising 1107 hexameters and divided into 64 chapters. Despite some displacement of material the poem generally respects the *a capite ad calcem* order in the sequence of ailments. Most of the receipts are drawn from popular medicine as already published by Pliny, who together with the so-called *Medicina Plinii* is a major source. The titles or rubrics vary in the different MSS and give the appearance of having been altered by later writers. Under each heading many receipts, usually very short and often consisting merely of a list of simples, are coordinated by *aut, vel* or *sive*. The *Liber Medicinalis* enjoyed considerable popularity in the ninth and tenth centuries, but was eclipsed by other texts in the next two centuries, only to be subject to a revival in the Renaissance.[28] Quintus Serenus was not, it seems, himself a doctor, but a practical writer, sympathising with the needs of the poor and chastising the *medici* for their expensive prescriptions with an excessive number of ingredients. The *Liber* is a kind of formulary of practical medicine for laymen, wholly didactic and never theoretical in tone or matter.

Perhaps contemporary with Quintus Serenus is the third-century North African Quintus Gargilius Martialis, a soldier, born in Auzia, and evidently a reader of Dioscorides and Galen.[29] He is known to have written an agricultural treatise, which included the surviving *De hortis*, a set of remedies for cattle (*Curae boum*), and a collection of about 60 receipts or *compositiones*, the *Medicinae*. Gargilius is greatly indebted to Pliny whom he often cites. His approach is brisk and practical, especially with regard to the availability of drugs. He lists ingredients, gives directions for mixing them, and describes their administration. He does not speculate on the manner in which they achieve their effects or mention observed side-effects. His *materia medica* comprises approximately 60 different plants or vegetable products.[30] His vegetable remedies make considerable use of leafy vegetables (especially cabbage, lettuce and endive), bulbs, aromatic herbs (especially fennel, rue, sorrel and mint), orchard fruits and nuts. He deals mostly with simples and provides some discussion of substitutes. Amongst the ailments dealt with bites, stings and poisons are prominent. Digestive disorders affecting the alimentary canal, liver and spleen, are the subject of almost half the remedies and urinary problems are also given special attention. The influence of folk medicine is everywhere apparent and includes the presence of gibberish, chants, prayers, the use of magic colours and numbers, rituals concerning the gathering of plants, and references to phases of the moon. From Pliny comes the understanding of homeopathy.

Folk medicine also plays a considerable role in the *Liber de medicamentis* dedicated to the Emperor Theodosius by Marcellus ('Empiricus') of Bordeaux and written c. 395–410 AD.[31] Much of his work, including his selection and description of simples, is entirely traditional. The collection of receipts which constitutes the *Liber* is distributed over 36 chapters, following the *a capite ad calcem* sequence, and is entirely empirical. Nevertheless, in his frequently bizarre, gallicized Latin Marcellus reports many rustic practices and beliefs and is a source of precious information for folklorists. He uses something like 350 plant names and there remain many unsolved lexical problems.[32] His own lexical interest in the *synonyma herbarum*, not just in the plants themselves, foreshadows medieval developments (the rise of synonymies), as does Marcellus's emphasis on *indigenes*. A third way in which he anticipates the characteristics of medieval receipt collections is in his adherence to polypharmacy – the ingredients of his receipts rarely number less than ten and may exceed twenty (to a maximum of 73!) The preparation of the *composita* is often described in considerable detail. We do not know whether Marcellus was a Christian, but he includes in the *Liber* some 65 incantations, charms and magic formulas ranging from gibberish to complex rituals. Magic tokens such as amulets, phylacteries and rings are also frequently mentioned, as is a variety of apotropaic devices.[33] The directions for the collection of herbs are often extremely detailed and complex.[34] Of all the medical writers of the first five centuries of the Christian era Marcellus is the most conspicuous forerunner of the medieval composers of receipt collections.

Marcellus's sources include Scribonius Largus and the so-called *Medicina Plinii*. Whole sections of Scribonius are copied out without acknowledgement, a not uncommon practice in the history of medical literature. The *Medicina Plinii* is an epitome of the relevant parts of Pliny made in the fourth century.[35] It was extremely influential.[36]

In the middle of the fifth century the Christian Cassius Felix[37] wrote his compendium *Medicinae Liber*, a work dominated by Hippocratic-Galenic humoral pathology and totally devoid (with perhaps four exceptions) of magic elements. The chapters on each disorder take the form etymology, definition, aetiology, symptomatology, incidence, therapy. Whilst any of these sections may sometimes be omitted or radically abbreviated, the section on therapy is often expanded to form a sequence of receipts. Throughout there is a pragmatic concern for the circumstances of the individual patient. The *a capite ad calcem* pattern is carefully maintained.

Similar in arrangement are the *Celerum atque tardarum passionum libri* of Cassius's predecessor Caelius Aurelianus,[38] who through his translations transmitted to the West the important writings of the great representative of the Methodist school of medicine, Soranus of Ephesus. Caelius Aurelianus himself was a member of the Methodist sect and one of a number of North African writers on medicine who are sometimes held to constitute a 'school'. Unfortunately the translations of Caelius Aurelianus are known only through early printed editions and fragments of a MS from Lorsch. In them the account of each disease usually comprises the etymology of the name, definition of the disease, description of symptoms, methods of distinguishing other similar diseases, naming the part affected, an account of the treatment practised by the Methodists followed by that of the treatment by others together with a refutation of such treatment.

In addition to the popular tradition of receipt collections represented by the writers discussed above there is a second important tradition illustrated by a series of treatises on *materia medica*, stemming from the ancient *rhizotomika* and owing much to Pliny the Elder. Pliny (c. 23–79 AD)[39] is, indeed, a major influence on subsequent medical writers including the compilers of receipt collections. His encyclopaedic *Historia Naturalis* in 37 Books (nos 20–32 of which treat animals and plants) maintained an unbroken tradition of popularity for 1500 years. Pliny records a great deal of magic and superstition and is more than a little credulous, and yet the very fact that he records so voluminously makes him a valuable witness to contemporary practices. For *reportage* he has few rivals. Over 1000 trees and herbs are mentioned by him and a very large number of therapeutic activities.[40] He himself remarks (Book 19, 189) that one can only understand the nature of plants through studying their medicinal effects. Thus the receipts in the *Natural History* are intended to illustrate the properties of individual plants. Already we find the doctrine which Paracelsus was later to elaborate as the 'Doctrine of Signatures', an extension of the principle of 'sympathetic' therapy or 'similia similibus curantur'. Thus some outward feature of the plant is perceived to resemble some symptom of human disorder and consequently held to be efficacious in the treatment of that disorder. Many passages in the *Natural History* illustrate or presuppose such a doctrine. So, whilst we should not look to Pliny for structural features of the medical receipt, we discover in him much about the attitudes and beliefs which guided the medicinal use of plants.

From the purely scientific point of view Pedanius Dioscorides of Anazarbos (fl. 40–65 AD) is of much greater importance.[41] He is the standard authority on *materia medica* for 1500 years, an essential pharmacopeia to which almost all subsequent works on drug therapy are heavily indebted, and the fountainhead of the Western tradition of herbals (even though the Latin Dioscorides was not illustrated). Books 3 and 4 of his *De materia medica*, composed c. 64 AD, describe some 500 plants,[42] many from overseas,[43] and in all Dioscorides refers to over 1000 natural products,[44] in, it has been calculated, approximately 4700 medical usages. The scope, reliability and empiricism of the *De materia medica* ensured for it a far-reaching success.[45] By the second century a revisor had introduced alphabetical ordering of the materials and a set of lexical glosses consisting of *synonyma* in various languages was early on affixed to the beginning of most chapters. A Latin translation had appeared by the sixth century, but it was superseded by a new translation, the *Dioscorides alphabeticus* of c.1100, with stricter alphabetical arrangement. As a treatise on the medicinal properties of various products it naturally includes receipts by way of illustration.

Much of Dioscorides was disseminated in the fourth century by Oribasius (325–404 AD) who as court physician was commissioned by the Emperor Julian to assemble a compendium of medical writings. His *Synagogai* in 70 books he reduced to a *Synopsis* for the use of his son and this work was twice translated into Latin, probably in or around Ravenna at the beginning of the sixth century, together with the *Euporista*.[46] Many of the medical receipts so transmitted were exploited by later writers.

Another influential work was Pseudo-Apuleius, *Herbarius*, a book of simples which illustrates some 130 plants. It was written in the fourth century and the name Apuleius was probably attached to it because of an association between Apuleius and the cult of Aesculapius.[47] The work is transmitted in over 50 MSS, very often in the company of Pseudo-Musa, *De vettonica*, the anonymous *De taxone* and Sextus Placitus, *Medicina ex animalibus*.[48]

Equally influential was the *Ex herbis femininis*, transmitted in approximately 30 MSS, 13 of which are dated to before 1200.[49] There are 71 chapters, 19 of which are translated directly from Dioscorides with minimal changes. On the other hand, 14 chapters appear to be completely new. Lavishly illustrated in most of the MSS, the *Ex herbis femininis* was obviously much easier to use than the vast *De materia medica* and contained more detailed medicinal directions of a practical nature. It contains very few supernatural elements. Many of the receipts seem to have been drawn from an anonymous *receptarius*, possibly of African origin. Chapter headings were added and later expanded. There is an important translation in Old English. The original

Ex herbis was probably produced in southern Europe towards the end of the fifth century.

At the end of this early Christian era we have the last representative of the Alexandrian school in Paul of Aegina (625–690),[50] an important mediator of Greco-Roman medical knowledge to the Arab physicians of three centuries later. Book 7 of his *Pragmateia* contains a considerable number of receipts and catalogues 600 plants.

From the sixth century medicine moves into the monasteries. As the gloom of the so-called 'Dark Ages' is gradually dispelled, so we are led to a revaluation of *Mönchs-medizin*.[51] The obligations set forth in ch. 36 (*De infirmis fratribus*) of the Rule of St Benedict gave a considerable impetus to the acquisition of medical knowledge by the monks. The monasteries became the repositories of large numbers of medical MSS.[52] Already in the time of Cassiodorus Ravenna had become the 'Western Roman Alexandria' and a canon of translations of Hippocratic works was already emerging.[53] Cassiodorus himself mentions Dioscorides, Hippocrates, Galen and Caelius Aurelianus. Isidore of Seville in Book 4 of his *Etymologiae* provided a summary of the principal doctrines and terminology of Greco-Roman medicine.[54] The famous monastery school of St Gallen was active in the production or collection of medical receipts[55] and its celebrated monastic plan depicts a *herbularius* which was given literary embodiment in Walahfrid Strabo's poem *Hortulus*, composed c. 842.[56] The monastic catalogues reveal a wide range of pharmaceutical literature including treatises on *materia medica*, receipt collections, hermeneumata and treatises on weights and measures, all of them the legacy of the Greco-Roman tradition.[57] In a series of short medical and botanical treatises, it is true, we witness some attempts at revising and reworking ancient materials. In a ninth-century 'Botanicus',[58] for example, 36 of its 62 chapters are lifted straight from Pseudo-Apuleius, 10 of them being freely adapted. The sources of 26 chapters have not been identified. The whole text is a collection of receipts arranged under the name of an individual plant, as in Pseudo-Apuleius. A notable number of receipts relate to superstitions. Also in the ninth century a number of modest medical compendia emerge[59] and continue to be produced until the school of Salerno makes its great impact. The period from 600–1100 AD is essentially an age of conservation, of copying, of consolidation. There is little innovation. Most of the medical works produced are anonymous, many of them being *receptaria* and *antidotaria*. There are also treatises relating to the virtues of *materia medica* and certain natural conditions (winds, natural location etc.) known as *dynamidia*.[60] It is rare to find a treatise by a named author.[61] Such a case is that of Crispus, a deacon in the Milanese church, who died almost a century before the Carolingian revival of learning, and who composed a therapeutic compendium, *Medicinae Libellus*.[62] This consists of a prose introduction and 241 hexameters in which the author leans heavily on Serenus Sammonicus and the *Medicina Plinii*.[63] According to his own testimony the purpose of the work is to initiate the dedicatee, Maurus praepositus in Mantua, in the uses of medicinal herbs. It is divided into 26 chapters subdivided according to various disorders taken *a capite ad calcem*. For each disorder Crispus offers a brief symptomatology and a therapy. In such limited space he confines himself to the practical description of the drugs and their administration without any theory or speculation. There are clear traces of folk medicine, but little of the magical or superstitious practices that are found in Serenus or Pliny. Crispus's work is isolated and does not seem to have exercised any influence on later writers. The opposite is true of the most characteristic productions of the period, the *receptaria* and *antidotaria*, published by Jörimann and Sigerist.[64] In the Greco-Roman tradition receipts are found embedded in therapeutic treatises rather than being assembled in collections. There are about 200 in Celsus and even more, albeit very short, in Galen, where they are to all intents and purposes concentrated in three treatises. The practical needs of the monasteries, however, resulted in a demand for receipt collections large and small and there remains a vast mass of unedited material. The division into *receptaria* and *antidotaria* indicates some important distinctions. The *receptaria* belong, strictly speaking, to medical rather than pharmaceutical literature; that is to say, they deal largely with simples, are arranged according to indication i.e. the disorder for which they are efficacious, they are usually anonymous and without any title or rubric (other than the indication), and they are of a generally popular character. Many of the *receptaria* do not strictly observe the *a capite ad calcem* sequence. The *antidotaria* are more complex and belong more properly to pharmaceutical literature. Although the term 'antidote' was at first used to indicate a remedy for poisonous drinks, it was soon extended in use to cover all types of poisons and by Galen's time might be used in the most general sense of remedy against any kind of disorder. Whilst in the *receptaria* the receipts are arranged in consideration of their effects (and hence aptness for treating certain diseases), in the *antidotaria* the arrangement is normally by medicinal form (e.g. electuary, plaster, pill, trochisk), in other words in consideration of their preparation, and the multiple indications are therefore contained within the receipt. These compounded *medicamenta* are frequently of considerable complexity and it may be doubted whether some of them were either practical or efficacious – some may have been intended largely for teaching purposes. With the passage of time an alphabetical arrangement was often introduced (especially at Salerno). In the *antidotaria* the prescriptions are given names or titles according either to their presumed inventor, a famous patient, their main ingredient, their principal purpose or some other salient characteristic. Then follow indications, the list of ingredients and their measures, their preparation, and finally application. Monastic medicine naturally emphasized *indigenes* rather than *exotica* but the *antidotaria* frequently offer long receipts of great complexity. The remedies proposed are entirely pharmacological and there is nothing of the folk medicine which sometimes infiltrates the *receptaria*, nor gynaecological treatments and prognostic methods concerning childbirth which somewhat surprisingly occur in monastic *receptaria* and hint at the increasing scope within the community of *Mönchsmedizin*. In the *antidotaria* weights and measures are normally precise and detailed, whilst the *receptaria* often replace the *siliquae*, *oboli*, *scrupuli*, *drachmae*, *unciae*, *denarii* etc. with more popular and indeterminate measures like *pugna plena*, *quantum tres digitis levare potes*, a nutshell, an eggshell etc. The ingredients are principally *vegetabilia* and monastic medicine shows a considerable diminution in the use of *animalia* (it retains milk, butter and cheese, of course) and an even greater reduction in *chimica* and *mineralia*. In all types of receipts a great deal is taken for granted and presupposes a sound knowledge of plant morphology or recourse to a herbal. Thus many receipts make no attempt to specify which parts of the plants recorded are to be used. There is little on their collection or preservation. Dosage is rarely specified and dietary considerations play a small role. Directions concerning possible reactions of the patient and subsequent precautions are very infrequent. From time to time a receipt is found to present full details on these matters whilst others offer nothing but a list of ingredients. This startling variety reflects the heterogeneous nature of the collections, many receipts being traceable to Antiquity whilst others appear to be entirely without analogues. The treatment of illness itself is often confined to the simple indication, there being nothing on diagnosis or symptomatology. The collections of receipts are anonymous and there is never any formal introduction and statement of aims as were found in earlier writers. The period from 600 to 1100 represents a very minor chapter in the history of medicine and an essentially conservative one in the evolution of pharmacotherapy.[65] Historically it marks the transition from Greco-Roman medicine to the great developments at Salerno which transmit the advances and discoveries of Arabic medicine.

The period 800–1100 marks the Golden Age of Arabic pharmacology.[66] The importance of Arabic medicine has long been recognised[67] and the assimilation in the West of its guiding principles and progressive ideas has been the subject of a number of studies.[68] Less well known to medieval scholars are the advances made by Arabic writers in the field of *materia medica*[69] and pharmacotherapy. The speed with which the debt to the Greco-Roman tradition was consolidated and then superseded is a remarkable phenomenon.[70] Despite varied Oriental and central Asian influences from China, India and Persia and indigenous traditions of Iraq, Syria, Palestine and Egypt, Arabic pharmacology was firmly based on Greek models, notably Dioscorides. The legacy of Antiquity was then reworked and refined by Syriac Christian scholars and physicians working under the auspices of caliphs and private patrons. Outstanding among them was Ḥunain ibn Is'hāq (809–73)[71] who translated into Arabic the most important of the available Greek medical writers. Ḥunain and his associates represent a powerhouse in the generation of scientific attitudes to medicine and, more specifically, to pharmacology. Dioscorides was first translated into Arabic by Iṣṭafan ibn Bāsīl under the supervision of Ḥunain and later revised by al-Nātilī.[72] Ḥunain was the first to explain and justify the proper use of compound drugs. It was inevitable that the expansion of the drug and spice trade, the influx of new medical works in translation, and the scientific advances due to scholars like Ḥunain in the gloriously rich ninth century should hasten the rise of licensed pharmacists (ṣayādila) alongside the more traditional figures of the spicers ('aṭṭārīn) and lead to the clear recognition of pharmacy as quite distinct from medicine.[73] This recognition is prominent in al-Rāzī (Rhazes) at the beginning of the tenth century but was not authorised in the West until the edict of the Emperor Frederick II in 1240. Arabic pharmacy bequeathed to the West a greatly expanded pharmacopeia and a strong lexical interest in botanical nomenclature[74] which influenced the production of collections of *synonyma* in the thirteenth century.

Pharmacological writing in Arabic is usually divided into the following categories: compendia, formularies, *synonyma*-lists, treatises on poisons, and lists of drug substitutes. The more specialised writings were little known in the West, whilst the *compendia*, the *pandectae* or comprehensive treatises on medicine, were celebrated. The popularity of al-Rāzī, Alī al-'Abbas al-Majūsi and al-Zahrāwī is indicated by the familiarity of their latinised names Rhazes, Haly Abbas and Abulcasis.[75] What needs to be emphasised in connection with the development of the medical receipt is the extension of *materia medica* and the evolving interest in compound medicines. The discussion which follows is necessarily selective and aims only to bring into relief the most significant writers of pharmacology about whose treatment of *materia medica* informed researches have been published.

Arabic medical compendia exhibit a considerable variety in subject matter and emphasis, yet certain consistent features are easily identified. Writing about the tenth-century *al-Mi'a*, a systematic encyclopaedia of medicine by al-Masīḥī, G. Karmi observes of the Arabic compendia,

> They all included at some point a section on diseases arranged from head to toe; many also included sections on medical theory, that is the nature of humours, temperaments, crisis, coction and so on. Diseases were described in a stereotyped way: cause, symptoms and signs, and therapy. The therapy section was usually the biggest part and often included a number of prescriptions . . . Many of them [i.e. compendia] had a section on simple and compound drugs, and on poisons of animal origin or otherwise . . .[76]

One of the earliest compendia was the 'Paradise of Wisdom' consisting of 358 chapters on medicine and natural history.[77] Its author, 'Alī ibn Rabban al-Ṭabarī, completed it c. 850. There is a detailed section on *materia medica*.[78] Al-Ṭabarī included Indian and Persian drugs that were generally unknown, whilst at the same time exhibiting caution about the administration of all that were not tried and tested.[79] Although the 'Canon' (al-Qānūn) of Avicenna (Ibn Sīnā) displays few original or innovative traits in its treatment of *materia medica*, it was a thorough and celebrated account in which over 760 drugs are described.[80] More interesting is his specialised treatise on cardiac drugs where he gives an account of 63 simples, discusses a number of compounds, and adds a section 'Some Tested Prescriptions'.[81] Here aromatic drugs are particularly favoured. Although originally composed in Arabic, the 'Book of the Foundations of Pharmacology' by Abū Manṣūr Muwaffaq, written between 965 and 975, survives only in a Persian version.[82] It is composed of 584 chapters and the author claims superiority for the indigenous flora of India to that of Greece. Interestingly, the plant names are given throughout in Arabic. This contrasts with the *Zahīra* of al-Jurjānī (d.1136) where the majority of plant names are Persian rather than Greco-Arabic and consequently of great importance for Persian lexicology.[83] Book 10 deals with *materia medica*, whilst Book 6 discusses illnesses listed *a capite ad calcem*. Two large compendia of al-Rāzī (Rhazes), the *al-Ḥāwī* and *al-Manṣūrī* were to become well known in the West as *Liber Continens* and *Liber ad Almansorem* respectively. The discussion of *materia medica* is still of interest.[84] Strictly pharmacological compendia naturally yield even more valuable material. For example, *al-Saydana* of al-Bīrūnī (973–1051) is described by Hamarneh as 'one of the finest contributions to our pharmaceutical knowledge during the Middle Ages'.[85] The second section is devoted to *materia medica* and describes over 700 simples in alphabetical order in 1197 entries. The author does not recoil from the complexity of synonyms with which he is presented, given the vast extent of territories covered by Islam, and as a result of his own travels he is able to report on a number of otherwise unknown drugs.[86] Personal knowledge of *materia medica* is a salient feature of many of the Arabic pharmacologists. In Spain (al-Andalus) al-Ghāfiqī (d.1165), a physician of Cordoba, displays a detailed knowledge of Spanish vegetable products in his *al-Jami* and greatly influenced the distinguished Cairo herbalist Ibn al-Baiṭār (d.1248) who in his own treatise on simples described more than 1400 drugs, 300 of which had not been mentioned before.[87] He had earlier composed a detailed commentary on Dioscorides (omitting Book 5). Compendia such as these[88] attest to the importance of pharmacology in Arabic medicine and to the significant extension of the knowledge of drugs which greatly exceeds all that could be derived from Dioscorides.

The *aqrābādhīn* or medical formulary is a traditional form which assembles receipts according to *medicamenta*. [89] As a compilation of compounded prescriptions for a wide variety of ailments it forms part of a tradition which reaches back to Galen's *De compositione medicamentorum* and forward to Peter of Abano's supplement to the work of Messue the Younger.[90] Its counterpart in the West is the *antidotarium*. The first exclusively medical formulary in Arabic appears to have been the 'Great Formulary' (*Aqrābādhīn al-Kabīr*) of Sābūr ibn Sahl (d. 869)[91] where the pharmaceutical preparations are duly classified according to medicinal forms, the entries dealing with dosage form, preparation, therapeutic uses, and the techniques used in the preparation. In ninth-century Baghdad al-Kindī (c. 800–870) produced his own *aqrābādhīn* which leaves no doubt about the increasing superiority of Arabic pharmacology.[92] Drawing a great deal on his own experience, al-Kindī deals almost exclusively with *vegetabilia*, of which there are some 320 items. A similar work by Sahlān ibn Kaysān (d. 990)[93] describes a great range of compounded drugs under headings such as myrobolan confections, electuaries, pills, hieras, pastilles, powders, syrups, lohochs, robs, gargles, collyria, suppositories, pessaries, cataplasms, oils, lotions etc. This work influenced the formulary produced by al-Bayān (d.1161) which also included poultices, epithems, kneaded preparations and others. Particularly interesting is the formulary of al-Samarqandī (d.1222)[94] whose extant works are almost all devoted to simple and compound drugs and their preparation. Through the tradition of the *aqrābādhīn*[95] we can follow the general trend to include simples drawn from outside the Mediterranean and understand the emergence of the twelfth-century *Antidotarium Nicolai*, which, as we shall see, was to have such a marked influence on the development of Western pharmacology.

A concomitant of the sheer size of the territories covered by Islam was the need to record and explain the numerous *synonyma* so that firm botanical identifications could be made.[96] Spain was particularly known for its field botanists. Ibn Juljul wrote a book c. 982 on the interpretation of names of plants in Dioscorides which is unfortunately now lost and added simples not found in the Greek authority. In his great pharmacopeia, already discussed, al-Bīrūnī, dictating his work at the age of 80, provides drug synonyms in Syriac, Persian, Greek, Baluchi, Afghan, Kurdi and various Indian dialects, whilst al-Baiṭār (1197–1248) covers 3000 terms in alphabetical order.[97] It was he who copied the sole surviving manuscript of the Glossary of Drug Names drawn up by the celebrated philosopher and physician Moses Maimonides (1135–1204).[98] Covering 405 products, he furnishes some 2000 names including Greek, Syrian, Persian, Berber and Spanish. Maimonides deliberately excluded from his work very well known drugs and drugs known by only one name. Writing in Egypt, he cites no fewer than five works on drugs by Spanish authors. Lexico-botanical treatises such as that produced in tenth-century Spain by Ibn Samagun offer largely unexplored sources for our knowledge of medieval botany.[99] The major source for the botanical nomenclature of classical Arabic remains Dīnawarī's 'Book of Plants' written towards the end of the ninth century.[100]

Treatises on poisons also provide useful pharmacological information.[101] Already in the ninth century Jabir had written his 'Book of Poisons' and al-Biṭrīq had translated Galen's work on theriacs. A series of treatises on poisons was produced in the succeeding centuries.[102]

Of a series of tabular, synoptic texts the most important is the *Kitāb al-Musta'īni* of Ibn Biklārish, a Jewish physician of Saragossa (fl.1106).[103] This yields an astounding richness of information about Arabic *materia medica*. The tabular section consists of over 121 folios with detailed treatment of the same subjects on the facing pages.[104] This treatment gives the name of the drug, its nature and degree,[105] its synonyms, its substitutes, its usefulness, properties and methods of use, together with synonyms in Syriac, Persian, Greek, Arabic, Latin and some in the Berber vernacular.

Because of the varying availability of many drugs and the fraudulent composition of various *medicamenta* by some druggists, there was a need to produce lists of drug substitutes like Galen's *Antibalomena* called *abdāl*. The vast area – from India to Spain – covered by the Islamic empire naturally meant that careful consideration had to be given to *synonyma* in order that the correct drugs and their substitutes might be selected, a particularly delicate task when, as so often happened, it was desired to substitute *indigenes* for the various *exotica* found in compound preparations. Often, too, cheaper drugs replaced expensive ones. About 190 substitutions taken from Galen, the major authority for the treatises on substitutes which came to be known by the name *Quid pro quo*, are recorded by Paul of Aegina and it is to the seventh century that we may trace the earliest Arabic treatise on substitutes, though the most famous is probably that of al-Rāzī.[106]

By the twelfth century the glorious period of Arabic pharmacology is drawing to a close.[107] There is a period of consolidation in which a number of compendia spread before us the impressive extent of the knowledge gained over three centuries[108] and then the Mongol invasions of the thirteenth century put an end to most scientific writing in the Near East. As the Arabs themselves had reached eagerly to Syriac, Greek and Persian authors for scientific knowledge, so the West now turned to Arab writers, through the intermediary of Muslim Spain, for inspiration and there begins, with the school of Salerno – which was to endure until closure under Napoleon in 1811 – a new chapter in the history of medieval medical writing.

Whilst the intellectual outlines of the school of Salerno have been brought into much sharper focus through the researches of Kristeller and others,[109] its origins remain shrouded in obscurity. Of the organisation of physicians in Salerno we know almost nothing and it is only the emergence of a curriculum of prescribed texts which encourages us to speak of a school at all. We simply have no records in which to seek enlightenment for the period before 950.[110] The heritage of Salernitan physicians was no doubt general rather than distinctive, being made up of works from the classical medical tradition available throughout northern Italy, in Africa and in Spain, which bore the stamp of Methodist therapeutics and Galenic anatomy and theory. The notion of a direct line of descent to the Roman medical college at Velia (some 80 km down the coast from Salerno) has rightly been rejected.[111] The medical curriculum at Alexandria in the sixth and seventh centuries gives us some idea of an organised corpus of medical texts which would be widely available.[112] By the late tenth century it is clear that Salerno enjoyed a considerable reputation as the home of practical medicine and successful therapy. Whether its fame is largely the result of the activities of laymen or clerics is still a much disputed issue. In the eleventh century there is increasing evidence of a teaching programme, albeit a conservative one, and two compilations of Galenic and other antique excerpts survive, the *Passionarius Galieni* of Gariopontus and the *Practica Petroncelli*.[113] A number of medical works are attributed to Alfanus, a monk of Montecassino and archbishop of Salerno 1058–1085.[114] Undoubtedly the most significant single figure at this time is Constantinus Africanus (c.1015–1087) who translated many medical works from the Arabic.[115] He seems to have arrived in Salerno c.1077 before going to Montecassino where he died about ten years later. A true assessment of the *Corpus Constantinum* (c. 25 works) has yet to be made. Amongst the most important translations are those of the *Pantegni* of Haly Abbas, the *Viaticum* of al-Jazzār and treatises on diet, urines and fevers by Isaac Judaeus. Whilst Sudhoff was inclined to exaggerate the importance of Constantinus,[116] more recently it has been observed that there was little immediate impact on Salerno from his translations[117] and that there are few signs of their influence before the middle of the next century.[118] The real importance of the school of Salerno lies in the introduction of a new philosophical and scholastic bias during the twelfth century and the elaboration of commentaries to a corpus of set texts in a way which anticipated university teaching and which achieved a new level of theory and learning.[119] The assimilation of the Aristotelian *libri naturales* in scientific and medical writing at Salerno marks one of the fundamental stages of the so-called renaissance of the twelfth century. By the end of the century there were four commentaries to the corpus of texts known as *Articella*.[120] This corpus comprised the *Isagoge* of Johannitius (i.e. Ḥunain ibn Is'hāq), which was an introduction to Galen's *Ars*, the Aphorisms and Prognostics of Hippocrates, the *De urinis* of Theophilus, the *De pulsibus* attributed to Philaretus, and the *Tegni* (i.e. Galen's *Ars parva*). The importance of natural philosophy is also reflected in the use of *quaestiones*, the tradition of which at Salerno has been investigated by Lawn.[121] In addition, we witness the rise of the term *physicus* which frequently replaces *medicus* in the course of the century. The figure of Urso of Calabria emerges as a prime mover in the history of Salernitan Aristotelianism. The celebrated 'Tables of Salerno' [122] receive a commentary from Bernardus Provincialis (fl.1150–75). We are no longer in the world of conservative compendia and receipt collections, but of systematic teaching through commentaries which are more theoretical, speculative and scholastic than anything found earlier at Salerno. And yet, by the thirteenth century the decline of the 'Civitas Hippocratica' has already begun and few works of any lasting importance – the *Regimen Sanitatis*[123] is, of course, celebrated – are to be produced.

In the more restricted field of *materia medica* Salerno is influential on account of three major works: *Antidotarium magnum*, *Antidotarium Nicolai*, and the *Circa Instans*. By the end of the eleventh century the emphasis on practical medicine at Salerno had produced a rich stock of medical receipts,[124] but a stock which was both heterogeneous and unorganised. It was natural that some attempt should be made to assemble a more standardised and structured corpus of receipts through which they would be more easily accessible. Many were embedded in large treatises on general medicine, others, like those constituting the tenth book (an *antidotarium*) of Haly Abbas's *Pantegni*, contained many unfamiliar drugs introduced by the Arabs and many unfamiliar names too. Already in the *Passionarius* of Gariopontus we see some attempt at a systematic presentation of the available materials. The exact circumstances in which the *Antidotarium magnum* was created are unclear. The basic plan may have been initiated by Constantinus Africanus and continued by his pupil Afflatius together with a team of collaborators. However that may be, the work seems to have been in existence by about 1100. It was only in 1960, thanks to the researches of Alfons Lutz, that a manuscript of the long-lost work was brought to light.[125] It contains almost 1200 receipts, over 30 of which are drawn from Galen and Alexander of Tralles. The arrangement is by alphabetical order of *medicamenta*, sometimes alternative receipts (marked *minus*, *minor*, *media* etc.) being provided under a single heading. Over 200 receipts simply begin with the formula 'medicamentum ad . . . ' They are largely drawn from *receptaria* and clearly indebted to Greek sources, the Greek names often being retained without any attempt to explain them. It is difficult to trace the influence of the *Antidotarium magnum*,[126] but it seems to have generated a set of glosses which are sometimes attributed to Matthaeus Platearius as if they were the accompaniment to the *Antidotarium Nicolai*, though such a view is erroneous.[127]

The *Antidotarium Nicolai* became the essential pharmacopeia of the Middle Ages.[128] It seems to have been the product of Salernitan teaching and was produced some hundred years after the *Antidotarium magnum*, at any rate by 1244 when there is an explicit reference to it in Vincent of Beauvais.[129] Like the afore-mentioned glosses (known as the *Liber iste*), which reduced the number of receipts to approximately 70, the *Antidotarium Nicolai* makes a radical selection from the available receipt literature. The earliest redactions contain no more than 110–115 receipts, rising to a maximum of 175 in late versions. Whoever the author 'Nicolaus' was, he was a medical teacher writing at the request of his students who desired a uniform, plain guide to the constitution of *medicamenta*. The 200 or so 'medicamenta ad . . . ' of the *Antidotarium magnum* are cast aside along with the various alternative prescriptions proposed. Largely ignored, too, are the more domestic remedies including gargles, pessaries, suppositories etc. The receipts are generally shortened, the list of indications being much reduced, and the experiments for testing the medicines generally discarded. Against this trend to a more discriminating selection which has produced a work considerably shorter than many of the preceding *antidotaria*, 'Nicolaus' has amplified the treatment of the names of the various preparations. Some 64 of these are named after their principal ingredients following the formula *dia-*.[130] Others are named after the effects they are designed to produce e.g. *unguentum laxativum*. A striking number take their name from proper names, the alleged inventors or celebrated patients associated with the remedy. There is a good deal of etymological material mostly drawn from Isidore of Seville. The use of names, of course, greatly facilitated the identification of the remedies. The essential purpose of the *Antidotarium Nicolai* was to provide a reliable guide to the ingredients required for well known remedies. As the latter are arranged alphabetically, and not according to indications, it is obvious that the user was expected already to possess the necessary nosological knowledge. It is also clear that the work presupposes familiarity with the various methods of preparation, since in over two thirds of the receipts no information is provided on this aspect of pharmacology.[131] Once the identity, number and sequence of ingredients were recorded,[132] the most significant feature remained the indication of quantities. Here the *Antidotarium Nicolai* had a signal contribution to make. The directions provided in the *Antidotarium magnum* envisaged heroic quantities of drug preparations ranging from 10 to 30 pounds. The author of the *Antidotarium Nicolai* appends to his work a section on weights and measures (see below p.60) in which he draws attention to the difficulty of converting from such large quantities to a much smaller scale. This practical need he has met by introducing the basic unit of the grain (*granum*), 20 of which constituted the Salernitan *scrupulum* (local variations abound throughout Europe) or gramm, and by reducing the quantities prescribed to 2 pounds. Of course, it was more economical for the pharmacist to make up reasonably large quantities and to store them, but the quantities had to be realistic and not in excess of true demand. The short-term *ad hoc* remedies such as the author of the *Antidotarium Nicolai* discarded could, along

Notes on pp.338–53

with simples, be made up by the physician himself. The domain of the *Antidotarium Nicolai* is therefore that of the more complicated *composita* or compound medicines which exceeded the resources of the physician in time, cost and expertise. As a manual or guide to the stocking of the medieval pharmacy the work was indispensable and was rapidly translated into the principal European vernaculars.[133] The author had made a conscious attempt to diminish the Greek linguistic elements of his sources and not a few names introduced by him reflect the influence of the vernacular e.g. Italian. By 1270 the work had become part of the prescribed syllabus in the medical faculty of the University of Paris. The new system of weights based on a decimal rather than duodecimal system and exploiting the natural unit of the *grain* had the great merit of adaptability, since it could be used at any time and in any place, whatever the local traditions and variations might be. Such a universal and easily calibrated system represented a crucial innovation in medieval pharmacology.

The third important work associated with Salerno is the *De simplicibus medicinis*, better known by its opening words as *Circa instans*, which describes over 270 drugs in alphabetical order, expounding both their properties and their uses.[134] It is generally believed to have been composed by a member of the celebrated Salernitan medical family of Platearius (Johannes or Matthaeus?) in the middle of the twelfth century. There are over 200 MSS (with varying configurations of contents), the earliest of which are only a few decades distant from the presumed date of composition. It remained a fundamental guide to simples throughout the Middle Ages and was heavily used by the compilers of the *Tractatus de herbis* in MS London, B. L. Egerton 747 (s.xiv) ff.1ra–106rb and the 'Grant Herbier en Francois' (*Arbolayre*), which was translated into English as *The Grete Herball* in 1526.[135]

Throughout the twelfth century, of course, the advances of Arabic science were becoming known not only through the work of Salernitan masters but also via Toledo.[136] At the head of a group of translators, Gerard of Cremona (1114–1187)[137] provided an *Antidotarium Rasis* (Lemay 58c) and a *Liber Galieni de medicina simplici* (Lemay 59). He also translated *Liber de gradibus medicinarum* (Lemay 62) of al-Kindī, *Liber de simplicium medicinarum virtutibus* of al-Lahmī, and the *Breviarium Serapionis* (or *Aggregator*, *Pandectae*, *Practica* etc.) (Lemay 60). The latter work was written by the Syriac physician Yaḥyā (Yūḥannā) ibn Sarābiyūn in the tenth century, was translated into Arabic, and then epitomised in a smaller edition or *Breviarium* consisting of 7 books in Latin. The field of *materia medica* was further enriched by the *Antidotarium* of Mesue (Abū Zakarīyā' Yūḥannā ibn Māsawaih, d. 857) and a *Liber medicinarum simplicium et ciborum*(Lemay 59) of al-Wāfīd. All this, following the establishment of an Aristotelian *corpus naturalium*, gave Western medicine a comprehensive and systematic structure which it had previously lacked.

Also important were a number of individual writers who had frequented the medical schools. Gilles de Corbeil (Aegidius Corboliensis) was born in Corbeil (Seine-et-Marne) c.1140, went to Paris to study with Adam of Petit Pont, and thence, c.1160, to Salerno where he spent some fifteen years.[138] Thereafter he was for a short while at Montpellier, where he was apparently poorly received, and he finally returned to Paris, becoming personal physician to Philippe Auguste and dying c.1224. His *De laudibus et virtutibus compositorum medicaminum*,[139] composed shortly before 1181, is a free, metrical adaptation of Matthaeus Platearius's *Glossae in Antidotarium* ('Liber Iste') and was rapidly revised, being issued nearly twenty years later with a new preface by Gilles himself.[140] A new edition of this useful work is an urgent desideratum.

A less well known figure is Johannes de Sancto Amando, born in Tournay, who taught in Paris. As well as writing a commentary on the *Antidotarium Nicolai*, (c.1260) he composed a massive, alphabetically arranged compendium of quotations from medical writers, especially Galen and Avicenna, on all aspects of medicine called the *Revocativum memoriae*. The second, most comprehensive part, dealing with pathology, was known as the *Concordantiae*, whilst the compilation dealing with therapy and materia medica was the *Areolae*.[141] They were composed in the late thirteenth century.

More important for the history of receipt collections is Peter of Spain. Born actually in Portugal, and educated at the beginning of the thirteenth century at the Cathedral school of Lisbon, he went to study in Paris in the 1220s and in Salerno (or possibly Montpellier) in the 1230s.[142] From 1245 he taught medicine at Sienna until about 1250 when he returned to Portugal for some fifteen years. In 1272 he became court physician to Pope Gregory X at Viterbo and was himself elected Pope as John XXI. Not long before his death in 1277 he composed his celebrated *Thesaurus pauperum*,[143] a compilation of popular (usually short) medical receipts which survives in over seventy MSS and which underwent various modifications including contamination with other collections. The short receipts, which resemble those of the old *receptaria*, are drawn from many sources, the most frequently cited of which are Dioscorides, Constantinus, Macer, the *Circa Instans*, and Gilbertus. In general the *a capite ad calcem* order is followed. The receipts assembled by Peter often recur in later collections and were translated.[144]

Form and Contents of the Medical Receipt[145]

The medical receipts which are the subject of the present study and which constitute the bulk of the medieval insular collections fall into six categories: therapeutic, prognostic, diagnostic, cosmetic, dietetic and eclectic.[146] The therapeutic receipt describes and prescribes a remedy, or remedies, against a stated disorder. The remedy may be pharmaceutical, religious or magical and hence be described as a prescription, a prayer, or a charm. By far the largest number of receipts edited in the following pages are therapeutic. The prognostic receipt outlines a method for determining in advance the answer to a given question, usually the outcome of some process which it is desired to know e.g. whether the child of a pregnant woman will be male or female, whether a man smitten with disease will survive or die etc. The diagnostic receipt offers a technique for identifying the nature of a particular ailment or for answering a question pertaining to it e.g. whether the patient's leprosy is inherited or has been contracted accidentally, whether a woman is barren etc. The cosmetic receipt largely deals with skin- and hair-care for women and may be attached to a set of therapeutic receipts or multiplied to form an independent treatise, in verse or prose, on cosmetics.[147] Receipts concerned with dental hygiene (e.g. PR 375 ff)[148] may sometimes be regarded as essentially cosmetic. The dietetic receipt provides advice on *regimen* and may sometimes be expanded to form a short treatise or *regimen sanitatis*. At any rate, it is concerned with general health matters rather than specific disorders. Finally, the eclectic receipt seeks to assemble diverse information on a specific topic such as hearing difficulties (PR 331ff), the value of a particular herb, or folkloric details (often from Pliny) about a bird or beast (e.g. on the nuthatch in Digby 69 no.14). Of course, there are other types of receipts which are not in any sense medical. They often deal with technical matters such as dyeing (see Sloane 3550 nos. 79–83), alchemy and practical tasks like getting rid of flies, removing stains from clothing etc. These non-medical receipts are often described as *secreta* or *experimenta.*[149] The medical receipt may be called *recette / receptum*, or *esperement / experimentum / esprove.* It displays what at first may appear to be a disconcerting linguistic variety, moving, in the case of insular collections, through three languages, often within the same sentence. One of the reasons for this, apart from the trilingualism which is now acknowledged to characterise thirteenth-century England,[150] is the need to check or verify details in manuals and compendia which themselves might be in any of the three languages displayed in the receipts.[151] Latin rubrics help to identify disorders and remedies as they are found in medical textbooks and the indices to large receipt collections (e.g. that to the collection in MS Add. 15236 below), whilst the vernacular translations of these rubrics aid the practical understanding of the receipts. Pre-Linnaean botanical nomenclature is so notoriously unstable that plant names would often have to be checked in *synonyma herbarum* which listed Latin, English and Anglo-Norman forms.[152] In MS Digby 69 f.10v a note is appended to the ingredient *succus de elfan* directing the user to an authority: 'herba elfan quere in libro de nigro et invenies qualis sit'.[153] Some plants were certainly most familiar in their indigenous name forms, whilst others seem to be referred to only by Latin names. Much of course depended on the culture of compiler and user and the auxiliary materials at their disposal. Often scraps of a Latin original seem to have been retained because of uncertainty concerning the identity of the plants mentioned. The plethora of trilingual *synonyma*-lists bears witness to the need for a ready-reference work which might render the identification of plants less precarious. A rare opportunity to compare a set of identical receipts in Anglo-Norman and Latin is provided by MSS of the so-called 'Lettre d'Hippocrate' discussed below. Compilation from multiple copies was also, no doubt, a cause for the thorough-going multilingualism of the receipt collections, the compilers of which lacked such systematic knowledge as would have permitted consistency in a single language. Some consistency is achieved, however, in the *form* of the medical receipt. In general it displays some or all of the following six components: rubric, indication, composition (ingredients), preparation, application, statement of efficacy (cure). Length varies from a few words ('Da ei bibere ditannum', 'Mangez ben letues') to whole pages of manuscript (see esp. Add. 15236[154] and Sloane 146).

Rubric:
In the strict sense, as distinguished from *indication* (see below), this applies to the type of remedy, the name by which it is known, or the enquiry of which it is part. In the first category come headings of the type *Pur fere syrup laxatif / oximel / unguentum sanativum* etc. Medical preparations known by the names of their alleged inventor, a celebrated patient, a distinguished practitioner and so on are most commonly found in the *antidotaria* and are well exemplified in the *Antidotarium Nicolai*, the *Compen-*

dium of Gilbertus Anglicus, and the collections edited in Ch.9 below. Thus we have *Agrippa, Marciaton, Arragon*. Many names are formed from the Greek *dia-* and the principal ingredient: *Diacalament, Diadragant, Diapenidion, Diamoron*. Etymological explanations are frequently given: '*Electuarium quod vocatur dyasaturion*: Dyasaturion dicitur a saturionibus qui ibi recipiuntur vel a saturis quos fama pronos in Venerem devulgavit . . . ' '*De diasaturionum radicibus*: Saturiacis enim grece, erectio virge dicitur latine . . . ' Vernacular rubrics involving proper names are *C'est l'emplastre le cunte Richard contre apostume el fundement . . .*; *Agrippe est un oygnement dunt le rey de Agrippe soloyt estre enoynt; La poysoun de Yrlande ke garist tut manere [de] playe; Ceo [est] l'emplastre seynt Cuthbert; La medicine Hubert Gernun de Ewardestouer.* Latin rubrics invoking the names of medieval practitioners include: *Emplastrum bonum m. J. de Lin; Experimentum secretum Gilberti; Cura m. Eruardi de opido contra fluxum lacrimarum cum rubore oculorum; Experimentum R. de Warwich ad visum accuendum.* The third category of rubrics is most commonly demonstrated by prognostic and diagnostic receipts, taking the form *Si vis scire . . . / Si vus volez saver . . . .* Undoubtedly the most unusual is that in MS Sloane 146 no. 207: *A saver si uone femme aime sun barun plus ke nul autre.* Usually rubrics are underlined (often in red) in the MSS and this is indicated by italicisation in the texts edited below. At other times the rubrics are set off from the text of the receipt and not infrequently they appear in the margins as an aid to ready reference. It is common to find a Latin rubric followed by its equivalent in Anglo-Norman and when there are several receipts under the same heading the rubric *Item / Aliud / Autre* is used. Receipts of a more popular character tend to adopt the indication as rubric.

Indication:
This is a statement in the rubric or at the beginning of the receipt of the medical condition for which the prescription is a remedy. The majority of vernacular receipts use the indication as a heading, employing formulae like *Pur cancre, (En)contre dolur de plaie, Pur garir de . . ., Ki a le . . ., Ki voudra garir de. . .* When Latin is employed it is often followed by a precise translation into Anglo-Norman: *Ad dislotionem pedis vel gambe vel alicuius, si pié ou jambe ou altre menbre seit aloché.* Sometimes the indication is placed at the end of the receipt, particularly when it represents an addition to the principal indication: *Icest meimes garist le poagre; Cest oignement est bon a plusurs dolurs e freid piz rechaufe e alasche e a pleuresi.* The principal indication may, in contrast, contain a restrictive clause: *Ki vodra fere un entrete pur totes maneres de gowtes fors de gowte enossé; Contra dolorem timporum non tamen provenientem ex calore.* Sometimes the indication is extremely comprehensive (see below MS Add. 15236 nos 3* & 12*) and in certain instances (see below ch.9, B 8, 13–16) constitutes the whole receipt on the assumption that the actual composition of the receipt is well known. Occasionally the indication contains a restriction concerning the stage of the illness or the duration of relief; *Pur la gute chaive al cumencement quant primes li vient; Ad hoc autem ut aliquid non sit totaliter impotens nisi tamen ad tempus videlicet pro uno anno vel dimidio.* It is often by indication that receipts are indexed (as in MS Add. 15236 below) and arranged in the collections (using the short form *Item / Aliud / Autre* after the first statement of the indication).

Composition:
The greater part of the medical receipt is usually taken up by a list of ingredients headed by the word *recipe / accipe / sume / collige / pernez / cuillez*. The number of

ingredients may range from one (PR 105 ff) to 66 (MS Add. 15236 no. 52*) and cover *vegetabilia, mineralia* and *chimica* or concentrate on a single type of ingredient (e.g. PR 1027 ff which enumerates 9 trees). Unusual ingredients include *crapout, fente de humme mort, sanguis hominis, fente de geline, teste de soriz, le cheel de levrer, .ii. ou .iii. huans blancs atirés en guise des gelines rosties, un vif cok, les os de morte gent arses, vieuz semeles de vieuz soulers, de .i. viel tacon .i. grant piece, lange de busard, terre del nid de arunde.* Mineral and chemical elements are unusual but include *calamine, neir plum, coperose, perre sanguin, poudre de veire, le neir ars ki est desoz le plum u chaudere as funz, faisil de ce qui est chaü de chaut fer quaunt om l'a batu.* Insects employed include flies and earwigs. Whilst earthworms were no doubt in plentiful supply, *oint de lion* was surely a luxury! Many of the ingredients, of course, had no therapeutic value whatsoever and simply represent the residue of popular traditions. The use of substitutes is readily acknowledged: *sepum ovinum, si sepum cervinum non poterit haberi; vinum album, si haberi potest; saxifragium, si habes; si par aventure foille de lorer ne seit trové, pernez oille de lorer; ki n'ad la grant malve, prenge la petite; sause de sel e de eawe, si vus n'avez sause de mer; gresse de thessun, si aver le porez, ou seym de porc male; castorie, si aver le poez; si vous n'avez blanche pois, si metez encens* It is interesting to note that proposed substitutions do not cover *exotica*, but perfectly familiar products, and are entirely practical rather than simply traditional.[155] In addition, recourse might be had to the numerous lists of drug substitutes which went under the name of *Quid pro quo*.[156] Herbal ingredients introduce the problem of botanical nomenclature and plant identification. It is not therefore surprising to find that the names of plants are often given in more than one language. Four different techniques may be distinguished. The first consists of introducing the vernacular name with a formula of the type *une herbe que nus apelum . . ., une herbe que est apelé . . ., herba que dicitur . . . une herbe qui ad num*, sometimes with the qualifying words *en engleis / anglice / gallice* (but not *en franceis!*). The second method is to provide an interlinear gloss e.g. *consolida minor / .i. briswort / .* An extension of this technique is the incorporation of the gloss in the text: *glajol, anglice gladen; parele, anglice redockes; pimpirnel .i. flewrt.* Finally, lists of vegetable ingredients often mingle Latin, English and Anglo-Norman in what seems a bewildering confusion, but which may reflect the relative familiarity of different plant name-forms. Some plants do not seem to have had any generally familiar vernacular name. As with all lexical glossing, some of the items surprise by their banality e.g. *ysopum .i. ysop.* A conspectus of the *materia medica* exploited in the vernacular receipts may be easily obtained by consulting the glossaries appended to the present study.

Less easy to tabulate or systematise is the use of weights and measures (for more detailed treatment see below pp.59 ff.), which are indicated in the receipts in a somewhat haphazard fashion. Purely relative indications are most commonly encountered: *equaliter, uniement, ouelement, ouele porcioun, par oel peis, equali mensura, ouele mesure, in equali porcione, altretant de l'un com de l'autre, duble de la premiere pudre, renablement.* Many of the measures reflect a popular rule-of-thumb method: *tant cum vus purrez enpuigner od une main; unius fabe quantitas; quantitas unius salsarii; muntant une feve; teste ovi plenitudo; deus escales de oef; autant cum entreit en dous oes; demi of de; treis feves; pugillum; demi poigne; vola manus; vint e set hanapees pleins; un quilere; quam duobus digitis levare poteris* and other natural measures introduced with the phrase *a la quantité de.* More scientific are: *un ferlinge; un dener pesant; le peis de un dener; quam denarius pensat; le peis de .iii. souz; ad pondus .iii. solidorum; ad pondus unius denarii.* It is difficult to determine the value of the most familiar scientifically calibrated measures, since they differed from place to place: *uncia / unce; manipulum; libra / livre; dragma / dragme* (explained in one receipt as 'asavoir le peis de deus [deners] e maille'); *quarteroun; sexterium; scrupulum*. Other quantities are indicated by *galun, hanapee, grein,* and *pinte*. The influence of the *Antidotarium Nicolai* with its emphasis on smaller quantities and on the basic unit of the *granum* does not seem to have been felt at the time these receipts were copied. A receipt for *popelion* specifies 'les burjuns .x. livres pesant', whilst in another the ingredients for a syrup include 'prunes de outre mer quarante quatre livres' (see below p.333 no. 8). There is only a very occasional reference to scales and much is left to the experience of the pharmacist or physician (e.g. *taunt com vous veez ke mestiers est*). Often the parts of the plants to be used are not specified, whilst at other times we have *flurs, foilles, racines, burjuns, ciuns, semences, copels, escorche, coperuns, tendruns, crops, greins* etc. Directions for the collection of plants are discussed below (pp.55 f.).

Preparation:
Instructions for what is usually known as the *confectiun* or *confision* of the ingredients may be given in the third person singular (fut. indic. and pres. subj.) or the second person plural (pres. indic.), the latter case being the commonest. There is no doubt that this is the area of the receipt where the greatest amount of knowledge and skill is assumed. The basic preparatory processes are indicated by the following verbs (citing vernacular examples only): *cuillir, boillir, culer, destemprer, tribler, frire, primer, priendre, escumer, estamper, braer, pestrer, buleter*. The essential apparatus is (in the vernacular): *vaissel de areim / quivre / estaim / veirre, morter, pestel, boiste, paele, esquiele, hanap, paellette, pot, picher, galun, sachel, ampulle, sarceyse, pouche, poteau, poke de canevaz, bage de canevaz, basin, possenet, puscette, furn, brasier, test;* (in Latin): *vas (eneum), olla, pixis, patella, potellus, lagena, discus, mortarium, sacculus (lineus), bursa (linea), scutella, pottus, furnus, ampulla, testa*. In addition to the forms of *medicamenta* discussed in the next section (application), we frequently encounter the preparation of *mortrels, niules, wastels, pulments, tisanes, chaudels, chaudelets, bruets, soupes, roeles, bature, past, morsels, coleice,* and countless beverages. The preparation time varies from a short period of the day to 40 days, depending on whether storage is involved. Some receipts call for the burial of ingredients in an earthenware pot in the ground for long periods, whilst others assume specific weather conditions such as sunshine for the drying of herbs. The preparation of the *medicamenta* depended a good deal on the availability of essential ingredients and especially on the recommended times for the gathering of fresh materials i.e. spring and early summer. A knowledge of the basic techniques of preparation is invariably assumed and sometimes explicitly indicated: *fetes eawe des flurs de feves com l'en fet eawe rose; de ces herbes seit ewe fete cum ewe rose; pus metez 'l'entrete as chivalers' sor le mal.*

Application:
This is the area of the receipt which contains the greatest variety of directions, for the administration of the *medicamenta* involves size and frequency of dose, form of treatment and nature of the medicament, preparation of the patient, place of application, and instructions for storage. Forms of treatment, besides the administration of medicines, include bleeding, vapour and steam baths, and minor surgery. The *medicamenta* comprise many different forms: *emplastre, entret, collirie, salve, oynement, papelotes, estrictorie, letuaire, silotre, stupha, gargarisme, clistere,* syrups, eye-

drops and so on, each requiring its own mode of application. The appropriate time of application is indicated in formulae like the following: *sero et mane, soir et matin, matin et soir, matin et tard, quando vadis cubitum, quando iterus es dormitum, sero ante cubitum, le soir avant coucher, quel hure que vodra dormir, au matin et au vespre, a noune et au seir, circa horam primam, ante horam prime, omni die hora prima, sero in aurora, omni tempore frigido, quando patiens surrexerit a sompno, ante prandium et post.* Particularly frequent is the formula *le soir chaud et le matin froid.* Dosage is usually limited to the number of applications rather than to quantities. A single application is sometimes specified, but far commoner are the general-purpose phrases like *donec sanus sit, donec curetur, joske seit gari, desque vus seez gari* or else *suvent, sepius in die, per aliquod spacium temporis.* The course of treatment may last for anything from one to forty days, though shorter periods of up to a week are the most usual. In the case of one remedy against *gutta caduca* mistletoe is to be hung round the patient's neck, to which is added the direction 'ke il le porte tute sa vie'. The following list illustrates the variety of instructions: *binis vicibus in die, per .iii. dies, pur .iiii. jurs e nent plus, dous fie le jor par noef jors, .iii. feiz le seyr e .iii. foiz le matin, per quadraginta dies* (charm), *per tres vel quatuor dies continuos, per diem naturalem, tote une nuith, tote la quinseyne.* Occasionally all the salient features of application are condensed in a short phrase: *checun jour en l'iver jun un quiller.*

The place of application is usually referred to in a general way with phrases like *là u le mal seit, sor le liu ke dout, de cele part ou le dolur est, là ou vus plerra, super malum* etc. The circumstances may be indicated with similar imprecision: *quando opus fuerit, quod necessitas deposcat, quotiens opus fuerit.* The following passage is exceptional for the detail with which it describes the process of application:

> Cum igitur uti volueris dictis unguentis pro scabie, primo sumatur modicum super digitum de unguento corosivo et ungatur tenue locus infirmitatis et statim corodet scabiem etiam usque ad crudam carnem. Hoc facto statim sumatur unguentum prescriptum sanativum et spisso modo ungatur dictus locus infirmitatis et citius quam credi poterit sanabitur. Cum etiam volueris pilos corporis deponere, fiat cum predictis unguentis prout dictum est de scabie et nunquam iterato crescent. (see below MS Add. 15236 no. 57*)

Many of the receipts lack any information about application, the preparation of the *medicamenta* being followed by instructions for storage: *estuer en boiste, metre en sauf, usui reservetur, reservetur in pixide, l'estuez par tut le an, in olla casui reservetur, in vase mundo reservetur, metre en sauf liu, metre en boystes que sunt encyrés, metre en un bel sachel de teile en sauf.* Occasionally there is added to such instructions an indication of the durability of the *medicamentum*: *semen per tres annos servari potest, per annum servari potest, durra en bone vertue plusurs anz, per annum servari potest − quanto recentior tanto melior.*

One of the most interesting aspects of application or administration in the receipts is the preparation of the patient − *le malade, le patient, li enfers, paciens, infirmus.* Very occasionally a distinction is made between male and female, and once between social classes: 'si il est gentil home, pernez lise de levrer, si vilain, pernez lise mastive' (MS Digby 69 no. 78). The treatment of head pains may involve shaving of the head. The internal use of medicines almost always takes place *jun, jejuno stomacho,* although in certain cases this is not advised because fasting 'le cervel fait troubler' (PR 151ff). Some medicines should be taken after evacuation of the bowels − *aprés ke il avera fet une sele.* Multiple treatments are sometimes prescribed, as in this instruction for a cough: 'Lavez vostre piz de ewe freide le seyr, si eschaufez les plauntes des pez e sovent versez l'ewe sur le piz, si bevez vetoine'. The administration of beverages is almost always accompanied by the formulae *calidus quam tolerari potest, ausi chaud cum il le put / purra suffrir, calidus sicut potest sustineri.* The possible reactions of the patient are only rarely alluded to: 'Quant le pacient deyt aler cocher metetz en le oyl e, mes ke il face graunt violence, ne seyt mie osté'; 's'il est issi ke age u enfermeté nel sufre pas, metez i du vin'. The dangers of weakening the patient are recognised, particularly in connection with bleeding:

> Hoc tamen habet intelligi: si in principio infirmitatis sue fecerit predictam medicinam, si vero per magnum tempus stetit in infirmitate, non minuat sibi paciens, quia per hoc forte nimis debilitaretur. (MS Add. 15236 no. 61*)

> Sequenti vero die de reliquo pede et iam extrahatur sanguis secundum virtutem eius, quoniam in omni egritudine respiciendum est ad virtutem pacientis et maxime timendum est de nimis debilitetur ... (MS Add. 15236 no.153*)

In contrast, illness may induce lack of docility in the patient, as in the case of the ague: 'si la maladie seit si forte ke il ne puse ne ne voille estre tenu u ausi cum il se arage, pernez ... ' A patient suffering from vertigo is to be kept still and in darkness for three or four days (PR 147 ff) and one suffering from a wound should refrain from anger (PR 979). The most detailed instructions concerning treatment deal with dietary control. One receipt states 'multo melius operabitur si a cenis vel saltim a superfluitate cenarum abstinuerit'. Another advises 'caveat a lacte, a salsis etiam piscibus et carnibus etiam salsis et caseo et a viscosis cibariis et potibus'; a third exhorts "vitet paciens per 9 dies carnes bovinas recentes, caseum, lac dulce, pisas, anguillas, ova, porros, alleum, sepas, novam serviciam, et breviter omne genus prandii guttosum, anglice goutouse'. Shorter prohibitions include 'faciat paciens abstinenciam per tres vel duos dies', 'le malade ne mange .iii. jurs ou quatre for pan alis e euue hu tisane', 'caveat a carne noctis precedentis, ut stomacus aliqualiter vacuus inveniatur' In MS Sloane 3550 no. 69 there is a receipt headed *La diete al malade* which appears in PR 971ff under the rubric *Por plaié garir.* Other details of *regimen* were derived from the highly influential 'Letter of Aristotle to Alexander' in the *Secretum Secretorum.* In a receipt designed to promote coitus we read 'post sumpcionem vero in mane laboret aliqualiter etiam si poterit, usque ad sudorem' and in another receipt 'post sumpcionem vadat spaciatum et moveat bene corpus suum ambulando'. A miniature *regimen sanitatis* opens a collection of receipts in Trinity College, Cambridge, MS 0.1.20 ff. (see below pp.330 f.) and is related to a plethora of small treatises on health matters (including the ubiquitous urologies) which circulated in the Middle Ages.

Finally, it must be admitted that the administration of *medicamenta* to the patient is often dealt with in the vaguest manner, omitting all reference to the site of application and not infrequently leaving room for doubt as to whether the medicine is designed for internal or external application! Very rarely we encounter practical suggestions to facilitate application. For example, in connection with ear complaints, 'metez la oreille vers val, k'il pusse bien entrer', 'si metez en l'altre oreille e issi gice une pose sor l'altre coste'.

Statement of efficacy:
Underlying the cure (*curaciun / cure*) was, of course, the Galenic theory of humoral

pathology.[157] Homoeopathy (*similia similibus curantur*) and allopathy (*contraria contrariis*) were frequently the basis of treatment. The receipts themselves have very little to say about the effects or side-effects of treatment. In almost all cases, on the other hand, they terminate with a formula asserting the value of the treatment. The stock of formulae is considerable: *ce guarra, si garra bien, ço est provee chose, esprové chose est, probatum est, sepe probatum est, probatur, ceo est aprové chose, ceo vus delivrera, si le sanera, salvus erit, la medcine est verraie e esprovee, si vus vaudra, istud veraciter est probatum, expertum est certe, sine dubio salvabitur, sanabitur paciens domino mediante, par la grace Deu garra, saunté avera li pacient par la grace Deu, sanabitur domino concedente, si estaunchera od l'aide de Deu, ki en Deus ferme creance a, tot certain seit, bien garira, si vus vaut / vaudra bien, multum prodest / proderit, ista medicina optime et pulcre vulnera sanat, ista medicina suaviter et celeriter sanat, experimentum optimum et probatum, istud est experimentum efficacissimum et probatissimum, infallibiliter . . . emittet se expellet, ista medicina cito sanat et optime prout sepius est probatum.* Superlatives abound: *sus ciel n'ad si bone medcine encuntre venim fors triacle, ice vaut sur tous autres kar il fu fet de part Nostre Seinur Jesu Crist, cest emplastre est mestre sur totes les autres pur rauncle, ce est le meillour bei[v]r[e] que seit pur poysoun, sachez ke c'est le meillur oignement que soit a froide gute, summa est medicina, suz ciel n'at meillure.* Sometimes the statement of efficacy is placed at the beginning of the receipt in combination with or before the indication: *A rancle ci orrez medcines esprovees, ci a esperment esprové contre festre et encontre cancre, medicinas probatas et veras.* Besides this general advertisement of the product, there are also references to specific effects which usually reflect the content of the indication: *en un nut despessera ou departera la maylle ou la teye, amendera le oie, tele medesine occira les lentes e les autres mals, dolor quamvis inveteratus sit tolletur, la gout s'en irra dedens treis jours.* Occasionally, effects and side-effects are mentioned in greater detail. In a receipt for constipation it is noted 'Ista medicina est valde suavis et sine periculo. Quidam vero dant succum radicis eiusdem cum alio liquore bene mixto, aliquando autem dant cum potagio, sed istud est aliqualiter periculosum eo quod nimis violenter laxat'. Another receipt observes 'si per duo vel tria emplastra talia cessaverit dolor et caro sive cutis dealbescat, signum est quod paciens est in convalescendo' with the corollary that the opposite symptoms – swelling and reddening of the flesh – require a new remedy. Symptoms rarely receive detailed description (though see PR 1247 ff), but the side-effects or secondary symptoms are sometimes acknowledged as a reason for modifying treatment. At the end of a receipt for constipation it is suggested that there be added 'comyn ou fenoyl ou anyse pur temprer la ventuosité'. The strength of the medicine prescribed may be adjusted to suit the circumstances: 'poterit etiam fieri sine turbentyn licet non fuerit tante virtutis sicut cum turbentyn'; 'ki vodra aguser cest oignement, si mette arubre e castor'; 'a agucer cest oignement metez fens de columb e de castorie, si aver le poez'; 'miel i metés por adoucir, se le poés donc le plus lonc tenir'.

The best advertisement for the efficacy of the receipt, of course, was the citing of specific cures: 'expertum est sepius per illum medicum de Lechlyn', 'de ce garit Robert de Neuport e le suppriur de colun de sa main', 'la Sarazine de Meschine garist une dame veont plusurs que tote fu calve e out perdu les sorcilz', 'sic enim curatus fuit frater N. de Credetoun in terra sancta', 'magister T. vidit quendam curatum de antrace solo succo iacee nigre'. At other times there are more general references to 'les dames de Salerne' (MS Digby 69 no. 4) or the opinion of 'bons mires' (PR 813).

There are a few references to anonymous written sources, notably in the *Physique rimee*, which has the only allusion to an ancient authority (107, 'Dauns Galiens').

This survey of the form and content of the medieval medical receipt should not be concluded without stressing an ubiquitous problem of interpretation, namely botanical identification.[158] The receipts contain none of the material furnished by the herbals, so that identification is perforce by name alone. The very few descriptive phrases to be found in the receipts (e.g. 'Lingua avis .i. semen fraxini . . . est herba que lingue avis similis est') are of little practical value. The notorious polysemy of medieval plant names makes certainty of identification a chimera. When, for example, a receipt specifies 'une herbe ke est apelé sanguinere' we are merely reminded that 'sanguinary' is the name given to several plants used for staunching blood and accorded to them on the homoeopathic principle or the so-called doctrine of signatures. Since the receipt in question is itself for the staunching of blood, any of these would be candidates in the present context. It follows that many plant identifications proposed in the following pages must be regarded as tentative and provisional.

The Medical Receipt in Medieval England

The reprinting in 1961 by the Holland Press of the Rev. Thomas Oswald Cockayne's *Leechdoms, Wortcunning and Starcraft of Early England* (1864–66) marked a long-overdue recognition of the importance of Anglo-Saxon medical manuscripts.[159] There are five major vernacular works all of which allot a considerable space to receipts. The *Laeceboc* (Leechbook of Bald) was written in the first half of the ninth century.[160] As C. H. Talbot has shown,[161] it contains a great deal of valuable material drawn from Greek medical writers via Latin translations and anticipates much that has been attributed to Gariopontus and Petroncellus and incorrectly dubbed 'Salernitan'. The *Peri-Didaxeon* (On Schools [of Medicine])[162] is a later work (first half of the twelfth century) based on a different translation of the same fundamental text as underlies the Leechbook. It contains 66 chapters of short receipts following the *a capite ad calcem* sequence and ends incomplete. The *Lacnunga* is a collection of about 200 receipts and charms, a work full of superstition and eclectic magic which has been used to denigrate Anglo-Saxon medicine,[163] but which is in reality not at all representative. The Old English *Herbarium*[164] survives in four MSS and in three of these it represents a translation of three originally independent Latin treatises – Ps.-Musa, *De Herba Vettonica*, Ps.-Apuleius, *Herbarium*, and *Liber medicinae ex herbis femininis*.[165] Its 185 chapters, each devoted to a medicinal plant, comprise a series of receipts. The *Medicina de Quadrupedibus* also consists of a translation of three originally distinct treatises: *Liber de taxone*, a treatise on the healing properties of the mulberry, and the short version of Ps.-Sextus Placitus *Liber Medicinae ex animalibus*.[166] It follows the Old English *Herbarium* in all 4 MSS and deals with the medical properties of various animal secretions or extracts.[167] Finally, besides heterogeneous scraps and glossaries, we have, from the first decade of the twelfth century, a set of Latin medical writings contained in a scientific encyclopaedia, St John's College, Oxford, MS 17 which represents the moment when Anglo-Saxon medicine gave way to the doctrines and practices of Salerno.[168]

The vernacular medical texts, especially the herbal remedies, of Anglo-Saxon England have recently been reassessed by Linda Voigts[169] and one cannot do better than to quote her summary of what amounts to the rehabilitation of the subject:

> We must rather look at the sophisticated handling of text by the Anglo-Saxon makers and users of medical books, at the vernacular revision in the *Herbarium Apulei* of the Latin tract on betony, for example, a reorganisation that deletes the nonessential, mostly magical section and unites the important material about habitat and preparation of the plant at the beginning of the chapter. We must also look at the way Anglo-Saxons attempted to make their books as useful as possible, by adding tables of contents and recipes, by marking recipes with marginal notations, by providing Latin-vernacular herbal glossaries to Latin remedy books and glossing Latin plant names with the vernacular labels. We must likewise acknowledge that Anglo-Saxon abbesses and kings acquired exotic drugs through informal exchange, largely through ecclesiastics, and similarly, we must consider that some exotic plants were likely obtained through trade. Most important, we must admit to the probability that Anglo-Saxon monks and nuns cultivated Mediterranean plants with great care and under more auspicious climatic conditions than exist today, remembering that plants like peony, formerly not native to Britain, were naturalised after cultivation during the pre-Conquest era. In short, we must grant that Anglo-Saxons valued healing plants, that they valued books about healing plants, and that they dealt with both intelligently. (p. 266)

After the Conquest receipt collections continue to be produced in Latin, often with great artistry,[170] and around the middle of the twelfth century the first Anglo-Norman receipts and charms appear.[171] In the thirteenth century the bulk of receipt collections is written in Latin and Anglo-Norman and forms the subject of the present study. By the fifteenth century, of course, collections of Middle English receipts are becoming common. A particularly neglected source of receipts, however, is a series of medical compendia, mostly in Latin, which were produced between 1240 and 1400, and these deserve to be described here.

The compendia in question fall somewhat between the purely scholastic compendia (which use authoritative sources in dialectical reasoning and assimilate much Aristotelian natural philosophy) and the more empirically therapeutic compilations with their sources in the Hippocratic-Galenic tradition of inductive reasoning.[172] The first compiler to be considered is Gilbertus Anglicus (Gilbert of Aquila) who, though mentioned by Chaucer, is an elusive figure. His *Compendium medicinae* (in MS Sloane 272 and the Geneva print known as *Laurea Anglicana*) is the first complete treatise on general medicine by an English author and was printed in Lyons in 1510 and Geneva in 1608. It was probably composed c.1240, the earliest MS dating from about thirty years later. Gilbertus certainly spent much time on the continent (possibly visiting Salerno and Montpellier) and may have been a contemporary of Gilles de Corbeil, on whose *De urinis* he wrote a commentary. A good analysis of the contents of the *Compendium* by H. E. Handerson was published posthumously in 1918.[173] By dint of copying out *in extenso* parts of Roger Frugardi's *Chirurgia* Gilbertus presents the fullest state of the art outside Italy, though he never actually names any surgeons. In more general terms he is a scholastic humoralist, fond of reporting distinctions and definitions in dialectical manner, and throughout is dominated by Avicenna whom he interprets in the light of Augustinianism.[174] He also shows interest in dietetics and is an enthusiastic polypharmacist. He includes much less superstition and magic than many of his successors. The *Compendium* is replete with receipts for compound medicines and some of these, drawn from Salernitan *materia medica* such as entered the *Antidotarium Nicolai*, are reflected in a set of receipts in MS Cambridge, Trinity College 0.1.20 discussed below.[175] Gilbertus's arrangement of material within each chapter of the 7 books of the *Compendium* is often confusing and difficult to follow.[176] The opening book, on fevers, is particularly prolix and was cut by the anonymous fifteenth-century adaptor of the work into Middle English.[177] Also cut were sections on skin diseases, women's illnesses, and an antidotary. On the other hand, the adaptor respected a large number of receipts, which are subsequently found in Middle English remedy books. In general the *a capite ad calcem* order, adopted by Gilbertus in Book Two, is continued thereafter. Although apologetic about the inclusion of the occasional charm, Gilbertus does not spurn popular remedies and he is regularly cited in the *Thesaurus pauperum*. It is clear that his *Compendium*, notwithstanding its exhausting complexity of exposition, was regarded as a rich repository of medical receipts. Curiously, it has almost no prefatory matter, such as would instruct us about the author's circumstances and ambitions.[178]

The second significant medical compendium is the *Rosa medicinae* or *Rosa Anglica* of John of Gaddesden,[179] probably composed at some time between 1305 and 1317. This is the first treatise by a physician wholly trained in England – John was a Fellow of Merton College, Oxford, with a degree in theology as well as a doctorate in medicine. He became court physician to Edward II (1307–27) and cured his son of smallpox, using a method already referred to by one of his sources, Gilbertus.[180] There are over a dozen manuscripts[181] and four printed editions: 1492 (Pavia), 1502 (Venice), 1517 (Pavia), 1595 (Augsburg).[182] John is heavily indebted to Arabic medicine and to Bernard Gordon's *Lilium medicinae*,[183] also to Henri de Mondeville. Primarily concerned, in his professional life, with clergy and students,[184] Gaddesden injects into his catch-all compendium personal anecdotes, charms, folk medicine, whilst at the same time offering a healthily critical conspectus of two centuries of continental medicine (there are references to over 46 authorities). He is more practical than Gilbertus and offers a more perspicuous arrangement of his materials, not following the *a capite ad calcem* order, but observing the sequence: description of disease, symptoms, causes, prognosis, cure.[185] The work ends with an *antidotarium*. Like Gilbertus's *Compendium*, the *Rosa* was plundered for receipts and also received a translation in the fifteenth century – this time into Irish.[186] There are frequent references to Galen, Averroes and Avicenna, and although the number of receipts is fairly modest, John displays a good knowledge of compound medicines as represented by the *Antidotarium Nicolai*.

Unlike Gilbertus, John of Gaddesden includes vernacular words in his text as an aid to understanding [quotations from MS Sloane 1067]:

[f.84r] punctelli . . . vocantur a laicis 'purples'
[f.84r] punctelli magni . . . vocantur anglice 'mesels'
[f.102r] pustule . . . 'burbeles' vocate a mulieribus
[f.105v] accipe salsamentum quod vocatur anglice 'gransil'
[f.156r] duricies splenis que vocatur gallice 'corten' [?], anglice 'elifcake' [MS Add. 33996 f.172r 'torten']
[f.162r] rapella anglice 'skirewit'

[f.208v] diabetica passio est immoderatus fluxus urine per renos . . . vocatur gallice 'chaudepisse'

John also glosses plant names:

[f.18r] succus albederagi .i. basilicon vel *columbine*
[f.34v] urtica mortua vel archangelica
[f.58v] rubei solsequii .i. calendule

The need for such glosses is amply attested by the lists of *synonyma herbarum* which appear in countless medical manuscripts throughout the Middle Ages in England.

John frequently refers to his own experiences or experiments, though a degree of caution is necessitated by the fact that he is so often copying out the work of predecessors:

[f.35r] viscus arboris cum calce contrita est medicina mea experta in duricie [corr. curatione] cuiuscumque duriciei sicut ego probavi in genu duro et splene et apostematibus

[f.57v] medicina mea specialissima ad omnem tumorem . . . sicut expertus sum frequenter

[f.79r] Frequenter operatus fui cum . . .

[f.101v] hoc est meum proprium experimentum et voco illud unguentum pineatum. . . . Istud est unguentum meum pro delicatis pro quo habui pecuniam et jocalia, nescio quot et qualia

[cf. MS Add. 33996 f.167r Istud est experimentum m. J. G. pro delicatis pro quo habuit jocalia, nescit quot nec qualia]

The famous cure for smallpox is related thus:

[f.86r] Deinde capiatur rubeum scarlatum et involvatur totaliter in eo variolosus vel in panno alio rubeo sicut ego feci de filio nobilissimo regis Anglie quando paciebatur istum morbum et feci omnia circa lectum esse rubea et tunc cum cura sequenti curavi eum sine vestigiis variolarum

Another interesting feature of John of Gaddesden's cures is that he recognises the need to fit the proposed cure to the patient's means:

[f.100r] De conservantibus de lepra et palliantibus videndum [est] quod quedam sunt pro pauperibus, quedam sunt pro divitibus

He gives detailed instructions for the *balneum* to be used to treat *febris ethica*, but realises that the bath of warm milk would be too costly for poor people ('quia esset sumptuosum pauperibus, possunt 4 lagene vel 3 lactis decoqui et linthiamen triplicatum inponi').

A fair idea of the charms and superstitious practices recorded by Gaddesden can be obtained from the following:

[f.19r] [for nosebleed] modo de empiricis videamus: Vade ad locum ubi crescit sanguinaria .i. bursa pastoris et genibus flexis dic Pater Noster et Ave Maria etc. Tunc istum versiculum dic: 'Te ergo quesumus, famulis tuis subveni quos precioso sanguine redemisti'. Et sic collige herbam unam vel duas. Sed si multas herbas colligas, oportet istas orationes iterare. Et tunc suspende illam herbam circa collum pacientis a quo fluit et ibi dimitte[t] et stringetur certissime.

Notes on pp.338–53

[f.19v] Experimentum Gilberti ad omnem fluxum sanguinis quod ponit tertio practice sue. Dic(it) 'In nomine Patris et Filii etc.' Caro cum calice confirma sanguinem Israelite novies versando aquam et colando per camisiam infirmi quam tribuas ipsi pacienti vel nuncio nomine infirmi . . . Item scribe hoc nomen Veronica in fronte pacientis cum sanguine eius et dic orationem istam: 'Deus qui solo tactu fimbrii vestimenti tui mulierem in fluxu sanguinis constitutam sanare dignatus es, te suppliciter exoramus, domine Jesu Criste, qui solus langores sanas, ut fluxum sanguinis istius pro quo vel pro qua preces infundimus restringere et sistere facias dextra tue potencie et pietatis extendendo: In nomine Patris et Filii et Spiritus Sancti, Amen.' Pater Noster et Ave Maria.

[f.248r] De dolore dentium . . . carmen pro dentibus: Scribe in maxillam pacientis ista nomina + In nomine Patris et Filii et Spiritus Sancti, Amen + rex + pax + nax + in Christo filio. Et statim cessabit, ut vidi frequenter.

Item quicumque dixerit orationem in honore Appolonie virginis, die illo non habebit dolorem dentis si ter dicitur de sancto Nigacio martire.

Item quamdiu legitur evangelium in missa quolibet die, dum audit homo missam, signet dentem et capud signo sancte crucis. Et dicat Pater Noster et Ave pro animabus [sic] patris et matris sancti Philippi. Et hoc continue et preservat a dolore futuro et cur(r)at presentem secundum veridicos.

[f.11v] [De vigilia] Item ex eis [=curis] que dormire faciunt febricitantes et alios est, ut extremitates in acutis habentium vigilias ligentur cum ligatione faciente dolorem cum nodis facilis solutionis et coram ipsis ponatur lampas vel ponantur candele ardentes. Et fiant coram pacientibus fabulaciones et sermones multi. Deinde solvantur ligamenta subito postquam clauserit paciens oculos. Removeantur candele et taceant ibi existentes repente et dormiet. Istud ponit Avicenna capitulo de acutibus febris.

Unlike Gilbertus, John of Gaddesden prefixes to his work an introduction to his aims and method:

[f.6r] Galienus primo de ingenio sanitatis, 'Non visites nimis curias et aulas principium', sicut nec ego feci quousque sciverim [libros], quia dicit Galienus septimo de ingenio sanitatis in prohemio non est possibile per aliquid fieri proximius Deo quam per scienciam. Ideo optavi humilibus istum librum facere, quia cum nullus liber est sine vituperio, ut dicit Galienus secundo de crisi, ideo nec iste liber sine vituperio erit. Rogo tamen ut istum librum videntes non dente canino mordeant, set humiliter pertractent, quia quicquid hic dicetur erit vel autenticum vel longa experientia probatum, quia omnia hic dicta ego Johannes de Gatisden septimo anno lecture mee compilavi. Circa quem librum talem volo processum habere, quia primo volo nomen investigare cuiuscumque morbi, secundo diffinitionem, tertio occasionem eius et causam. Iuxta illud Ysaac quarto febrium capitulo de ictericia, 'Omne quod volumus investigare tribus modis intelligimus: aut suo nomine, quod est placitum, aut diffinitione eius naturam ostendente, aut actione eius effectum demonstrante, et est ibi actio idem quod occasio vel causa'. Quarto signa generalia et specialia – accidentia infirmo sunt signa medico. Quinto dicam pronosticacionem. Sexto curam, et ibi sequendo Mesue dicta dicam que sunt facienda in cura cuiuslibet morbi periculosi et curabilis.

Antequam tamen ista fiant, volo nomen isti libro imponere vocando ipsum 'Rosam medicinae' propter quinque additamenta que sunt in rosa quasi quinque digiti tenentes rosam de quibus scribitur 'Tres sunt barbati, sine barba sunt duo nati' .i. tres articuli vel partes circumstantes rosam sunt cum pilositate, duo sunt sine, et ideo erunt quinque libri. Hic primi tres erunt barbati barba longa, quia extendent se ad multa, quia erunt de morbis communibus, et quot modis dicatur morbus communis vel universalis vide in prohemio secundi libri. Duo sequentes erunt de morbis particularibus cum declaracione alicorum omissorum in precedentibus et quasi sine barba. Et sicut rosa excellit omnes flores, ita iste liber excellit omnes practicas modernas, quia erit pro pauperibus et divitibus sirurgicis et medicis, de quo non oportet multum recurrere ad alios libros, quia hic videbitur satis de morbis curabilibus in speciali et similiter in generali.

This introduction provides an accurate enough picture of the work. Books 1–3 are massive, whilst 4 and 5 are short. Gaddesden does indeed provide a comprehensive range of medical extracts which would save physicians much labour, and he indicates alternative prescriptions for the poor, though not so frequently as does John Mirfield after him. Until a textual study is made of the MSS it is not possible to say how far Gaddesden's extensive aims were respected by the copyists. That he was both interpolated and abbreviated may be seen from the copy in MS B. L. Add. 33996 ff.149r–210v, which is acephalous, truncated and interpolated, ending 'Explicit rosula medicine secundum m. J. de Gatesden'. At the point where the copy begins there is a mixture of charms and vernacular receipts, some of which I print below:

[f.149r] A debrosure de pel de l'oyl: Pernez poudre de comyn e poudre de gyngere ana et distemprés od vyn blank. E fundez en le oyl une petite quantité . . .

In nomine Patris et Filii et Spiritus Sancti, Amen. Inter vestibulum et altare occisus est Zacharias sacerdos in testamentum domini nostri Jesu Christi. Extractus est sanguis eius. In nomine Patris sistat sanguis eius; in nomine Filii cesset sanguis eius; in nomine Spiritus Sancti non exiat sanguis eius. Ave Maria etc. Et similiter Pater Noster ter dicat et scribe de eodem sanguine in fronte eius, si sit masculus, Beronixus, si femina, Beronixa.

Item, alio modo sic: Dicas [f.149v] 'Longeus miles hebreus latus domini perforavit lancea et continuo exivit sanguis et aqua, sanguis redempcionis et aqua baptismatis + In nomine Patris cesset sanguis + In nomine Filii restet sanguis + In nomine Spiritus Sancti non exeat amplius sanguis. O Maria, credimus quod sancta Maria est mater Dei et verum infantem genuit, genuit Christum, et sicut Jordanis aqua in qua baptizatus est Christus restitit, sic restent tue vene que sanguine sunt plene . . .'

Ad sanandum vulnera primo dicatur istud carmen: Tres boni fratres iverunt ad montem Oliveti ad colligendum herbas et obviaverunt domino nostro Jesu Christo qui dixit eis 'Quo itis?' Tres boni fratres qui respondentes dixerunt 'Ad montem Oliveti ad colligendum herbas ad sanandum vulnera'. Et ait illis Jesus 'Conjuro vos, tres boni fratres, quod herbas dimittatis et oleum de oliva et lanam nigram sumatis dicentes "Conjuro te, vulnus, per vulnus Christi preciosum a Longeo milite perforatum, quod neque ranclescebat neque putrescebat nec vermem generabat nec dolorem amplius sentiebat, sic nec tu ranclescas, neque putrescas, nec vermem generes, nec dolorem inde sentias per virtutem olei et lane. In nomine Patris et Filii et Spiritus Sancti, Amen." Nec inde mercedem capiatis, sed in nomine Patris et Filii et Spiritus Sancti id faciatis'.

A totez playes: Batez plantayne et lancelé et medlez od le jus de l'aubun de l'oef, e en ceo moylez estupez e metez sur la playe et garra . . .

[f.150r] . . . Pur playe malement close: Pernez la crote de chevere e miel e oynt de pork, si en fetez une plastre, si metez al playe, si ele est malement close . . .

Pur fere entret sanatif: Cere virgine, oele de olyve, myel, oynt de porc, saym de berbys, rosyl, franc encens que peyse quatreble dez autres.

Pur checun playe curable pur fere entret sanative et attrative: Pernez rosyl e sere virgine, franc ensens, code, gummi arabic, galbanum, oynt de porc, bure de may, oyle de olyve, code peysé(r) a plus que les autres, e boy asemble e metez a playe . . .

[f.150v] . . . Dicas .iii. Pater Noster et Ave cum isto versu: 'Te ergo ques[o] domine fa t[?]'. Quot herbas colligas, tot Pater Noster .iii. dicas. Liga circum collum pacientis empericam.

Circa membrum a quo fluit sanguis frica eam inter manus ne homines cognoscant et pone in sindone vel panno lineo . . .

Pur morsure de chien: Pernez blank plom e arnement e corn [MS corf] de cerf (f)ars, e metez ces poudres ensemble e metez a mal.

Celi que ne put dormir: Escrivez ses nouns en foyl de lorere e si metez desus son cheff que yl ne sache: Exmael .iii. adiuro per archangelum Michaelem ut soporetur homo iste vel femina . . .

Pur morsure de l'yrayne[187] / n'est pas ben que fors remayne / graunt masse des muches purchasés / et de ceo la morsure [f.151r] oygnez. / Pus pernez foylez de rays / en vyn soient mult byen boylez. / Quant quit serra, byen les triblez / e sur la playe les metez. / La plaie overte se tendra / e le venym enchacera. / De foyls menuz pernez / e od miel estampez, / sur la playe pus metez, / si ert delyverement sané.

Pur poynture de eez: Pernez foyles de mauve, si triblez, sur la pointure lé fricez, e par meysmes garry serrez. . . .

Contra sanguinis fluxum: Scribe hec nomina [sic] Veronica cum sanguine pacientis in fronte et dic orationem istam: 'Deus qui solo tactu fimbrie vestimenti tui . . . [see above, MS Sloane 1067 f.19v]

Pur sanc estancher: 'Adiuro te, sanguis, per sanguinem domini nostri Jesu Christi et que vulnera que in cruce passus est, pro nobis cessa, sanguis. Adiuro te, sanguis, per hec sancta nomina domini nostri Jesu Christi, O, Emanuel, Sabooth, Adonay, Osa Dei, sicut mulierem in fluxu sanguinis cessare fecit, sic te cessare faciat dominus noster Jesus Christus'. .iii. Pater Noster dicatur . . .

[f.151v] . . .Oygnement sarsinés pur la goute ou que ele soit en le corps: Pren [MS pien] ravene e sareie e cerfoyl de checun un poigne, e triblez e metez en oyle. Pus pernez bure e sue de buc e de motoun e de cerf e myel quit en peiz, fetez toutz choses ensemble e colez parmy un drap e oygnez la goute . . .

Pur felon: Pernez matfeloun, ceo est 'cropwort' en engleys. Triblez mut bien, si donez a malade beyvere le jus e fetez emplastre de triblure, si metez sur le mal. Fetez ceo .iii. jours e donc gardés malade que .iii. jours manjwe nule chose for mye en ewe de payn de orge e de ceo poy e ne beyve nule chose que ewe. E s'il manjue autre chose, yl morra pur veir, e si ceo fet avant dit, garra.

Autre: Done a beyvre matfeloun en l'escale de un oeff. Pus ardez e od ycel [MS cyel] herbe user donez. Et ache et persyl pernez e fenil, ensemble boylez en bone cerveyse ou en vyn, e beyv[e]z a seyr e a matyn.

Autre pur feloun e pur rancle: Beyvez flour de orge e semence de lyn en eysel ou en vyn, si metez sur de motoun. Ceo ossit rancle e feloun.

Pur menesoun senglante: Pernez millefoyl e plantayne e fraser, si ert dil [MS sil] un cum de l'altre, estampé bien ensemble et distemprés od vyn e beyve a seir e a matyn.

Altre, uncore vous dirra[i] que mut vaut: Traiez un payn de furn tut chaud. Supez fetez en vyn vermayl, mangez, si garrez saunz fayl.

Uncore vous dirra[i] autre medicine: Centorie, estaunche e [f.152r] (e) terebentine. Ceo beyve, si avera santé en le noun de la seinte trinité.

A mal de coer a homme que toutz viaundes sount e[n]countre quer: Pernez centorie, si quisez bien en serveyse estale et quant ert mut quise, pernez le sus, si le distemprés bien e metz al pot, si lessét durement quire. E pus si le colez parmy un drap e fetz boyler ensemble jeskes yl soyt byen espés. E metz puz en boyste e fetz la malade manger pus de cete letuarie checun jour .iii. quilers jeske yl soyt garri. Ceo ly oustera glet de quer, si ly fra aver bon talent de manger.

Pur les enfirmetez que dames unt et sount [. . .] : Pernez pur femme que ad perdu ses flurs, pernez un herbe que est apele 'culrage', si le(s) quisez bien en vyn e metez sur la cuisse [MS cure] de la femme quant ele ert coché, si que la chalour cent. Fetz ceo sovent, si garra. . . .

A femme que [est] enseinte: Ne donez jammés puliol a manger, char mortele chose est. . . .

[f.152v] A ouster rancle de playe ou saun playe: Pernez ache, wymawe, ortie, senecion, chenelie, comfirie, matfeloun, herbe benet, de chescun ouel porcioun e pus batez bien. Quant yl ert bien triblez, pernez un neof pot ou payele [de] bon vyn ou estale servoyse bone ou eysel, si metez une poyne de gruel ou un de lino[i]s, si lessez bien boyler e byen quire. Pus si le batez bien. Quant yl ert triblez, fetez bien boyler ensemble que il soyt espés. Pus liez a l'emfflure sur le quir.

Pur rancle dedens [l]e corps: Pernez les grey[n]s de juniperie e blanc vyn e bev[ez] le seyr chaud e le matyn teve. . . .

Pur conustre festre e cancre:[188] Ore fet dunk a saver / a conustre cez maus pur veir, / quel est festre [MS fostret], quel noun, / e quel est [f.153r] cancre par resoun. / Un esp[ro]ve vous aprendray / itele cum apris le ay. / Le frés furmage dunk pernez, / od mel le oygnez, / si le metez (si) vus le primseir [MS pus seir], / l'en[de]ma(t)yn purrez ver / si le furmage soit entamé, / dunc i a le cancre esté. / Plusours dient que ceo est con[trov]e, / Pur ceo dirra[i] un autre esprove: / Pernez la arcille, si l'emplastrez / e le gros auk (?) si metez. / En une fourme serrunt mys, / net e ben sané et tut vifs, / e pus serra la playe liez. / Si l'endemayn seit mangé, / lors purrez saver de fi / ke goutefestre e[st], cet vous dy. / E de autre part garde(z) pernez / quant vou[s] lez playes engardez. / Le cancre mangue le quir / e si fet la playe neir. / Mes festre fet tut autrement: / la playe fet [MS est] parfunde[ment], / just les os [MS loes], juste lé nerfs, / lez jointes crossez en travers. / La festre est mult plu fort a garir, / kar bein vu (?) poez pruz [. . .] . . .

For schabbe on honden oþer clawyng: Tak þe rede dokke and do of þe rote and seth wel þe rote with botere of May and with old smere, and qwan yt ys wel sode, wring yt thur a cloth and do yt in to boxes and anoynte þe schabbes and þe clawyng aȝen þe fuir.

ȝyf þer ys yren oþer tre or thorn in ony stede of mannus body, tak egremoyne and stampe with colde smere and ley þerto.

Or tak ditayne and ley þerto or drink yt.

Or ellis tak þe rote of [f.153v] the rosel and poune yt wel with hony and do on a clout of flex and ley þerto and yt schal drawe out al þe ache. . . .

For man þat ys pykelyd: Seth peletre in wyn and ley on þe face.

A cely que ne put bien oyer: Pernez beau bure e mel e catapuces e vyn en ouele mesure e metez ensemble e chaufez que il soyt teve. E pus metz en les orailes [MS oraires] . . .

Ut mulier concipiat: Suspende circa collum has caracteres: 77 ct a n e ae gc x + x + c t h' ne anne p. Quod si volueris probare, suspende super arborem que numquam produxit fructum, et germinabit. . . .

[f.154r] . . . Ceo beyvere garist totz playes overtes: Batez ensemble waraunce e rouge cholete e plantayne e chawne vert ou sa semence, e distemprés en blanc vyn ou de serveyse de pur orge. E pus quisez mel e metz (e metz) eyns pur endocer quant vous avez pris lé herbis e ousté la drache. De ycel [MS cyel] beyvere beyve(re) ly naufré un hanap a matyn e autre a seyr jeskes yl soit garri. E kovere son pot de un crouste de payn que le odour ne isse e eyns que yl beyve, meove tut ensemble lez fundris [MS fundril] (lez) del pot od un bastoun fendu al chef ou quatre, que soit tutdys en le pot – pur ceo mesmes de cou(r)dre deyt estre fet. . . .

[f.154v] . . . For costif wombe: Tak lynsed and seth yt wel in water and þanne do out þat watur and nym þat lynsed and frie yt wel in a panne with fayr grece and lat hym eten.

For snelt of wombe: Poune ruwe in wyn oþer in ale and drink yt ofte. . . .

Pur feloun: Pernez solsecle e le mouel de oef e cel e triblez ensemble, si lez metez desus le mal. Esprové est.

Autre: Quisez en servoyse matfeloun e morele e avence od mel. Donez a beyvere.

A goutefestre e cancre: Pernez bure de may, herbe Water, bugle, pigle, sanicle, avence, consoude petit, egrimoyne, lancelé, sauge, osmund, senecion, melaundre et rue. Ceo garist. . . .

Ky ad beu venym beyve jus de horhoune od vyn, si garra. . . .

[f.159r] . . . Pur sausefleme en visage: Pernez un smere de grese de sengler, tant plu vel tant plus vaut, in le quarte partye de une unce de fraunc [f.159v] ensens e le peys de troys deners de vif argent e .x. quyler de jus de carsoun de funtayne. Toutes cestez chosez triblez ensemble en un morter net e pu(e)z lé quysez en un payle de quyvere. E pus pernez un bel hanap pleyn de euue de funtayne clere e(n) metz en ycel [MS cyel] ewe un poygne de cel blanc e net e lavez la visage sanz froter(e) encountre le fu auk[es] loynes. E pus pernez le quantité de une feve del dit oygnement e oygnez le dit visage. E pus le fetez segner deux fetez de la veyne capitale, si garra. E gardez cet oygnement en un vessel de ver. . . .

For bytyng of addre: Stampe centorie and drink oþer grene rue and fenyl and seth hem wel yn botere and ʒyf to drinke.

ʒyf addre or snake be withynne man or womman: Stampe rue and urine and ʒyf þe sike to drinke. Or tempre urine of þe sike [MS silue] man or beste and arnement and mak yt sum del hard and ʒyf hym to drinke and he schal casten hym with al þe venum.

For man þat ne may nat stalye: Seth in wel good wyn þe hokke and eysel and garlek altogeder to þe thrydde del, þe heved of þe garlek with þe braunches. ʒyf him to drynke.

For scabede hevedys: Poune garlek with hony and ley þer uppe or ellys tak þe blake bete and stampe and tak þe jus and ofte smere þe heved.

Forto makyn her growe: Seth þe levys of þe wythy and maydenher with oyle and ley þer þe her wanteth.

For scabbe of mannus body: Gadere fumytere and wasch yt wel and stampe and drink þe jus with ale. . . .

[f.165r] . . . Pur puour de bouche: Mangés puliol sek.[189]

Maungez betoyne jun, si vous ame[n]dra la vue.[190]

Pur sang estauncher: Pernez sangdragon, bol armoniac, franc ensens, mastik. . . .

Pur paralisie in les jambes ou in les pees: Pernez ambrosye, flour de geneste, eble, lavendre e faverole [MS laverole] .i. broklemke, e baynez in ces herbes boylez.

Pur poylez: Pernez le jus de rue, si oygnez.[191] . . .

[f.169r] . . . Si vis scire de suspecto an sit epilenticus vel demoniacus vel lunaticus, dic hoc nomen in aure eius: 'Recede demon, quia effimploy [corr. effimolei] tibi precipiunt'. Si [sit] lunaticus vel demoniacus, statim efficitur quasi mortuus fere per unam horam, et surgentem interoga eum de quacumque re volueris. Et dicet tibi et si non ceciderit audito hoc nomine, scias eum epilenticum esse. . . .

[f.169v] . . . Item: Cum est in paroxismo [= epileptic attack], ponat aliquis os super aurem pacientis et dicat ter istos versus, statim surget:

> Jasper fert mirram thus Melchior Baltazar aurum
> Hec tria qui secum portabit nomina regum
> Solvitur a morbo domini pietate caduco. . . .

[f.169v] . . . Pro pueris qui non possunt uti medicinis sive sit epilenticus, lunaticus vel demoniacus: Si patrem habeat puer et matrem, ducant eum ad ecclesiam facto jejuno trium dierum a parentibus [et] a paciente [MS pacientibus]. Si sint tante etatis quod sint compotes et confiteantur, (et) vadant die Veneris in jejunio quattuor temporum et audiant missam de die [et] similiter die sabbati dominica sequente. Sacerdos bonus vel vir religiosus legat supra caput pacientis in ecclesia evangelium quod legitur in Septembri tempore vindemearum post festum sancte crucis in diebus quatuor temporum. Et tunc scribat illud idem devote et portet paciens circa collum et curat. Et est evangelium ubi dicitur 'hoc genus demonii non eicitur [nisi] in jejunio et oratione etc.'[192] . . .

[f.181r] . . . Pur emflure de veyne capitale: Pernez vyn e oyle et clausez e lavez de bras[?]. Pus metez sur un plastre que est apelé dyaquilon.

Pur emflure de la mediane: Pernez foyles de betes e mye de payn e oyle e un poy de seel. E medlez e fetz emplastre e metz sur l'emflure.

Pur emflure de quele veyne que ceo soyt: Pernez semence de lyn e prendrés fyges secches, si vous volez, e grece de ferine e quisez touz treys ensemble en ewe. E pus triblez en un morter e pus lavez de cel ewe e metez l'emplastre desur.

This abbreviated and interpolated version of the *Rosa* also includes a number of vernacular glosses. At the beginning of the copy there are random glosses which seem to have been drawn from a *synonyma* list:

[f.149r] camyphiteos : medrattle; camedreos : klavre; [f.149v] enula : dokke; morsus galline : chikenmete; sanguinaria : noseblede; brionia : wylde nep; mentastrum : horse-mynte; lentigo aquatica : dokemete; grana solis : gromyl; speragus : mawewort; altea : wymawe; mellilotum : honysouke in prato; tapsus barba(r)stus : weltewort, lichelef, soft; ypoquistidos : taddestoles.

Vernacular glosses found within the text of receipts are as follows:

[f.160r] herba fullonis : *crousope*, borith [f.160v] nigella .i. *kockel; wy de cheyne* potatus idem facit [f.161r] succum centinodie .i. *swynescarsen* qui dicitur lingua passeris [f.161v] radix ciclaminis .i. *erthenote* [f.162r] radix altee .i. *wymawe*; recipe bractee .i. *savine* [f.164v] levisticum .i. *lovache* [f.165r] rostrum porcinum anglice *sowethistel* [f.168r] recipe tapsi barbasti .i. *lichelef* [f.172r] cura apostematis splenis gallice *torten* anglice *elfcake* [f.173r] rapella .i. *skyrewyt* [f.179r] pilosella .i. *musere* [f.182v] vocatur kevilla in oculo anglice *pyn* gallice *espyngle* [f.183r] pulvus albus communis gallice *blaunche poudre* . . . axungia coturnicis gallice *quayle* [f.196v] bedegar .i. *englenter* [f.197r] erebo [= orobus?] *wyche* [f.207r] antrax quasi antrum faciens .i. foveam anglice *feloun* [f.207v] picem liquidam .i. *tar pich.*

The third compendium of which mention must be made is the work of John of Greenborough and is found in MS London B. L. Royal 12 G IV (s.xiv) where it succeeds a copy of Gilbertus's *Compendium medicinae* (ff.5ra–127ra). The circum-stances of the juxtaposition are explained in a colophon:

[f.187vb] Frater Johannes de Grenborugh per triginta annos et plus nuper infirmarius emebat istum librum vocatum 'Gilbertinum' ad utilitatem infirmorum in ecclesia Coventre existente. Et ea que in novis quaternis sunt scripta compilavit a practicis phisicorum Anglie, Hibernie, Judeorum, Saracenorum, Lumbardorum et Salernitarum, et expendebat multa in medicos circa compilacionem illarum medicinarum. Multa in novis quaternis suprascriptis per practicam sunt vera, set plures phisici nolunt approbare ea quia multi illorum ignorant practicam, sed multa verba et vacua in ventum seminant.

Nothing seems to be known about John of Greenborough, although it is interesting to note that a Henry Greneburgh OFM is recorded as being at the Coventry convent from 1375 until his death in 1408.[193] Another problem is the extent of the 'quaterni' which form John's compilation. It is certain that ff.140va–157vb are part of the compendium, while ff.165ra–183vb would appear also to be part of the same collection of receipts.[194] More receipts follow on ff.185ra et seq. until the colophon quoted above.[195] There are receipts (some in Middle English) in a new hand on f.188ra–vb, and then on ff.188vb–199vb there is an incomplete collection headed 'Hic incipit practica Edwardi universitatis Oxonie qui fuit optimus in illis partibus cirurgicus'.[196] As far as f.194v the receipts are in Middle English, thereafter mostly in Latin. Whilst John of Greenborough's compilation, such as it is, includes sections *de scotomia, de emigranea, ad cerebrum confortandum, de reumate, de catarro* etc., it is principally made up of remedies, including charms,[197] under the rubric *medicina contra . . .* Some are drawn from the *Lettre d'Hippocrate*. There are a few in Anglo-Norman, and a number in Middle English. The Anglo-Norman examples are as follows:

[f.145vb] Item a homme que novelment est feru de pa[ra]lasie: Faistez fere une fosse en terre al longure de une homme et fetez prendre les ossez de toutz manere de bestes que vous poiez trover et eluminetz lé osse en ceo fosse. Quant serront bien elluminez, si est prest une cleie que soit coché sur le fosse e cele cleie seit couverte de foil e de here e de eble. E fetez le malade cocher sur e seit bien covert par desus et quant il avera tant esté comme il le purra suffre[r] sur une cost, se turne sur le autre tanque com il purra sufrer e puis gyse sur le autre tanque com il purra sufrer. E cele chalour trera hors le venim dé membres e degurdera les nerves e destupera les conduz que la maladie avera estupés. E chaud se tenge sur tut rein et sanez serra.

[f.148vb] Item potus pro omni dolore in corpore: Pernez cerfoil, sawge, tansey, aloyne, fenoil, planteyne, betoyn, centorie, e les foils de blanc maroil, ache, rue, cinkfoyle, centunque (?), la racine de gletoyner e ysope, mes dé amers herbes, c'est asavoir de aloyne, de ce[n]torie e maroil, meyn[s] en pernez que des autres. Ces quinze herbes bien lavez et mundez, triblez bien e puis les mettez en une beal vessel. E puis versetz sur de la clere cervoyse ou de vyn que suffitz. E puis le movetz ou quissetz ensemble e streignez par une streignour e clarifietz e donetz une bone quantité al pacient en matyne. Iste potus verus est et probatissimus. Quedam enim Sarazena docuit eum quendam militem pro cuius amore pervenit ad Christianitatem qui .s. miles multos egros fecit convalescere et sanos per usum illius cotidianum in sanitate permanere.

[f.170rb] Item pro homine infrigidato in omne loco corporis sui: Pernét une libre de gynger belentyn e tryét e fort si trenchét. E puys les mettez un jour e [MS cú] le nuyt en bon vinegre deske il seyt bien moyst. Pieus le colét e pernetz un potel de mel bien boylé e bien escumé e bulletz le mel e [MS a] le ginger ensemble desque a la terce partye. Puys pern[e]tz demi-livre de sucre de alizandre e mettez un coyler a cheste chose quant il bout e pieus a l'hour de syng Pater Noster e Ave mettez un autre, e si la tercie e quarte que tot soyt despendu que soyt espesse cum past. E mettez chaud en une boyste e maungez.

Vernacular words make a frequent appearance in the Latin text:[198]

[f.142rb] Pur *le blast* oculorum[199]
[f.144ra] succus de *wodebynd*; recipe *ribbe* cum omnibus radicibus
[f.144va] succus summitatis cini, anglice *hawthorn*
[f.144vb] unam herbam vocatam *spigurnell*
[f.145ra] aruina / *suwet* / ; unguentum langobardo, anglice *lombardes dewté*
[f.145va] succum de *larketong*[200]
[f.145vb] contra tetanum, anglice *craump*
[f.146rb] recipe alectorium .i. *chapone-stoun*[201]
[f.147va] recipe unum pomum vocatum *quynce*
[f.149vb] coque succum eius cum *lyf hony*[202]
[f.150ra] poma vocata *quincez*; pira vocata *wardones*[203]
[f.150rb] unum pomum vocatum *crab*[204]
[f.150vb] *mistel* crescent super *hawthorn* et non super alias arbores
[f.151ra] recipe senicion .i. *grounswily*, et *smerewort*; comede frequenter *skirwhites* et *pasteneps*; recipe morellam, *lemk* et *chikinmete*
[f.151va] unam herbam vocatam *walwort*
[f.151vb] lapides videlicet *grey pibel-stones*
[f.152rb] recipe vermes vocatos *anguthuuaches*;[205] recipe pisces vocatos *tenches*; recipe spodium vel *termetryne* . . . *termotryne*[206] invenitur *in bales of ginger*; piscis vocatus *tenche*
[f.153rb] recipe *laumbre*
[f.153vb] tragulidiructos[207] anglice *wagstre*; pisces qui vocantur *ostre*
[f.154ra] *knewholine*; unam herbam vocatam *cuylrage*
[f.154va] coque consolidam .i. *daisye*
[f.155ra] recipe *hawes*
[f.155rb] recipe semen herbe vocate *stanch*; recipe herbam vocatam *camboc*[208]
[f.155va] alligetur fortiter unum *wolvesfyst*
[f.157rb] contra morpheam: recipe *vertgres*, sulphur, *chedesope*;[209] item . . . *vertgres chedesope* . . . lappati acuti .i. *rede doc*
[f.162rb] vermes terre .i. *angultwiches* . . . recipe caseum ranarum .i. *padokchese*
[f.165vb] cardonis magni .i. anglice *fouthistell*
[f.172ra] alia herba vocata *perspere*;[210] aliam herbam vocatam *dauke*
[f.172va] tragulidirutos, anglice *waggestart*
[f.172vb] recipe . . . *brere* portantes *hepes*
[f.175rb] sinapium videlicet *grete grounden*
[f.176ra] recipe folia de *hertwort*
[f.176rb] consolida media .i. *dayeshye* j. . . . *hertwort* . . . pulver seminis de *lovehace*
[f.177ra] *chedesope* . . . misce cum *chedesope*
[f.179rb] instrumentum vocatum *chisel*
[f.179va] pinguedinem porci, *schepes talow* [sic]
[f.180va] recipe herbam vocatam *bonchawe*[211] vel *feltrik* crescentem in montibus vel petrosis locis . . . folias de *walwort* . . . recipe unam herbam vocatam *bonchawe* et *feltrik* . . .

Greenborough's compilation also includes a number of Latin verses, for example on the signs of death (f.185va),[212] from the *Schola Salernitana* (f.147ra–rb),[213] and on the plant scabious (f.151ra).[214] There are references to 'Gilbertinus' i.e. Gilbertus Anglicus (f.143rb) and in one receipt we read 'Hoc probatum est per magistrum Willelmum de Stafford' (f.145ra).

Finally, and most important of all, we have the *Breviarium Bartholomei* of John Mirfield who died in 1407. He was born probably in the village of Mirfield near

Leeds and was a clerk at the Austin priory of St Bartholomew, Smithfield, and subsequently at the hospital.[215] The *Breviarium* is probably a late work, written after John Arderne's treatise on *Fistula in ano* (1376), possibly in the period between 1380 and 1395. Nothing in the work is original, rather it represents a comprehensive *summa* of medieval English medicine, popular rather than learned, in the time of Chaucer and of the Black Prince. There is relatively little theory and almost no anatomy, the tenor of the whole work being therapeutic. The two surviving MSS, B. L. Harley 3[216] and Oxford, Pembroke College 2 were both written in, or very shortly after, John's lifetime. They are both considerable scribal accomplishments, given the vastness of the work which Hartley and Aldridge calculated would run to 2400 pages in translation. The Harley copy is extremely accurate and carefully rubricated. On f.21v we find the note 'ordine pretacto si connumeres capitales / nomen factoris demonstrabunt tibi tales'. In fact, by recording the first letter of each chapter, starting from part 2,[217] the reader discovers an extensive acrostich in the form of a prayer. This prayer has been written out on f.302va:

> Ora pro nobis sancte Bartholomee ait Johannes de Mirfelde, ut digni efficiamur promissionibus Cristi. Oremus: Deus qui mirabiliter creasti hominem et mirabilius redemisti et dedisti medicinam ad reparandam sanitatem humanorum corporum, da omnibus secundum tenorem huius voluminis fideliter operantibus prosperitatem et effectum bonum ad laudem nominis tui, domine, et ut famuli tui, quacumque infirmitate vexati, per modum medendi hic anotatum convalescant et perfectam sanitatem recipiant ut graciarum tibi referant actiones per Cristum dominum nostrum, Amen. Explicit.

The purpose of Mirfield's vast compilation is clearly expressed in the extensive preface:

> [f.6ra] In principio huius compilationis sicut in omnibus operibus nostris Deo gratias agamus sicut sui status celsitudo et beneficiorum ipsius exigit multitudo. De cuius bonitate confidens quasdam notabilitates medicinales quas in diversis locis textuum et glossarum artis medicine necnon et in opusculis plurimorum de ista scientia subtiliter et copiose tractantium inveni et collegi quas nunc tenet labilis memoria mea hortatu quorundam amicorum meorum iuxta ingenii mei modulum sub quodam compendio collocare disposui . . .

> Quoniam non decet me scribere tanquam docturum sed si velim ad labilitatem mee memorie supportandam quasdam notabilitates medicinales collectas in uno breviario conscribere quod tanquam promptuarium mihi fiat, non credo quod debeat aliquis rationabiliter inde mihi invidere. Sed si rudis sit lector sicut et ego mecum si velit participet de collectis, sin autem in ista scientia sit precellens qui rudem hanc collectam respexerit parcat oblivioso sibi providere volenti. Et evellat si velit inconvenientia et addat meliora. Quod enim tanti operis utilitatem temptavi tractare et ordine certo doctorum precedentium sententias sub compendio redigere desideravi, plus fuit ex [f.6rb] desiderio simplicioribus mihi similibus proficiendi quam ex cupiditate alicuius inanis iactancie procurande. Quo circa providus lector simplicitati compilatoris parcat corrigendo . . .

After these protestations of humility and the emphasis on the practical utility of the compilation as a vast aide-mémoire, Mirfield now copies out a passage already found in Marcellus on the malpractices of contemporary physicians:

> [f.6rb] Alia etiam subest causa scribendi presentia. Frequenter enim michi accidit ut aut propter meam aut propter amicorum meorum infirmitatem varias fraudes modernorum medicorum experirer. Quidam enim illorum ea que curare nesciebant cupiditatis causa

curare se promittebant. Quidam etiam pro medicinis modice valoris et efficacie multa impudenter exigebant. Nonnullos etiam comperi qui langores quos paucissimis diebus possent repellere in longum tempus protraxerunt, ut pacientes diu sibi tributarios haberent. Quare propter necessitatem michi videbatur et utile ut undique valetudinis remedia collecta velut in uno breviario, ut predictum est, conscriberem. Ut quocumque venirem huiusmodi impostores vitare possem et ut michi metipsi et Christi pauperibus scirem mederi si in langoribus curabilibus et levibus incidere oporteret.

Mirfield also comments on the importance of providing a choice of treatments and of keeping in mind the impatience of many sufferers:

[f.6rb] Hoc tamen considerare non omittas quoniam medicine actio secundum proprietatem subiecti frequenter immutatur. Propterea multas medicinas pro una et eadem infirmitate ponere propono in multis locis istius compilacionis. Quoniam de proprietate medicaminum est quod iuvabunt uno tempore et non alio. Et hoc est mirabile. Et forte facit hoc varietas proprietatis adquisite ex influencia orbis alicuius. Preterea scire te volo quod in multis locis opusculi huius experimentis uti propono, tum quia breviter expediunt, tum quia multi infirmi modernis temporibus valde impacientes sunt. Nolunt enim sicut antiquitus facere solebant expectare usque ad quartum vel quintum diem vel amplius si necesse fuerit, quousque materia peccans fuerit digesta et utiliter evacuata. Verum nisi statim in prima die sentiant alleviamen de medico diffidunt eiusque medicinas respuunt et contempnunt.

The epilogue of the *Breviarium* again provides a summary of the compilation's intended utility:

[f.301vb] Hic autem compilacionis huius facio finem gratias agens ei cuius magnitudinis non est finis. Protestor autem in fine huius opusculi quemadmodum et in principio quod de omnibus que in hoc tractaculo continentur nichil quod est ad propositum de meo apposui quia quod apponerem ex meipso in meipso non inveni. Sed simpliciter philosophorum et phisicorum autenticorum verba et practicorum sententias collegi et collectas conscripsi in summula una ut simplices et pauperes copiam librorum non habentes in promptu hic valeant invenire saltem superficialiter plurimorum egritudinum remedia non pauca. Quod cedat oro ad proximorum utilitatem et ad ipsius precipue honorem et gloriam qui est alpha et omega, principium et finis omnium bonorum, qui est deus benedictus sublimis et gloriosus vivens et regnans in secula seculorum. Amen.

Explicit compilacio ista que intitulatur Breviarium Bartholomei

Sit tibi celorum rex gloria culmen honorum
Quod conpletorum datur hic mihi meta laborum

Justus vir vividus equitat nunc equore lato
Gratia divinitus scriptori nomina dato

An adequate conspectus of the contents of the *Breviarium* can be given using Mirfield's own words:

[f.6rb] . . . presentem compilacionem quam Breviarium Bartholomei vocari cupio in quindecim partes principales [f.6va] dignum duxi dividendam. Et ponam unicuique parti propria capitula, ut quod inquiritur facilius possit inveniri.

1 Quarum in parte prima auxiliante gratia Christi tractabitur de febribus.
2 In secunda de morbis aliis universalibus ocupantibus totum corpus vel saltem maiorem partem corporis.
3 Pars tertia erit de infirmitatibus totius capitis, colli et gule usque ad superiorem partem pectoris.

Notes on pp.338–53

4 Pars quarta erit de infirmitatibus totius clibani pectoris et contentorum ibidem et etiam brachiorum et manuum.
5 Pars quinta erit de infirmitatibus corporis a pectore usque ad membra genitalia.
6 Pars sexta erit de infirmitatibus membrorum genitalium.
7 Pars septima erit de infirmitatibus ab uno usque ad extremam partem pedis utriusque.
8 Pars octava erit de apostematibus.
9 Pars nona erit de vulneribus cum suis pertinentiis.
10 Pars decima de fractura ossium.
11 Pars undecima de dislocatione iuncturarum.
12 Pars duodecima de medicinis simplicibus.
13 Pars tertia decima de medicinis compositis.
14 Pars quarta decima de laxativis et purgationibus humorum nocivorum.
15 Pars quinta decima de fleobotomia et regimine sanitatis et de multis aliis, ut inferius patebit.

Like his predecessors, Mirfield gives exhaustive treatment to fevers. In part 9 he copies out Roger Frugardi and Lanfranc of Milan (*Cirurgia magna*). Part 12 is essentially a herbal in the tradition of the *Circa instans* with an admixture of anecdotal material including this account of the way merchants select musk:

[f.226vb] Quidam mercatores cum volunt muscus emere obturant nares ne odorent vel iubent discooperiri muscum et currunt obturatis naribus per medium iactum lapidis flatum tenentes. Deinde attrahunt aerem per nares et os et si tunc sentient odorem musci, emunt, si non, non. Et ita probant muscum.

Mirfield describes over 420 simples, though some are dismissed with the phrase 'est satis nota'. Part 13 on compound medicines also covers over 400 items including 107 electuaries![218]

Mirfield's handling of his sources is twofold. He frequently cites an authority, antique or medieval, together with the title of his work. When copying out extensive passages, however, he tends to employ the verb *inquit* and substitute for the real identity of his source the phrase 'magister meus'. When in Lanfranc he finds the expression 'as I did', he replaces it with 'as my master did' and similarly when the source itself contains a source reference. A selection of Mirfield's own source references looks like this:

ait Johannes in suo Rosario; experimentum magistri Bernardi de Gordonia; experimentum Johannes de G.; Rogerus et etiam Rolandinus in opusculis suis dicunt; dicit enim Platearius in 'Amicum induit'; Saracena quedam scripsit regine Hispanie quod testiculi asinini comesti preservant a lepra; ipse de Chadesden in suo Rosario; sequitur de uno secreto Chaddesden pro scabie; est unum de secretis meis inquit Chaddesden; Bernardus de Gordonio dicit; Mesue in suo antidotario; Jo. Mesue; emplastrum ceroneum in antidotario Nicolai; Constantinus; auctoritate Philagorii; fiat experimentum quod ponit Consta[n]tinus .li. practice sue c. de epilenci et Galterus in practica sua et Gilbertus et alii; dicit Alexander quod didicit a quodam rustico in Tuscia qui habebat servum epilenticum secum in agro; in libro medicinali qui Rosa vocatur; Mesue ponit in antidotario suo; Mesue in practica sua; falsum esse experimento didici, ait Platearius; Bernardus ipse de Gordonia docet; Constantinus neopolitanus medicus; apud Lanfrancum; magister Rogerus de Villa Nova; unguentum calidum magistri Roberti de vico novo; Bernardus ipse de Gordonio in tractatu suo do pronosticationibus; frater Egidius et etiam venerabilis Lanfrancus pariter dicunt; cura tinee capitis secundum fratres de Fountayns; dicit Bristollensis; Rasis in suo antidotario; electuarium Bruni Lo[n]gobardi; Brunus Longoburgensis in prima parte cyrurgie sue; Rogerus in suo maiori; Rogerus

Salernitanus; Galenus in Megategni; experimentum magistri Odonis probatum; secundum Lanfrancum in maiori; teste Galieno in passionario; dicit magister Galterus Agilon; experimentum magistri G. Agilon; Rasis in experimentis; Averoys; Macer; secundum Haly; Galenus de ingenio sanitatis; secundum Diascorides; Galienus qui princeps dicitur medicorum; Galienus in Megategni; experimentum fratris Egidii ad frangendum lapidem in vesica; et dicitur hoc esse probatum per Robertum Grostest episcopum Lincolniensis ; quidam medicus regine francorum; quidam Saracenus; Diascorides dicit quod corallus portatus maleficia aufert; prout dicit magister Gilbertus; multum valet exhibucio trociscorum que fuerint magistri bone memorie W. de Salernia; curat oxirocrocium secundum Nicholaum; talem regulam tradit Albucasim; Nicholaus in antidotario suo; secundum P. Yspanum; ipse de Gordonia dicit in suo lilio; Ysaac in dietis particularibus; Ysaac in dietis universalibus; Lanfrancus in suo parvo tractatu de cyrurgia c. de antrace; Platearius autem dicit; Bartholomeus autem dicit; Lanfrancus in sua summula parva; multas alias laudes ipsius [= sinapis] predicat Plinius libro XX c.xxiiii; Johannes de sancto Amando dicit; electuarium Bruni Longobardorum; aqua cicerum secundum Arnaldum de Villa; secundum Johannitium; Arnaldus de Villa Nova; Albucasim dicit; de iudiciis urinarum secundum Galterum Agylon; dicit Bartholomeus in libro suo de proprietatibus rerum quod se lactuce tam silvestris quam domestice libidinosas ymaginaciones in sompnis compescit.

It will readily be understood from this list that Mirfield borrows from all the standard authorities of the late twelfth century and the thirteenth century. His *Breviarium* gives a reliable picture of medical knowledge in fourteenth-century England, not only in terms of formal teaching and relatively sophisticated medical receipts, but also in terms of more popular medical practices. For example, he transmits over thirty charms[219] and frequently invokes popular practices:

[f.113rb] baculus in quo suspenditur bufo ficum sanat solo tactu.

[f.116vb] agnus castus sparsus circa lectos monachorum eos a libidine retrahit.

[f.117ra] unge aliquam corrigiam cum succo vervene et porta ad carnem et eris effeminatus. Quidam dicunt quod vervena portata non sinit virgam erigi per .vii. dies.

[f.123ra] [retentio menstruorum] accipe mercurialem viridem et ita integra mulier per totam noctem in vulva teneat et statim habebit menstrua.

[f.126ra] De sterilitate mulieris . . . mulier transglutiat dextrum testiculum leporis in fine florum suorum et coeat.

[f.126va] Si ypericon teneatur in domo, omnes demones fugantur. Ideo dicitur a multis fuga demonum.

Item artemesia supra introitum domus posita vel suspensa facit ut nullum maleficium noceat illi domui.

Si quis maleficiatus fuerit ad amandum nimis aliquam vel aliquem, merda illius quam diligit ponatur recens mane in subtelari dextro amantis et calciet se et quam cito fetorem senserit, solvetur maleficium.

[f.128rb] mulieri ergo que multum laborat in pariendo fetum mortuum sic potest subveniri: pone in lintheamen parientem et fac .iiii. juvenes tenere .iiii. angulos linthiaminis et capite pacientis aliquantulum elevato, huc atque illuc ab oppositis angulis fortiter trahere lintheamen eos facias. Et statim pariet.

From his sources Mirfield also takes detailed accounts of popular cures:

[f.147vb] magistro meo adduxit quidam apotecarius juvenem quendam amicum suum habentem antracem in partibus faciei cuius malicia adeo acuta erat quod totum caput et collum et facies ultra credibile erant inflate. Et eger iam habebat signa mortis quia non erat in eo pulsus et sincopizabat. Et dixit magister ille apotecario quod duceret eum ad domum suam quia moriturus erat in brevi cui dixit apotecarius 'Numquid remedium amplius non est?' Et medicus 'Credo certissime quod si tu dederis ei tyriacam in magna quantitate forte posset adhuc vivere'. Apotecarius autem hoc auditu duxit illum in domum suam vix euntem et dedit ei de tyriaca approbata circa [f.148ra] dragmas duas et posuit eum in lecto suo et cooperuit eum. Et continue arripuit eum sudor incipiens circa capud et locum egritudinis. Et plus paululum erat sudor universalis et rediit in eo pulsus et confortatus est. Et post excitationem apotecarius proprio motu dedit ei iterum dragmam unam tyriace eiusdem et in eodem die factus est sanus nisi quod in eo remansit ulcus viscosum quod postea leviter erat curatum. Et dixit magister ille 'Numquam vidi alium qui postquam fuit in sincopi et tremore cordis sine pulsu evasit'. Sed de hiis quosdam loquentes et quasi nullum malum sentientes iudicati sunt, inquid, per me ad mortem et mortui sunt multum adiurantibus amicis de pronosticatione tali.

[f.148ra] Item aliam hic ostendam tibi curam ut in casibus aliis tibi sit exemplum. Quidam juvenis 30 annorum habuit antracem in dextra parte colli cuius malicia adeo fuerat augmentata per totum collum et gulam et adeo inflata fuerant quod mentum et spatule parum colli grossicis differebant. Virtus tamen in eo valida inventa est. Egritudinem autem cognovit medicus per quandam vesiculam que in parte colli dextra fuerat orta que erat principium egritudinis. Tunc medicus ipsum infirmum ex duobus brachiis flebotomari fecit satis extrahens de sanguine. Et iniunxit dietam sicut febrium acutissimarum pateretur. Crastina autem die mane evacuavit venenosam materiam illam. Super locum autem ubi erat vesica posuit scabiosam tritam cum auxungia, nam ille medicine nullam parem cognovit.

Receipts are often followed by references to successful cures:

[f.10va] Quidam quartanarius non potuit curari et tandem ministrato ei tribus diebus succo tapsi barbasti curatus est.

[f.26va] Hoc expertum erat in quodam abbate qui in prima nocte incredibile multum sudavit et sic liberabatur a scabie qui prius leprosus putabatur.

[f.38ra] Quedam vetula liberavit quendam qui tunc erat fere aschites vel tympanites factus propter ictericie diuturnitatem. Accepit enim vetula illa ollam et implevit eam succo plantaginis et decoxit usque ad medium. Et ex eo cotidie mane dedit patienti et eo solo experimento eum liberavit et multos alios.

Alia quedam vetula sanavit multos cum succo plantaginis bene decocto et syrupato et potui dato.

[f.38rb] Unde magister N. de Tyngewich narravit in cathedra sua Oxoniense quod equitavit .xl. miliaria ad unam vetulam que curavit per hoc quasi infinitos homines et dedit ei unam summam pecunie pro doctrina istius cure.[220]

[f.133rb] cancrenam in tibia habuit quidam delicatus quam sic curavit magister N.

[f.135ra] Dixit mihi quidam monachus etiam philosophus quod cum diu laboraverit circa cura socii sui podagrici nec tamen potuit proficere, apparuit ei Galienus in sompno et dixit ei 'Accipe . . . [receipt follows]'. In crastino executus est curam istam Galieni et infra triduum curatus est.

[f.138va] Et de isto casu habuit magister meus quodam tempore maximum honorem de filio cuiusdam magnatis qui habebat apostema in humero. Et erat ibi sanies in veritate et non inveniebatur aliquis medicus qui cognosceret illam infirmitatem. Et ille coram illis medicis stans et cum tactis et signis indicavit in loco saniem esse. Et incidit apostema coram eis et sanies emanavit.

[f.75vb] vocatus autem fuit magister meus ad quandam mulierem que amiserat loquelam et ut ei restitueretur loquela, fricavit palatum oris eius cum th[e]odoricon euperisticon et aliquantulum apposuit de dyacastor[i]um. Et recuperavit loquelam . . .

[f.98ra] Item mulier quedam apud Montem Pessulanum ita vexabatur a dolore stomachi quod vix duo homines poterant eam tenere. Tunc pulvis coralli datus fuit ei et statim convaluit.

References to surgery and surgeons are inevitably accompanied by expressions of caution!

[f.62vb] [eye complaint] non curatur nisi per cirurgiam sed operacio cirurgie in oculo est timorosa valde propter nobilitatem illius membri et teneritatem eius. Et ideo de tali cura non te intromittas, meo consilio. Cura enim talis potius pertinet ad dedecus quam ad honorem vel lucrum nec de levi potest duci ad bonum finem.

[f.132va] sed plenam, ut quidam dicunt, varices non recipiunt curacionem nisi per manum cirurgicam. Et hoc periculosum est valde nisi sapientem et discretam habeat incisorem. Sin autem leviter potest homo interfici.

Like Gaddesden before him Mirfield frequently distinguishes wealthy and poor patients:

[f.36va] Si patiens yposarcham sit puer . . . si vero patiens pauper fuerit, bibat omni die urinam suam mane.

[f.37ra] Si vero patiens sit pauper, herba nasturcium aquaticum et levisticum decoquantur in vino vel aqua et cum melle dulcoretur et potet mane et sero.

[f.121rb] De sanguine exeunte cum urina: [detailed receipt] . . . Pauperibus sufficit comedere de mane duos bolos pentafilon.

[f.141vb] vel sic pro rusticis et pauperibus: tere radicem agrimonie cum vino et exprime et bibe.

Finally, to complete this rapid survey of Mirfield's *Breviarium* mention should be made of the vernacular glosses encountered in the course of the work. These are far more numerous than was the case in Gaddesden:

[f.7ra]   morsus diaboli, anglice *forbyten*
[f.8vb]   radices lappacii maioris, anglice *clote*
[f.27rb] radix jari .i. *de cucukespintel*
[f.27vb] accipe frutex que anglice dicitur *misteltayn*
[f.29va] accipe picem albam .i. *rosin*, pinguedinem taxi animalis .i. *bauceyn*
[f.29vb] medicina probata contra guttam fistulam: accipe pisces qui dicuntur *roches*
[f.40rb] quedam muscilago que dicitur anglice *sterslim*
[f.45rb] sint solea de illo ligno levi quod dicitur *corke*
[f.47ra] cucumer agrestis, anglice *wilde nepe*
[f.54ra] picem liquidam .i. *tar pich* anglice
[f.54rb] de pustulis que nascuntur in capite quequidem infirmitas vulgo dicitur *roigne*
[f.57va] pisciculi qui vocantur anglice *baynstikelynges*
[f.62ra] auxungia coturnicis, gallice *quaille*
[f.62ra] prunelle nigre .i. *slou*
[f.62rb] pulvis albus communis vocatus gallice *blanche poudre*

[f.66ra] auxungia coturnicis anglice *quayle*

[f.70va] herba que dicitur *crowfote*

[f.78vb] contra grana in facie .i. *sorlecornes*

[f.78vb] accipe fel piscium aque dulcis sicut *breem* vel *tenche*

[f.80ra] medicamen bonum mulieribus nobilibus que cum ungant se in juvenili etate *blancheth*

[f.87va] De dolore pectoris quod anglice dicitur *stiche*

[f.91va] passionem sclirosam in splene que dicitur anglice *elfcake*

[f.97va] pone agrestam .i. *verjus of þe grape*

[f.103va] crusta panis que dicitur *wastel*

[f.104va] istud animal marinum pilosum . . . vocatur anglice *sele*

[f.106vb] semen de *cedewale*

[f.107ra] crassula minor anglice *stonehore*

[f.113va] herba que dicitur *foxglove*

[f.118ra] aqua facta de jaro .i. *yekesters*

[f.119rb] lapidis gagatis .i. *geet*

[f.121va] hasta regia .i. *wodrove*

[f.133ra] de infirmitate quadam in partibus istis que vulgo dicitur *bonschawe*

[f.134va] De passione crurium que vulgariter dicitur *bonshave*

[f.134va] est autem quedam alia passio que a quibusdam ruralibus dicitur *bonshawe*

[f.134va] succus cuiusdam herbe sive fruticis que vulgo dicitur *grete morel*

[f.135vb] est autem infirmitas quedam in pla[n]tis pedum que anglice a ruralibus dicitur *dagges*

[f.146ra] ippiam que anglice [dicitur] *chykenemete*

[f.146rb] tumorem qui vulgariter dicitur *rancle*

[f.146vb] pro apostemate intra corpus quod dicitur a quibusdam *elfcake*

[f.147va] contra antracem quod vulgariter a quibusdam dicitur *feloun*

[f.149va] . . . *tan-doust* [221] . . .

[f.152vb] cum succo rubi .s. *blakeberien*

[f.154va] serpigo . . . in alio idiomate dicitur *dertre*

[f.161rb] memithe .i. *cerflange*

[f.175va] bibat *muge dé bois* .i. *woderove*

[f.184vb] illa superfluitas que crescit super spinam que anglice dicitur *mosse*

[f.200va] instrumentum quod vocatur tornellus, anglice *a wyndas*

[f.201va] ippiam minorem .i. *chykenemete et lenke*

[f.202ra] foliorum lauri alexandri .i. *stanmerche*

[f.203vb] alleluya herba est que in lingua nostra dicitur *wodesoure*

[f.208va] bedegar . . . dicitur *eglenter*

[f.212ra] castor sive *bever*

[f.213vb] ciclamen . . . anglice dicitur *erthnote*

[f.220ra] succositas . . . que anglice a quibusdam dicitur *sappe*

[f.227ra] nuces . . . vocantur gallice *nugages*

[f.232vb] saliunca . . . dicitur gallice *calcatrappe*

[f.233ra] lignum quod dicitur *brasil*

[f.233rb] saponaria . . . anglice dicitur *crowsope*, gallice *savonele*

[f.239va] viticella quod anglice dicitur *smerenep*

[f.263ra] aqua citrina: aqua citrina sic potest fieri: recipe lexivie bone lagenam .i. *welde* tantum quantum potest convenienter decoqui in eadem lexivia.

[f.263va] herba muscata .i. *woderove*

[f.265va] de cineribus clavellatis .i. *wode aysches*

[f.273vb] unguentum quod comeditur quod vulgariter dicitur *save*

[f.273vb] senecionis .i. *groundeswilye* . . . viscis .i. *mousepese* . . . *chaunet*

[f.274ra] . . . *woderove* . . .

[f.278ra] Ad faciendum viscum per quem consolidabis pergamenum: recipe *soundes de stokfische*, coque ea in ciromello .i. *wort*
[f.278rb] viscus vocatur ab Avicenna lignum crucis, anglice a quibusdam dicitur *mistel*
[f.280vb] consolida maior, *stublewort*[222] .i. alleluia
[f.296ra] ... *lemke* ...
[f.298va] mora celtica .i. *mulbere*

Published Receipts in Middle English

BAIN, D. C. 'A Note on an English Manuscript Receipt Book', *Bull. Hist. Med.* 8 (1940), 1246–48 [MS Osler 7591]

BENSKIN, M. 'For a Wound in the Head: a Late Mediaeval View of the Brain', *Neuph. Mitt.* 86 (1985), 199–215 [Dublin, Trinity Coll. 158]

CAMERON, A. & SCHAUMAN, B. T. 'A Newly-Found Leaf of Old English from Louvain', *Anglia* 95 (1977), 289–312

DAWSON, W. R. *A Leechbook or Collection of Medical Recipes of the Fifteenth Century* (London, 1934) [Medical Society of London MS 136]

FORDYN, P. (ed.) *The 'Experimentes of Cophon, the leche of Salerne': Middle English Medical Recipes (MS Add. 34111, f. 218r–230v)* (Brussel, 1983)

GARRETT, R. M. 'Middle English Rimed Medical Treatise', *Anglia* 34 (1911), 163–93

HARGREAVES, H. 'Some Problems in Indexing Middle English Recipes' in A. S. G. Edwards & D. Pearsall (eds.), *Middle English Prose. Essays on Bibliographical Problems* (New York, 1981), pp. 91–113

HEINRICH, F. *Ein mittelenglisches Medizinbuch* (Halle a. S., 1896) [MS B. L. Add. 33996 collated with Sloane 3153, Royal 17 A III, Add. 674, Harley 1600, Sloane 405]

HENSLOW, G. *Medical Works of the Fourteenth Century together with a List of Plants recorded in Contemporary Writings, with their Identifications* (London, 1899)

HOLTHAUSEN, F. 'Medicinische Gedichte aus einer Stockholmer Handschrift', *Anglia* 18 (1896), 293–331

id. 'Zu den mittelenglischen medizinischen Gedichten', *Anglia* 44 (1920), 357–72

JONES, I. B. 'Popular Medical Knowledge in Fourteenth-Century Literature', *Bull. Hist. Med.* 5 (1937), 405–51, 538–88

LÖWENECK, M. *Peri Didaxeon. Eine Sammlung von Rezepten in englischer Sprache aus dem 11./12. Jahrhundert*, Erlanger Beiträge zur engl. Phil. XII (1896) [Harley 6258]

MAYER, C. F. 'A Medieval English Leechbook and its 14th Century Poem on Bloodletting' *Bull. Hist. Med.* 7 (1939), 381–91

MÜLLER, G. *Aus mittelenglischen Medizintexten. Die Prosarezepte des Stockholmer Miszellankodex X. 90*, Kölner Anglistische Arbeiten 10 (Leipzig, 1929)

OGDEN, M. S. (ed.) *The 'Liber de diversis medicinis'*, EETS 207 (London, 1938)

SCHÖFFLER, H. 'Gedruckte mittelenglisch-medizinische Texte', *Archiv für Geschichte der Medizin* 11 (1918), 107–9 *id. Beiträge zur mittelenglischen Medizinliteratur* (Halle a. S., 1919) [I. Lexikographische Studien zur mittelenglischen Medizin = pp.1–144 II. Practica phisicalia magistri Johannis de Burgundia = pp.145–260 = MS Oxford, Bodl. Libr. Rawl. D 251]

SUDHOFF, K. 'Die gedruckten mittelalterlichen medizinischen Texte in germanischen Sprachen', *Archiv für Geschichte der Medizin* 3 (1910) [273–303], 297–303

TORKAR, R. 'Zu den ae. Medizinaltexten in Otho B. XI und Royal 12 D XVII mit einer Edition der Unica', *Anglia* 94 (1976), 319–38

USSERY, H. E. *Chaucer's Physician. Medicine and Literature in Fourteenth-Century England* (New Orleans, 1971)

VOIGTS, L. 'Editing Middle English Medical Texts: Needs and Issues' in T. H. Levere (ed.), *Editing Texts in the History of Science and Medicine* (New York / London, 1982), pp. 39–68

For comparable Germanic materials see:

BRAEKMAN, W. L. *Middelnederlandse Geneeskundige Recepten* (Gent, 1970)

id. Medische en Technische Middelnederlandse Recepten (Gent, 1970)

id. Middelnederlandse Versrecepten voor miniaturen en alderhande substancien (Brussel, 1986)

LINDGREN, A. *Ein Stockholmer mittelniederdeutsches Arzneibuch aus der zweiten Hälfte des 15. Jahrhunderts* (Stockholm, 1967) (with good bibliography)

For French materials see:

GOLDBERG, A. & SAYE, H. 'An Index to Mediaeval French Medical Receipts', *Bull. Hist. Med.* 1 (1933), 435–66

CÉZARD, P. *La Littérature des recettes du XIIe au XVIe siècle*, Ec. Nat. des Chartes, Positions des Thèses, 1944, pp. 23–30

HAUST, J. *Médicinaire liégois du xiiie siècle et médicinaire namurois du xve* (Bruxelles/Liège, 1941)

The Preparation of Compound Medicines

The vernacular medical receipts refer to a variety of forms of *medicamenta* whilst offering little information about their preparation. Compound medicines (*compositae*) might conveniently be classified according to the principal vehicle used to facilitate their application. The celebrated *Flos medicinae scholae Salerni* lists the following under 'Nomina medicamentorum':

> Dicitur *emplastrum* quaevis confectio dura;
> Tunc *embrocamus* cum membra liquore roramus.
> De pannis madidis fit *fomentatio* sola;
> Estque *synapisma* superunctio pulvere solo;
> Quaevis *aposema* decoctio fertur acerba,
> Ex *catapasma* cum sessio fit super herbas.

Si fumum recipis sit *fumigatio* dicta;
Sacellatio fit cum sacco jure repleto;
Fertur *epithema* de succis unctio sola;
Sed *cataplasma* facis cum succum ponis et herbam;
Potio *syrupus*, ut dicit arabs, vocitatur;
Nomen ex electis capit *electuarium* speciebus;
Conficitus *pulvis* ex siccis fit speciebus;
Antidotum plures species sed dicere debes;
Ex opio vel ope dici debent *opiatae*;
Oximel est trinum: simplex, squillae, diureticum.
Oximel in morbis confert ex frigore natis;
Mel melius quod vernale fit, dulceque, spissum,
Quod rubet ut aurum, melius residens prope fundum.[223]

Many of these terms remain imprecise and English forms such as apozem, cata-pasm and epithem have not been maintained in use.[224] A much more practical conspectus of the principal forms in which compound medicines were administered is provided by part 13 of John Mirfield's *Breviarium Bartholomei* which represents a treatise describing over 400 compound medicines.

First to be described is the syrup, derived from the Arabic term *šarab* and equival-ent to Latin *potio* or drink. It was introduced to Salerno through Arabic medicine transmitted via Sicily and Southern Italy. Made from a solution of unrefined sugar or honey and water, it was freely combined with simples (*simplicia*), which were suspended in a sachet if they were spices, and then strained and fined. It was often used as a preservative and could be used as a vehicle for a wide range of medicines. Mirfield cites the authority of Johannes de Sancto Amando (presumably his com-mentary on the *Antidotarium Nicolai*) for preferring honey to sugar and advises physicians to make up the syrup themselves rather than buy it from an apothecary. The instructions given for judging the viscosity of the syrup during preparation are frequently reflected in the vernacular receipts.

Sugar and honey are also the main vehicles for the electuary (*electuarium* Grk. *ekleikton*, *ekleigma*) and the right consistency is again important for preservation. Mirfield lists seven spices commonly regarded as active ingredients and gives exam-ples of dosage according to the strength and vigour of the patient. After the elec-tuary it is usual to take an infusion of herbs or other substances appropriate to the complaint being treated and which can easily be looked up in an *antidotarium*.

Whatever may be compounded to form an electuary can also be made into pills. Pills were less frequently employed in ancient times but grew in popularity. On account of their frequently disagreeable taste they were taken with a variety of other substances and the pills themselves were to be neither too hard nor too soft.

Powders may be administered in a number of ways, with solids or liquids, and are particularly recommended for affected parts which lie far from the stomach. Laxa-tive medicines, however, lose their force when finely powdered and it is suggested that they be combined with sugar or honey to form small lozenges or trochisks. Powders when kept rapidly lose their effectiveness.

Oils and waters are easily produced and administered.

Salves (lat. *unguenta*) are preparations which include wax, animal fats or oils and are softer than plasters, being applied in the heat of a fire or of the sun and rubbed in to the affected part. They existed in a bewildering variety, often bearing splendid names, one of the oldest being *unguentum marciaton* and the most commonly cited *unguentum apostolicon.* Mirfield describes 69 such preparations. Whilst the salve often demanded much time and labour for its preparation, the plaster was even more elaborate. Minerals, powders, gums, fats etc were combined with wax or oil or soap to form a harder preparation for external application. The plaster (*emplastrum*) was laid on to the affected part with the aid of a piece of linen or a strip of leather. Sometimes the preparation was formed into cylindrical shapes like rolls known as *magdaleones* which were said to preserve it longer.

Nothing of what Mirfield puts in to his *Breviarium* is original. For the present purposes, however, this is not in the least a disadvantage and no attempt has been made to establish the sources of the passages cited below. Mirfield simply records for the practical use of those without access to a library what could be known in fourteenth-century England from the best authorities. In other words, the discussion of the basic forms of compound medicines which follows reflects accurately enough the assumptions which underlie the seemingly incomplete directions given in the receipt collections.

SYRUPS

[f.241ra] DE SYRUPIS IN GENERALI ET POTIONIBUS

Multi sunt syrupi, electuarii et alie confectiones in Antidotario Nicholai et alibi a multis satis note quas omnes hic inserere quamvis scirem nimis longa ocupatio esset necnon et fastidiosa, presertim cum multe earum raro a medicis componuntur, sed apud apotecarios atque pigmentarios quasi semper parate inveniuntur. Ideoque solummodo de precipuis et quibusdam quasi ignotis breviter aliquid dicere incipiam auxiliante domino.

General principles
Unde in primis circa confectionem syruporum notande sunt regule multe.
1. Una regula quod omnis syrupus confectus cum zuccara magis debet decoqui quam confectus cum melle.
2. Alia regula: omnis syrupus aut debet confici cum melle aut cum zuccara.
3. Item regula: omne mel quanto minus est coctum tanto magis est laxativum, et quanto magis est coctum tanto magis est nutritivum et tanto magis est constrictivum.
4. Item regula: omnis syrupus confectus cum melle magis durat quam confectus cum zuccara.
5. Item regula: omnis laxativis parum debet decoqui, constrictivis vero multum.
6. Item regula: nullum laxativum est ponendum in syrupo nisi in fine decoctionis.
7. Item regula: in omni syrupo facienda est decoctio usque ad consumptionem medietatis liquoris vel duarum partium, ita quod tertia pars remaneat – aliter enim nichil valet.
8. Item: nota quod omnis pulvis in panno debet decoqui in syrupo iam clarificato. In oximello autem, quod nunquam clarificatur, ab initio decoctionis in panno ligatus apponatur.

Preterea memoria retine quod si psillium vel dragagantum vel aliquid huiusmodi viscosum in syrupo apposueris, diu decoque ut quasi aduri videatur syrupus. Si vero signum perfecte decoctionis syrupi in hiis attenderis, non valeret, quia in principio decoctionis propter viscositatem facit filum et etiam adheret ipsi cacie.

Ingredients in composition
Flowers
Si vis syrupum facere de floribus, prius aquam mundam bene bullire facias. Deinde aqua sit cocta et bene colata. Prohiciatur super flores in aliquo vase et obturetur vas. Deinde iterum calefac eandem aquam et similiter prohiciatur super eosdem flores secundo, et post super alios, si habeantur flores multi. Et hoc fiat quousque aqua ista colorem florum habeat. Deinde huiusmodi aqua calefiat et fiat syrupus de floribus.

Roots
Syrupus autem de radicibus sic debet fieri: Radices primo debent contundi et postea decoqui in aqua vel aceto secundum syrupi exigenciam. Et huiusmodi radices multum debent decoqui, et post debent ab igne deponi et parum refrigerari, et postea bene exprimi. Et de illa decoctione fiat syrupus.

Spices
Syrupus de aromaticis [f.241rb] sic fit: Primo decoquatur aqua et zuccara. Deinde species pulverizate ponantur in sacculo lineo raro et sic debent poni in syrupo et parum bullire. Et quando removetur saccus, bene debet exprimi.

Juices
De succis autem sic debet fieri syrupus: Succus debet extrahi et post debet decoqui in mediocri quantitate et postea refrigerari. Et tunc bene coletur et post cum melle vel zuccara bene decoqui usque ad spissitudinem.

Variety of above
Aliquando autem fit syrupus de floribus, radicibus, et seminibus diureticis et de speciebus aromaticis. Hoc modo debent poni radices parum conquassati et bene decoqui. Postea semina diuretica et mediocriter debent coqui. Deinde debent apponi flores. Et syrupo quasi iam facto sunt posita aromatica.

Preparation
Doctrina ergo in conficiendum syrupos talis esse debet: Bulliant flores vel semina vel similia simul aliquantulum trita in aqua usque ad tertiam partem. Deinde cola, et colature adde zuccarum tali mensura ut ad unciam unam (zuccari) florum vel radicum vel pulveris apponatur libra una zuccari. Et in quocumque liquore volueris facere syrupum tantum pone de illo liquore ut possit zuccarum cooperire.

Judging the consistency
Signum decoctionis syrupi est quando accipitur cum spatula et distillat continuus sicut olium.
Aliud signum est quando adheret spatule.
Item aliud signum est si gutta syrupi bullientis super unguem vel marmor aut cultellum ponatur, si tunc digito apposito adhereat et non distillat huc neque illus, coctus est syrupus.
Dosis autem generalis syrupi est uncia una, vel sic: syrupus aut multum est coctus aut non. Si vero multum sit coctus, debent commisceri due partes aque et tertia syrupi; si autem non sit multum coctus, ponatur medietas aque et medietas syrupi. Et sic

exhibeatur. Et nota quod omnes syrupi debent dari longe a cibo, et cum aqua calida in yeme et cum frigida in estate.

Selection of ingredients

Item regula generalis est quod cum datur aliqua medicina, debet dari cum decoctione aliquarum herbarum vel medicinarum ad hoc valentium et membrum paciens confortantium. Et nota quod si vis facere syrupum contra aliquam egritudinem, considera in antidotario medicinam contra illam egritudinem, et, eisdem speciebus tritis et in aqua bullitis, fiat syrupus. Considera tamen que species debent bullire multum et que non. Pro quo sciendum est quod aromatica pauca indigent decoctione. Immo si multum decoquerentur, totam vim suam amitterent et propter hoc huiusmodi aromatica debent pulverizari et in sacculo poni. Et quando clarificatus est syrupus, tunc apponantur.

Clarification

1. Preterea, cum de succis feceris syrupum et vis ipsum clarum habere, bulli prius succum seorsum et bullitum permitte parum residere. Et quod quasi feculentum supernataverit vel ad fundum descenderit, caute remove. Et in residuo quod clarum est sicut aqua fac syrupum. Et sic clarior erit, sed non tante efficacie. Nec tamen hoc poteris facere cum succis quarundam herbarum frigidarum nisi virtutem constrictivam habuerit.
2. Vel cum huiusmodi succus fuerit per se bullitus [f.241va] et postea resideat, tunc quod feculentum fuerit residebit in fundo, quod vero clarum est supernatabit. Tunc cola per pannum suaviter, sed non exprimas ne turbetur succus. Et ex illa colatura, que videtur esse quasi aqua, addito zuccaro, fiat syrupus clarus.
3. Si vero volueris facere clariorem cum depositus fuerit ab igne, permitte aliquantulum infrigidare, deinde cape quinque vel sex albumina ovorum et bene contere et mitte in syrupo. Et postea iterum [pone] ad ignem et permitte bullire parum. Albumen enim ratione sue viscositatis omnes immundicias mellis vel zuccari et herbarum secum trahit et supernatando usque ad syrupi superficiem secum ducit. Quas immundicias cum penna vel huiusmodi caute remove et depone et si ex hoc non sufficienter clarificetur, iterum bene coletur. Et imponantur albumina ut prius.
4. Item syrupus clarificatus et colatus per pannum ubi crocus et pulvis liquericie sint magis clarificabitur et purificabitur. Et est sciendum quod clarificatur syrupus ut minus sit abhominabilis. Et licet clarificetur, non tamen est majoris efficacie propter hoc, sed minoris. Et nota quod nunquam continget quod clarus sit syrupus ex aceto et zuccaro nisi purissimum sit acetum et zuccarum albissimum.

Preterea notandum est quod syrupi, si competenter conficiantur, servari possunt per tres vel quatuor annos. Et hoc generale sit preceptum quod quotienscumque dabis syrupum ad digestionem sive ad divisionem semper danda est cum calida [aqua] sive diureticum est sive non.

Comparative virtues of sugar and honey

Item si syrupi facti de zuccaro emantur ab apotecariis, timendum est ne sint facti de zuccaro rubeo. Ideo melius est medico et egro quod eos faciat medicus quam eos emat ab apotecariis. Zuccara enim rubea calidior est melle, et ideo mel est melior illo.

Johannes autem de Sancto Amando dicit quod syrupus factus cum melle melius valet quam syrupus factus cum zuccaro et causa est quadruplex:

1. Prima quia mel, cum sit viscosum, melius conservat medicinas positas in syrupo quam zuccara quod est rare compositionis.
2. Secunda est quia mel tegit horribilitatem medicine melius quam zuccara quia mel est dulcius omni re.
3. Tertia est quia mel magis mundificat quam zuccara cum mel sit calida et sic communis in secundo gradu et zuccara in fine.
4. Quarta causa est quia mel melius digerit quam zuccara.

Sed licet syrupus confectus cum melle sit melior ad digerendum, tamen ad con-fortandum et infrigidandum plus valet syrupus confectus cum zuccaro quam cum melle. Sed quando syrupus cum melle confici debet, oportet mel album novum plenissime prius mundificari cui tantumdem aque vel alterius liquoris bulliti cum speciebus diligenter et colati misceatur, et fiat syrupus. Et debet minus bullire quam syrupus qui factus est cum zuccaro donec parum inspissetur.

ELECTUARIES

[f.246ra] DE ELECTUARIIS IN GENERALI

In electuariis et aliis confectionibus mel et zuccara non secundum arbitrium confi-cientis sed secundum certam proportionem sunt ponenda. Unde ad uncias duas specierum requiruntur libre quatuor mellis vel libre tres zuccare.

Judging the consistency
Item in confectione electuariorum primo debemus decoquere aquam cum zuccara ad spissitudinem et completam decoctionem quod sic potes cognoscere: Ponatur aliqua eius porcio supra marmor vel ferrum politum et si adhereat ut mel, coctum est. Et tunc deponatur ab igne et aliquantulum infrigidari permittatur. Deinde pulvis spe-cierum supraspergatur et cum spatula agitetur donec omnia bene incorporentur.

Comparative virtues of sugar and honey
Unde scire debes quod secundum quosdam ad libram unam zuccare debent poni uncie due pulveris, et ad libram unam mellis uncie tres pulveris. Quidam autem dicunt quod confectiones que fiunt cum melle sunt inepti saporis et liquefiunt et sunt abhominabiles. Et ideo, ut plurimi, conficimus, inquit, cum zuccara.

Johannes tamen de Sancto Amando dicit quod electuarium sive syrupus factus cum melle melius valet quam factum cum zuccara, quia mel melius conservat me-dicinas et melius tegit orribilitatem medicinarum, et quia mel magis mundificat et etiam mel magis digerit quam zuccara. Sed licet medicina confecta cum melle sit melior ad digerendum, tamen ad confortandum et infrigidandum melior est confec-tio facta cum zuccara quam cum melle. Unde si voluimus utrumque facere fiat in utroque.

Ingredients
Preterea notandum est quod septem sunt species in quibus est vis facienda in confectione et sunt iste: lapdanum et ambra, muscus, camphora, aurum et argentum atque margarite. In confectione autem lapdanum et ambra debent distemperari cum quolibet syrupo scilicet antequam ponatur in confectione. Muscus autem et cam-

phora teri debent cum aqua tepida vel cum aqua rosacea. Aurum vero et argentum atque margarite cum aliquo alio pulvere in mortario debent teri et pulvis cum ipsis apponatur ne aliquis istorum mortario adhereat. In quibusdam autem confectionibus invenitur quod margarite sic debent preparari: accipiantur margarite et super marmor bene politum et ablutum pona[n]tur et cum vino albo distemperentur et sic in electuario ponantur. In diamargariton autem confectione facta et decoctione preparata cum illa decoctione pulveres incorporari debent, et primo camphora, deinde margarite, deinde muscus per se vel cum aliquo liquore distemperatus.

Dosage

Dosis autem cuiuslibet electuarii triplex est secundum quod triplex est status hominum. Quidam vero fortes sunt et robusti et istis magis est tribuendum. Et quidam sunt debiles et illis minus est tribuendum vel minor dosis [f.246rb] exhibenda. Et quidam sunt mediocres et istis exhibenda est dosis media. Maior autem dosis est drachme sex, minor drachme tres, media drachme quatuor vel quinque.

Use

Item cum datur electuarium vel medicina alia, dari debet cum decoctione aliquarum herbarum vel medicinarum ad hoc idem valentium et membrum illud patiens confortantium. Non est tamen intelligendum quod aliquod electuarium distemperetur cum aliqua decoctione, sed sumpto electuario debet dari decoctio illa aut vinum vel aqua ordei et huiusmodi. Preterea electuaria et huiusmodi sumenda post prandium post intervallum modicum sumenda sunt ut zinziber conditum ad confortandum et huiusmodi. Si enim sumpto cibo statim accipiantur confusa per cibaria et dispersa, virtutem suam perdunt. Preterea quedam singula electuaria vel antidota acuunt et dantur exceptis opiatis et constrictivis electuariis quibus nullus utatur cum scamonia vel acumine aliquo, cito enim mortem inducerent. Item notandum est quod medicina purgans humores frigidos pectoris et membrorum spiritualium debet acui cum drachma una de agarico represso cum drachma una succi liquericie. Item medicina purgans humores frigidos stomachi et epatis debet acui cum drachma una pulveris piperis aut cum mirabolanis Inde et kebulis secundum suas proprias doses aut cum esula secundum suam dosim. Medicine autem evacuantes humores calidos debent acui cum mirabolanis citrinis aut reubarbe aut cum scamonia repressa. Si vero humores frigidi habundent in iuncturis, tunc acuantur medicine cum hermodactile aut cum turbith aut esula secundum suas doses. Si vero fuerint calidi in iuncturis, acuantur medicine cum scamonia aut cum reubarbe aut cum cassiafistula. Et notandum quod acumina que multum sunt violenta et venenosa, ut scamonia, turbith, agaricus et hiis similia, debent reprimi antequam misceantur medicinis compositis. Preterea sciendum est quod in hac compilacione non intendo loqui de omnibus electuariis et confectionibus in antidotario contentis, sed de aliquibus usualibus et non plane de illis et eorum receptionibus omnibus et confectione, sed transcurrendo assignare eorum virtutes in operationes et modum exhibitionis earundem in parte et quasdam magistrales confectiones inserere inter eos deo auxiliante propono . . .

PILLS

[f.257va] DE PILLULIS IN GENERALI

General rules
Notandum vero est quod de omni medicina que conficitur more electuarii pillule possunt fieri, exceptis illis que recipiunt electuarium in tanta quantitate ut virtus electuarii dominetur et exceptis vomitis medicinis. Electuaria autem et cetere vomite medicine vim habent resolvendi humores et ventositatem quos attingunt et ex longa sui mora in stomacho quandoque inducunt suffocationem. Unde semper virtus accipientis, complexio, vis medicine, tempus anni et huiusmodi que impedimenta esse possunt vigilanter sunt attendenda. Et preter hec qui accepturus est pillulas eodem modo preparari debet quo et ille qui potionem est accepturus et fere eadem accidencia que circa potionem evenire solent circa pillulas observari convenit, excepto hoc quod pillule in nocte dentur. Dari autem debent pillule in sero et superdormiendum est, ut confortato naturali calore in sompno resolvatur [f. 257vb] medicina interius. Si ergo purgandus aliquis pillulas acceperit, superdormire poterit quousque medicina dissolvatur et ducat potionatum. Hoc autem est generale preceptum, ut nulli medicine ex quo ceperit aliquam movere superdormiatur quousque purgatio compleatur. Vis enim medicaminis per sompnum perit et evacuatur. Calor enim qui in sompnis medicinarum dissoluit, si diu duraverit, eius vim consumit. Utiliter autem in principio noctis potest dari medicina laxativa in pillulis et hoc post parvam commestionem. Unde debet comedere ova sorbilia et huiusmodi. Medicina autem danda in liquida substantia in mane debet dari neque debet tunc potionatus superdormire. Qui vero pillulas vel potionem est accepturus, in die precedenti mane sufficienter refici debet cibis dumtaxat laxativis et sorbilibus. Sero vero abstineat. Pillulas quidem damus quando remotas partes volumus purgare et maxime ad purgandum caput. Sed scias quasdam pillulas non esse laxativas velud sunt pillule ad tussim et pillule ad asma et ad vocem clarificandum et huiusmodi que sub lingua sunt tenenda donec resolvantur.

Indications
Preterea sciendum est quod pillule laxative tribus de causis exhibentur:
1. Una causa est propter debilitatos. Sunt enim aliqui qui medicinam in liquida substantia non possunt accipere et propter hoc dantur eis pillule.
2. Secunda causa quare dantur pillule est quia sunt fortis attractionis.
3. Tertia causa dantur pillule quando materia est multa et grossa et indiget attractione forti.

Administration
Et propter horribilitatem saporis multis modis possunt dari:
1. Uno modo dantur cum nebula sic: accipiatur pars nebule et ponatur in vino et ibi involvatur pillula. Et sic involuta ponatur in cocleari et sic exhibeatur.
2. Alius modus dandi talis est: accipe mel bene despumatum et isto melle involvatur pillula et sic exhibeatur.
3. Tertio modo possunt dari cum pultibus: fiant enim pultes et ibi involvantur et in cocleari exhibeantur.
4. Quarto modo exhibeantur in ovo sorbili.
5. Quinto modo cum nectare bono.

6. Sexto modo, sed non in omni tempore, sic: accipiatur pellis cerasorum vel uvarum, remoto quod intus continetur, et in pelle ponatur pillula et sic detur. Et sic de aliis modis ab ingenioso medico inveniendis. Sed adhuc sunt aliqui qui nullo tali modo possunt recipere medicinam. Unde oportet quod fiant eis cibi laxativi vel nectar laxativum vel huiusmodi. Preterea sciendum est quod in medicinis pillulatis ad libram unam specierum requiruntur libre tres mellis vel libre due et semis zuccare. Et nota quod pillule omnes rite confecte servari possunt per biennium, sed pillule non debent esse nimis exsiccate neque nimis molles. Secundum enim quod vult Avicenna pillule non sunt dande postquam siccate fuerint et facte dure ut lapides, nec tamen sint nimis molles, sed sint sicut que modo siccari [f.258ra] cepint et que digitis sedant si comprimantur.

POWDERS

[f.260rb] DE PULVERIBUS IN GENERALI

Intelligendum est in primis quod de omni medicina que more electuarii vel in pillulis conficitur potest dari pulvis, sed si necesse fuerit, addatur scamonia in debita porcione. Quidam autem adeo abhorrent medicinas confectas ut nullo modo eas accipere volunt, quibus damus pulverem ad hoc valentem et forte laxativum et incautis offerimus in principio prandii in jure aliquo vel cibo vel potu. Et cum pulverem laxativum acceperint, revocentur a cibo ne nimia quantitate eius suffocetur virtus medicaminis. Et nota quod medicina in pulvere data valet plus contra vicia partium remotarum a stomacho quam pillule vel apozimata. Pulvis enim subtilitate sua profunde penetrat. Precipue autem diuretica et huiusmodi indigent subtili pulverizatione, ut citius penetrent ad membra. Unde quecumque medicina habet respectum ad partes remotas debet subtilissime pulverizari, sed, ut quidam dicunt, medicine laxative pulverizate cito virtutem amittunt. Unde melius est ut cum melle vel zuccara conficiantur vel saltem cum succo sibi competente in unum conglutinentur et in trociscos formentur. Et cum eis uti volueris, cum aliquo liquore ad hoc valente destemperentur et per os sumantur. Pulvis autem laxativus dari debet febricitantibus cum aqua, non febricitantibus cum vino. Pulvis enim propter subtilitatem cito amittit vim suam. Et ideo non debet fieri pulvis saltem laxativus nisi ad quindenam vel mensem ad plus nisi conficiantur ut predictum est. Preterea quando avis vel alius animal debet pulverizari, prius in olla rudi addito cooperculo circumlinitaque argilla in furno ferventi ponantur – non ut comburantur, sed ut desiccentur ut possint pulverizari.

WATERS

[f.261vb] DE AQUIS IN GENERALI

Contra diversas egritudines diverse sunt aque medicinales invente, alie de foliis, alie de floribus, alie de radicibus, et de multis aliis rebus diversimode, ut inferius patebit, de aliquibus gratia exempli. Et scire debes quod omnes aque ex herbis facte habent easdem virtutes quas habent herbe de quibus extrahuntur.

Preparation

Cum autem de floribus aut foliis vel huiusmodi aquam extrahere volueris, mane coligantur et abiectis stipitibus minutim incidantur et aliquantulum frangantur in mortario. Et inde repleatur vas inferius distillatorii usque ad medium et cooperiatur cum alia parte distillatorii. Et tunc vasa illa bene ligentur circa labia cum argilla, et tunc ponantur super fornacem terream que habeat orificium strictum. Et tunc apponantur carbones insensi sine fumo et distillabit aqua per rostrum stillatorii que recipiatur in fiala vitrea, et usui reservetur.

OILS

[f.267vb] DE OLEIS IN GENERALI

Olea humanis usibus utilia de multis rebus possunt fieri. Fiunt enim olea aliquando de floribus, aliquando de seminibus, aliquando de fructibus, aliquando de lignis, aliquando de radicibus, et aliquando de rebus aliis, ut inferius ostendetur.

Flowers

De floribus autem fit oleum hoc modo: accipiatur libra una florum, olei olivarum libre tres. Terantur flores aliquantulum, deinde cum oleo bene misceantur. Et ponantur simul in vase vitreo et opilato ore ad fervidum solem ponantur. Et sic per novem dies soli exponantur. Et hoc iterum vel tertio fiat si vis. Deinde colatum usui reservetur.

Potest etiam fieri alio modo sic: accipe florum libram unam, olei libras tres. Fac diu bullire in vase dupplici, deinde cola per pannum. Et proiectis floribus alios appone si vis, et fac ut prius.

Fruit

De fructibus autem fit oleum sic: tere eos et tritos per aliquot dies dimitte. Deinde aqua tepida manibus malaxa et oleum adde. Et in dupplici vase diutissime bullire permitte. Et per pannum cola. Qua infrigidata, quod supernataverit collige.

Seeds

De seminibus autem fit oleum sic: accipe semen sinapis vel aliud et in vase luteo pone et panno superposito fode in terra humida et dimitte ibi per novem dies. Postea tere fortiter et in sacello mitte et per caceam cola et quod emanat colige et reserva.

Fit autem oleum aliter de seminibus et de baccis: redige in pulverem et fac bullire in vino et cola. Et colature adde libram unam olei. Et bulliat ad vini consumpcionem et usui reserva.

Herbs

Item de herbis et radicibus sic potest fieri oleum: calefiat oleum commune et herbe et radices dimittantur ibi ad minus per septimanam. Et cotidie moveantur herbe et radices. Deinde totum fac bullire in dupplici vase. Et cola et usui reserva.

Woods
Generaliter autem de lignis fiunt olea sic: dividantur ligna in minutissima frusta et ponantur in olla foramen habente in fundo. Et superponatur cooperculum de terra tenaci scilicet argilla, et sigilletur cum pasta ne fumus exeat. Et fiat fossa in terra in qua ponatur olla alia non perforata. Et circa latera olle superioris fiat ignis et quod resudabit a lignis in ollam inferiorem cadet, et usui reservetur.

Roots & herbs
Olea de radicibus et herbis possunt fieri: decoquantur in aqua et vino parum conquassate et postquam videbitur virtus earum liquori esse mandata coletur. Et colature addatur oleum. Et sic totum bulliat usque ad consumptionem colature et olium usui reservetur. Vel cum succo radicum vel herbarum bulliat oleum usque ad consumptionem succi. Deinde coletur et usui reservetur.

Spices
Similiter quaslibet species pulverizatas possumus in vino vel aqua decoquere et post decoctionem coletur. Et colature addito oleo decoquatur usque ad consumptionem colature et usui reservetur.

Powders
Item pulveres in vino simul et oleo mixtis bullimus decoctoque vino et consumpto colamus, et quod per colatura exibit, oleum erit.

OINTMENTS

[f.271vb] DE UNGUENTIS IN GENERALI

Unguentorum quedam calida et quedam sunt frigida. Calida sunt ut dialtea, Agrippa, unguentum aureum, unguentum Arrogon, marciaton, unguentum fuscum, unguentum ad salsum flegma et huiusmodi. Frigida autem sunt ut popileon, unguentum citrinum, unguentum album et huiusmodi.

Et nota quod quando de pulveribus cum oleo etc. vis facere unguentum, tunc ad unciam unam pulveris pone olei uncias quatuor, cere unciam unam in estate, in yeme unciam semis.

Si vero unguentum recipit gummas que resolvuntur et non teruntur, non debent gumme in predicta mensura ponderis computari quoniam non addunt in spissitudine neque in mollicie. Sed si unguentum recipit pinguedines porci, galline, anseris vel alias huiusmodi que in substantiam oleaginam dissolvuntur, tunc debet pinguedo dissoluta computari pro oleo et predictam quantitatem debes ponere de pulveribus et de cera.

Preparation
Modus autem faciendi unguenta de quibuscumque herbis [si] volueris: primo herbas pone in olla sive in cacabeo et ad summum impleatur aqua. Deinde cooperiatur os olle cum panno lineo forti et sigilletur cum argilla ne fumus exeat, et apponatur igni usque ad consumptionem aque. Et tunc iterum impleatur olla aqua et iterum bulliant tritis tamen herbis ante decoctionem. Deinde ponantur ille herbe cum tota

decoctione in panno lineo forti et exprimatur succus et succo illo utere in unguentis faciendis. Quod si volueris decoctionem illam reservare, confice cum cera et reservetur in pixide.

Et nota quod omnes medicine redigi possunt in unguenta, si frigide fuerint medicine cum frigidis oleis, si calide cum calidis distemperentur. Et modicum cere addatur et bulliant aliquantulum et sic fiat [f.272ra] unguentum. Ex unguentis sic operamur et maxime calidis. Ponatur unguentum in testa ovi et ad ignem resolvatur. Et tunc cum illo unguento ungatur membrum paciens ad ignem vel ad solem. Et tunc post inunctionem ponatur pellis aliqua vel aliquod tale super inunctum membrum ut virtus unguenti conservetur.

PLASTERS

[f.278vb] DE EMPLASTRIS IN GENERALI

Emplastrum dicitur ab *en*, quod est 'in', et *plastes*, 'forma', eo quod super formam morbi inducitur. Item emplastrum dicitur quando multa simplicia diversarum naturarum, ut pulveres, gumme, pinguedines, cum cera, sepo et oleo usque ad perfectionem decoquuntur et in magdaleonibus conservantur. Postea super corium distendatur et loco cui est necessarium applicetur sicut diaquilon et apostolicon et multa alia.

Vel sic emplastrum dicitur dura confectio ex diversis rebus et conglutinosis que manibus malaxari possunt. Emplastrum autem et cathaplasma multociens ponuntur unum pro alio. Et nota quod emplastra servari possunt donec amittant odorem.

Collection of herbs

We shall later see that many of the rituals recorded by Delatte involve the time and manner of collecting herbs.[225] Storage was also an important consideration. Yet the early herbals provide few directions about such questions.[226] In Dioscorides the introductory letter to Areius offers a number of common-sense observations which show an awareness of the factors of phenology and climate: 'It must also not be forgotten that herbs frequently ripen earlier or later according to the characteristics of the country and the temperature of the year'.[227] Branches should be gathered 'whilst great with seed', flowers 'before they fall', fruits 'when they are ripe', and seeds 'when they begin to be dry and before they fall out'. Few herbs, with the exception of White and Black Hellebore, will last for more than three years. They should be carefully stored:

> Flowers and sweet-scented things should be laid up in dry boxes of limewood: but there are some herbs which do well enough if wrapped up in papers or leaves for the preservation of their seeds. For moist medicines some thicker material such as silver or glass or horn will agree best. Yes, and earthenware if it be not thin is fitting enough,

and so is wood, particularly if it be boxwood. Vessels of brass will be suitable for eye-medicines and for liquids and for all that are compounded of vinegar or of liquid pitch or of Cedria, but fats and marrows ought to be put up in vessels of tin.[228]

There are scattered indications in herbals like the *Circa Instans*, but surprisingly little attention is given to the question of collection until there appear in the fifteenth century a number of individual treatises *de collectione herbarum*, in both Latin and the vernacular. In the present state of our knowledge we must assume that these treatises were based on earlier sources. Some account of them therefore seems in place in the present study.

In the remedy-book edited by W. R. Dawson[229] a section on collecting herbs is translated (from the Middle English) by him thus:

> Gathering of seeds should be when they be full ripe, and the moistness be dried somewhat away. Flowers should be taken [when] they be somewhat open, before they begin to wither or fade. Stems should be gathered when they be full of moistness before they begin to shrink. Roots should be gathered when the leaves have fallen. Fruits should be gathered when they be at their fullest size before they fall, and the heavier the fruits are and the sadder (denser), the better they be: and those that be large and light thou shalt not choose. And those be better that have been gathered in fair weather than those that have been gathered in rain; and those herbs that have been gathered in the field be better than those that grow in the town and in gardens. And [of] those that grow in the field, those that grow on hills be best; and commonly the field-herbs be smaller than the town-herbs. Many herbs there be that have a special time to be gathered, and in that time they have the virtue, and they be gathered in any other time, they have not the virtue, or else not so good. Some help whensoever they be gathered, and some be harmful if they be gathered out of time.

There follows a list of 42 herbs with an indication of the best time for gathering e.g. origanum in June, solsecle 'in the same monyth þe xvi day before the rysynge of the sunne withowte reyne', saffron before sunrise etc.

MS B. L. Sloane 2584 (c.1400) ff.87r–89v contains a short treatise on the best times for gathering specific herbs, prefaced by a general section (*[M]edicynes ben don sum bi leves, sum bi seed . . .*) on leaves, seeds, roots, stems, flowers etc. Leaves should be gathered 'whanne þei ben at here ful wexyng or þat here coloure chaunge or þat thei welowe or fade ony þyng'; seeds 'whanne þei ben ful ripe and þe moystnesse be dried away'; flowers 'whanne þei ben fully opene or þei begynne to fade or welowe'; stems (ȝerdes) 'whanne þei ben fulle of moistnesse or þei begynne to schrynke'; roots 'whanne þe leves fallen'; fruits 'whanne þei ben at here ful gretnesse or þat þei falle'. The information is almost identical with that given in the remedy-book edited by Dawson and the description of town and country herbs is the same as that quoted above. Similarly there follows a list of plants with specific suggestions: 'swinegrass' may be gathered 'whanne so evere a man nediþ hym', camomile in April, betony 'principali in Lammas moneþe with þe seed and þe rootis and wiþouten yrune . . . and before þe sunne risynge', pennywort 'in þe begynyng of wynter', groundsel 'after mydday', marigold 'þe xvi day of þe monþe bifore þe sunne risyng wiþouten irune', gourds when ripe at the end of September or the beginning of October and dried 'in suche a place þat þei myȝtten have þe sonne al day', the berries of 'wild neep' 'whanne þei wexen zelowe', flax dodder 'in somer whanne he bigynneþ to floure and it may be kept .ii. ȝeer'.

In MS B. L. Sloane 3535 (s.xv) ff.11r–12r the same preface as in the above treatise appears in Latin, whilst the times of gathering for different herbs are given in English ('unde sequitur doctrina in anglicis'). There are many similarities with the directions given in MS Sloane 2584, but zodiacal influences have been included e.g. 'golde or solsecall shal be gadred in signo Virginis, for hit is apropriate to that signe' (f.12r).

Sometimes the number of herbs listed is reduced to seven, each corresponding with a day of the week. A treatise in MS B. L. Sloane 962 (s.xv) ff.85v–86r begins '*Ypocras de erbis colligendis:* Nunquam nisi in fine Aprilis colligas radices omnium herbarum quarum radices sunt medicinales, quia radices tales omnes maioris sunt virtutis pro tunc quam alio anni tempore', and is followed by a list of seven herbs each of which has its particular day of the week for gathering. Similarly, in MS B. L. Sloane 2584 (s.xv) f.85r–v we read:

> Seven daies þer ben in þe weke. Ry3t so þer ben seven principal herbis of þe whiche iche haþ his day and certayn hour of þe day. The first herbe is archemesie and þat herbe schal be takyn and gaderyd on þe sonday next aftir seven daies of þe prime of þe mone and þat herbe so takyn and in to poudre made makeþ men to dispoilen hemself of hure cloþes and to castyn hem fro hem. The secunde herbe is hertistunge and þat herbe schal be gaderid on þe monday þat is to wecyn þe secunde monday aftir þe prime . . .

A detailed investigation is needed of the Latin treatises which must have preceded such vernacular works. Flower published Irish verses from MS B. L. Add. 30512 which dealt with the times for the collection of herbs and suggested that they reflected a twelfth-century composition.[230] Yet Wickersheimer, who did valuable work on such treatises,[231] could find only manuscripts of the fifteenth century. A *Tractatus de collectione herbarum*, found in MS B. L. Arundel 369 f.48ra/vb and elsewhere,[232] begins with a general introduction in which we read:

> Flores vero herbarum et semina earum in saccellis vel in loculis ligneis, in archa aut in soliis ubi bonus et mundus sit aer, reponi debent. Succus vero de recenti herba cum fiat, in vasis vitreis vel corneis reponatur et ad oculorum causas cum fiat succus aliquis, in vasis eneis aut stagneis debet recondi.

Not only are plants allocated appropriate months, but medical preparations are treated in the same way:

> In Februario et in Marcio collige violas et de recentibus fac trociscos et oleum violaceum et sirupum violaceum et oximel et triferam sarracenicam . . . oculos eciam populorum collige et infra quinque dies cum auxugia contere et fac trociscos et serva donec omnia illa habeas que intrant populeon et tunc populeon facias.[233]

Wickersheimer also drew attention to an *Epistola Ypocratis ad Alexandrum de tempore herbarum*,[234] possibly of the twelfth century though the date is very uncertain, which begins 'Memento cavere ad herbas coligendas et conficiendas in lune diminucione, per quam minus eas valere te scire oportet'. Each month is the subject of a separate section.

Daems and Keil have published another text from two fifteenth-century Bavarian MSS with the title *Tractatulus de collectione medicinarum*, beginning 'Consideracio collectionis medicinarum simplicium medico est necessaria ut sciat quando radices, quando folia, quando flores vel semina sunt colligenda . . .'[235] A total of 143 herbs are mentioned, distributed over nine periods of the year. Styptics, we are told, are more efficacious before maturity, laxatives should be gathered 'in diebus canicularibus'. Much of this text must be very much earlier, as the introduction is found in MS Oxford, Bodl. Libr. Digby 69 (s.xiii²) f.137r:

De collectione

Collectionis etiam consideratio et scientia medico sunt necessaria, ut sciat quando radices, quando folia, quando flores vel semina sint colligenda. Incompetens enim medicinarum collectio plurimum operatur experimentorum fallaciam. Collecte enim medicine quodam tempore plurimum sunt laxative, alio vero tempore collecte parum vel nichil laxant. Item quedam ex collectionis tempore vim suam retinent, quedam vero vim suam omnino amittunt, ut ille que colligentur ante tempus sue maturitatis. Colligende sunt hec herbe quando ad suam pervenerint maturitatem. Si herbe florifere fuerint, cum flore sunt colligende ut pulegium, origanum, calamentum, sticados et similia. Flores vero colligende sunt cum fuerint ad plenitudinem adulti et sue maturitatis pervenerint ad incrementum, ut non in principio sue generationis nec nimis tarde, sed cum mature fuerint, colligantur. Semina vero et fructus cum ad plenam pervenerint maturitatem sunt colligenda, folia vero et frondes cum ad sui incrementi [MS-um] [plenitudinem] pervenerint, quando scilicet humiditatem combiberint nec adhuc a stipite cadunt. Nec ea quando sint matura [corr. viridia?] nec nimis tenera colligere aliquis presumat. Radices autem tunc colligendas censemus quando foliis delictis succositatem suam in se retinent et nutrimentum ad folia et stipitem non transmittunt. Notandum quod stiptica ante tempus sue maturitatis collecta sunt stipticiora. Laxativa autem in canicularibus sunt colligenda. / f.137v / Hec autem secundum herbarum varietatem sunt intelligenda. Quedam enim flores citius producunt, quedam vero tardius. Collecte autem medicine hoc modo conserventur ut neque in siccis locis ne ex siccitate virtutes earum varientur neque in nimis humidis ne ex humiditate citius putrefiant. Radices vero collecte et semina ad solem siccentur, non tamen nimis ferventem, ne virtus earum ex nimio calore dissolvatur. Frondes vero et folia et flores in umbra desiccentur soli vicina vel in sole parum calido. Semina vero que habent folliculos in ei(u)sdem conserventur. Medicine desiccate in vasis vel cistis cipressinis vel fraxineis vel lignis similibus non putribilibus ponantur. Confecte vero medicine conserventur in pixidibus, colliria in vasis cipressinis vel cupreis, auxugie in vasis testeis.

A representative set of directions is given by John Mirfield at the beginning of part 12 (De medicinis simplicibus in generali) of his Breviarium Bartholomei in MS B. L. Harley 3 f.202rb:

Simplices etiam dicimus que licet aliquod artificium [f. 202va] receperint alterius tamen medicine admixtionem non admittunt ut scamonia, elacterium, tamarindi et similia.

Et, ut dicit beatus Augustinus, scire debes quod multe sunt utilitates manifeste vel occulte omnium que radi[ci]tus alit, sed incompetens medicinarum collectio vel collectarum indebita conservatio plurimum operatur experimentorum fallaciam. Pro quo sciendum est quod colligende sunt herbe medicinales quando ad suam maturitatem pervenerint.

Si autem flores habeant, cum flore sunt colligende, ut origanum, pulegium, calamentum et similia. Flores colligendi sunt quando fuerint adulti et ad plenitudinem sui pervenerint incrementi. Et hoc priusquam incipiant marcessere et cadere.

Semina vero colligenda sunt cum ad plenitudinem pervenerint maturitatis videlicet quando prope matura sunt.

Folia quoque et frondes tunc debent colligi cum ad sui incrementi [MS incrementum] [plenitudinem] pervenerint nec adhuc a stipite cadunt.

Radices autem tunc colligende sunt quando discussis foliis succositatem suam in se retinent et nutrimentum ad folia vel ad stipitem non transmittunt, quia tunc humiditas
colligitur circa radicem.

Fructus autem colligendi sunt antequam cadant vel sunt preparati ad cadendum et postquam finitur complementum eorum, quia oportet ut coligantur cum habeant plenitudinem
fortitudinis.

Et scire te volo quod herbe medicinales in silvis montuosis precipue reperiuntur. Collecte
autem medicine hoc modo serventur ut neque in nimis siccis serventur locis ne ex siccitate
virtus earum exhauriatur neque in nimis humidis ne ex humiditate citius putrefiant.

John also provides clear instructions for the treatment and storage of plants once
gathered:

[f.202va] Radices autem et semina collecta ad solem possunt desiccari, non tamen ad
nimium ferventem solem ne virtus earum ex nimio calore dissolvatur.

Frondes vero et folia et flores in umbra desiccentur soli vicina vel in sole parum calido.

Semina vero que folliculos habent in eisdem conserventur.

Desiccate vero medicine reponantur in cistis fraxineis vel ex lignis aliis inputressibilibus
compositis.

Electuaria et etiam medicine perfecte reponantur in ceratis pixidibus.

Colliria vero melius in vasis cupreis conservantur.

Auxugia et unguenta in vasis terreis sed vitreatis vel plumbatis.

Weights and Measures

Although most of the popular medical receipts do not specify quantities, many of
the manuscripts which transmit them include notes or a small treatise on weights
and measures, *de ponderibus et mensuris*. In general, it may be said that there are
three variables: the system being used; the value of the measure indicated; the use of
abbreviations. All three were rendered complex by the existence of local variations.
Whilst we find the Roman system in Galen and Isidore,[236] this was gradually
modified in the early medieval period and Salerno introduced a more standardized
system based on the unit of the grain (*granum*). The core of both systems was the
following set of equivalents: [237]

> 1 libra = 12 unciae
> 1 uncia = 8 drachmae
> 1 drachma = 3 scripula
> 1 scripulum = 2 oboli
> 1 obolus = 3 siliquae

The problems of metrology and posology remain so great[238] that there is no sure
agreement on the exact weights represented by these indications[239] and it seems

beyond practicality to seek to reproduce the receipts volumetrically in today's terms. The principal variation in the above table is that at Salerno the *uncia* comprised nine *drachmae*. This is clear from verses in the *Flos medicinae scholae Salerni*[240] which are frequently found in receipt collections and copies of *antidotaria*. In MS B. L. Add. 33996 f.163v they are part of a small treatise on weights and measurements:

> Pondera in arte medicine hec sunt per grana frumenti collecta. A scrupulis igitur sumamus initium. Scrupulus est pondus .xx. granorum. Duo scrupuli sunt pondus quatraginta granorum que insimul faciunt dragmam unam et est hec .3.. Exagium pondus nonaginta granorum que faciunt dragmam et semis et ex totidem granis constat solidus. Exagia .vi. vel solidi sex faciunt unciam unam et est uncia duodecima pars libre. Item ex dragme faciunt unciam unam. Item centum et octo dragme faciunt libram unam. Item .xii. uncie faciunt libram unam. Item medicinale sexterium vini vel olei quod intrat in unguentis sive medicinis est pondus duarum librarum et semis. Inter cotilam et sextarium nulla est differencia nisi in vocabulo. Et hec omnia possunt hiis versibus denotari:

> > Collige triticeis medicine pondera granis,
> > Grana quater quinque scrupuli pro pondere sume.
> > [f.164r] In dragmam scrupulus surgit ter multiplicatus,[241]
> > Si solidum queris, tres dragmas dim[id]iabis,
> > Exagium solido differt in nomine solo.
> > Constat sex solidis, vel ter tribus uncia dragmis,
> > Uncia pars libre duodena quis ambigit inde?
> > Et libram quarta cum parte tenebis emina.
> > Si queris pondus, quod habet sextarius unus,
> > Librarum quinque debes pondus mediare . . .

The prose section of this little treatise is taken straight from the end of the *Antidotarium Nicolai*. What is missing is the symbols or abbreviations which are so often employed in the receipts themselves. These are often supplied in annotations to medical MSS, as in MS Oxford, Bodl. Lib. Auct. F. 5. 31 (s.xiii ex) f.60r:

> Sciendum quod nomen minimi est scrupulus quod sic scribitur ꝫ qui est pondus .xx. granorum tritici non minimorum nec maximorum sed mediorum. Scrupulus triplicatus facit dragmam quod sic scribitur .3. Novem dragme faciunt unciam[242] unam quod sic scribitur ÷. Dragma una et semis faciunt exagium .i. solidum. Quindecim ÷ faciunt libram maiorem per quam[243] omnia humida vendi debent ut sunt syrupi, olea et huiusmodi. Duodecim ÷ faciunt minorem libram per quam vendi debent omnia sicca sicud zinziber, gariofili, macis et huiusmodi. Uncia habet grana .cccccxl., libra habet grana octo milia etc.

Another variation in the accounts of quantities or weights is the number of *scrupuli* constituting an *uncia*, which may be three, as in the above passages, or two, as in the account below taken from MS B. L. Royal 12 G IV:

> [f.140va] Siliqua habet ordei grana .iii. ꝫ quod est scrupulus habet siliquas .vi. Obulus habet ꝫ et semis. 3 quod est dragma habet scripulos .ii. ÷ quod est uncia habet 3 .viii. Cratus habet 3 .ix. Emina habet libram et semis . . .

An interesting passage on weights and measures is appended to John Mirfield's *Breviarium Bartholomei* in MS Oxford, Pembroke College 2 f.349v:

> Oportet modo pondera medicaminum mensurasque eorundem cognoscere. Intellige

ergo secundum doctrinam auctorum quod .xx. grana frumenti faciunt ɜ .i. Et ɜ .iii. faciunt 3 .i. Sed in pecunia nostra non possumus accipere pondus certum. Tamen apotecarii ponunt denarium pro ɜ .i., sed ɜ .i. non ponderat denarium sed .iii. quadrantes cum tercia parte unius quadrantis. Quis ɜ .iii. faciunt 3 .i. Et 3 .i. ponderat .ii. denarios et obulus. Et 3 .i. cum dimidio facit solidum, exagium et aureum, que tria idem sunt in pondere licet nomina diversificentur. Et secundum doctrinam antiquorum 3 .ix. faciunt ÷ .i. Et ÷ 12 libram .i. Et libre .ii. cum dimidio faciunt sextarium .i.

Sed nostri apotecarii qui emunt ad unam mensuram et vendunt ad aliam habent ut dicitur libre .ii., scilicet libra magna et libra minima. Libra magna ponderat .xxvi. solidos et .viii. denarios sterlingorum. Et habet ÷ .16. Sed libra parva non ponderat nisi .xx. solidos sterlingorum et habet ÷ 12. Et sic ÷ ponderat .xx. denarios sterlingorum. Et .x. denarii faciunt 3 .iiii. Apotecarii autem ponunt pro ɜ .i. denarium .i. Et pro 3 .i. ponunt .ii. denarios et obulus. Et ɜ .iii. ponunt pro 3 .i. Et pro solido ponunt 3 .i. et semisse. Et per libram magnam deberent venderi omnia liquida scilicet syrupos, olera et huiusmodi. Et per libram minorem omnia sicca ut zinziber, gariofili et huiusmodi.[245]

This makes the clear distinction between Troy or Apothecaries' measures for dry substances and Avoirdupois measures for weighing liquids.

In the MSS transmitting Middle English receipts brief indications of weights and measures duly appear in the vernacular:

[MS B. L. Sloane 2584 (c.1400) f. 90r]
A pound is written þus lī. Half a pound þus lī ſ oþer ellis þus lī dī. A quartroun þus qᵃrt⁹. Half a qᵃrt⁹ qᵃrt⁹ ſ oþer þus qᵃrt⁹ dī. An ounce þus ÷. Half an ounce ÷ ſ oþer þus ÷ dī. A dragme þus .3. Half a dragme .3. ſ or þus .3. dī. A scrupul þus .ɜ. Half a scrupil .ɜ. ſ or .ɜ. dī. A scrupil weieþ a peny. .iii. scrupil maken a dragme. .viii. dragmes maken an ounce and .xvi. ouncis maken a pound. An handful is writen þus .m̄. Half an handful þus .m̄. ſ or þus .m̄. dī. Take .xx. wheete cornes and þei weien a scrupil.

[MS B. L. Sloane 347 (s.xv) f. 98r]
A pownde is wrytten thys £ .i. £ .ii. and so forth
Halfe a pownde . . . £ſ   £ᵍ
An unce . . . ÷ ʒ
Halfe an unce . . . ʒſ or ʒᵍ
A drame . . . 3
Halfe a drame . . . 3ſ or 3ᵍ
A scrypull . . . ɜ .i. ɜ .ii.
A handfull . . . .m. .i. .m. .ii.
Halfe a handfull . . . m.ſ   mᵍ
Lyke moche is wrytten thus ana or anᵃ
ʒ ʒ this figure afore standeþ all ways for gynger
The weight of .lx. corns of whete is a drame and þe weight of .xx. whete corns is a scripull.

The mixture of Greek and Latin terms and systems, the existence of numerous local traditions, the variety of symbols used all render the exact identification or duplication of weights in medieval medical receipts an extremely hazardous enterprise. Moreover, with the influence of Arabic medicine further variables were introduced.[246] There, too, there were fluctuations in the use of Greek and Arabic systems and in the reflection of local traditions.[247] Latin translators of Arabic works tended to latinize the Arabic names rather than convert to Western terminology, so that many words quickly became unintelligible.

Archaeological Evidence

In concluding this introduction to the medical receipt in medieval England brief mention must be made of the evidence provided by archaeology for the study of both diet and medicine in the Middle Ages. Particular attention has naturally been paid to early food plants and a survey of charred seed finds in the Netherlands covering the period from about 2350 BC to 900 AD together with the remains of crop plants recovered from coastal settlement sites from c. 500 BC to 1000 AD showed how it was possible to chart the gradual replacement of one species by another and to demonstrate the real significance of certain plants, such as Chenopodium album, in early times.[248] Medieval sites proved even more productive. Material drawn from a cesspit in Chester and dating from the end of the thirteenth century[249] consisted largely of the comminuted stones of bullace (Prunus domestica ssp. insititia (L.) C. K. Schneid) and sloe (Prunus spinosa L.) and the seeds of corncockle (Agrostemma githago L.). Twenty-eight taxa were identified and further evidence of the use as a food of Polygonium lapathifolium and Chenopodium album was found. The appearance of poisonous plants such as Agrostemma githago may in part be explained by the terminological confusion which existed in the Middle Ages and which must have led to many errors, some of them having serious consequences.[250] Carefully controlled dosage (rarely indicated in the receipts!) and selection of the right parts of the plant would usually be adequate safeguards against poisoning during medicinal use, but mistakes must often have been made. The remains found at Chester include corncockle, stinking mayweed, orache, black mustard, mosses, cornflower, goosefoot (fat hen), corn marigold, hazel, hawthorn, hemp-nettle, grasses, rushes, vetches, black bindweed, persicaria, hair-moss, sloe, bullace, bracken, dock (sorrel), field penny-cress, bilberry and various umbellifers. In York were found sloes and cultivated plums, hazel nuts, flax, hops, spinach, cabbage, sorrel, chickweed, nettle, mugwort, groundsel, poppy and devil's bit scabious.[251] In Southampton pit fills from the period 1200 to 1350 AD yielded conspicuous traces of wild strawberry (Fragaria vesca L.) and imported figs.[252] The house of the Austin friars at Leicester[253] yielded seeds from various pond and stream-bank plants including black mustard (Brassica nigra L. (Koch)), water mint (Mentha aquatica L.), water plantain (Alisma plantago-aquatica L.) and reeds and sedges. Again Agrostemma githago was much in evidence and weeds from cultivated land were knotted hedge-parsley (Torilis nodosa L.), corn gromwell (Lithospermum arvense L.) and plantain (Plantago major (L.) Gaertner). Turning to the palaeobotany of medieval urban sites, we find rich deposits in the Queen Street Midden area of Aberdeen,[254] where once more figs are evidence of imported food. Dye plants such as weld (Reseda luteola L.), madder (Rubia tinctoria L.) and woad (Isatis tinctorum L.) were common, as was bog myrtle (Myrica gale L.), which as well as being a dye was used in brewing. Yet again Agrostemma githago was found in considerable quantities and it is evident that the medicinal use of its seeds was well established. Reporting on an excavation in Dublin B. O'Riordain reveals that 'Examination of seeds and fragments of plants from different levels shows that the townspeople ate strawberries, apples, cherries, plums, sloes, blackberries, rowan berries and hazel nuts. Fig seeds were found in 13th-Century levels. It also appears that the seeds of goosefoot

(Chenopodium) and three species of Polygonum (knotgrass, black bindweed and pale persicaria) were extensively used as food'.[255]

One of the most ambitious projects based on the belief that the physical residues of medieval medical treatments, notably infirmary waste, repay careful analysis and have much to tell us about medical practice is SHARP (Soutra Hospital Archaeoethnopharmacological Research Project) under the directorship of Dr Brian Moffat.[256] Using Macer's *De viribus herbarum* as a guide, the project has examined carefully the evidence for Augustinian houses in Britain, including Jedburgh Abbey where a major excavation took place.[257] At Waltham Abbey, Essex, in a pit of c.1540 considerable traces of black henbane (Hyoscyamus niger L.) and hemlock (Conium maculatum L.) were found. The major focus of SHARP's investigations, however, remains Soutra on the northernmost edge of the Lammermuir hills and it is anticipated that many interesting discoveries will be made so far as medical botany is concerned.

Notes on pp.338–53

Chapter Two

MISCELLANEOUS RECEIPTS AND CHARMS

Receipts

When studying the pharmacotherapy of the Middle Ages it is obviously more interesting and profitable to examine whole collections of receipts, especially those which, carefully indexed and rubricated, display the signs of having been a vademecum for practising physicians,[1] than to record isolated receipts many of which have the status merely of flyleaf literature. Pharmacognosy is a subject best studied in the fullest medical context that can be retrieved and the copying of single receipts – often for simply antiquarian reasons – cannot be expected to yield much reliable information about medical practices and the general level of pharmacological knowledge. Nevertheless, it would be foolish to leave the copying of miscellaneous receipts out of consideration altogether. It is through the smaller collections and individual instances that charms and incantatory verses are most frequently encountered, for they were not assembled as collections but remain scattered amongst conventional medical receipts or are left to stand on their own. Most important of all, the earliest recorded receipts in the vernacular are mostly sporadic and they must necessarily be of value on account of their early date. It is therefore natural to open the present study – the rest of which will be devoted to major receipt collections – with a brief survey of miscellaneous receipts, followed by a presentation of the charms. In order to give as full a picture as possible of this much smaller corpus of material the chronological limits of our study are here relaxed.

The earliest receipts in Anglo-Norman date from the twelfth century. MS London, British Library Sloane 2839 was written in England c.1100. It consists of a series of medical texts and is notable for its inclusion of a set of cautery illustrations which are amongst the earliest of their kind.[2] On f.78v, which was left blank, a twelfth-century hand has entered the following receipt:

1. [K]i at la guttefestre si irat en sultiu lieu, si frat un fu, si prendrat un test de pot, si frat sun aisement enz, si metrat plein puin de peivre, si l'ardrat tut ensenble, si face puldre, si prendrat de cele puldre, si metrat là u le mal li tient, si guarrat. Pur icel mal pernét turmentine e genest e de la tanesie salvage e de bete e de mater herbarum, si pernez de cascun uniement, si dunez a beivre le matin e le vespre par .iii. jurs.

At the end of the MS, after the Hippocratic 'Epistola ad Antiochum [sic] regem'[3] (ff.111v–12v) the same twelfth-century hand has written another receipt for the same ailment:

2. Ki at la gutefestre, jubarbe e arrement e ail si estamperat tut ensenble, si ferat un emplas[tre], si lierat u le mal li tient. Se il i at pertuis, si metez enz le jus s. . . de m. . . [4] Ce guarrat.

MS London, British Library, Royal 5 E VI is a late-twelfth-century codex which contains on ff.45v–71v a text of the pseudo-Isidorean *De numero*. Beginning on f. 69v a hand contemporary with that of the main text has entered a number of Anglo-Norman medical receipts in the space surrounding the writing block.[5] Some elements have been lost as a result of the cropping of the pages, but 33 receipts remain more or less intact. They cover a wide range of conditions[6] and are not arranged in the customary *a capite ad calcem* order. The first two receipts are as follows:

3. [f.69v] Pur le fi ki seine: Quisez la mariul en ewe e quant ele ert quite, siece sur une sele percee, si metet le pot desuz le fundement, si que la chalur vienge amunt e face issi suvent.

4. Pur la gute chaive al cumencement quant primes li vient: Se ço seit madle, tuez un chien, si li dunez le fiel a beivre. Se ço seit femele, dunez li a beivre d'une lisse le fiel u dunez li a beivre le jus de rue e de valeriane e de sanicle, d'un herbe ki at nun *aquileia* en latin. Ço li faites al cumencement, si garrat bien. [7]

Receipts are often added on blank pages at the end of a MS whatever the nature of the principal text. MS London, British Library, Royal 8 D V is a carefully executed, twelfth-century copy of Book II of Hugh of St Victor's *De sacramentis* at the end of which the hand of the text has entered (f.147r/v) a number of medical receipts, the headings for which are placed in the margins. The coloured initials were never executed.

5. [f.147r] A *entrait faire*: [P]ernez iunt[8] de ver e iunt de porc e siu de mutun tuit a un peis. Si en faites saun e si metez un peis de cire e un altre de peiz raisine e mellez tut ensemble. Si en faites entrait a plaie.

6. A *collerie fe[re] as oilz*: [P]ernez le jus de ruge fonuil e de la rue altretan de l'un cum de l'altre. Si metez al soleil en plusurs vaissals tresque il seit dur. Si metez pudre de l'aloen.

7. *Cuntre le oscur[té] des oilz*: [P]erneiz le jus de rue . . .[9] e de ruge fonuil e mel e fiel de coc.

8. Ad *unguentum mitigati[vum] faciendum*: [A]ccipe lilie, aloigne, fonuil, viole, plantaine, lancelee, surele dé bois e surele des chans, cunsoude, senezun, milfuil, ortie, fraser, sanicle, bugle, pimpre, egrimonie, reine, vetonie, avance, cerflange, chienlange e halne, kenillee, le tendre des runces, la racine de ruge parele, peletre, quinquefoille, crespe mave, cerfoil, luvesche, ruge aguille, cumfirie, fumetere, morele, [f.147v] ache, primorele, fevrefuie. Pernez virgine cire e fuille

de nuer, et iunt de ver e de porc, siu de cerf, bure de mai, blanc vin e encens e olie de olive e buillez ensemble. E puis sil cuillez, sil wardez a vostre dolur.

9. [P]ernez mirabola[n]s citrins dous unces e une unce de cassiafistre.

10. [P]ernez le jus de l'eble e altretant de vin e un poi de saun u bure. E puis si l'es- chalfez.

[T]anacetum, caulis, warantia, canvre, coctum diu in vino rubeo.

More impressive is the whole collection of Anglo-Norman medical receipts found in MS London, British Library, Royal 12 C XIX which provide the earliest attestations of many plant names.[10] The MS is a volume of 112 folios written in England in the second half of the twelfth century. It includes an illustrated bestiary and a series of excerpts from Isidore of Seville. Following a sermon on ff.100r–102v come the vernacular medical receipts (ff.102v–108r) in turn succeeded by a collec- tion of Latin receipts (ff.108v–112r).[11] The 40 vernacular receipts are written out continuously with simply a paragraph mark to distinguish them. The first two receipts are as follows:

11. [f.102v] Jute a sain e a emferm pur estre soluble: Pernez les arraces e la plan- taine e la centoine e la morele e le fenuil e des cenillés e des orties e des ciuns de la runce e des cherlokes e metez buillir ensemble. E cum il avrat builli un undee, trahez les, sis hachez sur un ais e lavez. E pernez puis, sis metez buillir od char fresche, sis mangez devant les autres viandes e serez tut solubles e sains.

12. Altre pur cursun: Pernez le bren del furment, sil lavez en un vaisel e sil culez en un autre vaisel e laissez aseer. Puis si purez l'eue. De ço que remaindra faites mortrels e dunez al malade a manger par treis feiz u par quatre.

The collection is not ordered according to any system. A series of items on ff.105v– 106r which begin with plant names have evidently been drawn from a list of simples. A few of the receipts recur in the Peterborough fragment published by Alexander Bell.[12]

Elsewhere individual vernacular receipts are added to Latin collections. MS Oxford, Bodleian Library, Bodley 567 (s.xiii²)[13] has an interesting set of Latin receipts on ff.133ra–140vb. At the bottom of f.136ra a contemporary hand has added,

13. A feire pudre constrictive: Pernez un uf e oste lle aubun e leisez le muel. Si l'emplez de peivre e mettez desuz les breises. Sil leisés la desque seit pudre e dunez a beivre pur la meneisun.

This is certainly an insular MS, for a number of English glosses have been written at the bottom of the page, as follows: f.134va corigiola .i. restebuf; f.135vb neir prun, grana ebuli. The receipt at the bottom of f.134rb includes 'consolidam minorem .i. daiseche, et maiorem .i. confiria, et mediam .i. siwardeswurt'.

The receipts in MS London, Royal College of Physicians 227 (s.xiv)[14] freely mingle vernacular plant names with Latin prescriptions. There is a vernacular receipt, alone amongst the Latin items, on f.180v:

14. Ky garir voudra de gutefestre face iceste medicine: Herbe Robert e matefelon, puis si prenge un beu morter, puis si face destempere[r] solonc çoe k'il est a ese e le soir avaunt couchier. E mette sur la play pur ky garir voudra de gutfestre. Et [ki] du mal gari volt estre prenge avence e columbine et ambroise ke nus apelum [. . .] E les face tutes tribler de bon vin u bon cerveise. Boive le matin avant diner. Prenge la drache de la tribuler, de ceste chose se face mestre.

The receipt shows obvious signs of corruption and the English name of *ambroise* ('hindheal') is omitted.[15]

MS London, British Library, Add. 33996 (s.xv) contains an abbreviated version of John of Gaddesden's *Rosa medicinae* (here 'Rosula medicine') on ff.149r–210v [16] which is followed by a Latin receipt, an Anglo-Norman one, and a charm for the farcy.[17] The lengthy Anglo-Norman receipt runs as follows:

15. A fere save:[18] Pernez burnette, dauke, tormentille, croysé, bugle, sanicle, herbe Johan, herbe Walter, herbe Robert, comfirye, ceo est la grein[dr]e consolde, e pernez le meindre consolde e la petite, e chanvere e la rouge cholet e warance, epparge [sic], chardon, diamant, ceo est lupyes, ceneçhoun e violet, verge de pastour, melilote e egremoyne e melice e plantayne, lancelé, pulusette, sptuere [sic],[19] vesces e muge dé boys, betoyne, croplesewort e pigle, e de touz yceus perniét ouele porcioun e de avance ataunt com de totes les autres herbes, e ceoes herbes seount quillez en may e nettement aparailés e triblés bien en un mortier. E puis perniez bure de may e metez ensemble ataunt com vous quidiez que vous ppussiez frier. E fetez pelettes ataunt gros com vous poyez poygnier e puis lessyez estre .v. jours e aprés metiez a fu e friez si chaut com vous poez co- lier parmy un canevas. E puis le cler metiez en boiste e les foundris ostiez. Puys donez cest a beivre od vin ou a cervoyse ou a ewe a matyn e au seir ataunt com .iii. greyns de furment pur totes playez sanier.

Isolated vernacular receipts added to a Latin collection are frequently received into the collection through subsequent copying. The important collection of medical texts which make up MS London, British Library, Royal 12 B XII (s.xiii) includes an extensive set of medical receipts (ff.105r–179r) in a variety of thirteenth-century hands.[20] Amongst these are found the following vernacular items:

16. [f.136r] Item ad tineam capitis: Pernez graunt novel test, si l'emplez tut de eue, si metez bone partie de glan de chesne e lessez buillir autresi lungement kum ço feust char de vache. Pernez cel bru del glan, sil metez enz un vessel u eit autretaunt . . . Si l'estuez. Si lavez bien la teine jeske al saunt cheun jur. De cel laverez autresi chaud cum li malade pura bien suffrir e li chief seit einz res, si le faciez joske la teine seit amortie e le chief tut bel e net. Ço est pruvee chose.

17. Item ad tineam capitis: Pernez la urine del buef u de la vache, si lavez la teinne e puis si l'oinnez bien de cest oinement ke jo dirai. Pernez la racine de la raiz e la racine de eaune .i. horselen [21] e les fiens de l'owe e trublez tut ensemblez od vieuz oint de porc. Puis si fetis bien frire enz une paele, si culez parmi un linge

drap, si l'estuez enz un vessel, si uinez la teinn(l)e [22] teste joske seit gari. Chescun jur seit lavé de cele urine e de l'oinement bien oint.

18. **[f.140r]** Contra wen. A oster cel mal ke l'em apele wen: Pernez un anel d'or, si croisez sovent cele boce de cel anel e fetes cerne entur cel mal **[f.140v]** chescun jur, si defiera cele boce. Esprovee chose est.

19. **[f.176v]** C'est l'emplastre le cunte Richard contre apostume el fundement: Herbe Robert, milfoil, lingua avis, panis cuculi, primula veris, sanicle, pes leporina /.i. avance/, tapsus barbastus .i. moleine, bugle, de ces herbes covient treire le jus e prendre autretant del jus de faverole /.i. limeke [23]/ cume de tuz ces autres e mettre ambedeus les jus emsemble e pus mettre utre le feu e mettre siu de mutun renablement e miel e pus eschaufer e pus mettre flur de pur orge, k'il seit bien espés.

There remain for consideration a number of MSS which contain modest groups of vernacular receipts, to be printed below. MS Oxford, Bodleian Library, Auct. F. 5. 31 (S. C. 3637) is an important medical MS dating from the second half of the thirteenth century. It contains a copy (ff.62vb–73va) of a collection of versified receipts in Anglo-Norman which is elsewhere given the title *Novele Cirurgerie*.[24] This is followed by a miscellaneous set of prose receipts (f.73va) and then the fragment of a medical treatise in Anglo-Norman called in a colophon *Gardein de Cors* (f.78rb). There are more vernacular prose receipts on ff.78va–79rb.

MS London, British Library, Stowe 948 is a volume of only 16 folios executed in England at the beginning of the fourteenth century. It contains, besides a calendar (ff.1r–6v), a series of devotional poems in Anglo-Norman interspersed with full-page illustrations (ff.8r–16v).[25] Between these two sections there appears, on f.7r/v, a set of vernacular receipts. There are only two rubrics and no colour is employed.

MS Cambridge, Trinity College 0. 1. 20 (s.xiii) is an extremely important medical MS offering a great variety of vernacular texts and a beautiful set of line drawings accompanying an Anglo-Norman translation of Roger Frugardi's *Chirurgia*.[26] A number of miscellaneous prose receipts appear on ff.23rb–24va, the first being a charm which we shall encounter again later.

MS London, British Library, Royal 9 A XIV is a volume of theological works, saints' lives and canon law texts executed in England towards the end of the thirteenth century.[27] The only vernacular work, a set of medical receipts (f.192ra/vb), is inserted between the heretical propositions from the Lombard's *Sententiae* and Grosseteste's *Constitutions*. It has been written by a hand not represented elsewhere in the MS on the last surviving folio of a quire. There is no colouring, decoration or rubrics and the receipts are simply distinguished by a paragraph mark in the ink of the text.

MS Cambridge, Trinity College 0. 8. 27 (s.xiii) pt. 2 contains a fragment of the 'Physique rimee'[28] followed (f.3ra/rc) by a number of Anglo-Norman prose receipts and then (ff.6ra–19vb) by a collection of Latin receipts.

Finally, MS Exeter Cathedral Library 3519 (s.xv)[29] offers a vast compendium of miscellaneous receipts including many from the so-called 'Lettre d'Hippocrate' (see below p.105). I have extracted a small number of the more interesting receipts for purely illustrative purposes.[30]

As an example of a longer receipt I have taken from MS British Library, Sloane

1754 (s.xiv[1]), an anthology of Latin and French medical and alchemical texts, an isolated vernacular receipt from ff.17v/18r.

MS AUCT. F. 5.31

20. **[f.73va]** *Pur le jauniz bevere:* [31] Pernez celidoynne e endivie e copere, lé deus parties de celidone, la tirz partie de les avant dites herbes e lé detemprez o ewe benete e donez al malad a bevere tres jors jun. E fetez li dire checun jor tres 'Pater Noster' e tres 'Ave Maria' e garrira tost.

21. *Autre:* Pernez une herbe ke l'em apele collecreie, si la taillez en oblees, si la quisez mut ben en serveise, si li donez a beivere chescun seir chaud e le matin freid.

22. *Autre:* Pernez yvure, sil raez od un kutel e pus pernez ceo ke vus avez raez el metez en un hanap e atant de safran par oel peis. Sil destemprez od let de chevre u od vin, si lui donez a beivere.

23. *Autre:* Pernez aloine, si la quisez mut bien en ewe e de ceo planez tut le cors treis feiz, si garra.

24. *Autre:* Pernez safran, si destemprez od le jus de plantoine e le donez a manger. E pernez la pudre de yvure e le metez sur le manger e sur ses beiveres e manguce le cok od les jaune peiz e femme la geline. Triasandaly valez.[32]

25. *Pur gute enosé:* Pernez jus de eyble e ferine de aveine, sil quisez mult bien ensemble e pus sil metez sur le mal ausi chaud cum il le put suffrir, si garra. Ceo est aprové chose.

26. Hoynement a checune gute, u ke ele seit: Pernez deus ponnees de rue e de ere terrestre e une ponne de savyne. Triblez bien, pus le mellez od oille u od bure u suy de mouton. Si quisez bien, pus le colez e de ceo honnez la gote.

27. **[f.78va]** *Pur gute kayve:* Le malade face une chandele, ke seit si lunge de l'ortil del destre pié deskes a l'haterel, de cire e pus la cope en set parties oeles e en la primer copun escrivez le primer ferié e en la secunde copun la secunde ferié e si(l) des autres feriis e pus auge a moter tut jun. E il seit bien confés de tuz ses pechez e ke il seit mult contrit. E aprés ke il prenge discipline e a chescun cop ke le prestre moil la verge en ewe beneite e pus le prestre auge chanter une messe de Seint Esperit. Mes deprimes le malade deit offrir sur l'autel les chandeles. Aprés si prendra le prestre, si lui baudra une des chandeles e le malade verra le nun ke est en la chandele ke il avera e tuz jurs aprés junera cel jur en pain e en ewe. E pus serunt les chandeles aluminez a tote la messe e cele en sa mein, aprés la messe il la deit offrir al prestre e un dener.

28. *Autre:* Pernez lé pijuns de corfbin tuz vif en lur ni, si les ardez enz un noef pot et pus si en fetes pudre e donez lui a bevere od ewe benite e il gara. Icest meimes garist le poagre.[33]

29. *Autre:* Pernez herbe Johan e l'erbe seint Cristofere, sil fetes manger chescun jur, si garra.

30. *Encuntre parlesie dé jambes*: Pernez oinuns, si les cavez bien parfund. E pus les emplez de peivre molu e pus metez sel sure e pus lé estupez de la covercle e les metez en breizes, si les quisét deskes il sein tuz mol. E pus les pernez, si les metez en un fort drap linge e les premez e l[é] metez en voz boistes e de ceo oignez le malade.

31. [f.78vb] Pernez le herbe de senevey quant ele est verde, si la molez mult bien en un morter e pus le friez en oille de olive. E pus fetez une enplastre sur un quir tenve el metez teve sur le mal u seir e un autre al matin.

32. V[ersus]: Salgea, castorium, lavendula, primula veris, naster, avencia, sanant paralitica membra.

33. *Pur crampe*: Pernez la racine de ortie e la quisez e pus triblez la bien. E pus le friez bien en oille de olive e pus oignez le liu.

34. *Pur dertre*: Pernez aloigne e herbe Roberd e les triblez mult bien en un morter e pus les friez en une paele od oint de sengler mult bien e pus lé primez parmi un drap linge el metez en un net vessel e de ceo en oignez le mal.

35. *Pur la variole*: Quant il commencent de nestre, bevez pur jus de pulegii e de tanesi oelement e ceo vus delivera. S'il est issi ke age u enfermeté nel sufre pas, metez i du vin.

36. *Pur roigne u grature u manjue*: Pernez la racine de la roge parelle e triblez bien od bure de may e od vel oint de pork. E pus lé quisez mult bien ensemble. Pus lé culez parmi un drap, sil gardez en boistes e de ceo enoignez le mal encontre le fu. Triblez fumetere od serveise, sis bevez sovent.

37. *Pur la mangue*: Pernez ortie e kersun ewage, faverole, e triblez cheskun par sei oelement e metez le jus ensemble bien entremellez. Pus pernez oint de pork male [f.79ra] e vif argent bien entremellez el metez en une esquiele el tenez encontre le feu u contre le solail tant ke tut seit deguté en un vessel. Pus si pernez le jus de voz herbes e metez ovek eles entremellez bien el metez en voz boistes, si lessez refreidir.

38. Mutun en la seisun,[34] porc e nomement lé pesteus, les peiz e les orailes e le chaudun, mortrous, coliz. De ses herbes fetes jotes: borage, bete, mave, mercurie, persil, carsun de funtayne; od chars – boef tendre e joeune, vel, cheveroil, conis; dé oiseus – gelines, chapuns, pocins, ouez mous, perdriz, fesaunz. Usez le bré. Od vostre char seit quite, e nom[em]ent boef, motun, chapun, geline. Petit de sauge, plus de persil fetes mettre solum vostre pover, seez en joie. Estuvez vus ene ces herbes: fumeterre, eble e lovesche, paritare, mentastre, fenoil, foles del blanc pruner. Gardez vus de manger viande sur autre deskes la premere seyt defite. Si maschés bien kant ke vus mangez. Ne mangez nul pain alis ne trop dur ne trop poy quit. Ne junez mie trop ne velez mye trop. De freid vus gardez, [de] chaud vus gardez e de ire, de trop parfund pensers. Ne travelez mie trop aprés manger, de tard suppers vus gardez.

39. [f.79rb] Pernez herbe Jon, herbe Water, herbe Roberd, bugle, sanicle, pigle, surele dé bois, egrimone, burnet, consode, plantayne, lancelee, pimpernelee, milfoil, tormentine, pigre, coperon de ronce. Pernez de checune od uele

porciun, mes de herbe Water pernez plus ke dé autres. Si pernez bure de may,
si fetes oinement.

MS STOWE 948

40. **[f.7r]** Pernetz endive, violette, coupere, cerflange, de chescune deus poines;
ssaundres blaunches et rouges et rasure de yvere, de chescune un demy unce;
semences freides moundies, semence de letuse, semence de endive, de chescune treis dragmes; et euwe de endive demi livere; flurs de violette, de borage,
flurs de ninifar, de chescun demi unce; vyn de pomme garnés egre, demi livere;
prunes damaciens trente; liqueris moundie, un unce; ssugre, une livere et
demye; juis de scabiouse, un quartroun. Çoe est le beivere pur la ffaye.

41. Pernetz roses deus unces; ssaundres blaunches et rouges, de chescun treis dragmes; juis de plauntaine, juis de jubarbe, vin egre, de chescun ouwele porcioun.
Ceste euwette est pur le ffoie.

42. Pernetz aloigne, mente, de chescun une poigne; de giloffre deus dragmes;
comyn, un unce; galingale, une dragme; pain de orge ou farine de orge, un
quartroun. Fetes emplastre ové vin egre. Çoe est pur le estomak.

43. Pernetz opopanak, demi unce; terebentine, g[al]banum, mastik, de chescun
demi unce; clouwe de gilofre, deus dragmes; cire, un quartroun. Çoe est le emplastre pur le estomak. Ceo est pur le yve[r?].

44. **[f.7v]** Pernetz deus baies de lorer et les transglutez quaunt vous aletz dormir.

45. Pernetz un grein de fraunk encens et le transglutez et la fumee ressu par la
bouche restreint reoume: pomme de ambre flerré restreint roeme.

46. Quaunt vous avez reoume de quei vous sentez estopé, pernez dragagant,
gomme arabik, juis de liqueris, de chescun ouwelement dragme et demi; ysope,
horhune, de chescun un dragme; yringes et elena campana, de chescun deus
dragmes; figes, deus unces; liqueris moundie, un quartroun; sucre, demi lyvere.
Fetes quire deus lyveres et demy taunt qe a deus lyveres. Et tastiez de une
quilere cis foiz ou seet al matin et al vespre quant vous aletz cocher.

47. Pur le yver diapenidion et diairis medlé ensemble; pur le esté diagragant, jufus
et penites.

48. Pur menesoun: Pernetz sucre roset, une lyvere; saunk de dragoun, seool, ouwelement de chescun une dragme, çoe est asavoir le peis de deus et maille, et
medlez ensemble et ceste chose usez aprés dormir et quant vous estes pluis
voed.

49. Autre pur menesoun: Pernetz le juis de plauntaigne la greindre et la meindre,
euwe rose, de chescun ouwelement un quartroun de la lyvere; sumak, deus
unces.

MS TRINITY 0. 1. 20

50. **[f.23rb]** ESPERMENT A PLAIES
Treis bons freres estoient ke aloient al mont d'Olivet por coillir herbes bones a
plaie et a garison. Et ancontrerent Nostre Seignor Jesu Crist et Nostre Seignor
lor demaunda: 'Treis bons freres, ou alez vous?' Et il responderent: 'Al mont
d'Olivet por coiller herbes de plaie et de garison'. Et Nostre Sire dit a eus
'Venez o mai et me grantez **[f.23va]** en bone fei ke vous nel diez a nul home
ne a femme ne aprendrez. Pernez oile d'olive et leine ke unkes ne fust lavee et
metez sor la plaie'. Quaunt Longius l'ebreu aficha la launce en le coste Nostre
Seignor Jesu Crist, cele plaie ne seigna, ele n'emfla point, ele ne puoit mie, ele
ne doloit mie, ele ne rancla mie. Ausi ceste plaie ne seine mes, n'emfle point,
ne pue mie, ne doile mie, ne rancle point, n'eschaufe mie. En le nun del Piere,
el nun del Fiz, el nun del Seint Espirit, Pater Noster treis fois.

51. POR MALADE AVEILLER
Pernez le castor et ardez le et quaunt il est ars affumez le malade de cele fumee
[f.23vb] ki trop dort et il aveillera maintenaunt.

52. Pernez launcelee, plauntein, flor de trumel, tanesie .i. mirfoil, le couperon de
le coudre, jus de morele, jubarbe, herbe Robert, ortie griesche et lusalveon.
Ces herbes pernez et triblez chescun par sei ou .ii. ensemble. Et quaunt tous seront triblez, si les metez ens une paele, si i metez oint et siu et harpois et vin
blaunc ou aisil. Si le quisez taunt ki il ne fume plus, adonc ert assez quit. Puis si
metez virge cire o cire novele, si l'oste l'en de la paele par cloteus, si le metez
en .i. blaunche tuaille, si premez hors le jus et metez en boistes.

53 DECOCTION
Pernez racines de peresil, d'a**[f.24ra]**che, de fenoil, de ravele, si les lavez et
raez, si les fetes nes et puis les mincez et metez temprer en aisil .i. jor et une
nuit. Et puis metez i le tierç ewe et faites boillir deske a la meité. Et puis le
colés et aprés pernez miel une pinte ou plus taunt com vous plerra et quisez
bien. Et aprés le metez ovec l'aisil et quisez tot ensemble taunt ke tot reviegne
a la quantité del miel.

54. AUTRE
Pernez encens et mastic et roses et fetes poudre, si boillez tot ensemble en
megue et teve le tenez en vostre bouche ausi longuement com vous poez et
puis getez hors et issi faites sovent.

55. POR RESTREINDRE LE MARRIS
Por restreindre le marris mirre et encens seient pestri **[f.24rb]** ensemble et quit
en vin blaunc et foilles de roses et mente ovec et donez a boivre al matin et al
vespre.

56. AUTRE
Autre: Pernez foilles de vignee, de mente et de rose et de morele. Tot seit frit
en oile ens une paele. Aprés seit oint li malades premerment de oile d'olive et
puis seit cele friture mise sor le liu ke dout.

57. AUTRE
Autre: Warance .ii. poine, fenoil, tanesie, caunvre, blaunc bibuef et rouge

cholet, oile de olive et ambre destempree ensemble, ermoise avec. Et aprés oigne om là ou ele set par le ventre tot entor (oar tot), amont et aval.

58. POR ENTOUNEMENT D'OREILLE
Por entounement d'oreille saim d'anguille soit boilli [f.24va] en la paiele et puis refreidi. Et puis i metez jus de jubarbe et la poudre de nois muscade triblee et oile de lorier. Tot ce seit quit ensemble et mis en net veire. Et de ceste oignement oignez l'oraile là ou ele dout par la quel oignement oïe est recovré et le nerf retrait en oint aloins.[?]

59. AUTRE
Pernez aloine et vif argent estaint et aubun de l'oef et viel oint et triblez tot ensemble et por le sowef flairer, si vous volez, si i metez encens.

60. [f.324vb] Pro gutta caduca: + Appacion + + Appria + Appremont et qua settanua + e puis pendez cest escrit entur le col.

61. Encuntre sausefleme e roine: Pernez oint de sengler une livere, silium un unce, sufre deus unces, vif argent un unce, fel de pesun de duz eawe deus dragmes, canfer tres dragmes, ceruze demi unce.

62. Por garir de roigne: Lavez le primes de bone lesive de favaz, pus triblez ensemble peivre et vert de grece et arrement et blanc plum. Si friez en viez oint de porc, si le oignez de ces et le daubez de miel chescun jor et de jus de cerfel entre les daubes, si garra.

63. Por garir de gote: Pernez une poignee de cauquetrepe et de herbe ive et de plantein et de matefelun, de chescun demie poigne et quesez en .i. jalun de blanc vin duques au terz. Donez li a beivre.

MS ROYAL 9 A XIV

64. [f.192ra] C'est l'entrete au chevalers: [35] Pernez demi livere de peys reysine, un quarterun de franc ensens, un quarterun de dragan, un quarterun de gowme arabich, demi quarterun de aloen apatich, un quarterun de mastich, un quarterun de fenegrec, un quarterun de comin, un quarterun de noir poiz, un unce de sarcacol. Primes metez en la paiele peys reyseine et puis cyre et puis gowme arabich et puis noir poiz et puis aloen apatich et puis franc encens et puis fenegrec et puis sarcacol et puis dragan et puis mastich et puis comin et puis vos semences au derein et puis les colez parmi un drap en eawe freide et puis lé tenez au few come cyre et puis lé metez en eawe chawde et lavez bien dedeinz et puis lé tenez au few et puis lé metez en sawf.

65. A totes plaies saner: Pernez erbe Water, erbe Robert, bugle, senicle, avance, burnette, violette, plawinteyne, petite consewde, milfoil, quintefoile, trifoil, frasere, surele, rowge ortie, cowperun de runce, celidoyne, oumunde, temprez od cyre virgine et franc encens et bure de may.

66. Ki voust estre gari de meneson prenge la plantayne une grant partie, si le face mult bien laver en un eawe corante et puis face prendre hors le eawe nette-

ment et cuiller hors totes les foiles et puis tribler lé bien en un morter ou en un net vessel et prendre hors le jus. Et puis aprés prendre la drache et bele grese de porc malle et frire le ensemble et puis mettre le sur un es et le malade par matin en jun aprés ke il avera fet une sele, si ascese sus si chaut com il purra renablement suffrir. E tant com il serra, si beive le jus ke avant fu preenz de la plawnteyne et issi face treis jurs, si garira.

67. **[f.192rb]** Encontre dolur del chief: Pernez betoyne et camamille, puliol, erre terestre, fete les quire en eawe, si lavez le chief ou quant il sunt quites, fete[s] les bien batre emsemble, si fetes emplastre sur le chief.

68. Pur clows et pur emflures et pur le mormal et pur le felun quant il est depescé: Pernez biaw flowr de furment et eawe freide et le medlez ensemble et le fetes ausi espés cum tenve past et puis le metez en une paele et le bollez et le movez desque il seit espés, si ke il teigne ensemble et puis si le ostez tot del few et metez i bure de may et le movez ensemble desque le bure seit tut fundu et le metez en sauf.

69. Ki vodra fere un entrete pur totes maneres de gowtes fors de gowte enossé prenge adeprimes le peys de .xii. d.[36] de agrippe et puis le peys de .xii. d. de ungeunt aurin et le peys de .xii. d. de oint de tessun et le peys de .xii. d. de blanc encens et puis de un vert unement le peys de .xii. s. et puis prenge blanche grese .vii. cuillerez, si le fundez ensemble et un blanch quir cunraiez de furmage, si le metez atut et le averez amendé.

70. Ki vodra fere un vert oignement ki est bon a totes maneres des plaies et de sourvenues prenge plein poin de egremoine et poigne de primerole et poigne de saxifrage et poigne de pigle et poigne de frasere et poigne de violette et poigne de milfoil et poigne de trifoil et poigne de matfelun malle et poigne de femeterre et poigne de cunseude le greindre et poigne del meindre et poigne de erbe yve et poigne de planteine et poigne de launcelé et poigne de pié de levre et poigne de cressun d'eawe et poigne de mader et poigne de linois et poigne de semence de chaunvre et poigne de sawge et poigne de persil et partie de sew de beste; et festes tribler ensemble **[f.192va]** en un morter de arem mult bien od un demi galun de bure fres de may, et puis le fetes boiller en un galun de eysil mult bien, et puis le fetes coler parmi un drap et pernez la gresse de tut quant il est refreidi, si le fetes enfundrer et le metez en boistes et les averez bons.

71. Encontre dolur de denz: Pernez morele et sawge et fetes batre ensemble et prendre hors le jus et medler ovec levein et fetes emplastre et metez de cele part ou le dolur est.

72. A estreinture de piz: Pernez .vi. figes ou .vii. et licoriz paré et un poy de ysope et fetes le quasser et quire en eawe ou en tysanne et ce beive au seir et al matin tieve. Autre a riches homes: Deus letuaries diadragaunt freit et diapennidion medle[z] ensemble et usez de ce au matin et au vespere.

73. Encontre la tousse: Pernez racin de fenoil et de persil et de ache[37] et lur semences et ysope et esclarie et dragant e gowme arabich, figes secches, uves passes et prunes damascenes, de chescun une poigne, cestes choses faces quire en eawe de orge ou le orge seit quise en deus galuns et demi deques le demi galun

seit gasté et puis eschawdés lenz .ii. poignez de bren et puis si le colez et puis en cel eawe facez quire vos erbes et vos gowmes, si ke le demi galun seit gasté et metez atant de licoriz ke il seit asez douz de licoriz. Et de autre part facét quire en vos beiveres et en vos mangers solom vostre poer sawge, ysope, puliol, calamente, lavendre et la flur de betoine.

74. A oster peil et chevelure: Pernez les eofs de furmies et gowme de edre et orpiment rowge a owel peys et medlez od vin et oynez.

MS TRINITY 0. 8. 27

75. **[f.3ra]** A . . . *arit hume de(l) la taupe*: Pernez la plaunteine, lancelé, les foilles en esté et les racines en ivern, et freis uint de porc madle a madle e freis uint de truie a femele, et triblés les mut bien ensemble. Emplastrez le ben espés. Espruvé chose est.

76. *Pur pointure de serpent u de tuz venimuse verms*: Demandez cler ewe et dites trei fié utre le ewe In nomine Patris et Filii et Spiritus Sancti, amen, et trei Pater Nosters en le nun del Pere et del Fiz et del Seint Espirit. Et dites ces nuns utre: poro, poro, poro, pota, zaba, zaro, zarai, per Mariai paraclitus, in nomine Patris et Filii et Spiritus Sancti, amen. Donez a bevre a celui ke porte le message. Leque[l] ke ço seit, de hume u de beste, **[f.3rb]** guarra. Espruvé est.

77. *Pur lé boces que crescent entur le col sicume glanbres et depecent hors sicume plaies*: Pernez ces herbes et quise les en bone cerveise u en vin et bevez le jus, aut matin freid et aud vepres chaud: avenz et planteine et consoude et herbe ive. Et puis fetes ceste entret: pernez cire virgine et peiz reisin et seu de mutun et bure de mai et un herbe ke hume apele [en] engleis 'feltris' et fetes lé buillir ensemble et mettre lé freiid desure lé plaies.

78. *Pur teyne*: La racine de aune quit e la ruge parele, la racine quit e veil oynt e demi unce de vif argent e de coperose un unce e alum demi unce e sufre un ferlinge e olibanum e mirre e mastik. De cetes choses avant numés primes seint batuz ensemble le coperose e le alum e sufre e olibanum e mirre e mastik mut ben, e puis le vif argent mulu mut ben o tut, e puis le aune e la parele mis o tut e ben triblez ensemble, e puis le oint o tut e ben muluz ensemble. E puis seint mis en buistes e dunc prenge hom un unce de coperose e face arder en un **[f.3rc]** test e seit dunc fet en pudre e seit batu o tut un unce de sufre e seit destempré o duz leit. La teste al malade de ço seit oint deske le ordeure seit treit hors quatre jors u cinc. E quant le ordeure seit tret hors, si seit la teste oint de l'oiniement avant numé deske seit sein.

MS EXETER CATHEDRAL 3519

79. **[f.125v]** Pur garer de feloun: Bevez morele et oculescunse et osemound. Et ceo garra.

80. **[f.126r]** A la pere freyndre: Pernez osemunde, ache, betoyne, persile, lymer-che, alisandre, bayes d'ere, gromyle, jazere. Si estampez et boylez bien en vyn et culez. Si mettez la poudre d'un levre que seit ars en un furn dedeinz un pot bien covert. Si donez a boyre parmy un chalemel.

81. **[f.127r]** Pur roine de cheval: Triblez herbe benoyt et quysez en urine de vache jesqe al terce part et puis en lavez le cheval.[38]

82. **[f.129v]** Pur estauncher: . . . Quysez en vyn ou en ewe prunettes sauvages, si bevez, si maungez, et si estauncherez.

83. Item ad idem: Fetez papilotz de flour de frument et de let, si mettez flour de blaunche creis, si maungez.

84. **[f.137r]** Pur fort gute: Quysetz ensemble aukes ben les racynes de panwhet .i. uude[th]onge[39] e de gueschei .i. ortye salvage[40] par owele porcioun e pus les triblét ensemble tut menu e metetz ceste chose chaude sovent le jour là ou la gute est.

85. **[f.138r]** Pur maille en oyl oster u teye: Pernetz une anguoylle tute entere, si rostét mut ben e quant ele serra mut ben rosté, pernetz hors le fiel e de cel li-cour ke est en le foil une gute quaunt le pacient deyt aler cocher metetz en le oyl, e mes ke il face graunt violence ne seyt mie osté, kar en un nut despessera ou departera la maylle ou la teye.

86. **[f.143r]** Pur le fy e pur cancre: Pernetz un novele pot de tere e metetz une poygne de waide e ataunt e demy poygne de brasyl e un pece de veil quir e de fente de humme e autaunt de syu de buc e .viii. testes u dis de ayl e un graunt crapout neir e une poygne de cerfoil e escales de .x. eofs ou de .xii. e un pé de un humme mort.

87. **[f.146r]** Ad plagam sanandam: Herbes a medecyne, foeles, letues, sclariol, por-tulac, jubarbe, morele, hennemawe, popie, mirtus, planteyne, cerflange, chen-lange, coupere, maydenher, cey[n]torie, ceterac, mylfoyl, trifoyl, sanguinarie, launcelé, conseude le un e l'autre, solsecle, oseles, persyl, fenoil, carewy, ache, sauge, wymauve, kersun l'un e l'autre, senevey, vane, ysope, clareye, eble, hor-hund, lynoys, ortilles vermayles, ditaundre, rays, primerole, anyse, betoyne, camamille, neyre mente, flur de geneste, pelettre, cumferie, sanicle, bugle, centorie, eufras, pimpernele, veþervoye .i. fevrefeue, tansye, turmentyne.

88. **[f.155r]** Pur fere oygnement a sursanure de playe: Cest oygnement ad a noun cytrine. Mychel wrth is wormele of berecheve trou þat is drie in huse to drye horie woundes e sy mut vaut la pudre de launcelé.

MS SLOANE 1754

89. **[f.17v]** *Unguentum commestibile pro plagis curandis*
Ceo est la manere de fere unguentum commestibile et est bon pur garir nettement totes maneres playes et overtures et esprové [est]. R[ecipe] burnette,
dauke, tormentille, croysé, bugle, pigle, sanicle, herbe Robert, herbe Water,
herbe Jon, la grant consoude et la mene et la petite, chanvre, ruge cholet,
warence, sparge, vert chardun, senesciun / .i. groundswilie / violette, virga pastoris / .i. wylde tesel / melice / .i. modorwort / egremoyne, chevrefoyl, plantayne, launcelé, peluette, saponere, uesses verde [sic], flur de genette **[f.18r]** de
checun ouele porciun peysés par balance, et de avence autretant de tous les
autres avont només. Ses herbes seyent quilis in mai et soyent medlés ové bure
de may freche, que unkes ne tocha ewe. Et seit la bure primes fundue en une
bele paele sur un cler fu lent et ben ecumee de une penne de owe et ben puree.
Et pus de cete bure issint puree pernét plus ou meyns, solum ceo que la quantité de vos herbes est, issi que asét suffise, et metez en la vessele ové la bure
totes les herbes avont nomez. Mes primes seyent byen batuz en un morter de
areym. Pus lessét les byen quire sur un fu lent et cler longement jekes a la
tierce partie du bure ou a poy la moyté seyt degasté. Pus hostez les du fu et
lessét lé refroyder. Et pus soyt exprimé parmi un colour ou un net canevas en
une nette vessele de tere byen plumee et kaunt il est froyd soyt mis en violes
de verre. Et seyent toutdis les violes ben estopés que heyr ne entre. Et taunt
cum plus vel, meus vaut. Et done a malade a boyre a matyn et a soyr la quantité graunt de une blank peys et nyent plus, car si vous ly donez plus, yl garireyt
trop tost. Et metez le sur le coste del hanap et lessét le humer ens ov un poy de
serveyse estale ou blanc vin et coverez la playe de une foyle de rounce ou de
ruge cholet et il garira pur veyr byen et nettement saunz dote saunz ryens de
autre chose fere. Et ceste chose est byen et cortoysement provee de plusours
bone gens.

It is interesting to compare the Middle English version of the same receipt in MS
British Library, Sloane 2584 (s.xv¹) f.13r:

90. *For to make save in hys kynde*: Take burnet, dauc, turmentylle, maidenheer,
bugle, pigle, sanycle, herbe Jon, her[be] Robard, herbe Water, þe grete con-
saund, þat is comferi, þe mene consaunde, þat is daisie, þe grete [consaunde],
hempe croppes, **[f.13v]** þe reed cool croope, þe reed brere crooppe, mader, col-
verfot, sowþistil, groundeswillye, violet, þe wyld tesel, moderwort, egremoyne,
wodebynde, rybwort, mousere, mouspese, floure of brome, beteyne, vervayne,
croppe of þe white þorn, sowþerynwode, sauge, þe crope of þe rede nettel, os-
mound, fyveleved-gras, scabiose, strauberiewise, mylfoyle, pympernel, sel-
vehele, avans, as moche of avans as of alle þe oþere herbis be even
proporcioun and þei schulen be gadered in May before seynt Johannes daie.
And bray3e hem in a morter and medle hem wit may de tere[41] fresch and
clene made as þe melke comeþ fro þe cow3e. 3if þu have no may butter, take
oþur botter and purge it clene and lat it kele and medlet in a vessel and covere
it .6. daies or .7. til it begynne to hore. And aftur frie it in a panne and clense
it þro a cloth in a vessel til it be colde and seþen chaunge it. And do away þe
grounde and seþen do it over þe feer and clere it and lat it kele and do it in

boxys. And þe wounded man schal drynke þerof with ale oþer wit w[ine] as moche at ones as a barly corne or as a whete furst and laste eche daye til he be hool. And cover þe wounde wit þe leef of a calstok and ȝif þu ne myȝht noȝt fynde alle þese herbes, take 32 of þe furst and of avans as moche as of alle þe oþere wit mader for it nedeþ noon oþer save ne treyte.

Charms

Religion, medicine and magic have long been associated in therapeutic methods and their potent relationship investigated by students of both early Greek and early Christian medicine.[42] The results are similar in both cases: the rational has not totally assimilated the prerational nor neutralized its power and the two coexist. The image of Christus Medicus reflects the Old Testament view of God as the physician of His people and the beliefs which accompany it continue Old Testament ideas, namely that there should be no recourse to magic or pagan methods of healing, but natural methods might be used as part of the provision made by the Creator for the well-being of His creation. The discussion of medicine in Ecclesiasticus 38, 1–15 is a fair illustration of what became a common Christian position: ready acceptance of natural medicine, on the one hand, and a more cautious attitude to medical practitioners on the other.[43] Roman medicine had, of course, contained much magic and superstition – one has only to consider the material recorded in Pliny[44] – and late imperial writers, and those who drew on them, bequeathed to early Christian Europe much medical lore which was of a frankly superstitious nature. At the end of the fourth century Marcellus of Bordeaux transmits a great deal of popular medical practices in his *De medicamentis*.[45] The Church, fully conscious of the close ties between *medicina magica* and medieval botany,[46] sought to reconcile popular beliefs with the overriding recognition of God as the true source of cures. In one of his homilies Aelfric declares 'We should not set our hope in medicinal herbs, but in the Almighty Creator who has given that virtue to those herbs. Noone shall enchant a herb with magic, but with God's word shall bless it, and so eat it.'[47] Similarly, Chaucer's Parson argues 'charmes for woundes or maladie of men or of beestes, if they taken any effect, it may be peraventure that God suffreth it, for folk sholden yeve the moore feith and reverence to his name'.[48] The evidence of the medieval charms shows clearly how the Church, recognizing the deeply rooted belief in their power, assimilated them to orthodox faith by the simple expedient of substituting Christian for pagan names and prescribing the recitation of the Pater Noster, Ave Maria etc. innumerable times. Thus Bonser pointed out 'the Church's method of converting a pagan charm into a Christian remedy was by adding a few words of Church Latin, or by substituting the name of Christ or of a saint for that of a heathen deity – accompanied by the ever efficacious addition of the sign of the cross'.[49] Without the Christianising elements the charms might be universal.[50] Certainly, the Anglo-Saxon materials, which have been carefully studied,[51] can be traced to an impressive variety of sources. Grattan and Singer identified these as Greek medicine, formularies of the late Empire, Roman magic,

'Pythagorean' devices, Latin liturgical elements, Byzantine theurgy, pagan teutonic magic, Christianised teutonic ritual, Christianised Celtic magic and theurgy, Hisperic elements, south Italian classical survivals. Grattan and Singer had a rather contemptuous regard for the material of the *Lacnunga*, but Charles Talbot has shown[52] how the leechdoms anticipate 'Gariopontus' and 'Petroncellus' by two centuries, so that what is often regarded as the achievement of writers deemed to be the earliest Salernitan authorities is in fact the work of a much earlier period and shows exceptional knowledge of Greek medicine. For Talbot Anglo-Saxon medicine was far from being the 'hotch-potch of incantations, charms, magic and old wives's recipes' that it is sometimes made out to be. Despite this important corrective, however, it has to be recognized that the Anglo-Saxon charms lived on long into the Middle Ages. Their classification brings some problems. J. F. Payne took as his headings: (i) prayers, invocations, or other verbal formulae addressed to the herbs, and special observances used when gathering them or other natural remedies (ii) prayers and mystical words repeated over the patient, or written and applied to some part of his body as an amulet (iii) direct conjurations or exorcisms addressed to diseases as if they were evil spirits (iv) narrative charms, that is, anecdotes relating to sacred or legendary personages who suffered or had something analogous to what the patient is suffering from (v) material magic, that is, the attribution of magical powers to certain objects, such as plants or parts of animals, stones and engraved gems (vi) transference of disease by a verbal formula, or a ceremony, to some animal or material object. Grendon subsequently selected five classes; (i) exorcisms (ii) herbal charms (iii) transferential charms (iv) amulet charms (v) charm remedies. Whilst Storms correctly observes that none of these classes is discrete, Payne's classification will serve as a practical guide to the charms printed below.[53]

The first category, observances and addresses relating to herbs themselves, has been the subject of a comprehensive (for Antiquity) survey by A. Delatte,[54] whose sources include Theophrastus (lib.IX), Dioscorides, Pliny, Scribonius Largus and his followers, and, so far as astrological herbalism is concerned, a variety of treatises attributed to Hermes Trismegistus, Salomon, Ptolemy etc. The continuity of transmission is striking, many rituals recurring in MSS from the tenth century to the eighteenth. The first consistent element in these magical observances is the stipulation of the time propitious for gathering herbs.[55] This is often at night at a particular stage in the waxing or waning of the moon, also frequently just before sunrise. The influence of astrology is strong and there are innumerable variations. In Christianised receipts the time of picking herbs is often specified as St John's Eve (Midsummer's Eve), but many liturgical festivals are represented. The vernacular receipts sometimes stipulate that herbs are to be gathered just before sunrise.[56] Another set of directions concerns the preparation or condition of the herb-gatherer, who may be required to be a virgin, a boy not yet entered on puberty, to be naked, to be dressed in white, to be alone etc.[57] The range of cathartic and apotropaic rites is vast.[58] A frequently represented example is the *circumitio* or *ambitus* (Roman *lustratio*) which involves walking round the plant whilst singing. Prophylactic rites involve bringing the plant into contact with a particular substance such as gold or silver, or with an object such as a ring, knife etc. In Christianised charms much space is given over to liturgical recitations and even the saying of whole masses.[59] In the Greco-Egyptian tradition incantations were particularly prominent. These *carmina* might be magical formulae with no decipherable sense, as still sometimes occurs in the medieval charms,[60] though it is often difficult to say whether the gibberish is intentional or the product of miscopying. In the sixth century the Council of Braga condemned the incantations and rituals of herbalists, and in the next century a sermon of St Eligius contains strong criticism of the enchantment of herbs.[61] As usual, the Church found that the most effective way of dealing with such practices was simply to Christianise the form of words used.[62] The *Decreta* of Burchard of Worms contains the following statement; '*De arte magica*: . . . collegisti herbas medicinales, cum aliis incantationibus cum Symbolo et Dominica oratione, id est cum Credo in Deum et Pater Noster cantando. Si aliter fecisti, decem dies in pane et aqua poeniteas'.[63] In the older pagan charms the simples are regarded as powerful agents with personalities, dignity, will-power and so forth, attributes which are recognised by a wide variety of addresses including prayers, invocations, exorcisms, conjurations and declarations of every kind. Originally, the gathering of the plant was regarded as a sort of theft and offerings were made to Terrae Mater in recompense. Later these offerings were misinterpreted as being made to the plants themselves![64] Pliny speaks of the practice of offerings and sacrifices, which might consist in the placing of grains of corn, or wine, or a coin on the spot where the plant was picked.[65] The manner of the picking was also specified.[66] The taboo on the plant coming into contact with iron was very widespread and survives in some of the medieval charms.[67] Similarly, it was often stated that the plant should not touch the ground.[68] The gatherer was instructed to use a particular hand, and even certain fingers of that hand.[69] Finally, in a smaller number of cases there might be directions for the treatment of the plant after harvesting:[70] it was not to be placed on the ground, its roots were to be washed in wine, it was to be blessed and placed on the altar and masses said etc.

Payne's second category of charms comprised the words and formulae addressed to the patient, or else applied through some writing medium to the patient's body as an amulet.[71] The combination of magical letters or words[72] is often constitutive of the medieval charm. Whilst gibberish might sometimes be the result of misunderstanding or miscopying, there was certainly an attempt in the older charms to create mystery.[73] The languages employed were Greek, Latin, Hebrew and Irish.[74] Christian formulae were almost invariably tripartite.[75] They might be written on wood, parchment, traced on some part of the patient's body, or applied to objects both vegetable (apple) and mineral (lead).[76] Christian periapts were frequently accompanied by signs of the cross or by another symbol such as the tetragrammaton.[77]

The third category of charms described by Payne is that of exorcisms, commands to the disease and/or an evil spirit to depart.[78] These are often of considerable length and, as they are not so well illustrated in printed studies of charms, it is worth giving three examples which are found in MS B. L. Sloane 962 (s.xv[1]) ff.9v–10r:

In nomine Patris et Filii et Spiritus Sancti, amen. 'Conjuro vos, clues et omnia genera demonum nocturna sive diuturna per Patrem et Filium et Spiritum Sanctum atque individuam Trinitatem et per intercessionem beatissime et gloriose semperque virginis Marie, per orationes prophetarum, per merita patriarcharum, per suffragia angelorum et archangelorum, per interventum apostolorum, per passionem martirum, per fidem confessorum, per castitatem virginum, et per intercessionem omnium sanctorum et per septem dormientes, hos quorum nomina sunt hec: Malthus, Maximianus, Dionisius, Johannes, Constantinus, Seraphion, Martinianus, et per nomen Dei quod est benedictum in secula + a + g + l + a + ut non noceatis neque aliquid mali faciatis vel inferatis huic famulo Dei .N. neque dormiendo neque vigilando + Christus vi[n]cit + Christus regnat + Christus imperat + Christus nos benedicat et ab omni malo deffendat + amen.'

In nomine Patris et Filii et Spiritus Sancti, amen. In nomine meo demonia eicient, linguis loquentes novis serpentes tollent, et si mortiferum quid biberint non eis nocebit, super egros manus inponent et bene habebunt + crux admirabilis, evacuatio doloris, restitutio sanitatis + ecce crucem domine, fugite, partes adverse + vicit leo de tribu Juda, radix David, allelulia + Christus vincit + Christus regnat + Christus imperat + Christus hunc famulum Dei .N. ab omni fantasia et ab omni vexatione diaboli + ab omni malo omni hora + ubique per virtutem sancte crucis deffendat + amen + agios + hyskyros + athanatos + eleyson + [cf. MS Sloane 3160 f.168v]

[f.10r] Contra malignos spiritos: Audi, maledicte Sathana. Adiuro te per nomen eterni Dei et salvatoris nostri, filii eius, Jesu Christi, cum tua victus invidia tremens gemensque, discede. Nichil tibi neque angelis tuis sit comune cum famulo Dei .N. Neque noceas ei neque appareas coram illo visibiliter sompniendo neque vigilando. Et iterum conjuro vos, demones sive spiritos malignos, quicumque sitis, per aspercionem sanguinis Jesu Christi in cruce et eius vulnera cruentata. Et iterum conjuro vos per mortem Jesu Christi in cruce et spiritus emissionem qui ad infernum descendit et illum spoliavit, ut nunc et a modo semper fugiatis ab hoc famulo Dei .N. et nunquam in eum introeatis sed exeatis et recedatis ab eo. Et iterum conjuro vos per virtutem verborum istorum infrascriptorum hoc: si infra eum sis vel sitis, ut exeas vel exeatis, si plures sitis, ab illo ut ullum a modo habeat terrorem neque vexationem. Hoc vos cogat verbum caro factum + crux Christi, lancea, clavi, corona spinea in sanguine agni Dei in cruce perfusa. Salvent et deffendant hic et ubique ferentem ista ab omni adversitate diabolica et perversa. In Nomine Patris et Filii et Spiritus Sancti.

The commonest type of charm is the narrative charm, usually wholly Christian, with a clear bipartite structure, namely the 'epic precedent' or anecdote concerning the sickness or suffering of Christ or one of the saints, followed by a comparison and prayer according to the formula 'Just as ... in the past, so now may ... in the present'.[79] Bonser comments 'It was thought that the telling of what had once happened in the case of gods might induce the same event to happen again for the benefit of mankind. The supernatural occurrence was thus intended to form a precedent. Later still stories dealing with the feats of Teutonic deities gave place to New Testament incidents (especially those relating to Christ) or narratives (either true or invented for the occasion) concerning apostles and saints'.[80] One of the most frequently encountered examples of this kind of Christian charm is that commonly used against worms which invokes the experience of Job and is a so-called diminishing charm in that it involves the ritual counting down from 9 to 0 (and occasionally augmenting again).[81] The narrative charm is also very often used for the staunching of blood. One version describes how the sword of Longinus pierced Christ's side[82] and dwells on one or more of the following details: blood and water flowed from the wound;[83] the wound did not bleed or fester;[84] Longinus wiped his eyes with Christ's blood and clearly perceived the true nature of Christ.[85] The charm was often employed in the case of injuries caused by iron or steel. Another narrative charm used for staunching blood tells of how the Jordan stood still at Christ's baptism.[86] In the Middle English versions there is frequently a play on the word *stande*. The charm was extended to extinguishing fires, stopping hostile pursuers etc. Another frequently encountered narrative charm is for toothache. In one version St Peter is sitting on a rock / at the gates of Galilee holding his hand to his jaw.[87] Christ enquires why he looks so miserable and Peter explains that his teeth hurt. Christ drives out the pain with a conjuration.[88] Another saint commonly invoked in charms against toothache is St Apollonia whose teeth were knocked out by her persecutors before she suffered martyrdom.[89] Other saints who regularly appear in charms are St Lawrence (against burns), St Blasius (against sore throat or toothache)[90] and St Veronica (for staunching blood).[91] In charms designed to promote sleep or to drive away fever there is often an allusion to the legend of the Seven Sleepers of Ephesus.[92] In charms for childbirth there is usually a sequence of figures drawn from the New Testament and beginning 'Anna peperit Mariam . . .'.[93] For the healing of wounds there is an anecdote concerning the meeting of *tres boni fratres* with Christ.[94] In a class of its own there is the celebrated letter from Christ, sometimes attributed to St Eustace or envisaged as being given to St Susanna or St William.[95]

Payne's fifth category of charms, dealing with material magic i.e. objects held to possess magical powers is naturally scarcely represented in the period of Christianized charms, healing powers being more frequently associated with Christian rituals like the Mass.[96] The role of candles is perhaps the closest Christianized equivalent to the magic object.[97] Payne's sixth category, transferential charms, is illustrated below by charms for fevers.[98]

Miscellaneous charms which have received some study are charms for thieves[99] and the celebrated 'Sator arepo tenet opera rotas', which is a palindrome, forms a magic square, and which can be arranged in the form of a cross, and which has also been interpreted in terms of anagram and acrostich.[100]

MS London, B. L. Sloane 475 is made up of two parts, the second of which (ff.125–231) dates from the end of the eleventh century.[101] The first part (ff.1–124) is written in a minuscule of the first quarter of the twelfth century. It consists of a medical compendium of various texts, divided into five books, but which is unfortunately acephalous owing to the loss of folios at the beginning of the MS. It is likely that the MS was written in England.[102] The fifth book of the compendium (ff.85v–124v) consists of receipts and charms. Among the latter are found two vernacular items, as follows:[103]

1. [rubric] Ad superos carmen
   In nomine Patris et Filii et Spiritus Sancti pone pollicem super ossa et dic: 'Si cist souros ci est venuz par dialbe [sic] inchantesun, tollet l'en Deus par sa magne resurectium; si veirement cum Deus fut nez et el presepie fut mis et retrovez si veirement seit cis cavals de cest souros livrez e(n) icez verues'. Pater Noster (f.109r/v).

2. [rubric] Ad claudum equum
   Pissun par mar nodat, la destre ale s'esloisat, esloisat, et resoldat. Si facét li pez de cest caval de cuius colore sit. Dic Pater Noster (f.109v)

Also from the twelfth century is the earliest Anglo-Norman example I have found of the diminishing charm concerning Job and his worms. It is found on the last folio (f.40v) of MS London, B. L. Sloane 84, which was left blank after four lines of the ps.-Hippocratic *De dieta*.[104] The rest of the page has been filled by a large, angular twelfth-century hand which has noted several charms. The vernacular entry is the first:

3. Carmen contra guttam: In nomine Patris et Filii et Spiritus Sancti. Jop vers
hout. Quanz en hout? .IX. en hout, de .IX. .VIII., de .VIII. .VIIe. [sic], de .VII.
.VI., de .VI. .V., de .V. .IIII., de .IIII. .III., de .II[I]. .II., de .II. .I., de .I. nul. Si
verreiment cum Deus uuarit seint Job, si uuarisse il icest hume vel ista mulier de
cest enfermeté u de fes[tre] hu de gute. In nomine Patris et Filii. Christus natus,
Christus passus, et Christus resurectus a mortuis. Ego sum Alfa et Omega, primus et novissimus, initium et fin[is] mundi et consumacio seculi et vita et pax +
In nomine Patris et Filii et Spiritus Sancti.

This charm is frequently found amongst prescribed treatments for the farcy in
horses,[105] as, for example, in MS Sloane 962 (s.xv) f.133v:

4. A charme for þo farciouns: In nomine Patris et Filii et Spiritus Sancti, amen. In
þo honour of oure lord Jesu Criste and of oure ladi seynt Mari and of sen Jop
and for sent Jopes fadur soule and moder soule and all his auncetures soules, sey
.iii. Pater Noster and .iii. Ave. 'Seynt Jop had .ix. wormes, had .viii. worm, had
.vii. worm, had .vi. wormes, had .v. w., had .iiii. w., had .iii. w., had .ii. w., had
.i. worme þat had no heved'. Sey þis aboute þo hors and he chal be hole be þo
grace of God.

A French version, also for the farcy, is given in MS Digby 86 (see below), but the
same MS contains another French version for the treatment of *goute festre*. In MS
Exeter Cathedral 3519 (s.xv) f.124r the charm has been entirely Christianised as a
simple prayer:

5. Charme de seint Job pur lez vermez ou [e]lez sount; 'Com a Dieu ployt par la vol-
unté de Dieu et par la grace de Dieu et par la creaunce de luy, si en garist et auxi
garisez tu de tez mayus et de tez dolours, de ceo en avant ja mal te ne facent'. In
nomine Patris et Filii et Spiritus Sancti trois foitz soit dit ove .iii. Pater Noster
et .iii. Ave Maria et .iii. Credo.

A small collection of charms is found in MS Oxford, Bodleian Library, Digby 86
(s.xiii²)[106] following the expanded text of the so-called 'Lettre d'Hippocrate' on
ff.8v–21r. The vernacular charms are found scattered among various Latin charms
and remedies which follow an 'Oratio ad Dominum' (f.27v) and an 'Oratio ad
sanctam Mariam' (f.28r). Many of the Latin receipts have Anglo-Norman rubrics.
The collection ends (f.34r) with a set of Latin remedies or, more precisely, experiments or *secreta*: *Ut apareat aliquibus quod flumen sit in domibus; Si vis eligere meliorem
porcellum; Ad muscas necandas; Si vis facere aliqua mortua cantare; Si vis haboundare
apibus*. The vernacular charms are as follows:

6. [f.28r] *Pur saunc estauncher*: Pur saunc estauncher dites cest oreisun: 'Nostre
Seignur fu pris / e en la croyz fu mis, / Longis i vint a lui / e de la launce li feri; /
Saunc e ewe en issi tret, / ses oilz leve e cler veit. Pur la vertu ki Deus i fist, conjur les veines e le saunc ki ne seine plus avaunt, Deu veray Pere'. Pater Noster
.iii. fez le dirrez.

7. *Pur farcin*: Pur farcin dites ceste charme: Seint Job verms out. Quanz out? Noef
out, de noef a uit, de uit a set, de set a sis, de sis a cink, de cink a quatre, de

quatre a treis, de treis a deus, de deus a un, de un a nul. Jesu Crist, si veraiement cum tu garises seint Job de vermine, si veraiment guaris feraunt de farcin e dites trai feze Pater Noster, si guarrad.

8. *Pur enpledement:* Si un houme seit apleidé en la court le rey ou en autre liu de mes ou de tere ou de chatel e il eit bon dreit en sun defens, si die checun jour de l'an par bone devoscioun la plus procheine saume devaunt 'Dixit Dominus' qui est en le sauter .iii. feze e si sera vengé de sun aversere dedenz le an coment ki ceo seit.[107] Si comence la saume issi : 'Deus laudem meam ne tacueris quia os pecatoris et os dolosi super me apertum est'.[108] En meimes la manere si un houme apleide un autre en la court le rey ou en autre luy de mes ou de tere [f.28v] ou de chatel e il eit bon dreit en sun apel, si die meimes cele saume par bone devoscioun checun jour de l'an .iii. feze, si avera la meitrie de sun averseire dedens l'an coment ki ceo seyt.

9. *Pur fevres charme:* Pur fefres querez ou seit herbive e quanz vous l'averez trové, pernez des herbives .xii. od toutes les foilles e od toutes la [sic] racines, si les manjez .xii. jours e nul jour fors une. Le premer jour pernez une erbive, si la mangez, si endiez .xii. Pater Nosters en le noun del Pere e del Fiz e del Seint Esperit. Le secund jour manjue un autre herbive e die .xi. Pater Nostres en la manere cum au premer jour. Le terz jour manjue le terz erbive e die .x. Pater Nostres en meimes la manere cum au premer jour. Le quart jour manjue le quart erbive e die .ix. Pater Nostres en la manere avaunt dite e issi de jour en jour desques les herbives seient touz mangez e veie qui ne manjue nul jour fors une herbive. E amenuse les Pater Nostres a la manere avaunt dite e si face de jour en jour desques les herbives seient touz mangez.

10. *Autre,* pur fevres bone charme: Pernez la main destre al malade e fetes une croiz de vostre pouz dextre en cele main e dites 'In nomine Patris + et Filii + et Spiritus sannti, amen'. Pur treis feze le seynez de memes le pouz e a checune feze dites '+ Cristus vincit + Cristus rengnad + Cristus imperad +' e pus escrivez od enke le premer jour en cele main au malade '+ on Pater + on Filius + on Spiritus Sanntus'. E le secund jour fetes cum au premer e escrivez '+ on ovis + on aries + on angnus'. E le terz jour fetes cum au premer e si escrivez '+ on leo + on vitu[lu]s + on vermis'. E si estaunchera l'accés par la grace Deu e a checune manere de fevre est bone charme e esprove. Mes ne charmez de ceste nuli si ne vous prie par charité.

11. *Autre,* pur fevres: In nomine Patris + et Filii + et Spiritus Sanctus + amen. Ante portam Galilee jacebat Petrus febri[ci]tans . . .[109]

12. [f.29r] . . . *Autre:* Icest bref est bon a guarir les gent ki ount les fevres e comence issi: '+ Cristus + arex + yre + artifex + ranx + yriorum +'. Ici comence un autre bref qui bon est a fevres e a ces qui sunt travaillez de nuit. [f.29v] 'In monte Elion in civitate Effesiorum dormierunt .vii. dormientes + Maltus + Martinianus + Dionisius + Johannes + Maximianus + Serafion + Constantinus + Et sicut Dominus requievit super illos, sic requiescat super hunc famulum tuum .N.' Pus die .iii. Pater Noster el noun del Pere e del Fiz e del Seint Esperit.

13. *Pur houme ki avera wen:* In nomine Patris et Filii et Spiritus Sannti, amen.

Celui ki avera wen sur lui si le deit seigner de sun pucer e issi dire en l'ano-
raunz de Jesu Crist, ki char e saunc prist en la seinte virgine, e de seint Lo. E
deit comencer en creisaunt e veer k'il eit .ix. nuz devaunt le descours e nent
plus e .ix. nuz en le decurs aneire aprés e nent plus. E die 'seint Lo wens hot' e
issi dire desque a .ix. e pus dire Pater Noster. E quant la Pater Nostre seit dite,
si recomencez In nomine Patris et F[ilii] et S[piritus] S[ancti], amen. E pus dire
'seint Lo wens out' e issi tot a reburs desque a un. E pus Pater Noster e aprés la
Pater Nostre terce feiz. In nomine Patris et F[ilii] et S[piritus] S[ancti], amen. E
pus comencera 'seint Lo wens out. Quant en out? Un en hout', e issi desque a
.ix. e pus Pater Noster. E taunt dire chescun jour e nent plus . . . .

14. **[f.30r]** . . . **[f.30v]** . . .[110] *Pur rauncle*: In nomine Patris et F[ilii] et S[piritus]
S[ancti], amen, Pater Noster treis feiz, seint Cosme e seint **[f.31r]** Damien[111]
en veie alerent [e] Nostre Dame seinte Marie encountrerent. Dist la dame
'Chosme e Damien, ou en alez?' 'Dame, en ost alum, plaies i ferum. Dites dunc
coment nous les sanerum'. 'De vostre main destre les seignez, del quart dey les
tochez si que goute ne rauncle n'i acoille ne Nostre Sire Jesu Crist del cel nel
voille'.

15. *Pur pors medicine*: Jutus e Arnes enchausceent. Munt pluruent, se depleinount
pur lur pors ke moreynt. Seint Owrs i survint, si lur dist 'Beuz enfaunz, pur quei
plurez, pur quei vous despleit?' 'Sire, ci seum e plurum pur nos pors qui merent
de arch e de arech e de tuz mauz dount pors merent'. Seint Owrs lur dist 'De
par Deu, pernez ael e orge e triblez ensemble en un auge, si lur donez a manger.
Par la force de Deu gari seint vos pors de arch e de arech e de touz maus dunt
pors merent, amen'. E dites .iii. Pater Nostres e .iii. Ave Maries en l'onou-
raunce del Seint Esperit . . . .

16. **[f.31v]** . . . *Pur goutefestre*, pur gutefestre: Pernez un herbe c'um apele *revenes-*
fot e pernez la racine de cel erbe, si metez a checun pertus ke court une racine
ou deus, si ki le pertus seit covert de la racine e fetes le lier ferm al mal, ke la
racine ne se remue mie deques l'endemain a cel oure cum vous l'averez mis. E
a cel oure l'osterez, si n'i mettrez ren a la plaie for une foille de rounse. E dirrez
ceste charme: 'Deu fist Jop, Jop verms out. Quanz out? Noes i out, de noef out
uit, de uit out set, de set out sis, de sis out cink, de cink out quatre, de quatre
out treis, de treis out deus, de deus out un, de un out nul. Ausi vereiment cum
Deu garist Jop des verms, si garise .N. ke ci est des verms', Pater Noster. E dirrez ceste charme neof fez e neof Pater Nostres e dirrez al malade k'il eit bone
creaunce en Deu e ki il die sa Pater Nostre e k'il desporte aprés ceo k'il seit
charmé neof jours checune manere de [vin] blaunc e pain de segle e gutuse
viaundes, si la k'il seit gari e femme, s'il eit, ki il la desporte ou, si ceo seit
femme, desporte sun seignur si la ki ele seit garie. Kaunt vous averez ben lié les
racines as plaies e seingné(re) lé de vostre main . . . .

17. **[f.32r]** . . . *Charme pur soriz*, charme pur soriz:[112] Pernez autretauntes peres de
creye cum il i ad us en vostre graunge e corneres e fetes checune pere creuse e
mettez en creus seyl, sein e savun ouelement batu ensemble. E pus pernez de la
premere charettee ki vendra a l'us de la graunge (e) tauntes garbes cum vous
avez peres e alez par dehors le us e metez en checune garbe une des peres, si ke
vous ne espaundez ceo ke il i ad **[f.32v]** einz. E quant vous pernez la premere

garbe dites In nomine P[atris] et F[ilii] et S[piritus] S[ancti], amen. E si le em-
portez enmi la graunge e dites une Pater Noster, si le fetes tenir .i. let saunz parler e issi le fetes de tutes les autres garbes e donez pus celes garbes pur l'amour
Deu. Si fetes mestre desus le us de la graunge ou le blé entera une pere ou li eyt
escrit einz 'Jesu', sus les quatre corners les quatre peres ou en checune pere eyt
escrit un des nouns des quatre ewangelistes e fetes jettre ewe beneite par la
meisun. E pus alez a l'us ou le blé entera e dites a vostre cumpainun ki dedens
serra 'Jeo vous co[n]jur en noun del Pere e del Fiz e del Seint Esperit ki me diez
de quey viverunt les raz e les sorices ouan en ceste graunge'. E il respoundera
'Jeo vous di par le Pere e le Fiz e le Seint Esperit ki ne viverount for del seyl e
de creye e syu e savun'. E ceo dites treis feiz e treis fez dites vostre Pater Noster. E pus seit le blé mis eins e dient In nomine Patris et F[ilii] et S[piritus]
S[ancti], amen. Mes plus ne meins ne seit dit.[113]

The compendium of medical receipts assembled by John of Greenborough (see
above pp.33ff.) also contains a number of charms in the vernacular with an admixture of Latin. The first is *Contra dolorem dentium* and is an abbreviated version of a
frequently attested charm, followed in turn by the celebrated narrative charm about
Peter sitting on the rock and being cured by Christ of toothache:

18. Item aliud carmen dicat paciens: Ego .N. dolens peto pro amore Dei medicamen. Auxi vereiment comme Dieu suffrit peyne en le seint croice pur pechours rechater de mort en vie, auxi vereiment garrez cest cristien de dolours
de dentz si Dieus le plest (f.143va).[114]

Equally well known are the charms for staunching blood:

19. Ad sanguinem restringendum: . . . Estanchés sanc, estanchez en le honour de
Pier et de Fiz et de Seint Espirit et de la seynt crois. Auxi vereiment comme
Nostre Seignur Jhesu Crist suffrist mort en la crois le bon venderdy pur nous et
pur touz pechours, et auxi vereiment comme il releva le tiers jour de mort a
vie, et auxi vereiment comme Longius persa le quere et le coste Nostre Seignur Jhesu Crist et prist sanc de soun precious quere et coste, en la honorance
et en la vertue de cel precious sanc, estaunchés, sanc, estanchez. Amen.
(f.156ra)

20. Aliud carmen: Primo inquire nomen hominis et dic quinquies Pater Noster et
Ave et tunc dic: 'For þe woundes þat God sofrid on þe crois for to by us out of
al þe world, stanch, blod; in the worship of five blodi teres þat Our Lady lete
for Cristes love, stanch, blod; als wis as Longius went to his hert with his
spere, as wis as he died for mannes sake and nouth for his owne, stanch, blod;
for þe blode þat Crist bled on þe crois in þe worship of þat blode, stanch,
blode'. Et tunc dicat quinquies Pater et Ave Maria. (f.156ra)

Less common is the charm against fevers:

21. Carmen contra febres: . . . 'Lady seint Marie, I prey þe in þe worship of þe
seven cosses þat þou cussid þi son on þe rode, so save þis man of þis evel þe
which men clepe þe fevre, be it hot oþer cold, and þat in tokenyng of his hele

þis 3erd of hasil mote joyne togidre'. Et dic .vii. Pater et Ave in honore osculorum et crucis et fac celebrare unam missam de Sancto Spiritu et quando virga se conju[n]xerit, tolle unam partem illius conjunctionis ad quantitatem pollicis et pone in potu tuo per novem dies cum biberis et sanaberis. Ista virga erit ubi tantum[?] unius anni crescens (f.156va)[115]

The next vernacular charm is for toothache:

22. Contra dolorem dentium: . . . 'Sire Jhesu Crist par vostre vertue et par vostre pussancz diliverez cest cristiene de le dolour de son denz et de tutz altrez grevances, amen, pur seinte charité'. Et pete ubi dentes dolent et scribe istas litteras ubi volueris, *ililili*, et iterum pete et scribe et dic carmen bis, ter vel quater si necessitas fuerit, vel pluries (f.157va/b)

In what seems to be the second part of the compendium[116] there are a further three charms:

23. *Ad restringendum sanguinem:* 'Godde als witturly als þou wast in Bedleem born and houen in flum Jordan and made þe salt watur for to stond, stawnch þe blode of þis man or woman'. Et dic Pater Noster ter (f.162vb)[117]

24. *Item ad virgam jungendam:* Dic 'auxi vereiment come le prestre feit Dieu entre soun maynes, et auxi vereiment comme le moundi Die fuist de virgine nee et baisa sa tresdouce mere, Roy, vous conjure, virgine verge de coudre qe vous enbesét ensemble et eustés cest mal febre par charité de cest homme o(d) de cest femme. In nomine Patris etc.' Alpha + Omega + via + veritas + virtus + spes est remedium. Et celebrentur tres misse, una de trinitate, secunda de cruce, tercia de annunciatione (f.162vb)[118]

25. Ad sanguinem restringendum: Dic ista verba: 'God þat was boren in Bedlem and follet in flem Jordan, he steined þe flod, he steine þis blod .N.' Et dic quinquies Pater Noster et Ave (f.179vb)[119]

In the same MS a new set of receipts begins (f.188vb) 'Hic incipit practica Edwardi universitatis Oxonie qui fuit optimus in illis partibus cirurgicus' and occupies ff.188vb–199vb (as far as f.194v all the receipts are in English). It contains the following vernacular charm:

26. Item conjuratio pro sanguine: In nomine Patris etc. 'Oure lord was borne in Bethleem + he was howen in Jerusalem + he was bapteste in flum Jordane + whan he was bapteste þerynne + þe flode hit stod + so stynte þe blode + thorowe þe vertue of hem and of þe fyve woundes þat he suffred + on þe verray cros + and þerto I worchip þe fyve woundes with fyve Pater Noster þat he hele þis wounde and stynte þe blode and our lady whit .v. Ave in þe worchip of þe fyve blody terus þat scho weppud whan scho sye hym on þe verray cros' (f.197rb)[120]

Yet another collection of receipts is found on ff.201ra–202vb and includes a Latin charm for toothache which invokes the well known story of St Appolonia:

27. Contra dolorem dentium: Sancta Appolonia virgo fuit de cuius ore pro Christi amore dentes fuerunt extracti. Et deprecata fuit Christum dominum nostrum quod quicumque nomen suum super se portaverit, dolorem in dentibus non haberet + Alpha + Omega + primus + et novissimus + principium et finis me defendat a dolore dentium qui est sine principio et omnia creans ex nichilo. In nomine Patris et Filii et Spiritus Sancti, amen. (f.201va/b)

MS London, B. L. Harley 273 is an interesting fourteenth-century MS replete with Old French texts including the *Manuel des pechés* (ff.113r–190v), Richard de Fournival's *Bestiaire d'amour* (ff. 70ra–81ra) with moderately skilful line drawings, a French psalter (ff.8ra–59rb) and the Pseudo-Turpin Chronicle (ff.86ra–102vb).[121] The calendar on ff.1r–6v contains the entry (f.1v) 'Dedicacion de la eglise seint Laurence de Lodelawe' i.e. the parish church of St Lawrence, Ludlow. A fifteenth-century inscription on the flyleaf (f.1*r) reads 'Iste liber constat Johanni Clerk grocero ac ap[othe]cario regis Edwardi quarti post conquestum'. On f.85va/b, following a set of rules assuring love and friendship (inc. *Ky veut verrei amur aver il deit quatre choses regarder . . .*),[122] is inserted a charm in a contemporary (s.xiv[1]) hand:

28. Charme pur feistre, felun et playe: Pernez une piece de plum et la fetes batre, que eole [sic] seit si tenve cum ceo fust fueille, que vus la poez plyeer sa et la. Puis fetes desus le plum ov un cotel cinc croyz solum ceste furme:[123]

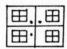

E tant cume vus fetes les cinc croiz dites cinc foyze Pater Noster en le honorance des cinc plaies Nostre Seignur Jhesu Crist. E quant vus fetes les treiz pertuz, deus a deistre et un a senestre, dites tres foize Pater Noster en le honorance de la seinte trinitee et des treis cloues dunt Nostre Seignur Jhesu Crist fust cloufichié. Et puis dites une foyze Pater Noster en le honorance de la passiun. Et puis dites ceste charme: 'Jeo vus cunjur .N. que vus garissez de feistre ou de feolun ou de playe en le nun des cinc playes que Nostre Seignur Jhesu Crist suffri, en le nun de la seinte trinitee et des treis cloues dunt Nostre Seignur Jhesu Crist fut clouefichié, en le nun de la seinte passioun sanz maheyn et sanz peril de maheyn'. Puis metez le plum au mal et turnez les croyz vers le mal et veiez que le plum seit chescun jur lavee et remis al mal. E puis que le plum seit charmee que il ne touche al tere et tant cum vus dirrez la charme tuz jurs le benesquiez. (f.85va/b)[124]

Following a passage in Anglo-Norman on the Seven Gifts of the Holy Spirit a later fourteenth-century hand has inserted three vernacular charms on f.112va/b:

29. Pur sang estauncher: In nomine Patris etc. Longes þe knyht him understod, to Cristes syde his spere he sette, þer com out water an blod. In þe nome of þe Vader astond, blod, in þe nome of þe Holy Gost asta, blod, at Cristes wille ne drople þe namore. Beau Sire Dieu, Jhesu Crist, auxi veroiement come Longes le chevaler vus fery de une launce a le coste destre, tannqe al cuer de quei il ne saneit dont il issist sang e eawe de quei sil recoverist la vewe, vus pri auxi ve-

roiement qe cest sang estanchez e vus comaund en soun seint noun, vus, sang, qe vus estannchez. Pater Noster etc. Ave etc. (f.112va/b)

30. Charme pur dolour de playe: 'Nostre Seigneur fust naufree e enoynt e lavee, oynt e puroynt, de une launce fust poynt. Longes la launce ly mist desqe al cuer. Dieux, auxi verroiement come myracle enfeites, e ce est veyr, garissez ceste playe qe ele ne oylle ne ne doyle ne ne rancle ne ne coille ne ne peille nient plus qe cele ne fist'. In nomine Patris etc. Si[n]t medicina tui pia crux et vulnera Christi. Sint medicina tui vulnera quinque Dei.¹²⁵ Pater et Ave etc. (f.112vb)

31. Charme pur fievre: In nomine Patris etc. 'Bieau Sire Dieu, Rey Omnipotent, pleyn de misericorde, je vus pri et requer qe vus garissez .N. le jour nomee de ces mals. Auxi veroyement come vus estes veroy Dieus e veroy reys plein de misericorde en le honorance de vostre seyntime noun e en le honoraunce de ma chere dame seinte Marie, vostre gloriouse mere, e en le honurance de trestous vos volers, amen'. Pater, Ave etc. (f.112vb)

Now, following Latin receipts on colouring (ff.209r–212v),¹²⁶ there is a set of charms, written like the receipts in a quite different fourteenth-century hand from those occurring before f.204, and mixing Latin and French. The vernacular charms are as follows:

32. Charme pur festre e pur cancre e pur gute: Dunc deprimes die la [sic] malade a celui ki deit garir .iii. Pater Noster en leu onnur de la trinité, e pus oie celui ki deit charmer preveement issi ke la [sic] malade ne oit pas cest oresun: 'Beau Sire Deu, ausi verement cum vus deliverastes seint Susanne hors de la prisun e de la claundre u ele fu enz, ausi verement deliverez cest malade .N. de festre e de gute e de cancre e de tuz mals'. E li malade face chaunter une messe de Seint Espirit, e une autre de Nostre Dame, e la terce pur les almes tuz cristiens e le malade veit ki il seit ben cunfés e ferme creaunce e verai charité etc. (f.213r)¹²⁷

33. Pur tuz felunz tuer: In nomine Patris et Filii, Spiritus Sancti, amen. 'Jo vus cunjur, mau felun, par Deu omnipotent de cel e de tere e del solail e de la lune e de tutes creatures e de cent abbés e de cent eveskes conreez ben cum de messe chaunter e de la nut de nowel e de la payle dunt Deu fu (fu) volupé, si tu eis, ne demorrez, si tu n'eis, n'entreez e al nun del Pere e del Fiz e del Seint Espirit vus cunjur ki t'en auges'. Ceo diés treis fiz ultre le mal là ke i(l) seit. E si est bone pur la farcine. (f.213r)¹²⁸

34. *Pur sanc etauncher*: Charme pur estancher saunc: 'La verei dame seit en sun baunc, sun verrei enfaunt seit en sun devaunt, verrei est la dame, verrei est l'enfaunt, verrei veine estaunche vostre saunc'. Dies ceo treis feis e treis feis Pater Noster (f.213r)¹²⁹

35. Ki ne pot dormir porte(s) ces nuns sor li: + Eugenius + Stephanus + Prochasius + Caudiscius + Dionisius + Chericius + et Quiracius + Malcus + Maximianus + Martinus + Dionisius + Constantinus + Johannes + Seraphion (f.213r)¹³⁰

36. Pur la mere maris: 'Jo te cunjur, mere mariz, de cent cinquant noratriz, de seinte Marie genitriz, ke al ventre ceste .N. mal ne feiz ne a sun quer ne a ses

veines ne a nul de ces membres, va en tu[n] liwe, si te lie bien en le nun del
Pere e del Fiz e del Seint Espirit'. Entre sun penil e sun umblil dites treis feiz e
treis feiz Pater Noster. (f.213r)[131]

37. [S]i acune femme travaille de enfaunter, acun prestre u acun clerc ki hordiné
seyt lise treis feiz set breve sur sa teste e le mette en sun seyn, e desur sun
umbre la tenge encuntre sun ventre, tout enfauntera e sun enfaunt ne perira
ne ele ne murra, amen: 'In nomine Patris et Filii et Spiritus Sancti, amen.
Anna peperit Mariam, Elizabet Johannem Baptistam, Sancta Maria dominum
nostrum Jhesum Cristum sine corde et absque dolore. In nomine illius meritis
et precibus sancte Marie virginis et sancti Johannis Baptiste exy, infans, sive
sis masculus sive femina, de utero matris tue absque dolore et absque morte tui
et absque illius. Pater Noster'. Et debes dicere has literas tribus vicibus super
capud eius: Pur dre chenge ... (f.213v)

This may be compared with the Latin version found in the *Breviarium Bartholomei*
[*De difficultate partus*, pars 6, dist. 3, c.xi] in MS Harley 3 f.128ra:

38. Quod si ista non sufficiant, tunc si sacerdos vel clericus presens sit, legat cedulam istam subscriptam ter ultra mulierem in partu laborantem. Deinde mulier
cedulam illam ponat super umbilicum suum et ibi ligetur suaviter. Et statim, si
Deus voluerit, pariet sine periculo sui aut infantis si cum bona fide aut devotione hec fiant + 'In nomine Patris + et Filii + et Spiritus Sancti, amen. Maria
peperit Christum, Anna peperit Mariam, Elizabeth peperit Johannem Baptistam, Maria peperit dominum nostrum Jhesum Christum sine inmundicia et
absque dolore. In nomine illius precipimus et meritis sancte Marie matris eius
et virginis et sancti Johannis Baptiste ut exeas, infans, sive masculus sis sive
femina, de utero matris tue absque morte tui vel illius + In nomine Patris +
Filii + Spiritus Sancti, amen'.

A number of well known charms are contained in the medical compendium formed
by MS Exeter Cathedral 3519 (s.xv):

39. Carmen: 'Longys ferist Nostre Seignur de la seynte lance e fist une seint playe.
Il y curust sanc e ewe. En cele plaie n'avint rancle ne dolur, ne en vostre ne
face .N.' Pater Noster. Ter dicatur carmen cum Pater Noster. (f.159v)

40 Cest charme qe seint Gabriel porta par Nostre Seignur pur charmer cristiens de
verme, de festre, de goute. Fetes premerement chaunter une messe de Seint Espirit e fetes le malade oyr la messe e dites cest charme: '+ In nomine Patris et
Filii et Spiritus Sancti, amen. Aucy verroyment cum Deus fust et est, aucy verroyment cum ceo ke il dist veir dyst, aucy verroyment cum ceo ke il fist bien
fist, aucy verroyment cum il de la virgine char prist, aucy verroyment cum en
sun corps synk playes suffrist pur tuz pecchours, auxi verroyment cum soun
seint corps en la croys estendist, auxi verroyment cum en ambez pars de ly furent deus larons penduz, auxi verroyment com en son destre coste fust la lance
ferue, auxi verr cum chyef fust des espines coronee, auxi verr cum soun seint
corps en sepulture reposa, auxi verr cum le tierce jour releva, auxi verroyment
cum les portes de enfern debresa, auxi verr cum les seins sus mena, auxi verr
cum a ciel munta, auxi verr com a destre soun pere se reposa, auxi verr coma a

jour de juge vendra e checun corage de trent anz matra, auxi verr cum nostre
[. . .] a soun plesir overa, auxi verr cum ceo est verys e jeo le crey, veyrs est e
veris serra, auxi verrment garri seit ceste .N. de goute, de rancle, de verm.
Mort est la goute, mort est la rancle, mort est la verm, mort est, mort seyt de
.N. si Deu plest'. Pater Noster dicatur. In nomine Patris et Filii et Spiritus
Sancti, amen. Dicatur ista conjuratio ter quolibet die ultra infirmum et sic dicatur quod nullam aliam faciat medicinam et comedat quicquid sibi placuerit
et ante novum diem per graciam Dei habebit sanitatem. (f.161r/v)

41. Nostre Seignor fust naffré e enoynt, de une launce fust poynt. Longeus sa
launce myst jesqes a poigne, le sanc se venist dens. Auxi verrement com ceo
est veirs jeo le crey garys. Ore cest playe, q'ele n'eit dolour ne poür ne puture
ne (ne) rancle ne cancre facet ne verm vent plus qe sole [sic] playe ne fist qe
vous mesmes soffratus. Pater Noster'. Credo dit e facetz le malade dire 'Auxi,
Deus, auxi verreyment cum avetz mis vertue en parole, en pere e en herbe,
auxi verreyment donez saunté a .N. par soun noun baptizé'. Pater Noster,
Credo, Ave Maria cum versibus istis: 'Sunt medicina tui quem Jhesu Cristus
qui pro nobis passus es in cruce et per quinque vulnera tua nos peccatores sanguine tuo precioso a languoribus sanasti et sicut ego veraciter hoc credo, ita
sanitatem da hinc famulo tuo .N. qui vivis et regnas Deus omnia secula seculorum, amen'. (f.162v)

The celebrated charm brought by Gabriel to Susanna is repeated in MS London,
B. L. Sloane 3564 (s.xv) f.41r with the following rubric in red: *La charme que seint
Gabriel porta du ciel par Nostre Seignur Jesu Crist et baylla a seint Susanne pur charmer
lez cristiens de verm, de festre, de goute et de cancre, de goute errant, de goute tremble, pur
toute maner et de rancle*. In this text there is a preamble beginning 'Faites adeprimes
chaunter un messe del Seynt Esprite . . .' The charm ends 'Mort est la goute, mort
est la cauncre, mort est la rauncle, mort est le verm, et festre et felon, mort est et
mort serra et mort soit de cesti .N. ové la eyde de la Piere et del Fitz et del Seynt
Esprit, si Dieux plest qe de cest cristien icest charme en vers fist. Pater Noster, Ave
Maria'. The final rubric, which follows the French text, runs (ff.43v/44r) *Ditez cest
charme par .iii. jours outre li malade chescun jour .iii. foitz par .iii. hours du jour et pur
voirs tust en soient il mile pertus, dedeyns le .ix. jours garra.*[132] The following Anglo-
Norman charms are found in the collection of receipts in which English and French
are often mixed:[133]

42. *Charme pur lé feveris:* Pernez un poume et le trenchez en .iii. partyes, si escrivez
en la primer partye 'In principio erat verbum', en la seconde partye 'et verbum
erat apud Deum', en la tierce partye 'et Deus erat verbum'. Et lessez li malade
manger chescun jour un partie jun par .iii. jours. (f.54r)[134]

43. *Item autre:* Pernez un poume et escrivez leyns ces treys vers 'Increatus Pater, inmensus Pater, eternus Pater etc.' Et escrivez le noun del malade en my lieu la
poume et escrivez cest noun Jhesus desus, si luy donez a manger. (f.54r/v)

44. *Item autre:* Pernez .iii. oblez et en le primer festes un croys, si escrivés 'Pater est
Alpha et Omega'; en le seconde festes .ii. croitz et escrivez 'Filius est veritas';
en la tirce 'Spiritus Sanctus est remedium' et jettez desuz ewe beneyte et le
donez li malade a manger le primer jour ceo que fust primez escrist et issi les
autres par ordre. (f.54v)

45. *Item autre:* Li malade dira, ou acun autre pur luy si il ne sache memes dire, par
.ix. jours cest 'Quicumque vult', c'est a savoir le primer jour .ix. foiz, le .ii. jour
ui(n)t foiz, le tierce jour set foiz, et issci chescun jour jun et li malade garra
bien. (f.55r)

Si mulier laboret in partu . . .[135]

46. *Item aliud:* Escrivez in parchemyn 'Sancta Maria peperit et mater illa non doluit, Christum regem genuit qui nos sanguine suo redemit'. Ceste chose lyez entour le destre flank de la femme. Et de ceste mesmes escrivez en un foille 'Quia
puer cest vrs[?] "iam nova progenies celo dimittitur alto"[136] + Christus +
Maria + Johannes + Elizabet + Remigius + Celina, Lazare veni foras, adjuro te,
creatura Dei utrum sis puer an puella, in nomine Patris etc., exi de utero.
Christus te appellat qui te creavit et redemit et in seculum judicabit, amen'.
Ceste lyez entre le destre dedeyns et tantost istera l'enfant vif u mort. (ff.55v–
56v)

47. *Charme pur fevere froide et chaude:* Hom doit prendre qe l'em apele *crowfote*, un
herbe, et quant hom doit prendre cele herbe, hom doit genulier et doit hom
prendre un foile et mettre le en vostre mayn en vos deus medluen [sic] deis
sanz plumer le herbe, et dire 'In nomine Patris etc.' et dic .iii. Pater Noster et
.iii. Ave Maria en le noun del Pere et del Fitz et del Seynt Esprist. Et pus dire
un autre foitz 'In nomine Patris' et donk plumer le herbe sur la mayn et issi le
face de .iii. foillez l'un aprés l'autre et a chescun die .iii. Pater Noster et .iii.
Ave Maria et In nomine Patris etc. et a chescun herbe plumer par desouz la
mayn et quant vous avez fait ceste charme de l'herbe, donk demaundés le malade coment il y a noun et lequel luy gref plus, le froide ou le chaude, et si il
die le froide, si devez dire 'Beau Sir Deux, issi vereyment cum vous tremblastez
de freyd quant vous fustes mis en la seynte verey crois pur pour de mort et donastez vertu en parole, en pere et en herbe, garrissez .N. de fevere, s'il vous
plest'. Et si il dist qe le chaud li grief plus quel froyde, si dites 'Beaux Sir Dieux,
auxi vereyment cum vous suastes quant vous fustes mys en la seynt verey croys
pur pour de mort et donastez vertu en parole, en pere et en herbe, garrissez cest
.N. de sa fevere, s'il vous plest'. Et pus pernez le herbe et mettez sur le pouz destre de homme, a senestre de femme, et celi qe fest la charme deit estre jun, et
le malade auxi, et le feverous ne doit poynt manger de oefs tanque il soit garry.
(ff.56v–58r)

MS Oxford, Bodleian Library, Digby 69 is a somewhat disorganized compilation of
medical extracts (see below Ch.8) which includes three Anglo-Norman charms, as
follows:

48. *Carmen ad fistulam:* In nomine Patris [et Filii] et Spiritus Sancti, amen. 'Seint
Job vermis out. Quanz en out? Noef en out, de nove uit et issi arere. Si veraiement cum Dex gari seint Job des verms et des mals ke il out, issi verraiement
garisse il cest home ou femme .N. de ces verms et de ses mals ke il ad. Pater
Noster. Ço face Dex pur quant il volt que l'um la sue merci deprit. Et requerre
que pur tuz les feialz Deu et pur tutes almes defunz cumfessés Deu verrai merci
lur face et Deu por l'amur de seint Job garisse cest crestien .N. de ces verms et

de ses mals que il ad'. Pater Noster. Omnia hec predicta sunt specialiter de fistula. (f.210r)

49. *Carmen ad idem* [i.e. guttam azaram]: 'Seel sustereins fu enmi fu salvage, gute euere ci te vi'. Istud ter dicatur. (f.211r)

50. *Ad fluxum sanguinis:* 'Quant Deu nez fud, quant k'il dist veir dist, quant k'il fist bien fist. Issi veirement cum veirs fu que Deu fud nez (fud), e veirs dist quant k'il dist, e bien fist quant k'il fist, issi vereiement estanche il cest hom .N. de seigner'. Pater Noster. Hoc totum ter dicatur. (f.211v)

As so few medieval insular charms are in print it is perhaps worth recording those – in Latin, Middle English and Anglo-Norman – found in MS British Library Sloane 962, a fifteenth-century copy of various receipts and medical extracts of much earlier date:

51. *Item pur fevers un charme:* 'Archidecline syttes on hye and holdes a vergyne ʒerde of hesil in his hande and seys "also soth os þo prest makes Godes bodi in his handes and also soth os God blessed is moder Mari and also soth, I conjure þe, vergin ʒerde of hesil, þat þu close and be bote of þis evel fever to þis man .N." ' In nomine Patris et Filii et Spiritus Sancti, amen. (f.38r)[137]

52. *For to staunche blode:* Firste ye most wite þo mannes name or þo wommannes and þen go to chirche and sey þis charme and loke þat þu sei it for no beste bot for man or womman.
    Carmen: 'Whan Oure Lorde Jesu Criste was done on þo croys, þan com Longius thider and stong him wit þo spere in þo syde. Blode and watur com out at þo wound. He wyped his yne and saw anone thorow þo holi vertu þat God did þere. I conjure þe, blod, þat þu come not out of þo cristen man .N.' and sey his name. In nomine Patris et Filii et Spiritus Sancti, amen.
    To sey þis charme ne (?) þar þe never rekke where þo man or þo womman be bot þat þu knowe her name. (f.38v)[138]

53. *An oþer:* 'Criste was borne in Bedlem, baptized in þo flem Jordan. Also þo flem astode, also astond þi blode .N.' In nomine Patris et Filii et Spiritus Sancti. (f.38v)[139]

54. *An oþer:* 'Longius hebreus cum lancea percuscit latus domini, sanguis exivit et aqua et lanceam ad se retraxit. Tetragramaton + Messias + Emanuel + Sabaoth. Ita cesset sanguis exire ab isto christiano sicud istud verum est'. In nomine Patris et Filii et Spiritus Sancti, amen. (ff.38v–39r)

55. *An oþer to stanche blod* . . . Conjuratio pro sanguine restringendo: 'God, also wisly as þu was in Bedlem borne and hoven in flom Jordan and made þo salt watur in þo see to stande, so wisly stanche þo blode of (of) þis .N. Longius lancea latum domini perforavit et inde exivit sanguis et aqua, sanguis redemptionis et aqua baptismatis. In nomine Patris + stet in nomine Filii + resistet sanguis in nomine Spiritus Sancti + non excedet sanguis amplius ab hoc famulo Dei .N.' (f.39r)

56. *Oratio:* 'Deus, qui in cruce fuisti positus et ad cuius pedes stetit Longius qui cum lancea eum percussit, [in] continuo exivit sanguis et aqua. Ita, vere dulce

Jesu, ceda sanguinem istius .N. pro tua vera misericordia'. Et dicitur ter Pater Noster et ter Ave Maria. (f.39v)

57. *Ad extrahendum ferrum carmen:* 'Nichodemus extraxit clavos plagarum domini nostri Jesu Christi et sanguis et aqua exivit, itaque sicut ista verba sunt vera, ita exeat iste carellus sive lancea sive ferrum de carne vel ab osse istius christiani'. In nomine Patris + et Filii + et Spiritus Sancti + amen. Et dicitur ter et qualibet vice Pater Noster et Ave Maria. (f.45v)

58. *Contra latrones carmen:* 'In Bedlehem God was borne, bytwene to bestes to rest he was leyde. In þat stede was nethur thef nor man bot þo holi trinite. Þat ilk self God þat þer was borne deffende oure bodies and oure catel fro fire, fro theves and all oþer harmes and eveles, amen'. Sey þis thre tymes and .iii. Pater Noster and Ave Maria. (f.51r)

59. *Item contra latrones ne noceant dicitur sic:* 'Dominus illuminatio mea et salus mea quem timebo? Dominus protector vite mee a quo trepidabo?'[140] Gloria Patri sicut erat. Dismas et Gesmas medio[141] divina magestas. Jesus autem transiens per medium illorum ibat. 'Fiant immobiles quasi lapis, donec pertranseat populus tuus iste quem possidisti. Irruat super eos formido et pavor in magnitudine brachii tui'.[142] (f.51r)

60. *Item contra latrones et cetera:* [143]
Disparibus meritis pendent tria corpora ramis
Dismas et Gesmas medio[144] divina magestas
Summa petit Jesmas infelix infima Dismas
Hos versus dicas ne per furtum tua perdas
'Jesus autem transiens per medium illorum ibat, sic nos per medium inimicorum nostrorum pertransire permittas. "Irruat super eos formido et pavor in magnitudine brachii tui. Fiant immobiles quasi lapis donec pertranseat populus tuus domine (po.) [nec] pertranseat populus tuus iste quem possedisti" usquequo, domine, oblivisceris me in finem'. Et ter cum gloria Patri sicut erat. Oremus. *Oratio:* 'Deus qui voluisti pro redemptione mundi a Judeis reprobari, a Jude osculo tradi, vinculis alligari et agnus innocens ad victimam duci atque conspectibus Pilati afferri, a falsis quoque testibus accusari, flagellis et ohprobriis vexari et conspui, spinis coronari, colaphis cedi, in cruce levari atque inter latrones deputari, clavorum quoque aculeis perforari, lancea vulnerari, felle et aceto potari, per has sanctissimas penas tuas ab inferni penis et periculis me libera et custodi et illuc perduc me peccatorem quo produxisti tecum crucifixum latronem, qui cum Deo Patri et Spiritu Sancto vivat et regnat Deus per omnia secula seculorum, amen. Sion + Maron + Saphert +'. (f.51r–v)

61. *For to stanche blod a charme:* 'En Bedlehem en la cité un dygne enfaunt i uut nee. Verray enfaunt, verrey veyne, tiengne [MS trengne] toun sanc'. In nomine Patris et Filii et Spiritus Sancti, amen. Pater Noster trey foyth. (f.53v)

62. *Item:* 'Veyne, tiengne [MS trengne] toun sank en toy sicome Dieu faet la ley'. Pater Noster .iii. foyth. (f.53v)

63. *Item:* 'Douce Dame, seynt Marie, requerez vostre chier filtz q'il pur le honour de vous et de soun douce sank q'il espaunda [145] en la croys et pur icele sank

que vous en plorant espaundites, estanche(s) le sank de cest homme .N.' Ditez cest orisoun .iii. feith ové .iii. Pater Noster et sachés qe averés vostre request. (f.53v)

64. *A charme for þo festur:* In nomine Patris et Filii et Spiritus Sancti, amen. 'Seynt Johan vermes out. Quant en oute? Nef de nef et oept de oept et sept de sept et sis de sis et cynk de cynk et quater de quater et treis de treys et dieus de deus et un de un et de un nule. Auxi vereyment come Dieu garrist sen Johan de festre et de feloun et de cancre, si garriseth cest cristien home ou femme .N. pur l'amour q'il avoyt adite sen Johan'. Et ditez Pater Noster et Ave Maria. (f.62r)

65. *A charme for a wounde:* Tres boni fratres ibant et per unam viam ambulabant, et obviavit eis Dominus Noster Jesus Christus et dixit eis 'Boni fratres, quo itis?' 'Domine et magister, nos imus ad montem Oliveti ad colligendum herbas et doloris et plagationis'. Et dixit eis 'Venite post me et jurate insignis maximis et per vulnera Christi ut non abscondite dicatis neque mercedem [quem] inde capiatis, set ite ad montem Oliveti et accipite oleum olive et lanam ovis et po- nite super plagam et dicite "sicud Longius hebreus percussit latus domini nos- tri Jesu Christi et plaga illa non diu sanguinavit nec putruit nec doluit nec guttam fecit nec tempestatem habuit ardoris, sic fiat ista plaga. In nomine Pa- tris + et Filii + et Spiritus Sancti + amen. Ut non sanguinet nec putriat nec do- leat nec guttam faciat nec senteat nec tumeat. In nomine Patris + et Filii + et Spiritus Sancti + amen" '. (f.63r)

66. *An oþer charme for a wounde þat it ake not:* 'Conjuro te, vulnus, per quinque vul- nera domini nostri Jesu Christi et per duas mamillas eiusdem sanctissime ma- tris (eius) ut a modo non doleas neque putrescas neque cicatriscas, set omni modo saneris'. In nomine Patris et Filii et Spiritus Sancti, amen. 'Quinque vul- nera Christi sint medicina tui'. Et dicitur versus ter. (f.63r)

67. *Carmen ad restringendum sanguinem:* + a + oo + initium mundi, consumatio se- culi, vita et pax Christi. Christus vincit + Christus regnat + Christus imperat + Christus natus est + Christus passus est + Christus crucifixus est + Christus lancea perforatus est + et continuo exivit sanguis et aqua in sua passione pro nostra redemptione, langores nostros tulit et dolores nostros ipse partavit Christus qui natus fuit de Maria matre et virgine mortuus et sepultus et sangui- nem dignetur, hunc delere et restringe hunc sanguinem qui exit de isto homine .N. Per Christum crucifixum te conjuro, sanguis, et per crucem qui corpus Christi sustinuit et per sanguinem de latere Christi cadentem ut nun- quam habeas potestatem emanare nec exire a corpore huius .N., amen'. (f.131r)

68. *Medicine pur sank estauncher verraie,* sive presens sit sive absens qui sanguinat de naribus vel de plaga: 'Ive e Eve e seynte Suene furent seorures. Ceo dist Ive: "scuche"; ceo dist Eve: "estupe", ceo dist seynt Suene: "meis nen isse gute". Ne place a Dieu ne a Nostre Dame seynt Marie que meis isse gute de sank de .N.' – nomez soun noun. Et puis Pater Noster. Et ita dic ter et curabitur ubi- cumque sit. Expertum est et probatum a multis. (f.138r)

69. *Carmen:* 'In þo name of þo Fader and Sone and Holi Gost and of þo Seynt

Spirit, þou ne bolne ne rancle ne affestre no more þan Cristes wounde was afestred upon þo rode and seynt Petrus armes ne oke not, ne alle martires ne oke not ne felth not, and in þo worchep of seynt Hermeredyn'. And say it .iii. wit .iii. Pater Noster and it chal never ake. Et hoc probatum est. (f.138r)

70. *For to sleen a kanker:* Sey to þo man 'What is þi name .N.? Has þu a canker? Mortuum est cancrum. Antea fuit Christus quam cancrum. Vivat Christus et moriatur cancrum'. Pater Noster .iii. times reherset, bot sey no more bot ones 'Man, has þu a canker? Bot has þu had a canker?' And sey þis charme and it chal sleen it, for it is proved for sothe. (f.138v)

71. *Ad dolorem dentium carmen:* In nomine domini nostri Jesu Christi fiant hec verba salubria huic servo suo .N. '+ on + in + in + in + on + bon + bin + bin + bon. Dominus opem ferat famulo suo super dolorem dentium'. Icest ditz treis foith sur les dentz que dolount et .iii. Pater Noster. Puys 'al' pendés entour soun cole escript en une escrow et absque dubio curabitur. (f.138v)

The following charms are drawn from a set of veterinary receipts in the same MS.[146]

72. *Item for cloyng of hors:* Sey þis charme. 'God, als wisseli as þu hang on þo rode and Longius stong þe to þo hert wit a spere, save þis hors'. And sey .iii. Pater Noster and .iii. Ave in þo name of Seynt Spirit. (f.134v)

73. *Farcioun. Item for þo farcioun:* Sey þis charme in his ere .iii. + .iii. Pater Noster: 'Mala, magubula, mala, magubula'. (f.134v)

74. *Item for þo farcioun:*[147] Aske þo mannes name þat owes þo hors and þo (þo) hew of þo hors and sey þis charme: 'Lord, als wissely as þis is þo first corne þat God let sow and setten on erthe, also stedfastliche, if þi wil be, delyver þis hors of festur, of worme (and of worme) and of rankel. Michael in þe hel cam to his brother Raphael þe archangele and seyde to him, 'Raphael, wher astou ben þat i ne mith þe þis day sen?' 'I have ben in þo land of worms'. 'Turne ageyn, Raphael, and sle þo .ix. wormes fro .i. tul .ii., fro .ii. tul .iii., fro .iii. til .iiii., fro .iiii. til .v., fro .v. til .vi., fro .vi. til .vii., fro .vii. til .viii., fro .viii. til .ix., fro .ix. til .viii., fro .viii. til .vii., fro .vii. til .vi., fro .vi. til .v., fro .v. tul .iv., fro .iv. tul .iii., fro .iii. til .ii., fro .ii. til .i., so þat þu not on live'. As Raphael delyvered þe .ix. wormes, als stedfastli, Lorde, if þi wil be, delyver þis hors fro farcioun and of þo rankel and of all wormes'. And þis is proved for soth. (f.135r)

75. *For an hors þat is wranch:* Take write þis scripture in parchemyne and hang it abouten his fote and he chal ben hol: + zinupt + anta + peranta + anta +. (f.135v)[148]

76. *For to staunche blode of hors:* 'God was borne of Bedlehem, done on þo rode-tre in Jerusalem, cristened he was in flum Jordan. Lord, as þo flod stode, so staunche þis blode, be it of man or of beest, if it be þi wille'. Pater Noster and .v. Ave. (f.135v)[149]

77. *An oþer:* Pone ista signa ad umbilicum scripta super aliquid. Fac pe. n. m. x. a. s. z. i. ii. iii. (f.135v)

78. *An oþer:* Tak þo knotte of a straw and wette it in þo blod and make .v. crosses in þo forhede and sey þis wordes at every crosse: 'bar and nex'. (f.135v)

79. *Item for an hors þat is wranch:* For to done a 3erd go togider. 'Seynt Architeclyn sat on his benche, in his left hand he held a 3erde of a brere and wit his rith hand he blessed þo 3erde. And Fader and Sone and sothfast Holi Gost, help þis hors þat is wranch'. Pater Noster and Ave and sei it til it go togider. (f.135v)

80. *Charme for foundyng:* 'Hinnitus quisitus vena vacca vane barra'. And sei it .iii. and Pater and Ave. For þis [is] proved for sothe of many marchall. (f.136v)

81. *Charmes and medicines for hors and for wormes and stranglioun:* 'Conjuro vos vermes malos per + Patrem et per + Filium et per + Spiritum Sanctum per + angelos, per + archangelos et per .xxiiii. seniores ut equum istum in pelle neque in sanguine neque in ullo pagine membrorum noceatis, sed fugite, omnes vermes mali, in nomine Patris et Filii et Spiritus Sancti, amen'. Et dic .v. Pater Noster et .v. Ave Maria. Et stare debes iuxta sinistram partem equi. Make þis signe in þis manere on þo erthe . . .[150] and sei In nomine Patris et Filii et Spiritus Sancti, amen. Take .ix. kernelles of pulled bere and sette in every ende of þo signe and þe last in þo myddel and as þu settes þo kyrnelles sey a Pater Noster and Ave. (f.137r/v)

82. *Pur les farcines:* Aske þan þo mannes name þat owes þe hors and þo hew of þo hors et cetera, ut supra, ad hoc signum. (f.137v)

83. *A charme for þo feloun:* In nomine Patris et Filii et Spiritus Sancti, amen. 'I conjure þe, wilked [sic] feloun, in þo name of God al-weldyng of heven, erthe and helle and of þo sonne and of þo mone and of þo .vii. sterres and of all creatures and of all aungeles and of all þe confessours, bisschopes and of all hundred abbotes redy to syng on mydwyntur nyght, þat þu ne entre ne no lenger dwell, in þo name of þo Fader and of þo Sonne and of þo Holy Gost'. Sey þus aboute þo hors. (f.137v)

With the passage of time the Christian element of the charms was often reinforced and the role of secular magic diminished. In MS B. L. Lansdowne 680 (s.xv), for example, magic letters in the small number of charms which it contains have been deliberately erased, probably during the medieval period. Conversely, the charms in MS B. L. Sloane 3160 (s.xv) display an augmented Christian element which make them little different from prayers:

84. Sanguis: Forst aske the name of him þat þu schal make þi charme, then go to þe kirke and say þi charm, but say it not for mon þat is seke. And begynne 'In nomine Patris et Filii etc. Quen Our Laurd was dragh on þe rod crose, þan com Longius þidur and smate him with is sper in þe syde. Water and blod com out at þe wounde. He wiput is en and sewe all son thurghe þe holi vertu of þe godhed. I conjur þe, blud, þat þu com not out of þis cristen mon' – neme þe name etc. Say þis .iii. and þe þar not rek quer þe mon be and þu have his name. (f.168v)

85. For fever: Architriclinus in alte sedens virgam coruli virginiam inter manus tenens dicebat 'Sicut sacerdos in altari verum corpus Christi ex divina magestate potestate sibi commissa conficit, et sicut beata virgo Maria suis mamillis ipsum Christum lactavit oreque virginio et impolluto osculabatur, sic conjuro te, virgam virginiarum, ut adiuvas et coniungas te in medio osculando et habeas potestatem per eius virtutem liberandi ac defendi famulum Dei .N. admodum crucis portatum ab omni vexatione febrium. In nomine patris et Filii et Spiritus Sancti, amen. Adiuro te, virgam virginiam, per virtutem sacratissimorum nominum Dei + Adaye + Sadaye + tetragramaton + Sother + Emanuel + Sabaoth + Adonay + ut adimplias tibi preceptum humiliter creatori obediendo. In nomine Patris et Filii et Spiritus Sancti, amen'. Et dicatur quinquies si sit necesse, hoc est si virga se non coniungat. (f.168v)

86. For wiccud wightus: In + n[omine] + P[atris] et + F[ilii] + et Spiritus Sancti + amen. Per virtutem Dei sint medicina mei Jhesu pia crux et passio Christi / Vulnera quinque sint medicina mei. Virgo Maria in .N. succurre et defende ab omni maligno spiritu, amen + a + g + l + a + tetra + gramaton + [f.169r] alpha + et o + Jesu Christus + nazarenus + rex + judeorum + fili + dei + miserere + mei + Marcus + Matheus + Lucas + Johannes + mihi succure et defende Jhesum, amen. Oremus: Omnipotens eterne Dei hunc famulum tuum .N. hoc scriptum super se portantem prospere salutis ab omni maligno demone et ab omni maligno spiritu et institionibus diabolicis custodi defende ne ab ullis illorum vexetur et amplius ad requiem et misericordiam tuam perducatur, amen. (ff.168v–69r)

87. For þe tothe warche: Virgo serinissima beata Appolonia, ora pro nobis ad dominum. Sancta Appolina pro domino grave sustinuerit martirium, tiranni eius dentes cum malleis ferreis fregerunt et in hoc tormento oravit ad dominum ut quicumque nomen eius portaverit secum, dolorem non habuerit in dentibus. Ora pro nobis, beata Appolina, ut Deus dolorem a dentibus famule sue .N. expellat. Oremus: Deus qui beatam Appolinam de manibus inimicorum liberasti et eius orationem exaudisti, te queso, domine, per eius intercessionem et beati Laurencii martiris tui, ut dolorem a dentibus meis expellas, sanum et incolumen me ipsum facias per Christum dominum nostrum, amen. (f.169r)

88. For erewigge: 'Conjuro te vermem per Patrem et Filium et Spiritum Sanctum et per victoriam passionis Dei + nostri + Jhesu + Christi + ut non habeas potestatem ulterius commorandi in hoc famulo Dei .N. nec in aliquo eius membro perforandi sive corrodendi licentiam habeas videlicet per virtutem glorissime Dei genitricis Marie et + domini + nostri + Jhesu Christi + et sanctorum martirum Dei Nicasii atque Casiani penitus confusus ab os decedas et contritus, amen'. Say þis charm in his ere and say .v. Pater Noster et .v. Ave in þe worship of þe fife woundez of Crist. (f.169r)

89. For a womon þat travels on child: Bind þis writt to hir theghe + in + nomine + Patris + et Filii + et Spiritus Sancti + amen et per virtutem Dei sint medicina mea. Sancta + Maria + peperit + Christum + Sancta Anna + peperit + Mariam + Sancta + Elizabeth + peperit + Johannem + Sancta Cecilia + peperit + Reonigium [corr. Remigium] + sator + arepo + tenet + opera + rotas + Christus + vincit + Christus + regnat + Christus + imperat + Christus + te + vocat

+ mundas + te + gaudet + lex + te + desiderat + Christus + dixit + Lazaro +
veni foras + deus ulcionum + dominus + deus ulcionum + libera famulam
tuam + .N. + dextra domini fecit virtutem + a + g + l + a + alpha + et o +
Anna + peperit + Mariam + Elizabet + precursorem + Maria + dominum + nostrum + Jhesum + Christum + sine dolore et tristicia. O infans, sive vivus sive
mortuus, exi foras, quia Christus vocat te ad lucem + agios + agios + agios +
Christus + vincit + Christus + regnat + Christus + imperat + sanctus + sanctus + sanctus + dominus + deus + omnipotens + qui + es et qui eras + et qui
venturus es, amen. Blrurcion + blrurun + blutanno + bluttiono + Jhesus + nazarenus + rex + judeorum + fili + dei + miserere + mei + etc. (f.169r)

90. Benedictio ordei propter porcos infirmos: Deus ineffabilis, Deus
[in]est[i]mabilis et invisibilis, qui de nichilo cunta creasti, pietatem et misericordiam tuam per sanctum et tremendum filii tui nomen suppliciter depreca-
mur, ut hanc creaturam ordii benedicas et ei potentiam invisibilis operationis
infundas ut animalia que necessitatibus humanis tribuere dignatus es cum ex
eo sumpserint aut gustaverint hec benedictio et sacrificatio illesa reddat et ab
omni temptationis incursu illibata custodiat per dominum. Et tunc legantur
ista quatuor evangelia super ordeum: 'In principio'; 'Maria Magdalene'; 'Re-
cumbentibus undecim discipulis'; 'Si quis diligit me'. Tunc aspergatur ordium
aqua benedicta et detur animalibus. (f.169r–v)

Chapter Three

THE 'LETTRE D'HIPPOCRATE'

One of many pseudo-Hippocratic treatises assembled in the Middle Ages, the so-called 'Lettre d'Hippocrate' was the most influential collection of vernacular medical receipts before 1300. A considerable number of the Old French receipts that have so far been published clearly derive from it, although their editors were for the most part unaware of the fact,[1] and many of those that remain in manuscript constitute as yet unrecorded witnesses to the work's popularity. When the detailed researches of Mme Claude de Tovar are put into print,[2] we shall be in a much better position to trace the genesis and evolution of the 'Lettre'. Although with this type of production the notion of a critical text is something of a chimaera, Mme de Trovar has already shown what can be done in the way of unravelling the skeins of textual contamination in other receipt collections.[3] For the present, we have two texts in print: that in Provençal published by Clovis Brunel from MS I 4066 (c.1441) in the Archives départementales du Gers[4]; and a Picard text edited by Östen Södergård from MS Vatican, Reg. lat. 1211 (s.xiv).[5] Neither of these copies has any claim to special status and there is no published account of the MSS and their relations. It is, in fact, the Anglo-Norman witnesses which are crucial to the reconstruction of the MS tradition, the most coherent and complete copy in Mme de Tovar's view being the text of MS London, British Library, Harley 2558 (s.xiv[1]) ff.175r–184v (see below).[6] The task of rescuing order from the complexity of the tradition is a difficult one which can only be undertaken by someone who is familiar with a wide range of receipt collections, for as Mme de Tovar observes, 'les contaminations d'un texte à l'autre, les interférences entre les manuscrits sont telles qu'il n'est guère possible d'étudier un réceptaire isolé sans tenir compte de ses apparentements multiples'.[7]

The 'Lettre d'Hippocrate' is an unsophisticated work. It begins with a short introduction, which varies considerably in the MSS, and continues with a more extended treatment of urines, which may also be more or less amplified according to the MS. There follows a corpus of receipts arranged in the traditional manner *a capite ad calcem*. In many of the MSS the exact limits of the work are ill-defined, there being no obvious conclusion or *explicit*, but rather a broadening out into a miscellany of completely heterogeneous receipts covering veterinary complaints, urinary disorders, gynaecological matters etc. A number of charms are included and many of the MSS mix Latin and French receipts.

This brings us to the question of sources. Although the 'Lettre d'Hippocrate' has sometimes been called 'Regimen sanitatis (salutis) ad Caesarem',[8] no Latin source has been recorded. It would be possible, without too much difficulty, to indicate antique sources for some of the individual receipts, but the collection as a whole has seemed to be an essentially vernacular work. Notable, therefore, is the compendium of medical receipts in MS London, B. L. Royal 12 B XII (s.xiii[2]) ff.105r–179r.[9] Within this collection, written in a variety of hands, ff.171v–175v (med. fol.lv–lx) contain a Latin text of the 'Lettre d'Hippocrate' which has so far escaped attention.[10] Whilst remaining close to the text of MS Harley 978, which we edit below, this Latin version seems to reflect a relatively expanded text of the 'Lettre', including many of the receipts found in MS Sloane 3550 which we print in the appendix. The question naturally arises whether the Latin is a source of the vernacular versions or is itself a translation from one of them. The second possibility seems to be confirmed by the presence of scraps of French in the text. For example, the intrusive French '.ix. baies de lorer' in no. 8 (see Latin text below) is actually found in the French text in some MSS. No.10 starts in French ('Al felun qui est . . .') and no. 44 has 'accipe jus de dragance'. Equally noteworthy, no.118 begins 'Puis li . . .' which has been expuncted and replaced with 'Post da ei . . .' The most striking clue to the origin of the Latin receipts resides in the title to no.145 'Contra ranculum dentium' which must be a mistranslation of the French 'Encuntre rancle dedenz le cors'! Finally, nos 163 and 164 are given in French. Elsewhere there are brief scraps of the vernacular e.g. 'Ad glandulas : fac cineres del trus caulis . . .', 'Contra retentionem medicina : accipe culrage . .' which help to confirm the hypothesis that what we have here is a Latin translation of the vernacular 'Lettre d'Hippocrate'.

A truly accurate account of the Latin text of MS Royal 12 B XII necessarily awaits a full study of the vernacular MSS. Amongst the latter, one of the earliest, which we print below, is MS Harley 978. Since the hand of the Latin text is of the first half of the thirteenth century, roughly contemporary with the Harley text, it is worthwhile making a brief comparison of the two versions. It is not to be forgotten that the Harley text has Latin rubrics and a number of Latin receipts too. The following Harley receipts are missing from the Royal MS: 17–20, 22–26, 40, 46, 52–55, 58, 63–64, 70, 73, 75, 77, 79, 81, 84–85, 87, 96, 108–13, 117, 123, 134, 138–139, 140, 141, 144, 146, 150, 155, 156, 159. The following Latin receipts are slightly abbreviated from the vernacular version: 7, 10, 29, 37, 41, 49, 50, 59, 60, 69, 91, 92, 101, 104, 107, 120, 127, 128, 132, 135, 143, 157. Conversely, a number of small additions occur in the Latin receipts as follows: 16, 51, 57, 90, 115, 125, 143, 161 with extra receipts after 66, 80, 82, 107, 116, 122, 133, 137. The rubrics in the Harley and Royal MSS are often identical e.g. 80, 82, 92, 99, 106, 137, though in the Latin no.122 seems to have been given the rubric of no.121. There are notably few divergences in the botanical elements. In no. 59 the Latin has *vetonica*, whilst the vernacular has 'wanteleine / .i. foxesglove/'. In no.133 'succum lanceolate' clearly differs from Harley's 'avence', but is confirmed by the 'lancelé' of other vernacular MSS. Below I print the Latin text of the Royal MS using the receipt numbers of the Harley MS.

I print the Harley copy, without prejudice to any theory of the genesis of the 'Lettre', because it is the earliest vernacular copy which I have seen and, further, is approximately contemporary with the Latin version of the Royal MS. MS B. L. Harley 978 is well known,[11] yet the collection of medical receipts which it contains (ff.27vb–34vb) has never been studied and remains about the only part of the volume not to have been printed. It is generally agreed that ff.1–34, including the collection of medical receipts, was written c.1240–50, whilst the rest of the MS belongs to a later period, in the second half of the thirteenth century.[12] It is worth giving a full description of the contents of this valuable MS, the more so since previous work on medical receipts has paid so little attention to the manuscripts themselves.

1 ff.2r–15r An antiphonary accompanied by neumes and including the celebrated Reading Rota 'Sumer is icumen in' (f.11v).[13]

2 ff.15v–21r Calendar with prognostications. Only ff.15v and 16r (January and February) have full entries. A fifteenth-century hand has supplied prognostications for May–August (ff.17v–19r), the rest is blank. The entry under Feb. Idus (Feb. 13) gives 'obit Sym. abb.', a reference to Abbot Simon of Reading who died in 1226. A similar entry is found in the Reading calendar transmitted in MS Cotton Vespasian E.v f.12r.[14] The Harley calendar is executed in red, blue and green and was probably produced at the Benedictine Abbey of the Blessed Virgin Mary at Reading in the period 1240–1250.

3 f.21v Blank, except for the following verses:

Allea vina venus ventus faba fumus et ignis[15]
Caseus et fletus piper ictus cepe cynapis
Ista nocent oculis set vigilare magis

4 ff.22ra–23rb Part of the medical section of the *Secretum secretorum* in the translation of John of Seville, [red rubr.] *Epistula Aristotelis ad Alexandrum Macedonem de conservacione sanitatis* inc. 'Oportet te o Alexander cum a sompno surrexeris . . .'[16]

5 ff.23rb–25vb Medical treatise, [red rubr.] *Item Avicenna de conservacione sanitatis* inc. 'Oportet quod conservator sanitatis studeat . . .'. It includes a description of various maladies, the four humours, the four seasons, the four elements, and articles *Quales mores efficiant de sanguine; De colera rubea; De melancolia,* followed by the explanation of various medical terms.

6 f.25vb The signs of death in Latin and French:[17]

Hiis signis moriens certis dinoscitur eger:
Fronte rubet primo, pedibus frigescit ab imo,
Decidit et mentum, nasus summotenus albet,
Decrescit venter, levus minuetur ocellus.
Excubias patitur juvenis de nocte dieque
Sique senex dormit, designat morte resolui.
Item
Par ces signes se mustera li malade ki tost murra:
Enmi le frunt enrovira, le quer del pé refreidira,
E le mentun decherra, le pynnun del nes emblanchira,
E le ventre decrestra, le oyl senestre emmenusera,
Si il est jufne, mult veillera, e jur e nuit traveillera,
Si il est velz, tost dormira, çoe signefi ke il murra.

7 ff.26ra–27va Bilingual glossaries of herbs (f.26ra *Chaudes herbes,* f.27ra *Freides herbes*)[18] followed on f.27va/b by a simple list under the heading *Des especes:* gingivre, canele, girofre, galingal, citewal, cardamomes, greins de Paris, peivere, cumin, lignum aloes, spikanard, spik celtic, bausme, terrebentin, carewy, sticados, ciremunteine, anise, crok, safran, castor, noiz mugét, maces, foilles, almaundes, riis, [f.27vb] figes, pelestre, manne, sucre, euforbie, carpobalsamum, caumfere, aristologia, asa fetida, ciperum, ermodacles, rubarbe, sene, esule, aloen patic, gumme de ere, jus de licoriz, dragagant, gumme arabic, mirabalauns, margarites, perles, turbit, palea camelorum.

8 ff.27vb–34vb A text of the 'Lettre d'Hippocrate', see below.

9 f.35ra/va A number of Latin receipts in a new hand, ending with the following verses: 'Gaudet epar spodio, mace cor, cerebrum quoque musco, / Pulmo liquiricia [sic], splen cappare, stoma galanga';[19] 'Cor sapit et pulmo loquitur, fel commovet iram, / Splen ridere facit, cogit amare iecur'.[20]

10 ff.35va–36vb Part of the medical section of the *Secretum secretorum* in the translation of

John of Seville (see above no. 4), including John's preface. There is a change of hand on f.35vb. There are various verses on f.36ra/b.[21]

11 f.37r 'Centum milia .xxvi. stadiorum a terra usque ad lunam, et bis tantum usque ad solem, et totidem habebuntur usque ad thronum Dei'.

12 f.37r Verses on the plant *scabiosa*:[22]

> Urbanus pro se nescit precium scabiose,
> Nam purgat pectus quod deprimit egra senectus,
> Rumpit apostemata levi virtute probata,
> Emplestrata foris necat antracem tribus horis,
> Intus potatur virus sic evacuatur,
> Languores pecudum tollit dirimendo venenum,
> Potata novies fit de languente boni spes.

The rest of the folio is blank.

13 After f.37v, which is blank, 22 folios have dropped out (the old foliation moves from 35 to 58). The note on f.162r (5 Martii 1595 sunt in hoc libro folia conscripta 182) suggests that this occurred after 1595. On f.38r occurs the following letter of commendation:

> Abbas Westmonasteriensis salutem et paratam semper ad beneplacita voluntatem cum dilectione sincera, pro dilecto clerico nostro magistro G. de N. presencium porti- tore(m) paternitatem vostram rogamus humiliter et attente quatinus in agendis eius penes vos ei exhibere amore nostri propensius gratiam et favorem, quod in hac parte sibi nostri contemplatione feceritis nobis fieri reputantes valeat paternitas vostra per tempora longiora.

Another letter follows:

> Viro venerabili et discreto R. Dei gratia abbati N. Ro. de N. salutem in domino. Quia vobis mandavimus quod hac die sabbati essentis [?] apud N. de negotiis vostris nobi- scum tractatur de quibus bene scitis et nos dicto die interesse non possumus signifi- camus vobis quatinus hac die dominica dicto loco intersitis [ad] dicta negotia expedienda. Dilectionem vostram rogamus quatinus credatis portitorem litterarum in hiis que vobis oretenus exponet. Credatis si placet uberius in hiis que dilectus clericus noster magister T.[23] vobis duxerit intimandum.   -

14 f.38va/b *Dicta cuidam Goliardi anglici* inc. 'Omnibus in Gallia anglus Goliardus . . .'[24]

15 f.38vb 'Quatuor ex puris vitam ducunt elementis'.[25]

16 f.38vb A note on the salamander inc. 'Salamandra vocata quod contra incendium valeat . . .'

17 f.39r/v Sixty-eight verses, beginning 'Nos aper auditu, linx visu, simea gustu . . .'[26]

18 ff.40ra–67va The *Fables* of Marie de France.[27] Folio 68r is blank.

19 ff.68v–74v (s.xiv) Poems of Walter Map.[28] Between ff.74 and 75 there is a blank folio (old fol.95).

20 ff.75ra–78ra *Apocalipsis Golye episcopi.*[29]

21 f.78ra/vb *Incipit confessio eiusdem.*[30]

22 ff.78vb–100va Miscellaneous poems by Map and others.[31]

23 ff.100va–102va *Methamorphosis Golye episcopi.*[32]

24 ff.103rb–104vb A text of the *Doctrinal Sauvage* ('short version').[33]

25 ff.104vb–106ra *De tribus angelis qui retraxerunt a nuptiis.*[34]

26 ff.106ra–107ra 'La Besturné', a series of nonsense verses by one Richard.[35]

27 ff.107ra–114rb The Latin poem on the Battle of Lewes.[36]

28 ff.114va–116rb *De conjugio patris ac matris beati Thome martiris.*[37]

29 f.116rb An incomplete Anglo-Norman translation of the above, beginning with a red rubric Ci comence coment Gilebert Beket le pere seint Thomas espusa sa femme la mere seint Thomas le martir. The fragment of text runs as follows:

> [G]ileber Beket, burgeis de Lundres, se croisa en la Tere Seinte pur penance fere, si ke il i vint e vint tant avant que il fu pris cum esclave en la prisun un amiraud . . .

30 ff.116va–117rb Part of an Anglo-Norman verse treatise on falconry.[38] Folio 117v is blank.

31 ff.118ra–160ra The Lais of Marie de France.[39] Folio 160rb is blank.

32 ff.160va–161rb A list of church antiphons.

The text of the 'Lettre d'Hippocrate' begins on f.27vb with an extended blue paragraph mark. The left-hand side of the column is already occupied by the continuation of the list 'des especes' and for approximately three quarters of the way down the page the first receipt is written in a space half the width of the column. To begin with there are alternating red and blue paragraph marks and red rubrics. The heading of each receipt is underlined in red. On f.29v the use of blue ceases and from f.34ra no colouring is used, the headings being underlined in brown ink. The 'Lettre' is apparently incomplete, a new hand appearing on f.35ra to provide a set of exclusively Latin receipts. The size of the page is approximately 188 x 128 mm, the vernacular receipts being contained in a writing block of c. 150 x 105 mm.

It is impossible here to study the many ramifications of the 'Lettre d'Hippocrate' tradition. There are many instances of excerpting, amplification and contamination. Some parts of the 'Lettre' were versified in the compilation of Jean Sauvage and much of it incorporated in a vernacular collection based on Peter of Spain's Thesaurus pauperum and known as 'Recettes de Philippe le Bel'.[40] Our main concern in the present context is to print the two early copies from the Harley and Royal MSS as characteristic examples of Anglo-Norman receipt collections. This task could not be accomplished without consultation of other Anglo-Norman copies the evidence of which is used in the notes. Since there is no printed identification of these copies, I describe them below.

C = Cambridge, Trinity College 0.1.20 (s.xiii²) ff.37r–44v (receipts), 53r–55r (introduction, sections on humours and urines).[41] This is an important collection of medical texts (see below pp.142ff.), but the text which it offers of the 'Lettre', though an example of the fuller version than that provided by the Harley MS, is scrappy and disordered. It gives the following receipts found in Harley:[42] 1, 2, 8c (Sd²), 8b (Sd²), 9, 8a (Sd²), 9a (Sd²), 10, 11–14, 16, 21, 28–33, 35, 37–39, 41–45, 88, 88a (Sd¹), 89, 90, 92, 94, 95, 97, 98, 130, 135–137, 142, *, 145–148, 102, 104, 47–49, *, 51, 56–60, *, 65, 66a (Sd³), 67–69, *, * (both 'pur face lentilluse'), *, 83, *, 86, 105–109, 114–116, * ('encontre meneison'), * ('encontre pressons'), * ('encontre totes gotes freides et chaudes'). There follow on ff.43v–44v a miscellany of receipts not found in Harley (with the exception of 3 and 27).

D = Oxford, Bodleian Library, Digby 86 (s.xiii²) ff.8v–21r.[43] A full text with extra material (see appendix), divided by red initials and rubrics, with some marginal red rubrics (often Autre or Autre manere). The incipit (in red) runs Ici comence le livre Ypocras ki il envead a Cesar l'emperour. The text offers the following receipts: 6 (short version), 7, 8, 8a (Sd³), 8b (Sd³), 21, 9, 8c (Sd³), 9a (Sd²), 10, 12, 11, 13, 14, 15, 16, 26, 27, *, 28 (conflated with 29), 30, 37–39, 31, 33–36, 47–51, 56–60, 62, 41–45, 65–69, 70, 72–74, 71, *, * (=Sd² bottom of f. 219r), 76, 78, *, 80, *, *, *, 82, *, *, 83, 83a (Sd¹), 88, 88a (Sd¹), 89–95, 97–101, *, 102–104, *, *, 105, 106, 106a (Sd³), *, 106b (Sd³), * (series of extra receipts for meneisoun), 114–116, *, 119, 118, 120, * (9 extra receipts on wounds imported from a text such as the 'Novele cirurgerie'), 124, 127, *, 125, *, 151, 152, 153, 154, 157–159, 160–162, *, 163, 164, 168, * (3 receipts). There now follow a series of receipts as found in Södergård's edition (MS Digby 86 ff.15r–18r; f.16 is an interpolated leaf in a 15th C. hand incl. some English). Then come 128, 130, 132, 133, * (various additions), 135–138, 147, 148. More additional receipts are found on ff.19v–21r, incl. some charms.

E = Exeter Cathedral Library 3519 (s.xv in.).[44] This is a medical compendium which includes an imperfect text of Macer, the Letter of Aristotle to Alexander 'De sanitate servanda', and a vast miscellany of medical receipts in Latin and French occupying ff.121–233. This miscellany contains many receipts from the 'Lettre' scattered amongst others on ff.142r/v, 151v, 152r, 162v, 163r/v, 165r–167v, 168v, 169r. The following Harley receipts are found: 28, 30, 38, 31–34, 36, 47–50, 56, 58–60, 44, 45, 65, 82, 7, 8, 8b (Sd³), 8c (Sd³), 9a (Sd²), 10, 12, 14–15 (conflated and written out twice), 15, 16, 26, 27, 7, 8, 8b (Sd³), 8a (Sd³), 21, 8b (Sd²), 9, 8c (Sd³), 9a (Sd²), 10, 11–13, 72–74, 76, 65, 66, 69, 26–30, 37, 38, 36, 47, 48, 51, 56–58, 62, 78, 80, 82, 83, 88–95, 99, 100, 102, 104 (in Latin), 103, 147, 150, 148, 101, 105, 159, 142, 108, 109.

H = London, British Library, Harley 2558 (s.xiv¹) ff.175r–184v.[45] According to Mme Claude de Tovar [46] this offers the most complete and coherent text of the 'Lettre'. The incipit runs 'Ceo est la livere ky joe Ypocras enveyé ay a Sesar qui joe a tey avoy promys. Peçha ore l'ay fet, od grant cure ajustee . . .' There are red and blue paragraph marks separating the receipts and some sections are distinguished by coloured capitals. A number of different scribes have been at work. The text ends 'Issi finist le libel Ypocras qui a Sesar promist de fere et par grant estudie le ad chevi, s'et asaver de la saunté des humes qui est numé en cel libel devaunt, primez de conustre urine et puys de la dolour de chef et des autre maus de cors'. The order of the receipts is as follows: 7, 8, 8a (Sd³), *, 8b (Sd³), 21, 8b (Sd²), 9, 8c (Sd³), 9a (Sd²), 10–15, *, 15, 16, 26–30, 37–39, 31–36, 47–50, 51, 56–58, 60, 59, 62, 41, 44, 43, 45, 65, 66, *, 67–70, 72, 73, 74, 71, * (3 receipts incl. that at the bottom of f.219r in Sd²), 76, 78, 79d (Sd²), 79b (Sd²), 79a (Sd²), 79c (Sd²), *, *, *, *, 80, 82, *, *, *, 83 (amplified), 86, 88, *, 89–91, 93–95, 97–101, 99b (Sd³), 102–108, *, 109, 110, 114–116, 119, 118, 120, *, *, *, *, 121, 122, 124, 127, *, 126, 128–130, *, *, 132, 133, 133a, 135, 136, *, 137, *, 138, 142, 143, 145–148, 150, 149, 151–154, 157–162, *, 163, 164, 168. Folios 181v–183r are then occupied by miscellaneous receipts more or less transmitted in Södergård, ending at Södergård p. 20 f.85r 1.16. Then comes a section 'Trente treys veynes sunt en le cors' and paragraphs on the ague and costiveness.

Sd = London, British Library, Sloane 3550 (c.1300) contains three copies of the 'Lettre':

Sd¹ = ff.89v–91v There is no introduction or treatise on the humours and urines. The text is divided by rubrics in red and by marginal headings, together with alternating red and blue paragraph marks. The truncated text transmits the following Harley receipts (for extra material see appendix): 26–39, 82, 82a, 82b, 83, 83a, 86, 88, 88a, 89, 90, 93, 94, 106, 106a, 106b, 105, 107, 114–116, 119, 118, 120, 121, 128, 129, 136. The end of f.91v and the whole of f.92r are taken up by Latin receipts (there is one short French entry on f.92r) and thereafter to f.98v there is an apparently new collection of receipts in French and Latin (see below p.299).

Sd² ff.217r–219r There is a red rubric Liber Ypocratis missus ad Cesarem quo eum de salutis [sic] instruxit inc. 'Ce est le livre ke yo Ipocras envei a tei Sesar ke jo ai od grant cure ajustee ki jo poi . . .' The text is very abbreviated, offering only a selection of receipts under the following rubrics: De signis urinarum, Pur dolur de chef, Pur puur de boche, Pur dolur de dens, Pur neir dens, Pur nariles puantes, Pur dolur des orailes, Pur fer cheveus crestre, Pur fer blanche face, Pur dolur de pis, Pur mal de cor, Pur saver si home playé pusse garir ou nun, Pur apine, Pur apine, Pur menesun astancher, Pur lé fevrs, Pur toute maner de fevre. Latin receipts follow on f.219r/v.[47]

Sd³ ff.220r–225r A full text introduced by a blue rubric Ici comense lé medecines ke Ypocras fit and beginning 'Ce est le livre ke yo Ypocras envea[i] a rei Cesar ke jo ai fet od grant cure . . .' There are alternating red and blue paragraph marks, and red rubrics (a few in brown). The text is amplified, there being, for example, far more entries under 'head' than in Harley, a section which ends (ff.220v/221r) 'Ore avét oï medesines encuntre dolurs de chef e si vus les fetes, si garrét munt de gens'. In a receipt *Pur totes vices de eus* (f.224v) we read 'Ice vaut sur tous autres, kar il fu fet de part Nostre Seinur Jesu Crist'.[48] The text of the collection ends with a Latin section (f.225r) *De splene* followed by 'Explicit', but this section is copied from another work, to be found on ff.225v–229v, which is incomplete, but transmits the first two lines of the *De splene* passage under the rubric *Nocent spleni.*

London, British Library, Sloane 146 (s.xiii²) see below p.265
Cambridge, St John's College D 4 (s.xiv¹) see below pp.149 and 367, n. 21.

There are a number of continental copies which are worth recording:

London, British Library, Sloane 1611 (s.xiv¹) ff.143r–147v.[49] A short, somewhat disordered text inc. 'Veés ci ço est li livres que jo Ypocras en[v]oiai a Cesar, car piece a que le lui pramis, ore l'ai fait a grant cure . . .'. After a short introduction there is a red rubric *La prologe* introducing the sections on humours and urines. The receipts are introduced by blue initials (decorated in red) and red rubrics. There is some interlinear glossing.[50]

London, British Library, Sloane 2412 (s.xiv) ff.2r–60r, partially printed by P. Meyer in *Bull.* *SATF* 1913, pp. 45–53.

London, British Library, Sloane 3126 (s.xiv ex.) ff.25r–64v. An amplified text inc. 'Cest livre envoia Ypocras a Cesar l'emperere de Rome, quar Cesar li avoit prié que il li enseignast . . ' The end of the Harley text corresponds to f.47v after which there is a great deal of extra material, with some repetition. There are no rubrics, but use is made of red and blue capitals. The text is preceded (ff.11r–24v) by another collection, divided into 19 'receptes' but incomplete, which has the red rubric *Ce sunt les receptes des oingnemenz et expiremenz les quiex furent aprins et enseigniez au roy Philippe le Bel et a Mons' de Val[ois].* [51]

Whilst a number of English texts offer the introductory section on the humours and on urines,[52] there is little evidence of complete translations. An exception is MS Cambridge, University Library Dd. X. 44 (s.xiv) ff.114r–117v. The opening red rubric runs *This booke did Ipocrase send unto Cezar for a gret tresour and therfor kepe it well as your owyn lyfe, ffor he made it for help and helth of his body, for all maner of ynyles for to exchew.* The opening paragraph reads:

> Ffyrst every man, beste and birde þat hath body hath four humours and namely humoris of mannys body, that is to say one is hote, another is colde . . . as in the hed to the wombe to the splene and to the bladder which thynge is nedfull to know.

The section on urines begins:

> If a man be hole, his uryn is by the morowe before mete and after mete rede. Urine fatt, whyte and trobilde and a litill in quantite is not gode. Urine mich thynne and not trobyld is goode. Urine feverous, yf it be trobele as it ware water, it signifieth mykell yvyll in the hed nygh to come . . .

The receipts are introduced by a red rubric *Here begynneth at the hed and so for to oþer menbire.* They occur as follows; 7, 8, 8a (Sd³), 8b (Sd²), 9, 8a (Sd²), 9a (Sd²), 10, 13, 27, 28, 38, 39, 41, 43, 47, 49, 50, 51, 56, 62, *, 68, 78, 79d (Sd²), *, 79b (Sd²), 79a (Sd²), 80, 82, 82b (Sd¹), 83, 83a (Sd¹), 88, 88a (Sd¹), *, *, *, (two in Latin), followed by extra material including receipts for wounds. The investigation of the vast number of Middle English medical manuscripts[53] will almost certainly reveal further copies.

    It is premature to describe the sources of the 'Lettre d'Hippocrate' whilst so much work remains to be done on the constitution of the text. Certainly some of the receipts are found in early medieval *antidotaria* and those listed below appear in the treatise of the so-called 'Petrocellus' printed by de Renzi in *Collectio Salernitana* 4 (Napoli, 1856), pp.185ff.

LH 8 Recipe rute fasciculum .i., edete terrestris fasciculum .i., foliorum lauri fasciculum .i. vel baccas lauri .xi., in aqua coques et oleo admixto caput inunges, sanabitur (p.193)

LH 13 Item blete nigre succo cerebrum et timpora illine, bonum est (p.195)

LH 23 Item ascinthium in aceto coctum fronti impones (p.193)

LH 28 Item ad lippitudines occulorum, atramentum et mel et albumen ovorum equa mensura terendo commisce et super oculos liga (p. 201)

LH 37 Item ad caliginem: hedere terrestris succi, pinpinele succi, feniculi succi et olei coclear commisce et oculos illini (p. 202)

LH 41 Item ad male olentes nares: mente et rute succum mitte, prodest (p. 206)

LH 42 Item ederam cum vino in nares mitte, fetorem tollit (p. 206)

LH 71 Cervina medulla imposita capillos fluentes confirmat (p.190)

LH 72 Item lini semen combure, adde oleum, commisce et perunge caput (p.190)

LH 73 Item ad capillos nutriendo[s] verbenam et ascinthium in lixivam coques et assidue caput lavabis (p.191)

LH 74 Item de cinere vitis vinee lixiva facta caput lavabis cum sapone gallico . . . (p.191)

LH 99 Herbe quinquefolii succi coclearia .ii. dabis; sine mora dolorem tollit (p. 258)

LH 100 Rutam tritam in potione frequenter bibat (p. 258)

LH 101 Aut cornu cervini combusti et triti coclear .i. cum mulsa potui da; lumbricos mire excludit (p. 260)

Some further sources are indicated in the notes.

THE TEXT OF MS HARLEY 978

PUR FERE SYRUP LAXATIF

1. **[f.27vb]** Pernez cerlange, coupere, centoire, ysope, esclareie, polipode, cicoreie, capillus Veneris, adiantos, andive, saxifrage, fanuil, persil, luvasche, puliol real, cettrake, letues salvage, malve orteilane, de chascune une poigne, e un unce des flurs dé violes e demi-unce de flurs des roses, e orge ben lavé e puré, e une livere e demi de sucre de alisandre – e si vus ne avez de cel, pernez sucre bogie .ii. liveres e demi – e un galun de eisil. Pus pernez une paele bele e clere e metez i treis galuns u .iiii. de bone cerveise estale e furmentale, e si i mettez vos herbes a quire. Si lessez boillir geskes au tierz. Pus metez i un potel de eisil, si le lessez bien boillir ensemble od les herbes, pus fetes culer parmi un drap e pus remetez cel jus arere en la paele **[f.28ra]** e pus vos freides semences e vos autres pudres e tiume e epetime e les avant dites violes e roses. Pus pernez les aubuns de .vi. oes, si medlez od l'autre potel de eisil, si medlez ensemble pur escurer. Mes veez ke vostre eisil seit deveite [?] e pus versez en la paele mult grelement e muvez durement que ne prenge a la paele. Pus fetes le culer parmi un drap, pus remetez arere cel decoctiun en la paele, pus vostre sucre, si le fetes boillir un petit, ben geskes a un galun u plus, pus si l'asseez aval, si le mettez enz un bel picher net, si le dunez a beivere le vespre tieve e le matin freit bon hanapé petit sulunc sa force.

A FERE OXIMEL

2. *A fere oximel:* Cuillez teles herbes: pren rascine de fanuil, persil, rascine de ache
e rascine de polipode, rascine de ditaundre e de careuy, e de eble e de reiz, e
meine escorce de seu, e lavez ces herbes mut nez, pus si les fetes trencher mut
menuz. Pus seient mis en eisil e seient iloekes .ii. nuiz e seient pus mis a boiller.
Pus si en fetes culer parmi un drap fort e prendre forment hors le jus, pus pernez
les .ii. parties de cel jus e le terz de bon mel quit e ben escumé, si medlez ensemble, sil fetes al tierz feiz boiller mult bien e muvez tuz jur e escumez tut jur e
le signe [f.28rb] de parfite coctiun est itele: pernez de vostre esclice, si degutez
sur vostre ungle, e s'il est si espés k'il ne decurget sur vostre ungle, si est assez.

DIOTÉ

3. *Uignement dioté:* Pernez la rascine de wymalve livere .ii., fenugrec e la semence
de linois u la rascine de luvasche u de burage, de ambes livere .i., squillis u oignuns livere demi. Raez les mut ben e lavez e batez tut ensemble od la semence
de lin e od le fenegrec e od lé squilles e metez a temprer .iii. nuiz en .vii. liveres
de ewe. Le quart jur met a quire utre le fu deske il cumencet espessir, pus metez
le enz .i. sacel petit (e petit) e quant vus le vulez prendre, metez i un poi de ewe
boillant pur en trere le meuz hors le jus e de cel jus pernez .v. liveres e .iiii.
liveres de oille u de bure e boillez ensemble tut deske a .v. liveres, si que les .iiii.
liveres seient quit einz, pus metez i vostre cire livere .i. e quant il ert defit, metez
i vostre terbentin e galbanum, gummi de erre, de chascun .ii. unces. Au derain
metez i vostre pudre de colofonie e de reisine, de chascun demi livere, e met a
quire e quant ert quit, seit osté del feu e quant il ert enfreidi e endurci, amiablement seit quilli sus e mis en boistes. E cest oignement est bon a plusurs dolurs
[f.28va] e freid piz rechaufe e alasche e a pleuresi: rechaufe .i. petit en .i. test al
feu e pus en oint le piz e tuz autres freid lius que sunt ensechi sanét e escaufét e
amoistét. La livere de cest vaut .iiii. deners.

CONFECTIUN

4. *Confectiun bon pur gute e pur cunforter l'estomac e que ben defit:* Pernez la rascine
de reiz ben paré blanc e pus hagé menu. Pus seit tempré treis nuiz e .iiii. jurz en
vin egre u plus. Pus pren bon mel, quit treis feiz e treis feis escumé, bone quantité e si il est gutus, pren le jus de neire mentes .i. bone quanteté e .ii. tant del
jus de l'herbe yve, si medlez ensemble e od vostre mel quit, si que les .ii. parz
seient mel e le tierz del devant dit jus. Pus seit autre feiz quit e escumé mut ben,
pus mis en boistes, bien en cire u enz un picher. Si mangue de cest leteweire
chescun jur une quilleree jun od la liqur e humez une feiz aprés de cele liqur. Si
l'estomac est enfreidi e ne defit mie ben, dunc pren les .ii. parties del jus de mentes e la tierce partie del jus de herbe yve aturné si cum est avant dit. Si il est reumatic, si pren les avant [f.28vb] dit jus des herbes par ouuele mesure e seint
aturné a l'avant dite manere.

---

2 Cf. the similar receipt in MS Cambridge, Trinity College 0.1.20 f.48v, below p.333 no.7.
For key to abbreviations see above pp.43f. and below p.362 n.1. References to Haust concern
MS Darmstadt 2769.
3 Essentially the same receipt as that in the Trinity MS above (f.51r/v), see below p.335
no.21.

Glossary on pp.396–403

YPOCRAS

5. *Des humurs:* Une est chaude, le autre freide, le tierz sec, le quart muiste. Par cha-lur sunt tutes choses sustenues par lesqueles nus vivums. Nos os sunt seccs, que il nus dunent force a suffrir travail. Freides sunt les entrailles, dunt nus espirums, e li sanc est muiste, lequel nurist la vie. Par les os e par les entrailles curent les veines ki guverne [sic] le sanc e le sanc la vie e la vie le cors sustient. Ore veez cum devez les maus cunustre. A quatre parties del cors est la cunuissance u l'en-fermeté est demustré; al chef, u al ventre, u a l'esplen u a la vessie, lesqueles choses covient issi cunustre.

DE URINIS

6. *Si hume est sein* sa urine est devant manger ruge, aprés manger blanche. Urine crasse e truble cum urine de asne signefie dolur del chef proceinement a venir. Urine enfievrés al setime jur terminee, si al quart jur est blanche e al secund jur ruge, signefie garisun. Urine que est crasse e mult blanche si cum cele que est de mutes humurs signefie a venir fevere quarteine. Urine que est sanglentee signefie la vessie estre **[f.29ra]** blescee de aucune purreture que ait dedenz lui. Urine carcive e blanche cum fust velue signefie le mal des reins. Urine que semble pudrus signefie la vessie blescee. Urine que chet par gutettes e si noue de-sure cum ampulles lunge enfermeté signefie. Urine que noue sure une crasse ree-lee ague [e] lunge enfermeté signefie. Urine a femme pure e clere, si al urinal lust cum argent e cele femme suvent vomist e si n'ad nul talent de manger, signefie la femme estre enceinte. Urine a femme blanche e pesante e puante signefie dolur des reins e le mariz plein de mal e de enfermeté de freit. Si urine a femme eit escume de sanc desure e est clere cum ewe, signefie dolur del chef e talent de dormir e de manger aver perdu pur le enfleure de l'estomac. Urine de femme que est del peis e de la colur de plum signefie la femme enceinte e signefie le mariz purri. Urine de femme que est enflé e que ad la tusse e la meni-sun, si ele est de colur de lin, signefie que la femme ne puet pas estre seine. Si devez cunustre par les urines les maus a jofne cors e quant vus les avez cunu, si purrez ver medscines encuntre. E pur ceo que hummes sunt **[f.29rb]** de divers qualitez, encuntre chescun mal i ad plusurs medscines e ore cumencerunt, primes al chief e pus as aultres membres.

PUR MAL DEL CHEF

7. *A dolur del chef:* Pernez puliol quit en eisil, sil metez as nariz, si que il sente le odur e fetes une corune de cel puliol quit e corunez le chef.

---

5 Sd^2 and Sd^3 read *alme* for *vie* in 'la vie le cors sustient' and *la nessance del sanc* (H = *la nesaunce de santé*) for *cunuissance,* followed by *de enfermete(z).* The passage is abbreviated in S p. 9, but has 'En quartes parties est la naissance de sanité ou d'enfermeté demoustree a l'home'. Wiese 664, 20 has *la isaunce de saunté.*

6 S pp.9f,; Wiese 664, 22ff. *Urine enfievrés* is corrected from MS *enfigures. Urine carcive* (see glossary) is probably an error, cf. *schamose*(C), *charnuse* (H), *camue* (S). For *une crasse reelee* (H *un crasse royle*) C has *une crasse roke,* Sd^2 *une grace coile.* In the next sentence the MS has *femme feie* (H *clere et roielee*) against *pure* in most of the MSS.

7 S 10; Wiese 664, 37ff.; Meyer 47,3; Reinsch 170; Haust 1; LM 1, 12ff; Sigerist 161. After *puliol quit* Sd^3 has '.i. hulwort' and E '.i. hulwurt'.

8. *A dolur del chef que lungement tient*: Pernez une poigne de rue e un autre de ere terestre e la tierce de foiles de lorer e de luvache, quisez tut cest ensemble en ewe u en vin e de ceo oigniez le chef.

9. Rue triblez ové sel e ové mel e mis cum est enplastre al chef e mult profite.

10. *Al felun que est el chef de humme, si fet le chef enfler*: Pernez la gresse de cerf e mel ové farine de orge e ere e morele e triblez tut ensemble e pus si raez le chef al malade, si metez cest enplastre en une almuce e si eschaufez le aumuz ové l'enplastre, si metez autresi chaud sur le chef que il seit ilocs deske il seit garri.

11. Rue e fenuil quisez ben ensemble ové ewe, si en lavez le chef.

12. Rue triblez ben, si metez en fort eisil, e de ceo oignez ben le chef desuz.

13. Pernez la neire bete, si l'estemprez ben e pernez le jus, si oignez ben le frunt e les temples [f.29va]

14. Pernez les moles foilles de l'ere, si les triblez mult ové eisil e ové oille e ové sel ars en pudre, si en oignez le chef.

15. Sauge ové eisil triblé e ové oille rosade, mellez e pernez, si oignez le chef.

16. Vetoine, verveine, aluine, celidoine, plantaine, rue, yeble, sauge e de l'escorce del seu, vint greins de peivere, e triblez tut ensemble, si le quisez ben en vin, si en bevez checun jur jun e autresi al cucher.

17. *Al dolur de la teste*: Pernez foille de ere terrestre e destemprez od oille e od eisil e oignez les narilles.

18. Foille de ere triblez od eisil e od le blanc de l'oef, de ceo oignez le frunt.

19. Fenoil e lovache e rue e peivere e mel destemprez od vin, si bevez jun.

20. Fenoil e aloine quit en eisil, de ceo lavez le chef e oignez le frunt sovent.

21. Item puliol chaut od sa flur bevez jun, si vus detenez de manger desque a nune.

22. Item pernez sauge, si triblez en vin, si en bevez suvent.

---

8 S 10; Wiese 664, 39ff.; Meyer 67,4; Brunel (1957) 104; Haust 2; Sigerist 161; Dawson 9. E has 'lorer e nef baies'. MS Harley 978 has *verniez le chef*.
9 Reinsch 171; Haust 7.
10 S 11; Wiese 665, 53ff; Meyer 50, 32; Reinsch 171; Haust 10; Brunel 516. MS Harley 978 has *autresi chaud sur le feu*. See also Dawson 352 and Bell 134.
11 S 11; Wiese 665, 59f; Meyer 47, 6; Reinsch 171; Haust 11; Dawson 450 (combined with 13).
12 S 11; Wiese 665, 58f; Meyer-Jor. 33; LDM 1,25f; Meyer 47, 5; Dawson 449; Haust 12.
13 S 11; Wiese 665, 60f; Dawson 450; Haust 13.
14 S 11; Wiese 665, 62ff.
15 S 11; Wiese 665, 65f.
16 S 11; Wiese 665, 67ff; Reinsch 171; Meyer 47, 6; LDM 2,11ff; Müller 117 ('.v. cornis of pepir'); Dawson 7 & 453 ('.v. cornes'); Reinsch 171 ('quatre grains'). Other MSS substitute *mel* for *vint*. MS Harley 978 has *aliverne* (for *aluisne*). On f.143v Sa reads *escorche de seuich*.
17 This receipt like several others is found in Peter of Spain's *Thesaurus pauperum*. Nos 17–20 are also found in MS Sloane 146, see below pp.271f., nos. 28–31.
21 Reinsch 171; Haust 5; Sigerist 160.

23. Item pernez aloigne, si quisez en eisil, si fetes emplastre, si liez al chef.

24. Item pernez betoigne, si quisez ben en ewe, si lavez le chef e sur le chef metez l'erbe chaude.

25. *Al chef purger e a la voiz esclarzir e al huvet desecher*: Pernez une poignee de aloigne e une de maruil e cent greins de peivere e treis coille[f.29vb]rees de farine de feves e un hanapee de mel, quisez tut ensemble en un pot, a la spes de mel, pus sil refreidez e metez en un ampolle e quant mester serraz, usez une cuilleree e endementers gardez vus de manger lard e oile e bure.

PUR MALADIES DES OILZ

26. *Dolur des oilz malades*: Avient a la fie od grant enflure, a la fie od perfusiun de sanc, a la fie od lermes, a la fie od grant buillissement, a la fie od manjue, a la fie od chacie. Encuntre tuz les mals des oilz ci orrez medcines.

27. *A tuz les mals des oilz*: Quisez mut ben le ruge limaçun en ewe, si en cuillez la gresse, si en oignez les oilz quant vus irrez dormir.

28. *Item a la chacie des oilz*: Triblez ensemble arrement, mel, aubun de l'oef, uelement, e metez l'emplastre sur les oilz.

29. Item triblez le cerfoil, sil destemprez od le aubun de l'oef e quant vus irrez dormir, sil metez sur les oilz e, s'il i ad ren de malveis sanc u de quiture, tut le juttera hors.

30. *Item as lermes des oilz*: Pernez une foille de cholet, si l'oignez de glere e metez la nuit sur les oilz.

31. *Item collirie bon as oilz*: Pernez eufrasie bone partie, si l'estampez mult durement, si en pernez ors le jus parmi un drap, si fetes saim en une paele de arreim de oignt de malle porc e autretant de saim de owe u de chapun, si [f.30ra] culez parmi un drap le seim, si metez en la paele, si eschaufez, pus metez le jus, si boillez ben ensemble e movez les funz de la paele ben od une ronde pere, pus le metez aval, sil lessez refreidir, sil gardez en une boiste, si metez as oilz quant vus irrez dormir un petit desque vus seez guari.

32. Item la gresse de tuz pessuns de fluvie eschaufe el solail deks i ait seim e cel seim mellez od mel, si vus en oignez les oilz, mult esclarirunt.

---

24 Cf. Dawson 14.

26 Reinsch 171 (*dolor de cuer!*) has *confusion de sanc* and *esvellement*; Brunel 518; Meyer 47,8; Brunel (1957) 23a conflates 26 and 27.

27 S 11; Wiese 665, 71ff; Meyer 48, 8; Reinsch 171; Haust 14; Salmon 55; Brunel 519 conflates 27 & 28; LDM 10,10ff; Dawson 476; Sigerist 161. Cf. Müller 55, 71ff.

28 S 11; Brunel (1957) 23b; Reinsch 171; Haust 15; LDM 9, 25ff; Dawson 473 (cf. 490). Some MSS conflate 28 and 29, as does Dawson 473.

29 S 11; Brunel 520.

30 S 11; Wiese 666, 75ff; Reinsch 171; Brunel 521; Dawson 469; Haust 16.

31 S 12; Meyer 48, 10; Brunel 522; Brunel (1957) 23c; Reinsch 171; LDM 11, 7ff; Dawson 501; Heinrich 68, 10ff; Schöffler 193, 15ff; Müller 110; Haust 17.

32 Brunel 525; Reinsch 171; Sigerist 171. Cf. 38r has *peissons de viver*. Sc has *de eue corrante*. The Latin is in MS Sloane 146 f.100v.

Glossary on pp.396–403

33. *Item as oilz que a la fie doillent e a la fie sunt seins:* Mellez ensemble mel e jus de centoire, si en oignez les oilz.

34. *Item as oilz sanglanz:* Maschez mente, si metez lungement sur les oilz.

35. Item mangez betoine jeun, si vus amendera mult la veue.

36. Item bevez chescun jur jun l'aune e mangez rue, si vus esclarzirunt les oilz que al soleil lusant verrez les esteiles.

37. *De la maele des oilz ne dei pas celer:* Cel mal avient de diverses humurs del cerveil, ceo est a saver, de melancolie e autres humurs. La curaciun de cest mal tele est: leissent le vin ruge e le baigner, si se forcent de chanter suvent e beivent leit de chevere suvent e blanc vin beive atemprément. Al comencement seignez le malade de la veine capitale, que vus eiez un petit sanc, e aprés pernez le jus [f.30rb] de l'here terrestre e le jus de pinpernele e le jus de olive uele mesure, si en oignez les oilz.

38. *Item oinement esprové a la maele e a la teie des oilz:* Metez eisil mut egre en un vessel de areim e le jus de purneles dé bois e plum e aloen e mellez tut ensemble e leisse le vessel ester ben covert longement e quant mester serra, metez as oilz.

39. *Item a la teye des oilz medcine esprovez:* Pernez le fel de lievre e mel uele mesure, si destemprez ensemble, si en oignez les oilz, si garra.

COLLIRIUM

40. *Ad clarificandum visum fiat tale collirium:* Accipiatur feniculum in aliqua quantitate, ruta in subdupla proporcione ad feniculum, et absinthium in subdupla proporcione ad rutam. Conteruntur omnia ista in mortario eneo. Postea accipiatur calamina et accendatur ad ignem et extinguatur in vino albo forti et subtili. Iterum accendatur et iterum extinguatur, sicut diximus, in vino albo et ita fiat decies vel pluries, deinde herbe predicte in mortario contrite distemperentur cum vino illo in quo extincta fuerit calamina. Coletur per pannum mundissimum et ponatur in patella cuprea munda et bulliatur ad ignem lentum et clarum et non fumentem et cum ceperit bullire, patella deponatur ab igne et cum penna aliqua vel pluma amoveatur spuma liquori [f.30va] super(e)natans. Postea dimittatur per unam horam vel duas residere, ut quod fuerit feculentum descendat in fundum patelle. Postea liquor ille reponatur in aliquod vas cupreum vel eneum mundissimum et usui reservetur. Si vero liquori illi postquam colatus fuerit et repositus in vas, sicut superius diximus, addatur sexta pars aque rosate – forcius operabi(bi)tur et melius erit. Liquor iste bis vel ter in die instilletur oculis et si in frequenti usu habeatur, potenter medetur obscuritati

33 S 12; Wiese 666, 79f; Brunel 526; Reinsch 171.
34 Salmon 56; Brunel 527 conflates 34 & 36; Haust 18.
35 S 12; Dawson 475 (cf. 504).
36 S 12; Brunel 527. Sc has *les fueilles d'aune.*
37 S 11; Reinsch 172. Some MSS have *ne s'esforcent* (E = *se forcent* my).
38 S 12; Reinsch 172; LDM 11, 3ff; Dawson 503 (cf. 473); Müller 112. MS Harley 978 has *finement esprove.*
39 Wiese 666,76ff; Reinsch 172; Salmon 59; LDM 11,26f; Dawson 502; Müller 112; Haust 19.

oculorum. Lapis vero ille in vino frequenter extinctus redigatur in pulverem minutissimum, tricocinetur pulvis et ponatur in panno mundissimo. De isto pulvere ponatur cum digito medico super inversionem palpebrarum. Istud miro modo deponit ruborem oculorum.

DE NARIBUS

41. *As narilles puantes laquele chose avient del cervel*: L'en trove richement verreies medcines encuntre, mes ore orrez medcines que ja ne faudrunt. Pernez le jus de mente e de rue, si mellez ensemble, si metez as nasrilles suvent, si amenderat mut le cervel e ostera tute la puur.

42. Item pernez le jus de l'here, si metez as nasrilles.

43. Item triblez la rose, si la quisez ben en vin e un poi de mel, si culez parmi un drap, si metez as narilles.

44. Item triblez le jus de dragance, si metez as narilles.

45. Item fetes poudre des [f.30vb] escales de oes de geline dunt les pucinz sunt issuz, sil sufflez es narilles e endementers que vus frez nules de ces medcines que jo ai devant dit, fetes le beivere aloigne triblé od mel.

46. *Item si nares fluunt sanguine*: Lumbricos terrenos super tegulam combure et facto pulvere in naribus suffla.

DE ORE PUTRIDO

47. *Puur de buche, si purrez oster*: Mangez le puliol sec u cerfoil u transglutez eisil quant vus irrez coucher.

48. Item mangez suvent les foilles de fou e lavez la buche de eisil.

49. Item bevez puliol destempré od vin aprés manger e ço mult suvent, si en jettera tute la puur e vus fra bone aleine aver.

50. Item destemprez peivere od blanc vin e si chaut cum poez suffrir en vostre buche tenez e par ces medcines la puur osterez.

CONTRA DOLOREM DENCIUM

51. *A dolur des denz*: Raez ben la corne de cerf, si quisez ben cele rasure en vin u en ewe, si humez de ço autresi chaut cum vus purrez suffrir, sil tenez en vostre buche desque seit refreidie. Pus le jetez fors, si humez plus e issi fetes suvent desque vus seez gari.

---

41 Salmon 60; Reinsch 172; Brunel 529 conflates 41–50; LDM 15,30f; Müller 116; Schöffler 196; Haust 20. H, Sd² and Sd³ have *trove relement*.
42 Reinsch 172; Haust 21.
43 Meyer 48,11; Reinsch 173; Salmon 61; Haust 22.
45 Reinsch 172; Salmon 62.
47 S 12; Brunel 531; Salmon 63 conflates 47–50; Haust 23.
48 S 12.
49 S 12; Haust 24.
50 S 12; Meyer 48,12; Haust 25.
51 S 12; Brunel 532; Salmon 64; cf. Brunel (1957) 71; Dawson 27; Haust 28.

Glossary on pp.396–403

52. Item pernez la pudre de baie de lorer od un poi de encens, triblez en vin, si tenez en la bouche.

53. Item rue quit en vin u en cerveise ben, tenez teve en la bouche.

54. Item mirifolium cum butiro tritum et ad dentes positum mirifice sanat.

55. Item granum[f.31ra] salis sub lingua jejunus pone et ibi dimitte donec liquescat. Dentes sanat nec putrescere sinit.

56. Item mangez le milfoil, si en bevez le jus suvent.

57. Item la racine pernez de la chanillee, si la quisez ben en breses, si la raez ben defors od un cutel. Si estampez ben la racine, si metez sur la dent desque seit refreidi e pus i metez aultre.

58. Item betoine quisez en eisil u en vin desque a la tierce part, si tenez ço ben chaut en vostre buche, e ço suvent, desque vus seez gari.

59. *Item a la dolur des denz que avient od enflure:* Pernez la wanteleine / .i. foxesglove / od sa racine e si la triblez ben, si fetes une emplastre, si metez sur l'emflure e seit iloques lunge pose e fetes ço suvent desque vus seez gari.

60. Item triblez ben la premerole desque vus en eez le jus, si metez le jus en sa narille, mes nient en cele part ou la dolur est, mes en l'autre.

61. Item triblez peivere e vin ensemble e chaut tenez en vostre buche.

62. *Item as neires denz:* Pernez les branches de la vigne, si en fetes carbun, si en furbez les denz od le carbun e od ewe e ço suvent.

63. *Item ad dentes confirmandos:* Maschez les racines de verveine e de agrimoine e quisez les avant dites racines ben en vin, si en lavez suvent les denz.

64. *Item pur denz dolur:* Pernez la entre-escorce de su e la [f.31rb] terce part de sel ars, si fetes une pelote e metez a la dent.

PUR DOLUR DES ORAILLES
65. *Pur la dolur des orailles:* Pernez le jus de mente, si fetes teve, si metez as orailles.

---

52 Sigerist 150.
54 Haust 29.
56 S 12; Haust 29.
57 S 12; Brunel 578; Meyer-Jor. 8 (*quanelle* is misinterpreted in the glossary); LDM 16, 22f & 18, 8ff; Haust 30; H f.176v has *la cheneleine.*
58 S 12.
59 S 12 (*wauertele!*); Haust 31 (*wauteloc*). E has *wasteline.* In Sd² *uuante beine* has been expuncted and replaced by *la plantaine.*
60 S 12; Schöffler 201, 21f.
61 Meyer-Jor. 10; LDM 16, 32ff; Schöffler 201, 9ff; Haust 32.
62 S 13 (*A oster toute doleur*); Salmon 65; Haust 33.
63 LDM 17,3f.
65 S 13; Meyer-Jor. 13 conflates 65 & 66 as does C f. 41v; Brunel 579; LDM 7,18f; Sigerist 167. MS Harley 978 has *metez as narilles.* See also Dawson 21; Haust 34.

66. *Item si il i ad verms as orailles*: Destemprez le mentastre od vin, si culez parmi un drap, sil fetes teve, si metez as orailles.

67. Item le jus de la semence de su metez as orailles, si amendera mult le oie.

68. Item le jus de fenuil teve mis as orailles oscist les verms.

69. Item le jus de eble metez as orailles auque teve, laquele chose dune oie a humme qui lung tens ad esté surd.

DE CAPILLIS CADENTIBUS

70. *De ço que les chevous cheent avient de la feblesce del cors u de males humurs. La curaciun est cete*: Pernez la cendre de peil de serpente e mellez od oignt de urs, si en oignez le chef.

71. Item de moele de cerf oignez le chef, si confermera les chevous.

72. Item ardez la semence de lin, si mellez od oille, si en oignez le chef.

73. Item verveine e aloigne quisez mult ben ensemble en lessive e assiduelement en lavez le chef de cest.

74. Item pernez la cendre de vigne e la cendre dé os de bestes i metez e veuz oignt, si en fetes oignement, si en oignez le chef .viii. jurs, chescun jur une feiz.

75. Item quisez saunsue en un noef pot e pernez le seim desus, si en oignez là ou vus plerra.

76. *Item que les chevous ne seient chanuz*: [f.31va] Quisez secces racines de cholet en clere ewe de fontaigne desque la meité, si en lavez le chef sovent en baign, ja ne serrunt chanuz.

77. Item a fere crestre cheveus que chaü sunt par teigne, mulez neele, sil mellez od crumel, si metez ou vus volez que chevuz cressent.

A FERE LA FACE BLANCHE

78. *A fere la face blanche e sueve*: Pernez le oint freis de porc e l'aubun de l'oef mi quit, si triblez cest ensemble od un poi de poudre de baies de lorer, si en oignez la face.

79. Item pernez en may la matinee les petiz blancs limaçuns un esquelee que vus truverez as prez e as gardins e pernez autretant des greins cum dosses d'ail de la racine de lis, e pus si pernez une geline, si la farsez ben de ces deus, pus quisez ben en ewe la geline e pus la metez einz un morter tute en tere od tuz les os, si

66 S 13; Brunel 580; Haust 35; LDM 7,12f.
67 S 13; cf. Meyer-Jor. 34.
68 S 13; LDM 7, 20f; Haust 37.
69 S 13; Brunel 581; Meyer-Jor. 14. Sd³ glosses *eble* 'anglice walurt'.
70 Meyer 49, 19; Haust 38.
71 Meyer 49, 19; Haust 39.
72 S 13; Meyer 49, 19; Haust 40.
74 S 13; Sc has *les branches .i. ossa des bestes*.
76 Meyer 49, 16; Salmon 66; Haust 41.
77 Meyer 51, 39.
78 S 13; Meyer-Jor. 4; Haust 42.

triblez mut ben, pus si premez parmi un drap la gresse e metez en boistes e oignez la face.

80. *Item merveilluse oignement a fere bele face e sueve e blanche*: Pernez seim de porc
e de geline uele mesure, si mellez ensemble, si en oignez la face e bevez fumeterre.

POCIUN PUR LE PIZ E PUR LES REINS E PUR LES ENFERMETEZ DEL CORS E DEL VENTRE

81. Pernez gingiber .x. d. pesant e .v. de peivere e un unce de lepre, un de pelestre
e un de semence de ache e un de lovesche [f.31vb] e un de fenuil e un de persil e un de carewy e un de espurge, escales .i. de scamoné e mel, que assez i ait,
e une dragme donez al fort humme.

ITEM PUR LE PIZ

82. *Item a la dolur del piz e la tusse e encuntre le mal del quer ci orrez medcines verreies
e esprovees*: Pernez un noef pot de tere, si fetes un lit es funz de maruil, e pus un
altre de lard novel, e si un e un desque le pot seit pleins, e pus versez tant de
cler blanc vin enz cum i purra entrer, e quisez ço tant desque a la tierce part, si
culez parmi un drap, sil gardez en boistes e quant mester serra, pernez une bone
coilleree, si metez en chaut vin u en chaude cerveise, cil bevez quant vus irrez
cocher e ensement en jun.

83. *Item a la secche tusse*: Pernez la semence de ache e la semence de fenuil, si estampez ben e medlez od vin e bevez en jun.

84. *Item ad tussim puerorum*: Oleum et vinum simul misces et de ipso ter comedat
statimque sanabitur.

85. *Item ad tussim que venit ex grosso humore et viscoso*: Valet cyropus violaceus et
zeucara violacea. Dieta sit panis azimus, pira cocta et mala cocta et lac amigda-
lorum.

86. *Item a la dolur e espurgement e encuntre tuz les maus del piz veez ci medcine esprovee e verreie*: Cuillez les purneles dé bois une bone partie e metez [f.32ra] en
un fort vessel, si les triblez ben ensemble e pernez la cerveise si tost cum ele est
culee, si mellez ensemble od les purneles e metez iço en un noef pot, si faites
en la tere une fosse e metez le pot iloques .ix. jurz e .ix. nuz e pus pernez de
cest une hanape[e] petite, si donez al malade le seir chaud e le matin freit e ço
fetes decs il seit gari. E ço sacez, que la medcine est verraie e esprove.

87. *Item fiat talis potus contra siccitatem et raucedinem et arteriacam passionem*: Accipiantur radices petrosilini, feniculi et apii, ysopus, marubium album, gummi
arabicum, dragagantum, ficus, uve passe, succus liquericie et liquericia in
magna quantitate. Omnia ista decoquantur in cervisia residenti et clara de
frumento vel avena et ordeo facta ad consumptionem tercie partis cervisie. De
isto potu actu calido bibat paciens cotidie, mane et sero, quantum capiat ci-
phus parvus. Item electuaria sunt eidem necessaria: diapenidion in mane, dia-

---

80 S 14; Haust 48.
82 S 14; Brunel (1957) 106; Haust 50. After *maruil* some MSS list further herbs. H has
grundeswylie anglice lastunwort. Sd² includes *grendessilie, hundestonge* and *heyhove*.
83 Cf. S 14; Meyer-Jor. 15 & 35; Haust 51.
86 S 14; Meyer-Jor. 37; Haust 53.

dragagantum calidum in yeme, frigidum in estate, et hoc post prandium, in sero electuarium ad restaurandam humiditatem.

DE VENENATIS

88. *A humme ki est enpoisuné ci orrez medcines esprovees*: Pernez une herbe que est apelé simphonie, si en pernez le peis de un dener, si destemprez od urine de femme, e donez lui a beivere, si vomera tost le mal e le venim hors e pus man [f.32rb] gez treis plantes de cerfoil e bevez leit u de anne u de chevere.

89. Item pernez luvesche e andre e anise, si triblez ben ensemble e quisez en vin, si li donez a beivere si chaut cum il purra suffrir e asseurement vomera hors la male poisun e tut le venim.

90. *Item encuntre tute poisuns e encuntre tuz maus venims oez ci medcine legere*: Quisez leit de chevre desque a la tierce part od semence de chanve / .i. henep / e bevez de cest treis jurz. Sus ciel n'ad si bone medcine encuntre venim fors triacle.

91. *Item ki ad beu venim*: Beive le jus de maroil od veuz vin, si jettra hors le venim e savera le pomun.

92. *Item al mal del quer ke fet que li humme ne poet manger, ainz li sunt tutes viandes encuntre quer*: Pernez centoire, si la quisez ben en cerveise estale e quant est mult quite, pernez la sus, si destemprez ben, si la remetez al pot, si lessez durement quire e pus si culez parmi un drap e pernez les deus parz de cest e la terce part de mel quit e escumez e culez parmi un drap e feistes boillir ensemble decs il seit mut espés e metez pus en une boiste bele e fetes le malade manger de cest lettueire chescun jur treis cuillerez desque il seit gari. E cest li ostera la glette entur le quer, si li frad aver talent de manger e de beivre.

DE VOMITU

93. [f.32va] *Encuntre ço que humme vomist e no puet retenir sa viande*: Pernez puliol e maruil e peivre e quisez ben ensemble en ewe, si li fetes beivre suvent.

94. *Item encuntre vomissement e encuntre glette*: Pernez les deus parz de jus de fenuil e la terce de mel e quisez desque il seit ben espés, si bevez al seir e al matin, si vus vaudra mult a l'esplen e al pomun e ostera glette e vomite.

95. *Item encuntre ço que homme vomist sanc u escopit*: Pernez la crote de chevre e fetes en pudre e pernez pure farine de orge, si en facez past en ewe e quant vus le quirrez, jetez une bone cuilleree de cel poudre enz. Si manguce de ço suvent e garra.

88 S 14; Brunel (1957) 108; Haust 54.
89 S 14; Dawson 212. Sd³ has *alisandre e avence*.
90 S 14; Meyer, *Romania* 37 (1908), 363 no.18; Haust 55. MS Harley 978 has *semence de chaume*.
91 Wiese 666, 81f. Some MSS have *sanera la poison*.
92 Wiese 666, 83ff; Meyer 51,41; Brunel 533; LDM 24,27ff; Haust 56; Schöffler 207, 17ff. Cf. Müller 98 and n.9.
93 S 15; Wiese 666, 90ff.
94 S 15; Brunel 534; Meyer-Jor. 7; Haust 57.
95 Wiese 666, 93ff; Haust 58.

Glossary on pp.396–403

96. *Item ad vomitum retinendum:* Dona bibere valerianam.

DE LOQUELA AMISSA

97. Si homme pert la parole en enfermeté: Pernez aloen, si destemprez od ewe, si versez en la buche.

98. Item destemprez savine e foilles del pin, si metez pionie e peivre, mellez ensemble, si li donez a beivre.

DE CONSTIPACIUN

99. A la dolur e a la duresce del ventre: Pernez deus cuillerez del jus de quintfoil, si li donez a humer.

100. Item a l'enflure del ventre: Triblez rue od vin u od estale cerveise, si la bevez suvent.

101. Item si vermes sunt el ventre de l'humme: Pernez la corne del cerf, si ardez en pudre e [f.32vb] destemprez od eisil, si li donez duvent a beivre, si osciraz les verms.

PUR COSTIVORE

102. *Encuntre costivure:* Pernez la semence de lin e quisez ben en ewe e pus si ostez l'ewe e pernez le linois e friez ben od seim en une paele, pus si lui fetes ço manger ben chaut.

103. Item pernez la racine de fugerole, si la taillez e lessez tute nut gesir en vin e l'endemein bevez ço jun.

104. *Item a costuvisun verrai medcine:* Pernez fugerole del chenne e lavez e estampez ben od lard e aparillez ben une geline pelé e uverte, si seit ben farsé de cel herbe estampé, si seit ben quit en ewe e une grant partie de cel herbe ofoec, e quant cele geline serra ben quite, si la raez ben dedenz e dehors e cele ewe humez a mesure, pus fetes une cominee ben espesse e grasse destempré od cele meimes ewe, e mangez dunc cele geline od cele cominee e si garrez sanz grevance.

ENCUNTRE MENEISUN

105. *Encuntre meneisun:* Pernez milfoil e estampez, si que vus en eez le jus, e pernez flur de farine de furment e fetes de la farine e del jus un turtel e quisez as breses e sil mangez ben chaut.

---

97 Wiese 666, 97ff; Salmon 71; Haust 62; Brunel (1957) 109; Meyer, *Romania* 37 (1908) 368 no. 61; Sigerist 166. Brunel 535 conflates 97 & 98; Dawson 839. MS Harley 978 *aloen* = wormwood.
98 Wiese 666, 99f; Dawson 841; Sigerist 166.
99 S 15; Wiese 666, 101f; Haust 59; Sigerist 165.
100 S 15; Wiese 666, 103f; Meyer-Jor. 38; Haust 60.
101 S 15; Wiese 666, 105ff; Haust 61.
102 S 15; Wiese 666, 108f; LDM 28,22ff.
103 S 15; Dawson 203; C has *fulgurole de cheine,* Sa *la feuchiere qui croist sur chaisne,* H *fuger de chene.*
104 S 15; Wiese 667, 109ff; LDM 28, 38ff. Cf. Dawson 183.
105 S 15; Brunel (1957) 110; Meyer-Jor. 17; Haust 63; Müller 87 (cf.111). Cf. Dawson 527.

106. *Item si vus volez saver si li homme qui ad la meneisun forte puisse garir:* Manjuce chescun jur de treis jurz le peis de un dener de semence **[f.33ra]** de kersun que crest en cortil e beive aprés un tret de vin teve u de ewe teve. Si cil estanche, si garra, s'il ne fet, il murra.

107. Item a la meneisun sanglante: Pernez milfoil e plantaine e fraser, si eit tant de l'un cum de l'autre, e estampez ben ensemble e sil gardez ben, e quant voldrez de cel, si destemprez od vin, si li donez treis jurz a beivre le seir e le matin, si garra pur veir.

AL FI

108. *Al fi veez ci medcines verraies:* Pur le fi sanglant pernez la moleine e triblez ben od cerveise e lessez estre si treis jurz e treis nuz, pus si en beive le malade jun e saul.

109. *Item al fi que est hors al fundement:* Estampez tresben la ameroche e bevez le jus e metez l'emplastre de menue l'erbe sure.

110. Item metez desure le poudre de aloen, si murra le fi.

111. *Item pur le fi qui est al fundement:* Pernez avence e fenuil, si triblez, si metez tut cru en novele cerveise, si leissez estre deus jurz u treis, si bevez chescun jur un poi, si desecchera le fi.

112. *Item pur le fi que anguisse le numblil:* Pernez un gros neir limaçun, si liez tut vif od une bende en la fosse del numblil, e quant il est mort e comence a defire, metez un aultre.

113. *Item pur le fi:* Pernez les rascines des orties, si triblez forment, sis metez en eisil un jur e une nut **[f.33rb]**, pus si culez parmi un drap, si metez od cel jus treis poignees de farine de segle e autretant de sel, e treis oes, e treis escales pleines de mel, si en fetes un tortel, Si ardez sur une chaude tiwele tut en pudre, si usez quant bosoigne serra, le jur, la nut, le matin, le seir u quant vus plerra.

CONTRA CANCRUM

114. *Encuntre le cancre:* Pernez le chef de la grue e les piez e les entrailles dedenz e fetes ben secchir en un fur desque vus en puissez fere pudre e metez sur le cancre; en poi de jurz le ocira e sanera e nient sulement est bon a cancre, mes a tutes (maladies) plaies del cors.

115. Item pernez le oef que est failli desuz la geline quant ele cove, si depescét cel oef e muillez dedenz estoupes deliés e metez sur le cancre; en poi de hure cil le ocira.

116. Item pernez mel e fel de chevre e triblez ensemble e oignez le cancre, si le sanera.

107 Meyer-Jor. 18; Haust 65.
108 S 15.
109 S 15. Corr. *de meme l'erbe?*
110 S 15.
114 S 16; LDM 81, 27ff. Brunel 538 conflates 114–116.
116 S 16.

Glossary on pp.396–403

117. *Item ad cancrum mamillarum*: Urticam cum sale modico mixtam inpone.

DE HOMME PLAÉ PRUVE DE VIE U DE MORT

118. *Si vus volez saver de humme plaé si il puisse vivre u nun*: Donez li a beivre chescun jur treis herbes triblez e destemprez od un poi de cerveise, ço est a saver,
pinpernele, bugle e sanicle, e quant il les avera bues, si li saudrunt hors a la
plaie [f.33va] e espurgerunt la dedenz e tresben le sanerunt dehors.

119. *Item si vus volez saver de humme plaé si il pusse vivre u nun*: Donez li a beivre
cerfoil; si il vomist, si garra.

120. *Item bone medcine a plaie*: Fetes saim de lard e pernez mel e farine de segle e
vin e quisez tut ensemble e metez sur la plaie e ben le espurgerat e sanerat.

121. *Item a tutes plaies, veilles e noveles*: Pernez le ruge cholet e quisez en ewe od tut
les truns, si en baignez les plaies. Mult par [est] beon medcine.

122. *Item a oster morte char de plaie*: Pernez dure siue e sel e la cruste de pain de
segle e un oef enter e la fiente de gars e les tresces de ail e metez en un pot e
ardez tut ensemble sur le fu, que vus en eiez pudre e metez sur la morte char,
si la mangera e ostera tute.

123. *Item ad omne vulnus*: Bibe succum herbe que dicitur bugle et succum sanicle
et herbe Roberti et succum avence. Et nota quod bugle claudit vulnus,
sanicle aperit, herba Roberti mundificat, avence curat.

PUR RANCLE OSCIRE

124. Pur rancle oscire; Pernez la mie de pain de furment od ewe e od gleire de
l'oef. Triblez e metez desure.

125. *Item a rancle*: Pernez aloigne e tanseie e triblez od mel e metez sure.

126. Item drap fet de chanve moillez en ewe e metez sure.

127. *Item a rancle de seignee*: [f.33vb] Liez sure les foilles de cholet e un drap de
chanve moillé en ewe.

PUR GUTE

128. *A la gute u que ele seit*: Pernez flur de seggle, si en fetes past od le jus de eble, e
de cel past fetes deus turteus, e quisez sur les breses e pernez une dé crustes si

118 S 16; Wiese 667, 141ff; Meyer, *Romania* 37 (1908) 364 no. 34; Haust 67; Dawson 524;
Müller 92. There is an English version in MS Sloane 2479 f.83r and a Latin version in MS
Sloane 146 f.100v.
119 Meyer, *Romania* 37 (1908) 364 no. 34. H, Sd$^{1-3}$ insert *ne* before *vomist*, as does Haust
66. The Latin in MS Sloane 146 f.100v has *non evadet*.
120 S 16; Wiese 668, 152ff; Meyer, *Romania* 37 (1908) 366 no. 44.
121 Wiese 668, 165ff.
122 Meyer, *Romania* 37 (1908) 366 no. 45.
124 S 16; Salmon 90; Haust 68.
125 S 16; Meyer-Jor. 39.
126 S 16.
127 Wiese 668, 170; Salmon 91; Haust 69.
128 Wiese 668, 173ff; Haust 26.

Glossary on pp.396–403

chaude cum piez suffrir, si liez sur le mal e quant serra refreidi, remetez i un aultre e issi desque vus seez gari.

129. Item pernez planteine e solsequie e suredockes que l'en apele porales, pernez od les racines e la lancelé od sa racine e les foilles de sauz e la racine del glettuner e triblez forment ensemble e quisez en ewe desque a la terce part e donez a beivre le seir chaud e le matin freid.

130. *Item veez ci merveillus oignement a gute*: Pernez le gars e sun oint e le chat masle e virgine cire le peis de .iii. souz e tant cum vus purrez enpuigner od une mein de kersuns, e treis oignuns e oint de porc sauvage. Mellez tut ensemble e triblez e pus metez el gars e quisez al fu le gars desque il seit ben quit e cuillez le seim que en curra, sil gardez e oignez la gute al fu. Esprovee chose est.

131. *Item si vus volez saver mun si la gute seit chaude u freide*: Pernez mel e farine de furment u de seggle e fai cum enplastre, si i metez la nut. Si ele est chaude, l'emplastre ert secche; si ele est freide, l'emplastre ert moiste.

132. **[f.34ra]** *A la gute festre, esprové mecine*: Pernez uns peissuns que sunt apelez roches, si ardez en un noef pot, si en fetes poudre. E pernez le jus de avence, si versez al pertus e emplez del pudre e fetes ço desque les pertuz seient ensecchiz e les plaies sanez. E endementers que vus frez cest, fetes lui beivre le jus de avence.

133. *Item a gute festre que est freide que fet les menuz pertus*: Pernez le jus de avence e le blanc de l'oef oele mesure e flur de seggle e do ço fetes past, si en fetes un enplastre e metez sur le mal e liez desur un drap e seit iloques desqu il chece par sei meimes e si remetez autre. Ço facez desque il seit gari.

134. *Pur le chaud mal .i. ague, medcine esprovee*: Pernez le coperun de bruere, sil fetes debatre tut menu, pus sil destemprez tut menu od ewe beneite, si donez al malade, si suera devant la .xii. hure.

135. *De guta caduca. Encuntre la gute chaive, medcines verraies*: Pernez les piguns del corf tut [vifs] en lur ni e gardez que il ne atuchent tere e que il ne veient nule meisun, si les ardez en noef pot, si en fetes poudre e donez a beivre od ewe beneite e par la grace Deu garra. Icest meimes garist le poagra.

136. Item pernez l'escorce del trus de ruge cholet e triblez ben e pernez del jus de kersun de ewe e eisil e mellez ensemble e bevez .ix. jurs ensemble en jun e garrez.

---

129 S 16; H f.179v separates the passage into two receipts. MS Harley 978 *porales* = 'pareles'.
130 S 16; Wiese 668, 178ff; Haust 27.
131 MS = *dutez*. Cf. Dawson 528.
132 S 16; Wiese 668, 185ff; Schöffler 235, 5ff.
133 S 17; Wiese 669, 190ff. Sd[2] has *le jus de lancelé .i. rubuurt*, H has *de la launceleye*.
135 S 17; Wiese 669, 201ff. For an English version see F. Holthausen, *Anglia* 19 (1897) 83 no. 21 and Müller 106–7.
136 S 17.

137. *Al felun que nest del cors par boces:* Bevez la plantaine **[f.34rb]** e metez l'enplastre sure.

138. Item pernez artemesie e oculusscunse, si en fetes pudre, si metez sure.

139. Item pernez le jus de la racine del neir cardun, si donez a beivre, si fetes enplastre e liez sure e garra.

140. Item scabiosa cum axungia contrita superposita expertissima est.

141. Item consolida minor cum radice inter duos silices contrita paciens eius succum bibat et de grosso circumligetur vulnus et infra unius diei spacium antracem ex toto curabit, ut non indigeat postea nisi cura vulnerum. Hoc in .c. expertum est hominibus.

142. *Si li fundement a homme est hors, medcines verraies:* Pernez la ruge ere e metez en un noef pot e versez vin sure desque li pot seit pleins e quisez al fu desque a la terce part. Pus le ostez del fu, si en bevez, le seir chaut e le matin freid. Pus pernez de l'ere quite les foilles e liez al mal.

143. Item pernez sanicle e viole e thanseie e chanve e la mere des herbes e quisez cerveise de brais e bevez.

144. Item pernez cerfoil, si l'envolupez en estupes, e pus sil cuverez en la brese, tant que il seit quit, pus sil liez al fundement si chaud.

145. *Encuntre rancle dedenz le cors:* Pernez les greins de junipre e boillez en blanc vin e pus bevez de ço chaud le seir e le matin freid.

146. Item medcine verraie: Pernez le chenlange e boillez en cerveise de brais en un noef pot, sil coverez ben, que la chaline ne puisset issir, e donez a beivre al malade, le seir chaut e le matin freit.

147. *Pur le mal des reins, medcines verraies:* Pernez la racine de gletuner e triblez ben e versez sure **[f.34va]** cerveise e bevez le seir chaut e le matin freit.

148. Item boillez chenlange e morele en cerveise de brais en un noef pot, si en bevez le seir chaut e le matin freid.

149. Item fetes quitures desuz les garez.

150. Item pernez mel e peiz e bure e boillez ensemble, si oignez le mal al fu.

---

137 Meyer-Jor. 40.
138 S 17. Sd³ has *occulus cuncere*, D has *oculoscounse*.
139 MS = *veir cardun*, which perhaps ought to stand [= vert chardon].
142 S 17; Meyer-Jor. 41; Meyer 52, 43; Haust 71.
143 S 17; LDM 43, 17ff.
145 S 17; Brunel (1957) 114.
146 S 17; Haust 72.
147 S 18 reads *rachine d'englenter*; Haust 73.
148 S 18.
149 S 18.
150 S 18. Sd² has *m.e.p. anglice pich.*

Glossary on pp.396–403

151. *Encuntre tutes maneres de fevres, medcine esprovez*: Quant le mal vus prendra, entrez en un chaut baigne e veez que voz braz ne atuchent l'ewe, e pernez ere terrestre e metez sur vostre teste, si vus fetes seigner de ambesdeus voz braz, si garrez.

152. *Item a freide fevre*: Pernez treis gutes de leit de femme que leite malle enfant e metez en un oef quit mol, si li donez a humer un poi devant iço que le mal li prenge.

153. *Item as terteines*: Cuillez treis plantes de planteine aprés le rescuns del solail e chantez vostre Pater Noster e donez li a beivre od ewe beneite quant il tremblera.

154. Item pernez le jus de artemesie e fetes tedve od oille, si en oignez par treis jurs sun cors.

155. *Item as quarteines*: Le jus de taneseie fetes tedve od oille, si oignez .iiii. jurs de ço sun cors, si garra sanz faille.

156. *Item in ombibus calidis febribus*: Bulli in aqua fontina cerlange, cycoré, coupere, morele, capillum Veneris, plantaine, viola, feniculum, persil, antos, sçucre vel licoriz, et bibe quociens volueris et interim cotidie lava pedes tuos in aqua ubi cocta sit plantago et folia rubee salicis et folia albe pruni et folia vinee.

157. *Si li homme ne puet dormir*: Triblez ben les moreles e bevez le jus e eschaufez [f.34vb] l'emplastre e liez entur le chef. Si dormira ben e suef.

158. Item escrivez icest en foilles de lorer e metez desuz sun chief que il ne sace mot, si dormira ben: 'Exmael, Exmael, Exmael, adiuro te per angelum Michaelem ut soporetur homa iste'.

159. Item mangez ben letues.

160. *Encuntre mors de serpent*: Triblez centoire e donez a beivre a l'homme u a quele beste que ço seit, si garra.

161. Item rue verte [e fenuil] quisez ben ensemble, si li donez a beivre.

162. Item si serpent u colevre est al cors de homme, triblez rue e destemprez od vostre urine meimes, si en bevez, si vus vaudra.

---

151 S 17; Meyer-Jor. 19; Haust 74.
152 S 17; Meyer-Jor. 20.
153 S 17; Brunel 641; Meyer-Jor. 21; Salmon 93; Haust 76. Some MSS have '.iii. Pater Noster'. Cf. LDM 60,1ff.
154 S 17 (under A *quartaine*); Haust 77. H glosses *artemesie* with *mugwed*.
157 S 18; Salmon 73; Meyer, *Romania* 37 (1908), 367 no. 59; Haust 78; Brunel (1957) 115; Brunel 540 conflates 157 & 158.
158 S 18; Meyer, *Romania* 37 (1908) 367 no. 58.
159 S 18.
160 S 18; Brunel 541; Haust 79.
161 Brunel 541.
162 S 18; Brunel 541.

Glossary on pp.396–403

163. *A estancher sanc:* Triblez ben les foilles de aune, si i metez. Icest meimes estanche la gute festre, si il est mis od sel e od ortie.

164. Item bevez le jus de sincfoil u bevez le jus de ache, si en frotez le frunt de ço: ço est encuntre le curs de narilles.

165. *Pur sanc estancher de plaie:* Accipe lineum pannum et cum vino et sale fac bene bullire et quam calidum pati potuerit inpone plage et fortiter liga et dei adiutorio sanguis stabit.

166. *Item ad sanguinem qui in corpore vel in plaga remanet:* Neptem terre et jus eiusdem bibe et absque mora sanguinem vomet.

167. Item medulla sambuci valet contra fluxum sanguinis intromissa in naribus.

168. Item escrivez icestes lettres en parchemin en deus lius, si li liez sur ambesdeus les quisses. Si vus nel creez, escrivez les lettres en un cutel, si en ociez un porc; ja gute de sanc ne li charra. Cestes sunt les lettres p.g.c.p.e.v.o.x.a.g.z.

THE LATIN TEXT OF MS LONDON, B. L. ROYAL 12 B XII [54]

[f.171v]
7. Ad dolorem capitis: Pulegium coctum in aceto pone in nares ut sentiat odorem. Et fac inde coronam capiti.
8. Item ad dolorem inveteratum: Rute, edere terestris, foliorum lauri ana manipulum .i., .ix. baies de lorer, coquantur in aqua vel vino et inunge capud vel lava.
[8a. cf. MS Sloane 3550 f.220v] Item ad vertiginem capitis: Abrotanum tritum cum melle et aceto jejunus bibat.
[8b. cf. MS Sloane 3550 f.220v] Item fel leporinum trituretur cum melle ana et inunge frontem et timpora.
21. Item pulegium cum flore trituretur et distemperetur cum vino et aqua calida et bibatur pro vertigine.
[8b. cf. MS Sloane 3550 f.217v] Item abrotanum, salvia, trifolium, edera terrestris distemperetur cum aqua et bibatur.
9. Item ruta trituretur cum sale et melle et positum sicut emplastrum super capud multum prodest.[55]
[8a. cf. MS Sloane 3550 f.217v] Item si videtur quod capud vulneretur in summitate tanquam fovea, folia agrimonie coquantur cum melle et emplastrentur super capud.
[9a. cf. MS Sloane 3550 f.218r] Item celidonia coquatur cum burro et coletur per pannum et [re]servetur in pixide et inunge capud et lava capud cum aqua in qua celidonia coquatur.
10. Item al felun qui est in capite ita quod capud infletur: Accipe sepum cervinum et mel et farinam de ordeo et ederam et morellam et triturentur insimul, capud radatur, et emplastretur capud calidum ut pati potest, et sit ibi quousque sanetur.

163 S 18; Meyer, *Romania* 37 (1908) 366 no. 48.
164 Brunel 642.
168 S 18; Salmon 74.

11. Item ruta, feniculus coquantur in aqua et lavetur capud.
12. Item ad omnem egritudinem capitis:[56] Ruta trituretur et ponatur in aceto et inunge capud superius.
13. Item nigra beta trituretur et exprime succum et inde inunge capud.
14/15. Item pro omni dolore capitis: Accipe folia mollia edere, triturentur cum aceto et oleo rosaceo, et inunge frontem et timpora.[57]

Item accipe succum cerfolii et misce cum oleo rosaceo et inunge capud.[58]
15. Item salvia trituretur et misceatur cum oleo rosaceo et inunge capud.
16. Item vetonica, verbena, absinthium, celidonia, ruta, plantago, ebulus, salvia, cortex sambuci, mel, .viii. grana piperis triturentur et coquantur in vino et bibatur jejuno stomacho et sero donec curetur.
21. Item pulegium cum flore ut superius dictum est.

AD DOLOREM OCULORUM

27. Ad dolorem oculorum omnem: Testudines rubee coquantur in aqua et collige pinguedinem et inunge oculos quando vadit dormitum.

[MS Sloane 146 f.9r] Ad omnes dolores et infirmitates oculorum subiunguntur curationes: Testudinem rubeam coque in aqua et pinguedinem supernatantem oculis cero inpone. Illud prodest catiosis.
28. Item ad caciam oculorum: Atramentum, mel et albumen ovi triturentur et emplastretur super oculos.

[MS Sloane 146 f.9r] Ad idem: Conmisce attramentum, mel et albumen ovi ana et inpone sero ante cubitum.
29. Item cerefolium trituretur cum albumine ovi et pone super oculos quando vadit [f.172r] dormitum.

[MS Sloane 146 f.9r] Si malus sanguis fuerit in oculo, delebitur si succum cerfolii sero inposueris, malos etiam tollit humores.
30. Item ad lacrimas: Accipe folium caulis et inunge glarea et pone per noctem super oculos.

[MS Sloane 146 f.9r] Contra lacrimas oculorum: Glarea ovi, folium caulis inunge et superpone.
31. Item collirium ad oculos: Accipe eufrasiam, distempera et exprime succum per pannum. Et accipe sagimen porcinum masculinum et tantumdem auce vel galline. Cola per pannum et ponatur in patella et calefiat et apponatur succus, bulliat et moveatur cum petra rotunda. Infrigdetur et in pixide custodiatur et in oculis ponatur parum, quando id dormitum donec curetur.

[MS Sloane 146 f.10r/v] Collirium bonum ad oculos non sanos: Accipe succum eufrasie in bona quantitate. Postea pone sagimen porci masculi et pinguedinem auce vel galline equali mensura in patellam eneam et calefac ultra ignem donec liquefiant. Postea cola et bulli simul succum cum pinguedine et move semper fundum patelle cum rubea petra donec spisum fiat, et cum opus fuerit, oculis inpone.
32. Item pinguedo omnium piscium de flumine calefacta in aceto donec ibi sit sagimen et cum melle admisceatur. Inunge oculos et clarificabuntur.

[MS Sloane 146 f.9r] Ad idem: Liquefac pinguedinem piscium fluvialium quoscumque habueris ad solem et appone mel prout videris expedire et oculis inpone.
33. Item oculis quandoque dolentibus quandoque non: Mel et jus centauree conmisceantur et inunge oculos.

[MS Sloane 146 f.9r] Ad oculos quandoque sanos quandoque dolentes: Conmisce succum centauree cum melle et oculos inunge.

34. Item ad oculos sanguinolentos: Mastica mentam et pone diu super oculos.
[MS Sloane 146 f.9r] Vel mastica mentam et super oculos ipsum emplastrum diu pone.
35. Item [betonicam] sepe tene inter manus jejunus et visus emendabitur.
37. Item macula oculorum sic curatur: In principio fleobotemetur a vena cefalica, deinde edere terestris jus et pimpernelle et jus olive ana conmisce, et inunge oculos.
38. Item unguentum probatum ad maculam et ad telam oculorum: Pone acetum acre in vase eneo et jus de purnellis de bosco et plumbum et aloen conmisce et cooperi vas diu. Et quando opus fuerit, pone in oculos.
39. Item ad telam oculorum probatum: Accipe fel leporinum et mel ana, distemperentur simul et inunge oculos.

AD NARES PUTRIDOS

41. Ad nares putridos: Accipe jus mente et rute, conmisce et sepe pone in nares et cerebrum emendabitur et auferet putorem.
42. Item accipe jus edere et pone in nares.
44. Item accipe jus de dragance et pone in nares.
43. Item rosa trituretur et in vino coquatur et parum de melle, cola per pannum et pone in nares.
45. Item pulveriza scalas ovorum unde pulli exierunt, insuffla in nares et interim dum predictas medicinas facis, bibat abscinthium cum melle trituratum.

AD FETOREM ORIS

47. [A]d fetorem oris: Tene sepe inter manus pulegium siccum vel cerefolium vel transgluti acetum quando vadis cubitum.
[MS Sloane 146 f.14v] Ad fetorem oris auferendum: Comede sepe pulegium siccum vel cerfolium aut gargariza sepe acetum ante cubitum.
48. Item sepe comede folia fagi et lava os aceto.
49. Item bibe pulegium distemperatum cum vino post prandium. Sepe probatum.
[MS Sloane 146 f.14v] Vel comede pulegium sepe post prandium cum vino tritum.
50. Item distempera piper cum albo vino calido [f.172v] et teneatur in ore.
[MS Sloane 146 f.14v] Vel tene in ore piper tritum in vino albo.

AD DOLOREM DENTIUM

51. Ad dolorem dentium: Rade cornu cervi et coque in aqua et vino et transgluti adeo calidum ut pati potes et tene diu in ore donec infrigdetur nec transseat guttur, et tunc eice ab ore et iterum huma et sepe sic facias.
[MS Sloane 146 f.12r] Contra dolorem dentium curaciones subiunguntur: Rade cornu cervinum et coque rasuram illam in vino vel aqua et tene in ore de illa decoctione quam calidum pati poteris donec infrigidetur. Postea expue et calidum resume donec cureris.
56. Item comede millefolium et bibe jus.
[MS Sloane 146 f.12r] Item manduca millefolium et bibe sepius succum eius.
57. Item accipe radicem jusquiami, coque sub cinere et corticem exteriorem rade. Tritura, pone super dentem vel coquatur in aqua et operare ut prius donec infrigdetur. Postmodum pone aliud emplastrum de eodem.
[MS Sloane 146 f.12r] Vel quoque radicem jusquiami sub prunis et emunda. Postea tere eam et pone super dentem dolentem donec infrigidata fuerit et deinde aliam appone.

59. Item ad dolorem cum inflatura: Accipe vetonicam, cum radice tritura bene et fac emplastrum et pone super inflaturam diu et sepe.

[MS Sloane 146 f.12r] Ad dolorem simul et inflationem dentium: Contere lanceolatam cum sua radice et superpone sepius donec saneris.

60. Item primula veris trituretur et coletur et jus ponatur in nare ex parte opposita.

[MS Sloane 146 f.12r] Vel contere primulam veris et exprime succum eius in narem pacientis, sed non ex parte dentis dolentis.

61. Item piper trituretur et cum vino teneatur in ore.

[MS Sloane 146 f.12r] Aliter distempera piper cum vino et bullitum calidum diu tene in ore tuo.

62. Item ad nigras dentes: Accipe ramos vitis, combure et cum carbone et aqua frica dentes sepe.

[MS Sloane 146 f.13v] Ad dentes dealbandos: Arde in pulverem vitis ramusculos et in pulverem redige et adde sal et aquam et dentes inde sepius confrica.

AD DOLOREM AURIUM

65. Ad dolorem aurium: Accipe jus mente et tepide auribus instilletur.

[MS Sloaen 146 f.13v] Contra dolorem aurium: Succum mente tepidum in aures mitte.

66. Item ad vermes in auribus: Distempera mentastrum cum vino, cola jus per pannum et tepide auribus instilla.

[MS Sloane 146 f.13v] Item contra vermes aurium et auditum adjuvandum mentastri succum tepidum inmitte.

–. Item jus vinee auribus instilla.

67. Item jus de semine sambuci auribus instilla et emendabitur auditus.

[MS Sloane 146 f.13v] Item ad auditum: Succum seminis sambuci inmitte.

68. Item jus feniculi tepide auribus instilla propter vermes.

[MS Sloane 146 f.13v] Succus etiam feniculi tepidus in aures missus vermes occidit.

69. Item jus ebuli auribus instilla tepide. Multum valet.

[MS Sloane 146 f.13v] Ad auditum diu amissum recuperandum: Succum ebuli tepidum inmitte.

AD CAPILLOS CADENTES

71. Ad capillos cadentes: Accipe medullam cervi, inunge capud et confirmabuntur.

[MS Sloane 146 f.15v] Aliter. Unge caput tuum medulla cervina et firmabuntur capilli.

72. Item semen lini combure et cum oleo conmisce et inunge capud.

[MS Sloane 146 f.15v] Aliter: Arde semen lini et misce cum oleo et unge.

74. Item accipe cinerem vitis et de cinere ossium animalium et unctum porcinum vetus et fac unguentum et inunge capud .viii. dies qualibet die semel.

[MS Sloane 146 f.15v] Aliter: Fac unguentum de cineribus vitis et ossibus bestiarum et de uncto veteri et unge per .viii. dies cotidie semel.

–. Item ad capillos longos faciendos: Pectina capud et in mense Maio rore madefac .iii. qualibet die.

–. Item ad capillos blavos faciendos: Accipe fructum qui crescit in quercu, coque diu in vino albo vel cervisia, inunge capud primo parum et postmodum inde lava.[59]

–. Item ad capillos longos faciendos: Accipe radicem ungule caballine, coque in aqua et inde lava capud et procul dubio capilli elongabuntur.

76. Item ne capilli canescant: Coque radices siccas caulium in aqua fontana ad medietatem et inde sepe lava capud in balneo, numquam canescent.
[MS Sloane 146 f.16r] Ne canescant capilli: Coque siccas radices caulis in aqua clara
usque ad medietatem et lava sepe caput inde in balneo.

AD FACIEM DEALBANDAM

78. Ad faciem dealbandam et suavem: Accipe sagimen /unctum/ porcinum sine
sale et albumen ovi coctum. Tritura simul cum parvo pulvere baccarum lauri
et faciem inunge.[60]
[79d. cf. MS Sloane 3550 f.218v] Item ad faciem dealbandam: Accipe radicem levistici et lilii, coque in aqua ad terciam partem, inunge faciem et lava sepe.
−. Item ad faciem lentulosam: Sepe inunge faciem sanguine leporino.
[79b/c cf. MS Sloane 3550 f.218v][61] Item ad caiem pulcriorem faciendam: Coque
in aqua peletricon (in aqua) cum sagimine gallinacea et inunge [f.173r] faciem cum oleo nucis et bibe plantaginem et inde lentigines de facie depones et
alias egritudines.
[79e. cf. MS Sloane 3550 f.218v] Item inunge faciem sanguine taurino et deponet
omnia vicia et faciem debellabit [sic].
80. Item mirabile unguentum ad faciem dealbandam et suavem: Accipe sagimen
porcinum et gallinaceum, conmisce, et faciem inunge, et bibe fumum terre.[62]
−. Item lardum sine sale, vinum, salviam et sepum et olibanum coque in olla
parva et quando infrigdatur, eice vinum et inunge faciem cum residuo, et faciem dealbaberit. Et post conmisce spumam marinam cum unguento et inunge
faciem et dabit colorem rubeum et pulcrum.[63]

AD PECTUS

82. Ad dolorem pectoris et ad tussim et ad malum cordis medicinas probatas et
veras: Accipe ollam novam et in fundo fac lectum de marubio et alium de
lardo et sic donec olla inpleatur. Et postmodum inpleatur vino. Coque ad terciam partem, cole per pannum et in pixide [re]serva. Et cum opus fuerit, accipe
unum coclear plenum et pone in vino calido vel cervisia et mane et sero bibe.
−. Item marubium et ysopum trituratum simul cum butiro in cervisia bibe jejunus.
−. Item ad pectus: Postmodum accipe tres baccas de lauro et coquantur in vino et
melle et bibe quando iterus es dormitum.
83. Item ad tussim siccam: Accipe semen apii et feniculi, tritura et cum vino conmisce et bibe.[64]
[83a. cf. MS Sloane 3550 f.90v and f.222r] Item ad tussim et ad pulmonem egrotum: Accipe semen apii et anisi et tritura simul cum pipere et melle et aliquantulum vini et simul distempera et coque ad spissitudinem et pone in pixidem
et mane et sero comede tria coclearia donec sanus sis.
86. Item ad dolorem et purgamentum et omnia mala pectoris medicina vera et
probata: Collige purnellas de bosco manipulum .i. et pone in vase forti et tritura, et novam cervisiam et cum purnellis misce et ponantur in olla nova. Et in
terra fac foveam et inpone ollam et cooperi et scutella cooperi, et postmodum
terra, per .ix. dies. Et inde parvum cifum cape et da egroto, sero calidum, mane
frigidum, donec curetur. Probatur.[65]

AD HOMINEM VENENATUM

88. Ad hominem venenatum midicina [sic] probata et vera: Accipe herbam que
vocatur simphonie ad pondus unius denarii et distempera cum urina feminea

et da illi in potu et vomet malum et venenum. Post manducet tres plantas cer-
efolii et bibat lac asininum vel capre.

[88a. cf. MS Sloane 3550 f.91r] Item accipe radicem dragancee et minutim incide.
Desiccatam ad solem pulveriza et pondus .v. denariorum pone in aqua tepida
per noctem et mane proice aquam [f.173v] et pone vinum et coque et bibe
tepidum.

89. Item accipe levisticum, anisum. Tritura, coque in vino. Bibat calidum et cito
vomet venenum.

90. Item contra omnes potiones et venenum: Coque lac caprinum cum semine
quercino vel *chanve* usque ad terciam partem et bibe per .iii. dies. Non est melior medicina preter triacle.⁶⁶

91. Item qui biberit venenum bibat morellam .s. jus, cum vino veteri et proicet
venenum.

92. Item ad malum cordis quod facit ne comedat et abominationem habet de omnibus cibis: Accipe centauream, coque in cervisia estala. Et accipe herbam et
tritura bene coctam et pone in olla et dimitte coquere et cola per pannum. Et
accipe tertiam partem mellis despumati contra liquorem et cole per pannum et
fac bullire simul ad spissitudinem et pone in pixidem et comedat tria coclearia.

CONTRA VOMITUM

93. [C]ontra vomitum qui non retinet cibum: Accipe marubium et pulegium et
piper, coque in aqua et bibat sepe.

94. Item contra vomitum et glettam: Accipe .ii. partes succi feniculi et tertiam
mellis. Coque ad spissitudinem et mane et sero sume et valet ad splenem et
pulmonem et vomitum.

95. Item ad vomitum sanguinis vel screatum: Accipe fimum capre, pulveriza, et
farinam ordei et fac pultes in aqua et dum coques inice .i. coclearium pulveris
illius et manducet.⁶⁷

CONTRA AMISSIONEM LOQUELE

97. [C]ontra amissionem loquele in infirmitate: Accipe aloen, distempera cum
aqua, versa in os.

98. Item savina distemperetur et folia pini et grana piperis et pionie et bibat.

CONTRA DOLOREM ET DURICIEM VENTRI

99. [A]d dolorem et duriciem ventris: Accipe .ii. coclearia de jure quinquefolie et
bibat.⁶⁸

100. Item ad inflationem ventris: Rutam cum vino tritura vel cervisia et bibat
sepe.⁶⁹

101. Item contra vermes in ventre: Accipe cornu cervinum et combure ad pulverem et cum aceto distempera et sepe bibat.

CONTRA CONSTIPATIONEM

102. [C]ontra constipationem: Accipe semen lini, coque in aqua, depone aquam
et semen bene frixa cum sagimine, et calidum manducet.

103. Item accipe radicem filiginis, scinde et per noctem jaceat in vino et mane
jejunus bibat illud.

104. Item accipe polipodium quercinum et lava et cum lardo tritura et pone in gallina. Et cum illa herba et gallina coquatur et bibe aquam et fac ciminatum

spissum et crassum cum illa aqua et man [f.174r] ducet gallinam cum illa ciminata.

CONTRA FLUXUM VENTRIS

105. [C]ontra fluxum ventris: Accipe millefolium, tritura, exprime jus et accipe farinam tritici et fac turtellum. Coque in cinere et calidum manducet.

106. Item si vis scire si homo qui habet dissinteriam fortem possit curari: Manducet qualibet die per .iii. dies pondus unius denarii de semine nasturcii ortolani et bibat vinum tepidum vel aquam. Si fluxus sistat, curari potest; si non, morietur.

107. Item ad dissinteriam sanguinolentam: Accipe millefolium et plantaginem et fragariam ana, triturentur, et cum vino distemperentur. Et bibat mane et sero.

–. Item ad dissinteriam: Accipe ova dura et jus plantaginis et comede vitellum cum jure illo.

–. Item: Accipe urticas rubeas, tritura, et coque in cervisia et utatur illo potu et non alio donec curetur et tamen moderate.

CONTRA CANCRUM

114. [C]ontra cancrum: Accipe capud gruis et pedes et intestina et in furno desiccentur. Pulveriza et pone super cancrum per paucos dies. Interficiet et curabit et valet non solum ad cancrum, sed ad omnes plagas corporis.

115. Item: Accipe ovum quod anglice appellatur 'adele' et frange et intinge stuppas et pone super cancrum.

116. Item accipe mel et fel de . . ., tritura simul et inunge cancrum.

–. Item saponem accipe et calcem et nigrum testudinem et tritura simul et fac emplastrum et pone super cancrum.

CONTRA VULNUS

118/119. [S]i vis scire utrum vulneratus possit vivere necne: Bibat cerefolium; si non vomit, curabitur. Post da ei bibere qualibet die tres herbas trituratas et cum cervisia distemperatas .s. pinpernellam, buglam, saniclam, et salient per plagam et mundificabunt et sanabunt.

120. Item medicina ad plagam: Fac sagimen de lardo et accipe mel et farinam siliginis et vinum et coque et pone super plagam.

121/122. Item ad veteras plagas et novas: Accipe de reisina et sal et crustam panis de siligine et ovum integrum et fimum garsi et tresciam allii et pone in olla. Combure, pulveriza, et pone super carnem mortuam et eam delebit.

–. Item accipe farinam frumenti et mel et sagimen porcinum et succum apii et in patella frixa et pone in pixide et est unguentum.

AD CANCRUM INTERFICIENDUM

124. [A]d cancrum interficiendum: Mica panis frumenti cum aqua et glarea ovi simul mixta et desuper posita.

127. Item ad ranculum post fleobotemiam: Accipe folia caulis et liga super vulnus.

125. Item ad ranculum: Accipe absinthium [f.174v] et tanacetum et cum melle tritura et pone supra locum dolentem.

[AD GUTTAM]

128. Item ad guttam ubicumque sit: Accipe farinam siliginis et fac pastam cum succo ebuli et inde fac turtullos et coque supra cinere[s]. Et accipe unam crustam calidam et liga supra locum dolentem. Illa infrigidata pone alteram.

129. Item accipe plantaginem et solsequium et acedulam vel parellam et lanceolatam cum radicibus et folia salicis et radicem bardane. Tritura simul et in
aqua coque ad terciam partem. Bibat sero calidum, mane frigidum.

130. Item unguentum mirabile ad guttam: Accipe gersam et eius ungtum et catti
masculi et ceram virgineam ad pondus .iii. solidorum et manipulum .i. nasturcii et ungtum porci silvestris, conmisce et .iii. cepe. Tritura et pone in ansere
et coque. Collige sagimen quod fluit. Inunge. Probatum est.

AD FISTULAM

132. [A]d fistulam: Accipe rochas .s. pisces in nova olla. Combure, fac pulverem,
et succo avencie superassperge foramina et pulvere illo imple et dum hoc
facis bibat succum avencie.

133. Item ad fistulam frigidam que facit minuta foramina: Accipe succum lanceolate et glaream ovi ana et farinam siliginis. Fac emplastrum et pone desuper
et drappo liga donec per se cadat, et aliud pone sic donec curetur.

–. Item accipe cornu cervi, minutim scinde, coque ad terciam partem
consu[m]ptam, infrigda, et eo inspissato inunge locum dolentem.

AD CADUCUM MORBUM

135. [C]ontra caducum morbum: Accipe pijones corvi vivos in nido et non tangant terram nec domum videant. Combure in nova olla, pulveriza, da bibere
cum aqua benedicta.

136. Item accipe corticem caulis rubei, tritura, et succum narsturcii aquatici et acetum et per .ix. dies bibe in vino et curabitur.

CONTRA LE FELUN

137. [A]d felonem que crescit per bozias: Bibe plantaginem et emplastrum desuper
pone.

–. Item morellam bibe et emplastrum desuper pone.

CONTRA EXITUM ANI

142. [A]d exitum ani: Accipe ederam rubeam et pone in olla nova et vinum infunde ad plenum. Coque ad terciam partem. Bibat sero calidum, mane frigidum. Et folia edere cocte liga super malum.

143. Item accipe saniclam et violas et tanacetum et canabum et radices earum.
Coque in cervisia et bibat.

CONTRA RANCULUM

145. [C]ontra ranculum dentium: Accipe grana juniperi et coque in vino albo et
bibat inde sero calidum, mane frigidum.

AD RENES

147. [C]ontra renes: Accipe radicem bardane, tritura, cervisiam infunde. Bibat
sero calidum, mane frigidum.

148/149. Item linguam caninam et morellam coque in cervisia. Bibat sero calidum, mane frigidum. Fac cauteria.

AD OMNES FEBRES

151. [A]d omnes febres: In accessione intret in balneum calidum [f.175r] et aqua
non tangat brachia et ederam terestrem pone super capud et fac fleobote-
mum de utroque brachio.

152. Item ad febres frigidas: Accipe .iii. guttas lactis mulieris masculum nutrientis et in ovo molli cocto pone. Da ad humandum ante accessionem.
153. Ad tercianam: Collige tres plantas plantaginis post occasum solis et dic Pater Noster et cum aqua benedicta da bibere in accessione.
154. Item ad quartanas: Inunge corpus cum succo arthemesie tepido et oleo per .iii. dies.

AD SOMPNUM PROVOCANDUM

157. [A]d provocandum sompnum: Jus morelle bibat et calefac herbam et inde fac emplastrum capiti.
158. Item scribe super folia lauri et pone sub capite ne sciat: 'Exmael, Exmael, Exmael, adjuro te per angelum Michaelem ut soporetur homo iste'.

CONTRA MORSUM SERPENTIS

160. [C]ontra morsum serpentis: Tritura centoriam et da in potu homini vel alii animali.
161. Item rutam et feniculum tritura et in butiro coque et da bibere.
162. Item si serpens vel coluber intret corpus hominis: Tritura rutam et cum urina propria distempera.

AD SANGUINEM STRINGENDUM

163. A estancher sanc: Triblez ben les foiles de aune, si i metez. Ice maimes la gutte festre estanche si il i est mis od sel [MS ser] e od ortie.
164. Item bevez le jus de cincfoille, bevez ache, si freez le frunt de ceo. Ceo est e[n]cuntre le curs des narilles.

CONTRA INFLATIONEM GUTTURIS[70]

–. [C]ontra inflationem gutturis: Equm fac ementulare et dextrum testiculum finde et sanguine illo unge et liga super testiculum illum et non deponatur ante tertium diem.
–. Item ad glandulas: Fac cineres del trus caulis et cum melle distempera et sepe inunge.

AD URINAM PROVOCANDAM

–. Ad urinam provocandam: Malvia coquatur in vino ad tertiam partem et allium et bibat sepe.
–. Item sanguinem mingentibus: Capud allii coquatur in vino ad tertiam partem cum radicibus et bibat.
–. [cf. MS Sloane 3550 f.223v] Item calculosi bibant cum aqua calida terram nidi arundinis.

AD PEDICULOS

–. Ad pediculos expellendos vel lendes: Fac cineres de vite silvestri et cum oleo misce et inunge corpus sepe.
–. Item accipe rutam et tritura et succo sepe capud inunge.

AD TINEAM

–. [cf. MS Sloane 3550 f.223v] [A]d tineam capitis: Accipe picem et ceram, simul funde et capud rade et in drapo pone emplastrum tepidum super capud et ante novum diem non deponatur.
–. Item mel tritura et superpone.

AD SCABIEM

–. [A]d scabiem: Accipe fumum terre et lava et cum cervisia tritura et bibat sepe.

–. Item contra pruriginem et scalporem: Accipe radicem parelle et cum butiro de mai cocta sub cinere, tritura et veteri uncto, cola per pannum et inunge.

AD FERRUM EXTRAHENDUM

–. [cf. MS Sloane 3550 f.224r] [A]d extrahendum ferrum vel lignum vel spinam: Agrimoniam cum veteri uncto tritura et desuper pone.

–. [f.175v] [cf. MS Sloane 3550 f.224r] Item: Accipe ditannum et tritura et pone super vulnus et comedat et bibat.

AD MULIEREM IN PARTU

–. [A]d mulierem in partu laborantem: Liga super ventrem istud scriptum: + Maria peperit Christum + Anna Mariam + Elizabet Johannem + Celina Remigium + sator + arepo + tenet + opere [sic] + rotas.[71]

–. Item scribe hunc versum et liga super magnum digitum pedis dextri: 'Deus deorum dominus locutus est et vocavit terram'.

–. Item da ei bibere ditannum.

SI INFANS MORTUU ...

[S]i infans mortuus est in utero, da ei bibere ysopum in aqua calida.

LAC DEFICIT

–. [cf. MS Sloane 3550 f. 224r] [S]i lac deficit mulieri accipe cristallum et minutim frange, pulveriza, da ei bibere cum lacte et habundabit lacte.

AD DOLOREM FEMORUM

–. [cf. MS Sloane 3550 f. 224r] [A]d dolorem femorum: Accipe crotam ovis et tritura cum aceto et inunge.

AD INFLATIONEM

–. [cf. MS Sloane 3550 f. 224r] Ad inflationem vel pellis fracturam: Bibe per .ix. dies ebulum cum cervisia.

SI HOMO AMITTIT SENSUM

–. [S]i homo amittit sensum et loquitur extranea, bibat semen rute distemperatum cum aceto et jus versa in nares.

–. Item: Da ei bibere gentianam et celidoniam et semen rute et cum aceto distempera.

CONTRA RETENTIONEM

–. [C]ontra retentionem medicina: Accipe culrage, coque in vino, et pone supra vulvam in lecto sepe.

–. Item accipe jus cerasarii quod est inter arborem et corticem et cum vino tepido per .iii. dies in potu.

CONTRA FLUXUM

–. [C]ontra fluxum medicina: Capillis suis liga aliquam arborem quam volueris que sit viridis, cornu cervinum combustum, redige in pulverem et cum vino veteri da in potu.

–. Item calefac fimum equinum cum aceto et super umbilicum calidum pone diu.

CONTRA GUTTAM INOSSATAM

–. [cf. MS Sloane 3550 f.224r] [C]ontra guttam inossatam: Ambrosiam in vino albo fac bullire et sepe inde bibat et oleo rosato contra ignem inunge sepe.

AD INFLATIONEM PEDOM

–. [A]d inflationem pedum: Cum apio triturato pone micam panis et vetus unctum et pone emplastrum super pedem.

–. Item: Plantaginem cum aceto distempera et superpone.

CONTRA FLUXUM

–. [C]ontra fluxum sanguinis menstrui: Fac fleobotemiam supra manum vel brachium.

AD SANGUINEM SURSUM TRAHENDUM

–. Ad sanguinem sursum attrahendum: Post accipe farinam frumenti, cum lacte coquatur et melle, et pone super umbilicum.

–. Item fac emplastra de consolida maiori et vino simul triturato, unum ventri apponatur et reliquum renibus.

–.' Item: Urtica viridis tritura cum uncto et liga ventri et renibus et si folium olive apponatur, melius est.

–. Item accipe scalas nucum magnorum, pulveriza et da in potu cum aqua de mara et postmodum fac emplastrum de crotis ovis cum uncto et ventri ligetur et aliud renibus.

–. Item scale ovi galline unde pulli exierunt pulverizentur. Detur in potu quantum cum tribus digitis capere potest qualibet die.

DE PUERO QUIS SIT

–. [A]d sciendum de quo puero mulier pregnans sit: Lac ipsius mulieris .s. una [f.176r] gutta ponatur in aqua fontis. Si petit fundum, masculus est; si supernatat, femina.

CONTRA MURES

–. Contra mures: Accipe .v. garbas primas que intrant in orreum et dic supra primam 'conjuro te, garba, ne habeas maiorem partem in hoc blado quam sacerdo(ti)s habet in missa dominicali'. Et dic ita per .iii. vices. Postmodum .iii. Pater Noster in nomine Patris et Filii et Spiritus Sancti. Et ita super unamquamque garbam.

AD APES

–. Ad apes: '[C]onjuro vos, apes, per ineffabile nomen domini nostri Jesu Christi ut non egrediamini et per sanctissimam matrem domini nostri Jhesu Christi ut filii nostri non fugiant de agro isto, Pater, Paraclitus, Consolator, Advocatus. Et dic hunc versum: 'Domine, dominus noster quam admiratum est nomen tuum in universa terra'.

AD COMBUSTIONEM IGNIS

–. [A]d combustionem ignis: Radix filiginis in mortario trituretur et quod supra lac non bullitum apponatur et conmisceantur et ponantur supra combustionem.

AD VIRGAM ESCHAUDÉ

–. [A]d virgam eschaudé: Radix altee coquatur in aqua et cum uncto porcino

Notes on pp.362–65

masculo trituretur et fiat emplastrum cum farina avene et cum folio populi in testa calefiat.

—. Item: eidem si habeat foramina: Plura ova in aqua coquantur et malve triturentur et cum ovis in testa supra ignem ponantur, moveantur et sagimen exprimatur et in foraminibus ponatur.

CONTRA VULNUS

—. Vulnerato potus: Rubea maior, tanacetum et canabus, folia rubei caulis simul triturentur et mel admisceatur. Bulliant in vino et da ei in potu. Et semper appone folium caulis rubei. Et si vulnus ranculetur vero audeas dare ei potum: radix consolide maioris coquatur in aqua et aquam tene. Radix trituretur et appona .ii. ova vel .iii. ita quod .ii. partes consolide et .iii. ovorum et admodum allii cum predicta aqua distempera ita quod non sit nimis spissum neque tepidum. Fac emplastrum. Pone super vulnus.

PRO BONO MALO DICAS HANC PRECEM

—. 'Ad te levavi oculos meos totum cum gloria P. + Ecce crucem domini', ter. 'Ha! fuge inimice' ter aspirando super malum. 'Salvum fac servum tuum. Esto ei domine .t. f. domine deus'. Oremus: 'Deus qui Eizechieli ter quinos annos ad vitam donasti et famulum tuum a lecto egritudinis tua potencia erigat ad salutem. Per Christum dominum nostrum, Amen'.

—. [I]n tali egritudine incontinenti post sudorem naturalem (sudorem) antequam comedat vel bibat eucaristiam accipiat et non recidivabit.

CONTRA VOMITUM CIBARIORUM

—. [C]ontra vomitum: Menta, absinthium, plantago triturentur, emplastrentur et cordi applicetur.

UNGUENTUM

—. [f.176v] Accipe cornu cervinum de venatione captum, minutim scinde, et in olla pone – in aqua purissima. Fac bullire a mane usque ad nonam vel amplius. Cola et pone in pixidem. Et fac ignem de sambuco non de alio ligno et iuxta ignem egrum inunge.

—. Si vis scire ex quo vel qua provenit quod homo non generat vel mulier non concipit: Fac hominem mingere in nova olla et inpone farinam avene et in alia olla similiter feminam. Cooperi ollas per .viii. dies et in qua olla vermes invenies in eo non peccat.

AD STRANGILONEM

—. Ad stranguilonem equi: Plantago, jovis barba, mel, butirum de maio simul triturentur et fac .ix. bucchettas et equs transglutiat et liga capud firmiter. Et cum stramine fabarum estuetur.

—. Item accipe capud allii et depone barbam que fuit in terra et trescam et accipe .iii. capita et folia enule caballine [corr. campane], et si non sint folia, summitates eius. Tritura simul. Fac duas buccatas et pone in aures et liga formiter per .iii. dies et noctes.

AD MALOS HUMORES

—. Ad malos humores destruendos: Absinthium, tanacetum, fumum terre ita quod tanacetum sit tertia pars aluminis [corr. absinthii] et fumus terre tertia pars tanaceti [. . .]

Notes on pp.362–65

AD DOLOREM DENTIUM

–.   Ad dolorem dentium: Atramentum combure, fac emplastrum, pone super
dentem.

–.   Olibanum et albumen ovi simul tritura et fac emplastrum in timporibus ex
parte opposita.

–.   Item tegula que in campis invenitur in igne incendatur et extracta in pelvi
ponatur ita quod dimidia pars aqua cooperiatur. Et superpone semen jusquiami et fumum recipe.

–.   Item radix jusquiami in aqua coquatur et supra dentem ponatur radix.

–.   Item tere lolium cum aqua benedicta et pone super dentem dolentem.

DE EQUO PERCUSSO IN OCULO

–.   Si equs in oculo percutiatur, fimus hominis combure et cum tuello pulvis in
oculo instilletur.

NE AUCULE ACAPIANTUR

–.   Auculas candela benedicta instilla super capud antequam terram tangant et
non capientur ave.

Appendix

RECEIPTS IN MS B. L. SLOANE 3550

Printed below are those receipts in the three texts of MS Sloane 3550 which are not
found in MS Harley 978.[72] Their approximate location is indicated by the use of
letters beside the number of the nearest Harley receipt and by a page reference to
the edition of Södergård [= S].

1. First copy, ff.89v–91v:

82a. [f.90v] Item: Triblét ben maruil e isope ensemble e quisét ben en serveise
estal e en bure freis, si en bevét checun jur gun. [not in S]

82b. Item al quer: Pernét .iii. baies de lorer, si quisét od vin e od mel, si en bevét
quant vus irret dormir. [S. p.14]

83a. [r–h. marg in red] Contra tussim et pulmonem. Item a la tusse e al pomun malada [sic]: Pernét semence de hache e semence de anis e triblét ben ensemble e
peivre e mel e auques de vin. Si destemprét ben tretut ensemble, si le quisét a
le feu desque il seit ben espés. Si le metét ben en boites e al ceir mangét .iii.
quilerés e le matin dekes il seit gari. [S p.14]

88a. [f.91r] Item: Pernét la racine de dragance, si le [MS de] taillét menue, si
sechét en le solail, si en fetes pudre. E pus pernét de le puidre le peis de .iiii.
deners, si metét en ewe teve e lessét etre tute nut. L'endemain jutét hors le
ewe e metét i del vin, sil quisét ben e lui fetes beivre ben teve e gara. [S p.14]

106a. Pus pernét une pa . . . Trincét en la furme de un dener, si li metét en paele
. . . Si li donét a manger. [not in S]

106b. Item: Pernét feves, si les metét en paele, si les friét en sein de motun, si les
lescét frider, si li donét a manger, si garra. [not in S]

136a. [f.91v] Pur gote enchacer: Facét un emplatre de postolicon [sic] e metét
desur, si trara hors la dolur. [not in S]

136b. Pur gecunne manere de gutte, chaute e freit: Pernét la flur de genet e gresse
de tessun ou de mastin e fetes un unnement e unnét la gutte. [not in S]

2. Second copy, ff.217r–219r:

8a. [f.217v] Item: Si vus estes avis ke le chef lasus seit enfundré enz cum une /f.
218r/ foce, lé foiles de agrimoine quisez od mel e metez une platre sure, si le
sanerét. [S p.11]

8b. [f.217v] Item pur dolur de chef: Averaig[n]e, sauge, cerfoille, er(b)e teretre od
euue detemprez, si li donét a beivre. [S p.10]

8c. Item: Triblét reu od oil, si ungnét ses temples.

9a. [f.218r] Item: Selidoine quisez ben en bure e pus si li colét parmi un drape e si
le gardét en boistes. E de ce oinez le chef e pus si le lavét od euue od la quele
celidoine fust quite. [S p.11]

74a. [f.218v] Item: Si volét longe chevelure aver, moilét votre chef .vii. jurs checun jur une fiet, si le moilét a le meis de mai de la rosee e se fetes treiz fiet
checun jor. [Cf. S p.13]

74b. Item: De la meule de cerf oinét le chef, si confe[r]mera le chev[el]ure. [not in
S]

79a. Item: Si la face est trobluse, pernét fumetere e plaintaine, destemprét ensemble, e donét a beivre. [S p.13: Harley 2558]

79b. Item [a] ambelir la face: Quisét plectrom en euue e od saim de geline, si en
oinét la face. [S p.13: Harley 2558 (plectrin)]

79c. Item a lenteluse face medesine; Oinét la face de oile de nugages, si bevét la
planteine e tele medesine occira les lentes e les autre mals. [S pp.13–14: Harley 2558]

79d. Item: Pernét la racine de lovasche e racine de lis / lilie /, si quisét en euue
desque a la terce part, si oinét la face. [not in S]

79e. Item: Unnét la face de sanc de tor, si ostera tutes vices, si embelit munt. [not
in S]

119a. [f.219r] [red] Pur apine. Si fer u fust u apine seit sailli en cors u en pié u al-
lurs: Pernét agrimoine et trembét od miel, si metét ou pernét ditane e triblét u
metét desure, si en bevét ou mangét ditan. [not in S]

[red] Pur menesun astancher. Pur astanger menesun: Pernét feves, si quisét en un
tete outre le fu, pus les friét en sui de muttun, si donét a manger. [not in S]

[red] Pur lé fevrs. Pur lé fevers: Bevét morele e persil e la scorce de su quit en servese u en vin, si en gara.

[bottom of f.219r]

Item a fere lunge ch[e]velure: Pernét la racine de ungle de cheval e un herbe ke est
apellé en englés 'colcreie', si li quisét ben en euue, si lavét ben le chef e de ce en-
lungerunt lé chivis saunt dote. [not in S: Harley 2558]

3. Third copy, ff.220v–225r:

8a. Item: Averoine od mel e od eisil triblét e bevét en vin sovent. [S p.10]

8b. Item: Fel de levere triblét od mel, si ke semblant eit de roge colur e tant eit de l'un cum de l'autre. E (de) oignét le frunt e les temples e sachét ke munt est bone. [not in S]

8c.   Si vus est avis ke le chef lasus seit enfundé cum en une fose, lé foiles de egrimoine quisét en mel e metét l'enplastre sure, si garra. [not in S]

66a. [f.221v] Item: Le jus de aloine si amendera munt la oie. [not in S]

83a. [f.222r] [red] *Pur la touse e le polmun* [MS plouũ] *malade*: Perne[z] la semence de ache e de avence e peivre e mel e un poi de vin e destemprét tut icet ensemble dekes il seit espés, si en mangét le matim [sic] treis quilers dekes vus set garri.

99a. [f.222v] Item: Pernét la perche de cerf, ci l'ardét en pudre e destemprét od eisil, si li donét a beivre. [not in S]

99b. Item quisét rue verte en vin, si li donét a beivre. [not in S]

106a. Item pernét pomes, si tailét en la manere de deners, si quisét en une paele od cire virgine ke il seit ben quites e freis en la cire, si li donét a manger si chaud cum il purat suffrir. [not in S]

106b. Item: Pernét forma(n)ge freis, si quisét munt en vin vermail, si donét a manger. [not in S]

120a. [red] *Pur plaie malement garie* : [f.223r] Pernét la grece de chevere e veil vin, si en fetes un plastre e metét sur la plaie: si ele est malement close, si overat, e si ele est malement overt, si clorat. [not in S]

[red] *Pur le chef esquaché de cop ou naufré*: Metét les (es)teiles de iraine od eisil e oile e ja ne partirunt ci ke l'averunt sanez. Pus pernét betoine, si triblét, si bevét le jus, si en icerunt les os e sanerunt la plaie. [not in S]

[red] *Pur les os depessés*: Per(e)nét les cholés [MS cloles] ruges e quisét en euue od tut le trus, si en baine lé pleis. Munt vaut. [not in S]

[red] *Pur gute ke ke il seit*: Pernét la malvve e lé escorces de sauz, si boilét en vin, si metét sur ben chaud. [not in S]

133a. [red] *Pur ardante gote*: Pernét flur de segle, si en fetes past od glere, gute de mel e pure, si fetes le past si dur cum vus purez, si fetes tauns de turteles cum il i ad de perteus. E metét a jecun pertus un turtel e quant il serunt enmoilés, otté[s] les e metét autres e ce fetes dekes il seit garri. [not in S]

147a. [f.223v] Item: Pernét semence de hache, si destemprét od vin, si levét sovent en vin, si garrat ben. [not in S]

160. (substitute) [red] *A home ke ne put ben dormir*: Triblé[t] sentorrie e donét li a beivre.

163. (replacement) [red] *Pur saunc astancher*: Pernét lé foiles de alissandre, si triblét od cel e od ortie.

164. (variant) Item: Bevét le jus de quintefoil ou le jus de ache ou pernét la roche ortie, si la triblét ben e liét desure, si estancherat. E bevét de meme le jus.

[red] *Pur estaler*: Quisét en bon vin la mauve, anglice hockes, e eisil ensemble dekes a la terce partie, si li donét a beivre. [not in S]

[red] *Pur la pere ke teut estaler*: Bevét la tere de nis de arunde od ewe chaude. [S p.18 and see below pp.277, no.78 and 293, no.234.]

[red] *Pur ottre teyne*: Pernét peis e ruue e fetes builer ensemble. E raét le chef ke tute la chevelure seit otté. E metét l'enplatre en un drap, si le metét teve sur le chef e ne l'ottét mie devant le .ix. jur, si garra. [S p.19]

Pur teine de tete: Triblét ail o mel, si metét sur le chef. [S p.19]

[f.224r] Item: Quisét foiles de saus od oile e metét la ou la chevelure faut, si cres-
cerat. [S p.19]

[red] *Pur fere chevelure*: Pernét fumiter, si lavét e triblét ben od cerveise e bevét. Si
vaudra al malade dedens. [S p.19]

[red] A *ki fer ou espine seit al cors ou en pé*: Pernét egrimoine, si triblét od veil oint
de porc, si metét al mal. [not in S]

Item: Pernét ditaine, si triblét e metét sur la plaie e mangét de la ditaine. [not in S]

Item: Pernét la racine de rosel e triblét [MS triben] ben od mel e metét sur la plaie,
si en iscerat sant dolur. [S p.19]

[red] *Pur mammeles enflé*: Pernét les pommes de cheine, si triblét od oile rosase e
metét sure. E anprés pernét le jus de morele, anglice chokenemete [sic], e de la
menue consoude, anglice brosewort, e de corianbre [sic] e de linoiz e les liés de eisil
e les oefs quis dures od les ascales. Si triblét e boillét ensemble o ferine de orge e
fetes un emplatre e metét sur le enflur.

[red] A *femme ke at faute de let*: Pernét letuse, si le fetes manger e humer bure od
vin. [not in S]

Item: Bevét semense de fonail [sic] od vin sovent. [not in S]

Item: Pernét le cristal, si le depessét en pudre e donét [MS deliet] li a beivre od let,
si avera asét de let. [not in S]

[red] *Pur dolur de quisez*: Trinblét les crotes de berbis od eisil, si oinét les quises sovent, si vus fetes une quiture desus le genil. [S p.19]

Item: Si les genuz sunt enflés desus ou la pel depescé, bevét eble triblé en cerveice
.ix. jurs, si garrat. [not in S]

[red] A *genuls dolens ou enflés*: Pernét rue e triblét ben od cel e mel e metét l'enplastre sure sovent. [S. p.19]

Item pur nerfs turtes: Pernét peis e cire virgine e metés ensemble, si enchafét e
metét sure. [S p.19]

[red] *Ke parole en dormant*: Destemprét averoine en vin, si donét a beivre. [S p.19]
Pernét un eof ke seit puns meime le jur k'il ad maladie, si escrivét sur sette lettres
.i. so. s. p. q. x. s. y. x. s. 9. o. Pus metét cel of là ors de[suz] le cel en saf liu [MS hu]
e pus l'endemein depescét cel of. Si sanc en ist, si murrat; si n'i ad nul signe de
sanc, si garrat. Esprové chose est. [S p.19]

(The Latin is given at the bottom of the page)
Ad probandum si eger possit evadere necne. Recipe ovum quod sit a gallina positum eadem die quo cepit egrotare et scribe super cum incausto has litteras + ygo. s.
ff. x. g. y. x. g. 9. Postea pone ovum per noctem foras sub libero aere. Et postea in
mane frange caute ovum; si sanguis inde exit, morietur; si nulla est ibi macula sanguinis, procul dubio evadet.

[red] *Pur gote enossé*: Pernét ambrosie, si boillét en vin blanc, si bevét sovent. U oignét la gute premerement de mel clere e depessét e debatét le blanc peis par tut en
pudre, si enchaufét ben e metét sur le mal. E liét [f.224v] od un long drap estupes
sure e l'emplastre portét dekes ele chece par sei. [S p. 20] [not in S]

[red] *Pur mal e pur enflure de pis*: Pernét ache e triblét e mellét od la mie de pain
blanc e od viel [MS veli] vin, si en fetes emplastre e metét a l'enflure. [S p. 20]

[red] *Pur vermes de le ventre*: Pernét amerok e culrage e mente e mel tut ouele mesure e metét en une paele de araim e builét munt ben e si le escumét. E pus si metét
en boites, si en donét le matin e seir, si garrat. [not in S]

Glossary on pp.402–03

[red] *Encuntre cancre*: Pernét un novel drap ke unkes n'eit esté ens ewe e le metét en un novel pot e ardét le en pudre e metét [MS metel] al mal. [not in S]

Item: Pernét vertegris e pudre de suffre e pernét fres forma(u)ge e raét desure e en liét, si garra. [not in S]

[red] *Pur fere bone atrete pur tote manere de playe, a fetre e a cancre puis ke il ne sunt morteles*: Pernét treis quarteruns de code, un peis reisine [MS deisine] e demi livere de cire virgine, un unce de galbanum e demi unce de heufrasie, e deus unces de gres de porc, e un ouncce de gresce de chapun, un partie de mel e un partie de acens [sic], demi unce de sauncdragun. E fiét tut ensemble e puis colét parmi un drap e puis metét en boites. [not in S]

[red] *Pur fere bone entrete*: Pernét le jus de eble e de cerfoil e de malve e de plan-taine e milfoil e lancelé ouelement de checun [MS clekun] e blanc de l'of, ferine de forment. Fetes une confectiun ensemble, si en fetes bone entrete. Icete chose est prové. [not in S]

[red] *Pur le mal ke est overt e ke ne poest estre garri sant grant metrie* [sic]: Pernét franc encens e de arnement, si triblét ben ensemble.. E pernét le poudre, si le metét en la pertus e garra ben. [not in S]

[red] *Pur garrir novele playe*: Perné[t] la racine de glajol, anglice gladen, e triblét ben en veil oint de porc sur la plaie, si garra ben. [not in S]

[red] *Pur totes vices dé eus*: Pernét milfoil, hache [MS bache], parele, anglice re-dockes, e su de motun o(d) de chevere. Friét, si mettét ensemble en une sarceyse. Puis si emplastrét linge drap, si metét desur. Ice vaut sur tous autres, kar il fu fet de part Nostre Seinur Jesu Crist.

[f.225r] [bifolium missing] . . . donét a beivre sovent. Oinét la face de oile de nug-ages, si bevét la plantaine, si otteras les lentes.

[red] *Pur gute aiguere*: [P]ernét orpiment e sufre e detemprét les ou mel, si metét l'emplatre sur dekes il seit gari. [not in S]

[red] *Pur gute currant*: [P]ernét lé racins de fenil e de persil e de ravene e radich e cerflanc, si lé triblét ensemble. Pernét comin e peyvere molu, quisét en vin e metét e fetes espés. [not in S]

[red] *Pur dolur de chef*: [P]ernét galbanum, si metét sur les temples del chef. Destem-prét ov gleire e ov flur de segle. Enplatrét sur linge drap, puis deit le chef estre ben lavé de ewe ou seit quit aloine dekes il seit garri. [not in S]

[red] *Pur entrair espine ou fer*: [P]ernét agrimoine e ditaine e savine e mel e flur de forment. Mellét ensemble e metét sure. [not in S]

I print below a selection of the additional receipts found in the text of the 'Lettre d'Hippocrate' in MS Digby 86, but missing from the Harley and Sloane MSS.

[f.11r] A bloye chevelure aver et longe: Pernez le fruit qui crest al fou, sil quisez mout en vin blaunc ou en cerveise. Si en lavez le chef sovent. Premerement un poy moillez et aprés le lavez sovent.

Pur lentiles ouster de la face: Oignez la face sovent de sanc de levre, sis ousterad.

Pur enbelir la face: Quisez plectrin en ewe od sanc de geline, si en oignez la face. Si la face est trubluse, fumeteire et plantein destemprez, si donez a beivre sovent.

A face lentillouse veray medicine: Oignez la face de l'oille de noiz gauges, si bevez le plantain, si en ousterad les lentilles et les autres maus.

[f.12v] Pur un mal que l'eum apele en engleis le vic: Pernez de estale cerveise e de fourment vint et set hanapees plains, si metez en un nof pot et taunt cum vous poez

enpoingner de une main des escorces de coudre, si taillez desus voustre mayn et
desouz, si les quisez si qui il n'i ayt que noef. Et puis si pernez farine de orge, si en
fetes noef turteus od le jus de milfoille et manjuce un des torteus. Et beive un plein
hanap de cel beivre en les noef jourz, si guarrad pur veir.

[Contre meneisun]
[f.13r] Ou pernez une tiwle, si l'eschaufez mout chaude qui ele seit toute vermayle.
Quant vous la trerrez del fu, si la metez en plain hanap de let de vache a muiller(e).
Si lessez ben boillir desque il seit mout espés. Puis si lui donez si chaut cel lart a
user et ceo sovent.
Ou pernez le restebos de la racine plain pot, sil quisez et boillez qui il soit ben quit.
Pus festes mettre les pez del malade dedenz cele ewe si chaut cum il le poest soffrir
desque a la chevile del pé longement. Et face laver ses genoilz et ses jaunbes de cel
ewe et ceo sovent, si estaunchira od l'aide de Deu.
Ou pernez le saunc del motoun, sil feites ben quire en ewe. Et pus pernez cel saunc
et del siu de motoun asez, si e[n] fetis une mule ben grase, si la quisez ben aprés.
Puis si donez al malade a manger toute chaude, si guarrad.
Ou pernez farine de forment et autretaunt de creie, si en feites viaunde de lait de
vache a muiller e si lui donez a manger chaut.
Countre menesun: Pernez prunes vertes et emplez un pot et metez en chaude
fourne et fetis secchir. Et fetes poudre et mellez od mel et od farine de furment et
lessez buillir desque il seit espés. Et fetes turteus et donez a manger al malade.
Countre meneisoun de sanc: Pernez une quillere plein de ruil de fer et metez en
ewe et lessez ester toute nuit. Le matin colez et bevez.
Countre meneisoun: Pernez plein poins de peivre et poudrez et mellez od le muel
de l'oef cru. Fetes cum dure paste et metez en une poume [f.13v] cresse et liez et
quisez desuz la brese. Et de ceo dounez al malade.
Countre cancre: Pernez crusie et secchiez et poudrez et de cel metez sur le cancre.
De l'herbe verte batez et fetes enplastre et metez sur la mal.

For staunching blood
[f.14v] Ou pernez un erbe qui est apelé en engleis swinekarse, si la tenez en voustre
main longement et la regardez ententivement, si estauncherad.

[f.20r] A sengle: Pernez del saunc a l'houme qui ad eu cel mal et en oignez la
sengle; si est houme, de houme; et si est femme, de feme. Si guarrad.

A number of receipts include English plant names:
[f.11r] un herbe qui l'um apele en engleis hundestunge . . .
[f.14v] mangez letues et popi mout sovent
[f.18r] pernez erbive, wilde tesle et brockarse et averoine . . .
pernez erbive et softe et les feus de sauz ruge
[f.18v] pernez de un erbe qui est apelé revenesfot
[f.20r] la racine de un erbe qui l'em apele hennebone

Chapter Four

VERSIFIED RECEIPTS (PHYSIQUE RIMEE)

MS Cambridge, Trinity College O.1.20 (1044) is one of the earliest and most important collections of medical texts in the vernacular that we possess, although its contents have remained entirely unedited. The MS is, in fact, best known for a series of fine drawings (occasionally washed with colour) which accompany an Anglo-Norman translation of Roger Frugardi's *Chirurgia* on ff. 240r–299v.[1] It consists of 331 folios (including f. 95bis) measuring approx. 198 x 155 mm, which compose four distinct sections, the work of different scribes. Whilst the main scribe of ff.1–237 was certainly Anglo-Norman and responsible for frequent metrical irregularities in the verse texts which he was copying, it is not at all certain that these texts are of insular origin.[2] Both M. R. James and Paul Meyer had trouble in establishing precisely the limits and identity of the various components of the MS,[3] so that a new description is essential:

1. ff.1ra–21rb a versified collection of medical receipts known for convenience as the 'Physique rimee', beginning 'Qui cest livre vodra entendre / bele raison il porreit aprendre'.[4] The text, of over 1700 lines, is written in double columns in a large clear hand which is difficult to date with precision but which probably belongs to the third quarter of the 13th C. There are usually 22 lines per column, though some of the receipts are written out as if they were in prose. There are red rubrics and alternating red and blue initials. Since the work is a collection of receipts drawn from a variety of sources, it is not easy to establish its exact extent. It leads without a break to the next item, which I judge to be of a different character and to have been originally distinct.

2. ff.21rb–23rb [red rubr.] *Les secrés de femmes* inc. 'Ypocras dit et enseigne / les raisons de femme baraigne'. A gynaecological treatise, possibly forming part of 13 below, which after 90 octosyllabic lines, punctuated by the red rubrics *Home de freide nature* and *Autre*, changes to alexandrines with the section headed *Autre* and beginning 'Le marris [et] le nature de lievre prendrés / Vous le seccherés bien et puis poudre ferés' (f.22rb). This section starts with a number of receipts and continues with the rubric *Espermen a femme a petite na[i]ssance* inc. 'Costentin defent femme a petite naissaunce / que od home ne couche ne receive semence' (f.22va/b). Then there is a return to octosyllables with sections headed *Por mort enfaunt* (f.23ra), *Autre* (three sections, f.23ra), *Por femme ke targe de enfaunter* (f.23ra), *Espeirement de enfaunt* (f.23rb).

3. ff.23rb–24va miscellaneous prose receipts (see above pp.72–3) beginning with *Esperment a plaies* inc. 'Treis bons freres estoient ke aloient al mont d'Olivet ...' followed by rubrics *Por malade aveiller* (f.23va), *Decoction* (f.23vb), *Autre*, *Por restreindre le marriz* (f.24ra), *Autre*, *Autre*, *Por entounement d'oreille* (f.24rb) and *Autre* (f.24va).[5]

4. ff.24va–30rb a fragment of a translation of Roger Frugardi's *Chirurgia* with red rubric *De tote manieres de froisseures* inc. 'Il avient ke li chief est naufrez en diverse manieres ...' The fragment covers Bk I, ch.1–3, 5–8, 11–22, 26 and Bk III, ch. 27.[6] At the bottom of f.24va

there is a contemporary drawing of a man with a mace being struck on the head by a man with a staff, which is obviously designed to illustrate the topic of head wounds with which the *Chirurgia* begins.

5. ff.30ra–32vb various receipts consisting initially in instructions for the preparation of ointments (see below pp.325ff.) beginning with a red rubric *Apostolicom cirurgicom*.

6. ff.33r–36v another set of medical receipts written in long lines across the page with red rubrics, beginning *Poudre por la piere* (see below pp.328ff.).

7. ff.37r–44v / 53r–55r the collection of prose receipts known as the *Lettre d'Hippocrate* (see above p.104) followed by the Introduction and the sections on humours and urines.

8. ff.45r–52v a medical treatise composed of receipts (see below pp.330ff.).[7] The introductory rubric in red is almost entirely effaced, as are the opening lines of the text.

9. ff.55r–194r a translation (acephalous) of the *Practica brevis* of Johannes Platearius II inc. 'Les signes iteles: l'urine roge ou sorroge . . .'[8] The explicit (f.194r) *Explicit Amicum induit* refers to the opening words of the *Practica*. This translation, which rarely abbreviates and makes few changes to the Latin original, seems to be unique and has never been studied. There are many coloured initials and a few rubrics. There is a change of hand at f.98v and a return to the first hand at f.105r.

10. f.194r a single prose receipt:

> Pernez une poine de cikoré et une de cerelaunge et la terce de coupere et une des racines de persil et une des racines de fenoil et une de menu ache et une de l'achun et une de la semence de aniz et une poine de l'escorche de saumbu et demi point de escroche [sic] de frene et deus poines de pollipode.

Folio 194v is blank.

11. ff.195r–213v a rather free translation of part of the Salernitan treatise *De instructione medici*[9] with an opening red rubric *Issi commence le sotil enseignement Ypocras a ces disciples que mult li aveient requis coment il deusent visiter li malades*, inc. 'Li auctor dist au comencement de cest livre et parole a ses disciples . . .' The rubrics are *Pur faire le malade enfier en vus* (f.199v), *Diete* (f.200v), *Issi parole de une maladie ke l'en apele crisis* (f.212r).

12. ff.213v–215v a new hand has written a series of brief descriptions of the properties of herbs, beginning 'Olibanum ceo est encens. Il est chaud e seche el secunde degrei . . .'[10]

13. ff.216r–235v a gynaecological treatise, possibly including (2) above, with a red rubric *Prologe* inc. 'Bien sachiés femmes, de ce n'aiés dotaunce, / ci est escrit por voir de lor science . . .' Written in decasyllabics and in alexandrines, it is based entirely on the *Trotula*.[11] Red rubrics are: *Teles i a que perdent lor flors* (f.219r), *Galiens* (f.220r), *Pudre a faire avoir les flors* (f.220v), *Autre* (f.221v), *Autre* (f.222r), *Autre* (f.222v), *Quant tel mal avient por aporter* (f.223v), *Pur abundance de fleumeine* (f.224r), *Por flors vermaux* (f.225v), *Galiens* (f.225v), *Ombaces* [sic] (f.227r), *A la marris* (f.227v), *A la marris issue medecine* (f.228v), *A la marris* (f.229v), *Del marris* (f.233r), *Por conceivre* (f.233v), *Ke ne se poent delivrer a l'enfanter* (f.234v), *A la marris* (f.235r). Meyer regarded the treatise as of continental origin.[12]

14. ff.236r–239v a set of 172 octosyllabic verses on beauty treatments for women, with a red rubric *Pur teches en le vis* inc. 'La quele que soit, dame ou pucele, / ki desire avoir la face bele . . .' Rubrics are: *Por faire clier vis* (f.236v), *Autre* (f.236v), *Por face lentilluse et froissie* (f.238r), *Lavement a dame par corteysie* (f.238v), *Por chanir* (f.239r), *Por jaune cheveus avoir* (f.239v) (see Appendix below)

15. ff.240r–299v a translation of Roger Frugardi's *Chirurgia* with initial red rubric *De tote manere de plaies ke avenent al chef* inc. 'A feiz avent que li chef est plaié en plusurs maneirs . . .'[12] The text is accompanied by many fine drawings.

16. ff.300ra–324va the Latin text of Roger Frugardi's *Chirurgia* as far as Bk III, ch.18 inc. 'Post mundi fabricam eiusque decorem . . .'

17. f.324vb a different hand has entered four receipts (including a charm):

Pro gutta caduca: + Appacion + + Appria + Appremont et qua settanua + E puis pendez cest escrit entur le col.

Encuntre sausefleme e roine: Pernez oint de sengler une livere, silium un unce, sufre deus unces, vif argent un unce, fel de pesun de duz eawe deus dragmes, canfer tres dragmes, ceruze demi unce.

Por garir de roigne: Lavez le primes de bone lesive de favaz, pus triblez ensemble peivre et vert de grece et arrement et blanc plum. Si friez en viez oint de porc, si le oignez de ces, et le daubez de miel chescun jor et de jus de cerfel entre les daubes, si garra.

Por garir de gote: Pernez une poignee de cauquetrepe et de herbe ive et de plantein et de matefelun, de chescun demie poigne. Et quesez en .i. jalun de blanc vin duques au terz. Donez li a beivre.

18. ff.325r–330v an incomplete treatise on confession inc. '[Q]ui vodra bel e beaus vestu apparer devant la face Jesu . . .' There are blank spaces for coloured initials which were never entered. Folio 329 is blank.

The versified receipts on ff.1ra–21rb represent a compilation known as the *Physique rimee* (see ll. 877, 1296) which has been studied by Professor Faribault.[13] The work is popular, designed to introduce those who have no Latin (l. 86) to the useful properties of herbs and plants the names of which may already be familiar to them. The translator observes that we are apt to take for granted what is commonly and freely available, but that common plants are greatly appreciated by those who know their true properties, for almost everyone, at some time or another, will be in need of them or benefit from them. The work is therefore a translation: 'En romauns dirai le latin' (l. 83), 'Ke en romauns l'ai translaté' (l. 89). Throughout the collection there are references to 'la lettre' (ll.200, 1194, 1328) and 'l'escrit' (ll.506, 1113, 1391, 1516, 1583), 'le livre' (ll.357, 971, 1580) and a written source which the translator had before him (ll.377, 632, 966). On one occasion (ll.1161f) the translator even refers to his own testing of a remedy. The written source was most probably various sets of Latin receipts from which the compiler made a selection. There is little obvious debt to the 'Lettre d'Hippocrate' or to that other versified collection, the 'Novele Cirurgerie'.[14] A few receipts are found in Peter of Spain's *Thesaurus pauperum*. Lines 165–280 represent a set of receipts which are found, reworked and 'derhymed' in an MS at Cambrai published by Amédée Salmon.[15] Extensive portions (ll.399–558, 1223–84, 1291–96, 1301–14, 1449–66, 1561–1658) are found in what appears to be a fragment of the same treatise in MS Cambridge, Trinity College 0.8.27 pt 3 (s.xiii[2]) ff.1ra–3ra which I have already published.[16] The whole text is also found in MS Cambridge, St Johns College D. 4 ff.83rb–99rb (see below). Other receipts are found individually in the collections contained in MSS Sloane 146 and Sloane 3550, and elsewhere.

In turn, the 'Physique rimee' was used by others. In the 14th C. Jean Sauvage, a native of Picquigny in Picardy and domiciled in Blois, translated the *Thesaurus pauperum* into French octosyllables, interpolating receipts from the 'Letter d'Hippocrate' and from a compilation very similar to the present one.[17] Three MSS survive, all of the 15th C. two of which are very closely related. Whilst retaining the verse form for two thirds of his work, Jean finally moved into prose, the quicker to dispatch his work. He freely acknowledged the 'Physique rimee' as one of his sources and his annexation of the prologue to that work: 'de la Physique rimee/ qui d'un autre fut translatee / vuil asseoir a ceste foiz / le prologue ci, quar c'est droiz'.

I list below the lines and distribution of receipts according to the various ailments. To begin with the collection follows the standard pattern *a capite ad calcem*, but rapidly becomes more random in its ordering of the receipts, like the 'Novele Cirurgerie'.

97–158	5 receipts dealing with vertigo and headache
159–280	15 receipts dealing with ocular complaints
281–344	10 receipts concerning diseases of the ear
345–398	6 receipts dealing with dental problems
399–456	5 receipts concerning vomiting
457–472	1 receipt for putting on weight
473–480	1 receipt for slimming
481–490	1 receipt concerning worms in children
491–554	6 receipts dealing with constipation
555–558	1 receipt dealing with a burst blood vessel
559–604	8 receipts concerning diarrhoea
605–630	4 receipts dealing with the fig which produces diarrhoea
631–704	5 receipts dealing with varieties of the fig
705–752	5 receipts concerning gout
753–772	2 receipts for staunching the blood of wounds
773–776	1 receipt for severed nerves
777–810	4 receipts dealing with the extraction of bone etc. from wounds
811–850	2 receipts providing a beverage for curing wounds
851–858	1 receipt dealing with scarring of wounds
867–872	1 receipt for the opening of wounds
873–898	3 receipts for healing wounds
899–912	1 receipt dealing with bone fracture
913–932	1 receipt for opening and cleansing wounds
933–964	2 ointments for wounds
965–1026	8 receipts for healing wounds
1027–1156	14 receipts for malignant tumours
1157–1202	3 receipts offering diagnostic tests for the differenciation of sores and tumours
1203–1222	a set of precautions for surgical intervention
1223–1246	4 receipts dealing with urinary problems
1247–1290	3 receipts for the stone
1291–1296	1 receipt dealing with incontinence
1297–1300	1 receipt concerning the kidneys
1301–1370	7 receipts concerning various fevers
1371–1386	1 receipt for confusion and loss of memory
1387–1426	6 receipts concerning hoarseness
1427–1448	1 receipt for inflammation of the liver
1449–1538	4 receipts for the fig
1539–1560	5 receipts for the staunching of blood
1561–1582	1 receipt for bleeding the patient
1583–1598	4 miscellaneous receipts concerning tumours
1599–1620	2 receipts concerning the delivery of a stillborn child
1621–1634	1 receipt for slimming
1635–1642	1 receipt for a substitute for nurse's milk
1643–1654	1 receipt for a soporific
1655–1658	1 receipt concerning swelling of the breasts
1663–1670	1 receipt for a depilatory

Notes on pp.366–67

1671–1678	1 receipt for curling hair
1679–1690	1 receipt for curing scurf
1691–1698	1 receipt for restoring hair
1699–1704	1 receipt for dyeing hair black
1705–1710	1 receipt for dyeing hair red
1711–1718	1 receipt for long hair
1719–1730	1 receipt for mange
1731–1744	1 receipt for a lotion for a woman's complexion

The shortest receipt is of 2 lines (ll.1597–98) and the longest of 52 lines (ll.1467–1518). The receipts are sometimes copied with a rubric *Autre* which is misleading in the new context in which the receipt has been included. For example, lines 1655–1658 headed *Autre* are not a soporific remedy, as indicated by *Por dormir* in the preceding remedy, but a treatment for painful and swollen breasts. The scribe has taken over *Autre* from his source.

The same problem occurs in the other, apparently complete, copy of the *Physique rimee* which I have been able to use. This is found in an important, though unstudied, medical manuscript of the first half of the fourteenth century, MS Cambridge, St John's College D. 4, ff.83rb–99rb.[18] On f.83ra there is a red rubric, as follows: *Incipit liber magistri Petri de Salerno transpositus a latino in romanum ad instanciam Margarum [corr. Margarete?] Fregille regine Yspanie de omnibus op[in]ionibus universorum magistrorum tunc salerine [corr. Salernie] commorancium.* This is followed by a short prose text in Old French on the four humours, the periods of their principal activity, and the salient effects which they exercise on the disposition of humans. Salvatore de Renzi, working from a copy furnished by Charles Daremberg, argued not only that the prose section was a translation of the treatise *De quatuor humoribus ex quibus constat humanum corpus*, which he had himself published, but that the succeeding set of versified remedies was essentially a rendering of the *Practica Petrocelli* attributed to a Salernitan physician.[19] This second claim is certainly false and seems to have been induced by the resemblance of a couple of receipts near the beginning of both works.[20] The verse text in the St John's MS is not preceded by any rubric, but begins with a large blue initial on f. 83rb. In this copy there is a larger number of receipts, often in a different order from that in MS Trinity O.1.20, with different rubrics, and including receipts which, whilst not found in MS O.1.20, are found in the fragment contained in MS Trinity O.8.27 which I have already published. Any future attempt to produce a full critical edition of the *Physique rimee* must involve a close examination of the St John's text, even though it contains many errors. I therefore provide a synopsis of its contents by citing the line numbers of MS O.1.20 and printing the rubrics offered by the St John's copy.

1–78	
79–96	(blue initial)
97–120	(*Autre medicine*)
121–40	(*Autre medicine*)
141–54	
155–58	(*A jaune cheveleure*, misplaced from next receipt)
f.84rb/va	new receipt of 14 lines – see Appendix
1699–1704	(*Autre medicine*)
1731–44	(*Bone laveure*)
1711–18	(*Pur ciruns*)
1719–30	(*Pur la grate e le manjue*)

1679–90	(*A ceus ki sunt teignus*)
1691–98 (+2)	(*As places u le peile defaut*)
1663–70	(*Ki voet fere letire*)
1671–78	(*A crespe chevelure*)
159–64	(*As oiz vermaus*)
165–70	(*Pur chacie*)
171–74	(*Autre medicine*)
175–86	
187–92	(*Pur la veue esclarir*)
193–96	(*Autre medicine*)
197–200	(*Pur la manjue*)
201–12 (+6)	(*Pur ciruns*)
213–24	(*Pur mal puis*)
257–66	(*Autre medicine*)
225–34	(*Autre medicine*)
235–42	(*Pur la maele*)
243–56	(*Autre medicine*)
267–72	(*A la m[a]elie*)
273–80	(*Pur malades oilz*)
ff. 85vb–86vb	cosmetic receipts - see Appendix
281–86	(*A dure oie*)
287–90	(*Autre medicine*)
291*–94*	(*Autre medicine*; different verses from MS 0.1.20)
295–98	
299–302	(*Autre medicine*)
307–16	(*Autre medicines*)
317–26 (+2)	(*Autre medicine*)
327–30	(*Autre medicine*)
331–44	(*Autre medicine*)
345–50	(*Encontre dolor de denz*)
351–54	(*Autre medicine*)
355–60	(*Autre medicine*)
361–64	(*Autre medicine*)
365–68	(*Autre medicine*)
369–74	(*Autre medicine*)
375–94	(*Pur denz enblanchir*)
395–98	(*Autre medicine*)
ff. 87vb–91ra	new receipts incl. T 1–192 – see Appendix
399–416	(*Pur home ki ad vumchesuns*)
417–26	(*Autre medicine*)
427–38	(*Ki voet aver medicine*)
439–44	(*Autre medicine*)
445–56	(*Autre medicine*)
457–72	(*Pur engrossier*)
473–80	(*Pur amegrer*)
481–90	(*A vermes dedenz le cors*)
1223–30	(*Pur estaler*)
1291–6 + 1231–8	(*Ki ne pot tenir sun estal*)
1239–44	(*Ki sanc estalent*)
1247–84	(*Ki ad peres en la vessie*)
1561–86	(*Pur le brace emflé*)
1587–90 + T 379–84	(*Autre medicine*)
1591–98	(*Autre medicine*)
1621–34	(*Pur damiseles saner*)

Notes on pp.366–67

1635–42	(Pur let a la norise)
1643–54	(Pur ben dormir)
1655–58	(As mameles)
1449–64	(Pur meneisun)
1599–1606	(Femme ki travail de enfant)
1607–20	(Autre medicine)
491–508	(Por encoistivure)
509–16	(Autre medicine)
519–54	(A solucion)
555–58	(A veine rumpé)
1301–14	(A fevre ague)
1315–18	(Uncore)
1319–28	(Autre medicine)
1329–34	(A fevre terciene)
1335–44	(A fevre cotidiene)
1345–58	(A fevre quartaine)
1359–70	(Pur fevre ague)
559–72	(Por meneisun)
573–78	(Autre medicine)
579–82	(Autre medicine)
583–86	(Autre medicine)
587–604	(Autre medicine)
705–32	(Por gute)
733–36	(Autre medicine)
737–42	(A gute aiguere)
743–52	(Oignement)
995–1008	(Entrait a plaie)
1009–14	(A la plaie ki ne veut saner)
753–60	(Pur estancher)
761–72	(Pur bature)
773–76	(A nerfs)
777–86	(A plaie munder)
787–96	(Bone entrait a plaie)
797–810	(Autre medicine)
811–50	(Bone boivre a plaie)
851–66	(A sursaneure)
867–72	(blue initial)
873–98	(Emplastre)
899–912	(A os fraint)
1371–78	(Ki pert sa memorie)
1379–86	(Autre medicine)
1073–76	(Al cancre)
1077–88	(Autre medicine)
1089–98	(Autre medicine)
1027–46	(Autre medicine)
1047–54	(Autre medicine)
1055–72	(Autre medicine)
1099–1114	(A cancre e a festre)
1115–22	(Autre medicine)
1125–30	(Pur cancre occire)
1131–34	(A gute festre)
1135–40	(Autre medicine)
1141–56	(Autre medicine)
1157–72, 1181–1222 + 1467–1512	(Autre medicine)

Notes on pp.366–67

1513–18	(*Autre medicine*)
1519–30	(*Autre medicine*)
1531–38	(*Autre medicine*)
697–704	(*Autre medicine*)
605–10	(*Al fie ke dune meneisun*)
611–14 + 4	(*Autre medicine*)
615–30	(*Autre medicine*)
631–56	(*Diverseté*)
657–74	(*Al fie ki fet emfler*)
675–84	(*Autre medicine*)
685–96	(*Autre medicine*)
913–32	(*A pleie overir*)
933–58	(*Oignement*)
959–64	(*Entrait*)
965–70	(*Beivre al plaie*)
971–88	(*Autre medicine*)
989–94	(*Autre medicine*)
1387–92	(*Autre medicine*)
1393–1402	(*Autre medicine*)
1403–10	(*Autre medicine*)
1411–20	(*Autre medicine*)
1421–26	(*Autre medicine*)
f.98vb	new receipt – see Appendix
1427–36 + 2	(*Pur eschaufisun*)

The *Physique rimee* is now followed (ff.99rb–100va) by a set of prose receipts in Anglo-Norman drawn from the 'Lettre d'Hippocrate',[21] ending with an explicit in red: *Explicit expliciat nobilis autor erat.*[22]

Qui cest livre vodra entendre   f.1ra
Bele raison il porreit aprendre,
Plusors choses il porreit oir
4   Ki mult font bien a retenir.
Ce vous di jo por cors humain
Ki longes ne poet estre sain,
Ne dure gueres en saunté,
8   Kar itele est sa qualité,
Le fais de quatre helemens,
De fu, de ewe, de tere et vens.
Ceus quatre que ci vous acont
12   De tele manere ensemble sont
Ke il sont entr'eus si muable
Ke il ne poent estre estable.
Le fu si degaste et confunt,
16   Ce sevent ceus ki veu l'ont;
De l'ewe vous dirai le voir,
En travail est jor et soir;
Le vent est en travail sovent
20   Et la tere, si com jo entent;   f.1rb
En travail sunt en tel endroit,
Chaut sunt, secche, moiste et froit.
Entr'eus a grant diversetés
24   Et si covient adversetés,
Divers maus et enfermetés
Dont mainte gent sont engrotés.
Vous entendez bien qu'ensi vait,
28   Mes Deus encontre ce nus fait
Mult grant solaz et grant confort,
Ke il garist maint home de mort
Par herbes, bien est coneu,
32   Ou Deus a mis grant vertu,
Chaudes et moistes, douces, ameres,
[. . .]
Ki bien la force conustroit
36   A maint home valer porroit.
Herbes ont mult tresgrant vertu
De bois, de pré et de palu,
Semence, flors, fuile, racine,
40   Mult par valent a medicine.

[J = MS Cambridge, St John's College D.4.]

[1] The prologue is found in the *réceptaire* of Jean Sauvage, see C. de Tovar, 'Contamination
. . .' (1974), pp.171–3. | [6] MS *poët*; gueres n.p. (J) | [9] Si est fait (J) | [17] de
verrur (J) | [19] forment (J) | [24] Pur ceo en vent a. (J) | [27] MS *que ce suhait*; b.
coment ceo vet (J) | [31] Ce sunt herbes, b.e. su (J) | [34] The missing line appears in
MS Paris, B. N. fr.1319 (see Tovar, *supra*) as *Seichez froidez maintez manierez* and in J as *Freides
seches muz de maneres*. | [35] conoistre les saveroit (J)

Maintes herbes poez voir
Ke multes maus poent garir.
Les herbes conustre poez,
44   Mes lor vertus pas ne savez.   f.1va
Voir poez des herbes plusors,
Foilles, semences et flors,
Vous ne savez lor qualitez
48   Ne lor vertuz ne lor bontez.
Et vous, por quei les priseroiez
Kant vous sol lor nons conusez?
Avis vous est n'ont nul poir
52   Kant chescun home les poet avoir.
Quant est plus chier achatee,
Tant est de vous plus desiree.
Eles crescent en bois et en prés,
56   En voies, en sentes et en blés.
Par ces fossés et par ces haies
Les troveras, poor nen aies.
Il i a homes plus de mil
60   Que por lor plenté les tenent vil,
Ke mult encrescent et tauns sont,
Les grant plentés plus viles ont,
Mes por ce qu(i)'il i a tauntes
64   Ne sont eles mie meins vaillauntes,
Ne le meins ne sont verteuses,
Profitables ne precioses.   f.1vb
Cil ki conust lor maneres
68   Les tient a bones et a chieres,
Mes cil qui la vertu ne siet
Ne poet chaloir si il les aime ou hiet.
Si n'est nul home al mien viaire
72   Ki n'ait de medicine afaire,
Ou por son ami ou por soi
Ou por aucun autre, come jo croi.
Mult vaut a proiser lor savoyr
76   Ke vous poet a bosoine valoyr,
Sen et savoir et riche fais,
Kar grant bien avienent aprés.
Ore vous voil par tant mostrer
80   Ke ai enpensé a translater,
Ce seroit eslit et scient

---

[42] A mult maus solen valere (J) | [49–50] om. (J; B.N. fr.1319) | [51] J inserts
before this line Nus est avis ki i ne sunt pruz /pur ce ki i sunt conuz a tuz. | [53–4] om. (J; B.
N. fr.1319) | [58] en herberes en places (J) en herbiers et en plasseis (B.N. fr.1319) |
[62] La multitude confunt (J) | [77] Bon est saver nest fes (J) Sens et savour n'est mie fes
(B.N. fr.1319) | [79] Blue initial (J) | [81–2] Ce ki truis en esperimenz / ki vaudrunt a
plusors de genz (J) |

Qui mult vaudroit a plusor gent.
En romauns dirai le latin,
84   Puis l'escrivrai en parchemin,
Ke plusors le puissent aprendre
Que ne sevent latin entendre.
Et si aucun home a envie
88   Qu(i)'il por ce de mai meisdie   f.2ra
Ke en romauns l'ai translaté,
Jo li dirai la verité.
Mon sen demostrer mult m'est bon
92   Et si li plaist, ce est bien saison;
Si envie a et il me hiet,
Moi ne chaut gueres, Deus le siet,
Kar en tele chose me delit
96   Ke tornera a graunt profit.

POR VERTIN

Por le vertin pernez la rue
O l'ere terrestre creue,
Triblez le bien, pressez le jus
100   Tant que ne poez traire plus.
Pernez miel et aubon de oef
Et un drap linge, viel ou noef,
Bien l'emplastrez, ne vous soit grief,
104   Si le metez sor vostre chief.

AUTRE

Autre medicine ai ici trovee
Ki de plusors est mult loe[e],
Dauns Galiens le nous tesmoigne.
108   En le mois de mai pernez vetoigne,   f.2rb
Triblez le, si li donez le jus
Plaine coupe ou auques plus.
Taunt com li mois de mai dura,
112   Guns usez, mult vous vaudra.
Tauns en faites cel mois quillier
Ke tot l'an le pussés tenir.
Et si vous verde les coillez,
116   En ewe cliere les boillés.
Vostre chief en faites laver,

[82] MS *vaudront*. | [91] Mun sen me lest ben amostrer / si en vie en ait ou il m'en het (J) | [97] Decorated initial. There is no rubric, but a post-medieval hand has written 'pour le vertin'. See MS Sloane 146 (hereafter S) no. 35 below, p.272 | [98] MS *ere enterre*. B. N. fr.1319 has l'erre de la terre. | [105] Decorated initial. | [107] En nostre escrit le testimonie (J) [110]   P. gubulet en plus (J) |

A graunt saunté vous poet torner.
Si ceste herbe volez secchir,
120   Tot l'an en poez estuer.

AUTRE

Rue et ierre pernez ensemble,
Aisil et oile, ce mai semble.
Vous devez tot ce assembler
124   Et de ce vostre chief laver.

AUTRE

Qui long tens a eu vertin
Mener le covient [a] dure fin.
Ore dirai mon conseil a ceus:
128   Tous facent riere lor cheveus,
Rue et vetoine facent coillir,
O vin egre en un pot boillir,
Al chief le doit om lier si chaut,
132   Boivre vetoine qui mult vaut,   f.2va
Ovec blaunc vin destempré soit,
Sages est ke geuns le boit.
Et si por taunt li mal [ne] fine,
136   Pernez de orge bele ferine,
A aisil fetes une emplastre,
Ne sera mie quit en astre,
Mes issi creu au chief soit mis,
140   Ensi porra estre garis.

AUTRE

Ki vertin a et mal el chief
Longues soffrir li est mult grief.
Il se doit sovent por cel mal
144   Seigner del veine capital
Et de son pié del gros ortel
Face seiner, ce li conseil.
En oscurté tresbien se gart
148   Tous les .iii. jors desi ke au quart,
En pais et en tranquillité,
Por nulle rin ne soit irré.
E si li defent a juner,
152   Qui le cervel fait troubler.

[119] secher (J) [120] estoier (J) | [121] Decorated initial. | [125] Decorated initial.
| [128] Ki sacent oster l.c. (J) | [134] Sein est (J) | [141] Decorated initial. | [146]
Tel seignur crat ki seit feis (J) | [147] En nostre cure t.s.g. (J) |

Glossary on pp.403–12

User doit itele viande   f.2vb
Come sa nature demande.
Foilles de saus et de popler
156 Mete en le sac de son orilier.
Graunt bien le fra le flaour
Ki assuage tel dolour.

AS EUZ LERMAUNS

As euz lermauns pernez la rue
160 Qui soit bien triblé et batue,
De une chievre pernez le fiel,
O tot ice si metez miel.
O une penne as euz li metez
164 A nuit quant vus coucherez.

POR CACHIE . . .

Vous por cachie ensement
Prendrez fenoil et arrement
E chievrefoil et miel et vin,
168 Triblez tot en un basin.
Parmi un drap bien le colés,
As euz le metés quant vous vodrés.

AUTRE

De celidoine me pernez,
172 O let de femme le mellez,
Ce garist lé euz cacheus,   f.3ra
Le manjue tout a estrous.

AS EUZ TENDRES

A tendres euz et a chalor
176 Ki de legier suffrent dolor
Le planteine o l'aisil triblés,
Le jus aprés fors me pressés.
L'aubun de l'oef metez o tot,
180 Ce garira les euz de bot.
Que vous diroi jo plus?
Le lin metez ens en cel jus.
La nuit quaunt vous coucherés

[155] J has red rubric A jaune cheveleure misplaced from 1699 which follows 158. | [156]
le teie d.s.o. (J) | [165ff] See Salmon, art. cit. no.10 and S no. 202 | [170] MS vodra |
[177ff] See Salmon no.10 (om. 174) | [175ff] See Salmon no.11 (om. 176). No rubric in
J. |

184   Vos euz de ce emplastrirés.
        Et ce vaut mult encontre calor
        Et encontre cachie et dolor.

        POR CLIER VEUE AVER

        A ceus ki ont trouble la veue:
188   Pernés fenoil et pernés rue,
        Pernez de la pertris le fiel,
        O tot ice si metés miel.
        A une penne degotés
192   Es euz quant couchier vodrés.

        AUTRE   f.3rb

        Uncore por autretele paine:
        Pernés le jus de la vervaine,
        Od let de femme le mellés
196   Et en vos euz le degotés.

        AUTRE

        Si vous avez es euz manjue,
        Si pernez celidoine et rue,
        Le jus devez en vos euz metre,
200   Si garirés, ce dit la lettre.

        POR SOIRONS

        Ki as chies des euz a soirons
        Si face ce que nos dirons:
        Un oef dur quit chaut doit peler
204   Et de un coutel quartilier.
        Aiez .i. drap linge aparillé,
        Blaunc et net et delié,
        As euz le doit mettre plus prés,
208   Puis le quarter aprés
        Si chaut com plus porra soffrir
        Et sor les euz doit tenir.
        Oez come la medecine vaut,
212   Les soirons istront por le chaut.

[187ff] See Salmon no.12. J has red rubric *Pur la veue esclarir*. | [193ff] See Salmon no.13
| [197ff] See Salmon no.14 | [201ff] See Salmon no.15. J has red rubric *Pur ciruns*. |
[201] Si as surcilz avera ciruns (J) | [210] sur les cilz (J) | [212] J adds six lines: Le drap
escuez as (as) charbuns / si orrez crustre les ciruns / ke ciruns i sunt mar / i manjuent la mort

AUTRE

Vermine i a de autre manere[s],
As chies sont et as paupieres,
Les euz lor enfle et manjue   f.3va
216   Et mult empirent la char nue.
Les euz lor covient froter,
Il ne se poent deporter.
Jo li dirai que m'en crera
220   Par quele medicine i[l] garra.
Pernez saugemme et arrement
Et bon aisil tot ensement,
Iceste emplastre metez i,
224   Si garrez, jo le vous di.

POR CACHIE ET ROJOR

Une medicine ai ici trovee
Ke de plusors est mult loee
Encontre cachie et roujor,
228   Encontre manjue et dolor.
Pernez freses en tens d'esté
Et bon miel chaut et escumé,
Ensemble les devez meller,
232   La goute en devés puis coler.
Icele goute es euz metez,
Si avra beus euz et cliers assés.

AUTRE

Autre medicine dire voil:
236   Cil ki la maile avra en l'oil
Et garis veut estre et delivre   f.3vb
Face batre gingimbre et poivre.
O sanc de anguile ou de fiel
240   Soit bien mellé trestot uwel,
Ou o le fiel de la partris,
Si ert hastivement garis.

AUTRE

Iceus qui l'ont eu grant pece
244   Si doivent prendre verdegrece
Mult delié et mult menu,

char / si od vos veez asez / de gent ki ont oilz verflez. | [213ff] See Salmon no.16. J has red
rubric *Pur mal puis*. | [215] Le cil suremfle (J) | [216] la veue (J) | [225ff] See Sal-
mon no.18. | [235ff] See Salmon no.19. J has red rubric *Pur la maele*. | [243ff] See
Salmon no. 20. |

Glossary on pp.403–12

Avaunt doit estre bien molu.
Ensemble soit tot amassé,
248 Parmi .i. drap delié passé
Plus menu que nule ferine.
Mellé soit o oint de geline,
En .i. bacin sor les carbons
252 Sera faite la confision.
Aprés ert mise por estuer
En .i. vassel de esteim por meuz garder.
Pernez ent quant il vous ert mester
256 [. . .]

AUTRE

Uncore dirai autre medicine
Ki mult est bone et fine
Encontre chacie et dolor
260 Ke tient es euz nuit et jor.   f.4ra
L'aluigne un petit me batez,
A les pauperes le metez
Et issi longuement i soit
264 Ke il eschaufe, ce est droit.
Dormez aprés, si reposez,
En le demain gari serrez.

POR LA MAILE ENCLOSE

Et por la maile que est enclose
268 Covient mult corosive chose.
Une linge csince pernez,
Sor une coigne la ardez.
L'oile que en ist pernez ataunt,
272 En l'oil le(i) metez meintenaunt.

BEIVRE POR LA MAILE

Por cel mal fait om .i. boivre
Ke la maile perce et desço[i]vre.
Eufrase, porpé et la termine,
276 Rue, vetoigne et tormentine,
Fetes icés prendre et coilir,

---

[252] confectiun (J) | [254] om. (J) [256] om. (J) | [257ff] See Salmon no.17. | [258] vaillant e f. (J) | [259] chalur (J) | [260] Ben garrir home sanz dolur. | [261] Le lowe entier pernez (J) | [267ff] See Salmon no. 21. | [269–70] Une linge coigne le ardez (J) | [273ff] See Salmon no. 21. | [274] depart e deseivre (J) | [275] Eufraise pinpre e la t. (J) |

En cervoise ou en vin boilir.
Donez cest boivre que vaut
280   Au matin froit, au vespre chaut.   f.4rb

POR CLIER OIR

As orailes de dure oie
Ke clierement nen oient mie:
Pernés urine de sengler
284   Et arrement o miel medler,
En l'oraile le degotés,
Si garis est tost, le saverés.
Et si il a escorcheure
288   En l'oraile par aventure,
L'urine metez d'un enfaunt,
Il garra solement par taunt.

AUTRE

Autre dirai; pernés beu miel
292   Et de un motun pernez le fiel,
O let de femme le mellés,
En les orailes le degotés.

AUTRE

Le jus pernés de la canelie,
296   Chaut le metés chescune fie,
Si ver i a, cil l'oscira
Et la dolor essuagera.

AUTRE

De vetoigne devés tribler
300   Et le jus un poi reposer.
Laine pernés, si le moillés,
En l'oreille puis le metés.   f.4va

AUTRE

De çaneson le jus pernés,
304   En l'oraille le degotés,

[281] The rubric in J reads A dure oie. | [287] J has red rubric Autre medicine. | [291–4]
Replaced in J by Pernez un herbe en sa seisun / ki l'em apele pie de liun / le jus de l'herbe
premes loes / e de formies pernez les oes / parmi un net drap cuillez / en le oriel degutez. The
rubric is Autre medicine. | [302] En les orielles degutez (J) | [303–6] om. (J) |

Glossary on pp. 403–12

Le ver oscira, ja nen doutés
[. . .]

AUTRE

As orailles qui dedens sonent,
308 Avis est a plusors que il tounent:
 Les branches de freine ardez,
 L'ewe que en ist me retenez,
 Jus de jubarbe autretant
312 Et vin o tot mult avenant,
 Saim de anguille i covient
 Ki mult bien sa vertu i tient,
 Es orailles le degotés,
316 Par itaunt recevra sauntés.

AUTRE

Dirai vous autre medicine
 Ke mult est vaillaunt et fine.
 Pernés l'oignon, si le eschufés
320 Et mult del miel dedens metés,
 Sor la brese le metés quire.
 Puis le premés com om fet cire,
 Mult tenuement et bien et bel
324 Le colés parmi un drapel,
 Et le nuit quaunt vous couchés   f.4vb
 En l'oraille le degoutés.

AUTRE

Si en l'oraille a nule vermine,
328 Je vous en dirai la medicine.
 Let d'ive i metés et aisil,
 Si garra de cel peril.

AUTRE

Il i a plusors acheisons
332 Par quei vienent les sordeissons.
 L'ewe entre ens et si remaint,
 Par quei meint home se plaint.
 Il i a vers come sirons
336 Mult petis, ne sont gueres longs,

---

[308] est is a superscript insertion by the scribe. | [319] sil me cavez (J) | [330–1] not separated in J. | [336] Un spiez (J) |

Ou il i a escorcheure
Por quei il est par aventure.

AUTRE

Si ordure i a, si l'entraiés,
340   Delivrement gari serrés.
Quaunt l'oraille est estopee,
Ne poet estre de leger sanee
Si cele ordure ne soit traite
344   Ke cele sordison a faite.

POR DOLOR DE DENS

Medicine contre dens dolor: f.5ra
Dé petis maus est la greinor.
Pernés racines de plantain,
348   Maschés les bien, si serés sain;
Ou noir soffoigne ov aisil,
Ce vaut encontre tel peril.
Pernés plauntaine et net le lavés
352   Et o siu de moton le destemprés.
Le face oignés de cele part,
Les vers istront, mult li ert tart.

[AUTRE]

Fetes autre medicine bele:
356   Pernés del lievre la cervele;
Si cum le livre nous endite,
Ele doit estre mult bien quite.
Endroit le mal oigniés adés
360   Et li vers morrunt tost aprés.

[AUTRE]

Un autre vous voil enseigner:
Pernés les foilles del pescher
Et finegrec quit et triblee,
364   Al mal soit mis et emplastré.
Puliol en vin boilliés
Et en la bouche le tenés.
A cele dolor por medicine   f.5rb

[338] U play ki seit (J) | [338–9] not separated in J. | [346] le peur (J) | [350–1] separated in J by red rubric *Autre medicine*. | [361] Uncore v. pusi e. (J) | [364–5] separated in J by red rubric *Autre medicine*. | [365] Pelester (J) | [367] Par le dolur del mal medicine (J) |

Glossary on pp.403–12

368   Poés bien faire gargarime.

AUTRE

Une herbe pernés que a non bete,
La racine me fetes nette,
Si le metés al mal de dent,
372   Mult vous vaudra a mien escient.
Ele en trera si graunt humor
Ke assuagera la dolor.

POR DENS ENBLANCHIER

Si home veut ses dens enblanchir
376   Et longuement blanches tenir,
Medicines truis ci escrites.
Les escales de nois petites
[A] poudre faites batre et moudre,
380   Puis pernés les foilles de coudre
Et mastic i mete om atot,
Si bien frotés les dens o tot.
Sor la foille la poudre metés,
384   Aprés vos dens bien frotés.
La nuit quant vous coucherés
Vostre bouche mult bien frotés,
L'endemain a vostre lever
388   Bouche et dens devés bien laver.   f.5va
Ce ostera le lumor des dens,
Si seront cliers come vif argent.
Chescun jor aprés manger
392   Tot sauz respit et sauns danger
De lange drap bien les frotés,
Net seront si cest us tenés.

AUTRE

Pernés ferine de orge et sel
396   Et mel metés i tot uwel,
Bon aisil soit ovesques mellé,
Les dens seront bien frotés.

ENCONTRE VOMIR

Cil qui avra vonques sovent

---

[369] amblete (J) | [379] Pernez si fetes b. (J) | [381] E le siel ars metez o tut (J) |
[385–6] om. (J) | [389] le limiun de d. (J) | [390] E mundre cum fiv argent (J) |
[399–490] correspond to MS Cambridge, Trinity College 0.8.27 (hereafter T), ll.193–280
in the edition of T. Hunt, *Romania* 106 (1985), [57–83], 66ff. | [399] MS *auques.* J has red

400   Et de vomir li prent talent
       Viaunde li siet mauveisement
       Qui il ne trove savourement;
       Ce fait le desdeing del ventrail.
404   De bon conseil doner ne fail:
       Por oster del ventrail le glette
       De humor porrie qui n'est pas nette
       Pernés aluigne ovesques rue
408   Et lovasche bien parcreue,
       En cervoise bien le quisés,   f.5vb
       Chaut le devés boivre, tot seras haités.
       Au chief de .viii. jors seras tot sain
412   Si bevés aloigne l'endemain.
       Au soir le bevés et au matin
       Et poliol flairaunt et fin.
       Tauntost com vous volés diner
416   Bon vin si devés user.

AUTRE

       Jubarbe et fenoil me pernés,
       Triblés le jus et espremés,
       Et puis si aiés bel miel quis
420   Ki o cest jus doit estre mis.
       Les .ii. pars deit estre del jus,
       De miel la tierce part ou plus.
       Aprés le laissés quire taunt
424   Que espés veigne en boillaunt,
       Et quaunt vous devés aler coucher,
       Si devés user un plein quiller.

AUTRE

       Ki veut aver bone vomite
428   Jo li dira[i] bone et eslite:
       Triblés evele et pernés del jus
       Pleins sis escales de oef ou plus,   f.6ra
       De clier saim de porc les treis,
432   Greins de peivre sinquante et treis,
       Et de gingembre la racine,

rubric *Pur home ki ad vunchesuns.* | [401–2] om. (T) Kar e li savur nient (J) | [404] A co covent prendre conseil (TJ) | [406] E le ordure ki n'est pas nette (TJ) | [407] P. a. anet e rue (TJ) | [408] lovasche corrected by scribe from lovesche (J, luvesche) | [410] Eissi chaudet le bevez (TJ) | [411–14] Aluisgne bevet l'endemain / e poliol serra sain / beivet al seir e al matin / descreaunt sei de pain e de vin (dejune seit de p. e de v, J) (TJ) | [415–6] om. (TJ) | [421] deivent (T) | [425] Encontre co ke hom deit cucher (T, hom om.) J) | [427ff] See S no. 55 below. J has red rubric *Ki voet aver medicine.* | [429] eble (J) l'eble (T) | [432] Cinquante g. de p. al meins (T) Cinkant g. de peivre (J) |

Molue soit come ferine.
Ensemble seient assemblé
436 Et mult bien quit et escumé.
Puis le devra chaut user
Ki bien se vodra delivrer.

AUTRE

Une autre qui n'est mie fause:
440 Faites une mult bone sause,
Sor le feu le faites boillir,
Bien escumer et puis refroidir.
Aukes chaut le devés user
444 Si bien vous vodrés delivrer.

AUTRE

Uncore vous dirai une,
Legere et aukes commune:
De seuz pernés l'entrerus,
448 A un coutel raés jus,
Od ewe chaude puis l'usés,
Bon vomite i prendrés,
Vomite o(d) solucion,
452 Si vous faites par raison.   f. 6rb
Si vous volés qu(i)'il vom[it]e doint,
Donc reés le contre mont,
Si vous aval le reés,
456 Bone solucion averés.

AUTRE

A megre home ou a femme esclendre
Por engrassier devés entendre:
Le fenugrec devés seccher,
460 Puis en un morter fruisser.
La poudre metés od ferrine
De pur forment et bele et fine,
Et une herbe que ad nun afodillus
464 Triblés, si empressés le jus.
O ce si me pernés anis

---

[434] En pudre fet c. f. (TJ) | [436] escure (J) | [443] Chaudet le devra puis user (T) Chaude le deit puis user (J) | [444] Ki bien se voldra d. (TJ) | [445ff] See Salmon no. 44 and S no. 56 below. | [447] MS *p. les tendrons* cf. 889. Salmon no. 44 also has tenrons. | [450] verrez (T) averez (J) | [453] Si volez ki vomist deiust (J) | [457] J has red rubric *Pur engrossier*. | [458] engrosir (T) | [462] Flur de f. (TJ) |

Glossary on pp.403–12

Et mastic si seit ovec mis.
Tot pastisiés a vostre main,
468   Bien broiés come om fait pain.
Puis seit bien quit et essuiés,
Cest pain e[s]t bon, bien le sachés.
Qui l'usera solonc reson
472   Gras serra com porc en pesson.

POR AMEGRIER

Une autre vous puis bien aprendre   f.6va
Ki fet home megre et esclendre,
Un beivre – qui bien l'usera,
476   Sachés bien, si s'enmegra.
Et saim et gresse et oint
Li vendra trestot a point.
Fenoil, fumitere en ewe quirés,
480   Au seir et au matin le beverés.

[PUR VERMS AS ENFANZ]

Ki vodra aprendre as enfans,
A ceus ki vers norissent ens,
Pernés kersons, si les triblés,
484   Emplastre al numblil metés.
Milfoil boive, quant ce ert fait,
Ki seit destemprés o le lait
De une norice receu,
488   Centoire seit ovesques beu.
Les vers s'en istront finement,
Li enfés garra hastivement.

POR ESCOSTIVEURE

Or vous dirai la dreiture
492   Ke vaut por acosteveure:
Aloine en cerveise boillés,
En la plus vele ke vous troverés,   f.6vb
La flame o tot et miel et bure.

---

[467] Tut le pessez (T) Tut prescez (J) | [468] E bien moulez (TJ) | [472] en seisun (T) p. u p. (J) | [476] Pur veir bien le semblera (semira, J) (TJ) | [477] A curt terme n'i larra point (TJ) | [478] Ne seim ne gresse ne oint (TJ) | [479] fumitere om. (TJ) | [481ff] See S no. 64 below. J has red rubric A *vermes dedenz le cors.* | [481] Ore voil a. (TJ) | [482] Pur verms k'il (ki, J) n. tanz (TJ) | [483] guersun (J) | [487] U la n. la receive (TJ) | [488] E od ço la centorie beive (T) E o c. beive (J) | [490] sauvement (TJ) | [491ff] See S no. 61 below. 491–558 correspond to T 471–534. | [491] dirum (T) dirrum (J) | [494] En cerveise egre e veuz (T) Cerveise fort egre e vieux (JS) | [495] Mellez o.t. (J) |

Glossary on pp.403–12

496   De l'eble pernés a dreiture,
               En un morter bien le triblés.
               Et pernés le jus et colés;
               Treis escales pernés del jus,
500   Une de saim et neient plus.
               Kaunt ert bien quit et escumé,
               Beivre le doit por aver saunté.

AUTRE

               De autre part l'oignon eschaufés
504   Et mult bel miel dedens metés,
               En chaude brese seit bien quit,
               Ce nous enseigne le escrit,
               Cele emplastre metre au numblil
508   Por tost garir de cel peril.

AUTRE

               Pernés clier lard et si taillés
               Un lard(r)on et si l'apareillés,
               De miel l'oinés et bel et gent.
512   Puis aiez poudre de arrement,
               Tot environ bien le poudrés,
               En le fundement puis le metés,
               Ileke le lerrés itaunt
516   Ke il remette illekes maintenant.   f.7ra
               Le megue cru li donés a boire,
               Kar de ce poet venir la foire.

AUTRE

               Ki veut aver solucion
520   Entendre deit ceste lesson:
               Le polipode devra prendre
               Et quire taunt ke tot seit tendre
               En bone cerveise novele.
524   Od saim metés en la paiele,
               Ou deus moeus ou .iii. ou .iiii.
               Et en net vassel le deit a jus batre.
               En la manere de chaudel
528   Seit fait et gentement et bel.
               Puis pernés mie de siur pain,

---

[496] MS *Del miel.* | [502–3] not separated in J. | [503] cavez (TJ) | [509ff] See S no. 61 below | [516] Ki jeo remette m. (J) | [517–18] om. (TJS) | [519] J has red rubric A *solucion.* | [520] Si entende (TJ) | [525] Treis moiels d'of prenge u quatre (TJ) | [526] a jus om. (TJ) |

Glossary on pp.403–12

Cil de forment est li plus sain,
Et le miés o cel manger
532   Et le mangés od un quiller.

AUTRE

Ou pernés la grasse geline
Por mieus faire la medicine,
Dedens metés la feukerole
536   Et la quisés tant que ele seit mole.
La geline devés puis prendre
Quant ele ert bien quite et tendre,   f.7rb
Cele [herbe] qui li est el cors
540   Devés coilir et metre fors.
Le grasse bruet devés retenir
Et tote la grasse cuillir.
Beus moeus de oes aiés assés
544   Dont vous le chaudelet ferés,
Et si aiés prest vostre esclice
A la geline coleice.
Sauge mettés en la saveur
548   Et comin por le mieudre odor.
Vostre chaudel humerés,
Puis vostre clistere metterés.

AUTRE

De mauves faites grasse joutes
552   Et puis si les humés trestotes.
Avaunt i metés gresse de porchet,
Mirsau(de) chaude un petitet.

POR VEINE RUMPUE

A veine rompue destreindre
556   Ne se doit om mie feindre.
De porchasser sa garison
Jus de plantaine beive o cresson.

[531] Miez euz quant voldrez manger (TJ) | [532–3] not separated in J. | [538] om. (JS) | [540] bel bro (TJ) | [544] la viande f. (TJ) | [549–50] om. (TJ) | [550–51] not separated in J. | [552] E (om. J) ki la voldra humer tute (TJ) | [553] Enz face quire (TJ) gresse om. (TJ) | [554] Mitsal de char un p. (T) Morsu de char u petite (J) | [555ff] See MS Sloane 3550 (hereafter S1) no. 56 below. | [555] restreindre (J) | [557] Por aver sa g. (TJS1) | [558] P. b. e jus de c. (TS1) P. b. e guersun (J) |

POR MENEISON

| | Ore entendés une reson | f.7va |
| 560 | Ke dirai por la meneison: | |

Icele ferrine prenderés
Ke entour le muele troverés,
Criblee seit et bien passee
564 Et aprés si seit bien bulletee.
Aprés si sera cele flour prise
Et en foille de cholet mise.
Issi deit quire en le brasier,
568 Ce deit le malade manger.

AUTRE

Une autre dirai qui mieus vaut:
Traiés del forn pain tot chaut,
Soupes face en rouge vin,
572 Ce manjue, si garra enfin.

AUTRE

L'arestboef ens el chaump querés,
Triblé sera, puis le quirés,
Puis le versés en une gate,
576 Les piés metés ens au malade.
Taunt com les piés la dedens tendra,
D'aler avaunt talent n'avra.

AUTRE

Ore vous dirai autre medicine:
580 Centoire, estance et tormentine,
Ce beive, si avra saunté, f.7vb
En le noun de la seinte Trinité.

AUTRE

Oncore dirai une autre bele:
584 Il deit beivre le pelu[s]ele
O lait ou o rouge vin fort,
Ce garist meint home de mort.

---

[567] en l'astre (J) | [568] E icel devez puis m. (J) | [568-9] not separated in J. |
[570] T. un pain de flur si c. (J) | [573ff] See S no. 67 below. | [578] Talent de ceo ne
li prendra (J) | [580] esthanche (J) | [583ff] See S no. 68 below. |

AUTRE

Vin rouge en un hanap metés,
588   En .i. autre chaut let pernés,
Et puis si averés .ii. tuaus,
Lé cors metés es .ii. vassaus.
O les tuiaus bevés issi,
592   Tost serés de cel mal gari.
Ou si il soit en tele saison
Que peussés trover boutons,
O lait de chievre les bevés,
596   Si garrirés, ce est voir provés.

AUTRE

Ou pernés grasse veneison
Od le sanc de mult gras moton,
Quit seit et od le grasse fait,
600   Tost garira, pas ne s'emait!

AUTRE

Autre pernés le frés formage
Net et bien fait et de jovene age,   f.8ra
En aisil le face boillir,
604   Ce manjust, si porra garir.

AU FI KI DONE MENEISON

Au fi ki done meneison
Vous dirai bele garison:
Les crotes de cerf devés prendre,
608   Arder et batre tot a cendre,
Cele poudre devés user,
Kar de tel mal vous poet saner.

AUTRE

La teste me pernés del lus,
612   Tous les os gros et les menus,
En .i. nuef pot tous les ardés
Et icele poudre userés.

[589–90] interverted in J. | [588] E autretant 1. repernez (J) | [597ff] See S no. 69
below. 596–7 not separated in J. | [600] Si garra bien mar s'en esmait (seet meat, J) (SJ) |
[601ff] See S no. 70 below. | [601] autre is probably mistakenly imported from an indica-
tion left for the rubricator. | [602] Bel e bien fait que soit (que soit om. J) de vache (SJ) |
[607] La perch de c. (J) | [614] J now adds E l'amerusche es chans quilliez / en une furn
ben le seckez / e poudre fetes frier / e ben garder e estuer. |

AUTRE

Oncore vous dirai plus
616   Ki plusors gent unt mult en us:
Ces poudres totes assemblés
Et o tot ce faisil metés,
Faisil de ce qui est chaü
620   De chaut fer quaunt om l'a batu.
Puis i metés miel par reson
A fere la confision.
Et si bien le volés faire,
624   Mangés de ceste lectuaire;   f.8rb
Par matin pleine une quiller
Devés a une fois manger.

AUTRE

Oncore dirons medicine bele:
628   Anblete pernés e frainele,
Mult bien lé quisés en blaunc vin,
Cest beivre usés au seir et al matin.

POR LE FI ARDAUNT

Multes maneres sont de fi,
632   Si com jo truis escrit ici.
Conustre devés fi ardant
En ceste guise, en cest semblant:
Tot environ il est enflé,
636   Gros et tesi et mult troublé,
Et pulens, rous, li fait router
Ne il ne sei poet delivrer
Deske au tiers jor ou al quart
640   Et donc li est avis qu(i)'il art.
Com espinis li poignent sovent,
Ce li est avis, el fundement.
A cel fi donc issi oez:
644   Semence de caunvre pernez,
Od siu de bouc le pestrisez
En .iii. torteles le(n) feré[s].   f.8va
Et puis si vous estuverés
648   Od chaudes tiules ou o pieres.
Faites une sege cum selette

---

[623] En vin quant averez a fiere (J) | [626–7] not separated in J. | [628] Amplette p. e frasnele (J) | [634] En tele sen (J) | [635] Tut ay iceo este hom e. (J) | [636] Gros et refet e mut casse (J) | [637] E pulenz rus li sait ruter (J) | [644] chenil (J) | [647] voz estues geres (J) | [649] A vostre oes poez fere sechk (J) |

Glossary on pp.403–12

De cel noiel de la carette,
Le un tortel seit en tele manere
652   Mis desor la chaude piere
Ke la chalor peust erraument
Munter desques el fundement.
Quant cest faudra, l'autre pernés
656   Et del tiers autretaunt en frés.

POR FI KI FAIT LE VENTRE EMFLER

Al fi qui fait le ventre enfler
Et le ventrail ruire et broiller:
En .i. pot ourine metés
660   Demi plain, .ix. jors le tenés.
Et une (es)sele aiés percee
Ki desor le pot seit fichee.
Ne serés puis ne fous ne lens,
664   Vos chaudes tiules metés ens,
Le malade deseur s'asese
Nues nages une grant piece.
Aiés donc prest nuef roelettes   f.8vb
668   Ne gueres grans, mes tenuettes,
Li ravenes ou rais a non,
En quareme s'en desjune om.
Pur miel aiés en un vassel,
672   En .i. hanap net et bel.
Les nuef roeles mangera
Totdis com il se estuvera.

POR FI KE FAIT VOMIR

A fi ke fait home vomir
676   Et del manger perdre le desir:
[. . .]
E jus de cou[d]re o tot metés
Et noef plauntes de bel plauntein,
680   Si li enfers desire est[re] sein.
Et bone cerveise boillir
Le doit, puis cole[r] par leisir.
Tous les noef jors le deit puis beivre
684   Si tost saunté veut receivre.

[650] Dedenz u moil de c. (J) | [653] arrement (J) | [658] reure e bugler (J) | [661] sele (J) | [662] pot cele fie (J) | [663] faus (J) | [664] c. peres (J) | [666] Iloc se tienge une p. (J) | [667] celetes (J) | [668] mes petites (J) | [669] De une herbe ki ad a nun raiz (J) | [670] Aces en crest par ces larreis (J) | [673] neueles (J) | [676] MS *pert* (=J) | [677] La cauketrape me pernez (J) | [678] E jus de coudre od ce mettez (J) | [681] Les face laver e cuillir (J) | [682] En bone cerveise buillir (J) |

AUTRE

Al fi qui rent lime el nomblil,
Por tost garir de cel peril:
Quere devés contre le seir
688   Un limaison vif et tot neir.
Al nomblil seit mis et lié;
Si il est l'endemain mangé,   f.9ra
Saver poez ki il est gari
692   De ceste manere de fi.
S'ensi n'est ne ne seit trové
Ke il ne soit mie entamé,
Autre fiez li remetés
696   Desi ke entamé le veés.

POR FI BRO[ÇO]NÉ

Dirai vous ke ai ci trové
Encontre le fi broçoné:
Un fil de seie vaut al mal
700   Et une seie de .i. cheval;
Ensemble mult bien torgiés
Et le broçone mult bien seonés,
Et de ceste medicine garirés.
704   . . .

POR GOUTE GARIR

Mainte fiez issi avient
Ke en aucun leu goute vous tient:
Querés une herbe en la saison
708   Ki kauketrappe a a non,
Triblés le bien, le jus primés,
Et o blaunc vin le destemprés,
Ou od cerveise qui n'a vin.   f.9rb
712   Chaut le beive plain mazelin
Au matin, a noune et au seir;
Encontre goute a graunt poir.

AUT[RE]

Puis pernés de segle ferrine,
716   Kar mult vaut a tele medicine,

[688] Une limance (J) | [693] Si sen est e seit trove (J) | [700] En une pel de cue de c. (J) | [701] l'escorcez (J) | [702] entur liez (J) | [703] Le brocun parmi coupera (J) | [704] E li malade en garra (J) | [705ff] See S no.18 below. | [711] Ou od cervoise ke vin vaut (S) | [712] Un maselin plein en beive chaut (S) | [713–4] om. (JS) | [714–5] not separated in J. | [715ff] See S no.18 below. | [716] Pestre soit od la m. (JS) |

Glossary on pp.403–12

O jus d'evele bien seit pestri
Et de bibuef autresi.
De cé trois torteles freés
720   Et en la brese(s) les quirés.
Quant seront quites, si traiés fors,
La croste desus taillés hors.
Cel tortel chaut al mal metés
724   Et tant longuement li tenés
Ki trestot refroidie sera.
L'autre tortel remetés ja.
Ausi freés du tiers aprés
728   Et si por ce garis n'en es,
Donc quer ke aiés oint de tesson
Ou de butor ou de lion,
Si la goute oignés de cel oint,
732   La goute n'i remaindra point.

AUTRE   f.9va

Ki tost vodra saunté receivre
Si devra polipode beivre,
Vetoine en cerveise ou en vin
736   Devés beivre chescun matin.

[A GOUTE AIUUERE]

A goute aiuuere pernés oés
Et des moeus oile freés.
Neire poiz prendrés e cire et sel
740   Et oint de char ou siu [de] vel.
Tot ce quisés et si le colés,
De une penne le mal oignés.

AUTRE

Ore vous aprendrons ensement
744   A fere .i. mult bon oignement:
Viel oint de ver et burre et mel
Et siu de bouc, puis cire et sel,
La rouge ortie et la sarree,
748   Cerfoil ovec seit ajostee.
Et kersons de ewe pernés

[717] eble (J) eblee (S) | [718] Pus freez ceo ke jeo vus di (SJ) | [719] Deus turtels fere devez (SJ) | [722] om. (J) hostez lors (S) | [724] Tut issi chaut bien le t. (SJ) | [725] E quant cel turtel freit serra (SJ) | [726] soit mis (SJ) | [727] Autrefoiz une pece a. (SJ) | [728] Si ne poez aver reles (SJ) | [733ff] See S no.18 below. | [743ff] See S no.19 below | [747] sacree (J) | [748] C. cigue i seit a. (J) | [749] Le gersun ewage (J) Le

Od les autres les triblés,
Puis seient quit et bien triblee,
752   Ce vaut a meint enfermeté.

POR ESTANCHER PLAIE

Por (plaie) estanche[r] tant mainte plaie
Dont maint ki est nauvrés s'amaie: f.9vb
A ce ne vous obliés mie
756   Les chions de la rouge ortie,
A un cotel tot demincés,
En fort aisil puis lé moillés.
Ki a la plaie ce mettra,
760   La plaie tost estaunchera.

AUTRE

Si home est quassés ne nauvrés
Ke ait membres quassés et froissés,
Prendre devés herbes plusors
764   . . ..
Pernés bugle, pernés confire,
Sanicle n'i seit mie a dire.
Consoude pernez et avaunce
768   Et vetoigne ke mult est franche,
Et lavandre et tanesie
Et osmonde n'obliés mie.
Tot ce en cerveise quisés,
772   Cest beivre usés, s'en sera liés.

POR LES NERS COUPÉS

Cest home qui ait coupé les ners
De tere prenge les gros vers,
Face les trébien esmier
776   Et puis sor la plaie lier.   f.10ra

POR OS PLAIÉ

Si aucun os est remis em plaie

---

kersun ewage (S) | [751] colez (S) cuille (J) | [753ff] See S1 no. 60 below | [753] A
stancher seynante playe (S1J) | [754] ki est om. (SiJ) | [760] Ja un sul gute ne seignera
(J) | [761ff] See S1 no. 61 below. J has red rubric *Pur bature.* | [761] Home ki est batue
u n. (J) | [762] Le membres li dolent assez (J) | [764] Por asuager si grant dolurs (S1J)
 | [768] ke munt l'avance (S1) | [772] Ces bones herbes beivre usez (J) Ces herbes he le
beivre usez (J) | [775] laver e esquaser (S1J) | [777ff] See S No.130 and S1 nos 3 & 62
below. J has red rubric A *plaie munder.* |

Et vous ne trovés ki l'en traie,
Ou fer ou fust qui dedens seit,
780   Ke nos ne veit ne aparceit,
De ditain deit beivre le jus
Et le pastel lier desus,
Ou la viole en ewe quite,
784   Ce est une herbe bone elite,
Sor les piés metés .i. pastel
Por oster ou os ou quar(t)el.

AUTRE

Emplastre querai que vous serve:
788   Pernés plantain et quinke[ne]rve,
Gote de miel, flour de forment,
Tot cru lé metés simplement.

AUTRE

Jo vous dirai .i. bon entrait
792   Ke en tel guise sera fait:
De segle pernés la ferrine,
Jus d'ache et miel en la medicine
Et l'aubun de l'oef i metés,
796   Bon entrait avrés, ne ne dotés.

AUTRE   f.10rb

Ore oiés ben a ceste fois:
Pernés cire et noire pois
Et siu de bouc par avenaunt
800   Et clier saim tot autretant,
Del saim autretaunt ou plus
Com des autres dunt di desus.
Deprimes fundés le saim
804   Et puis le pois en .i. bacin,
Aprés le siu et puis la cire,
Chescun par sei devés frire.
Aprés les devés assembler
808   Et metre en boistes et bien garder,
Ce sane plaie et fait le quir
Delié et bele revenir.

[780] Ki l'em ne seit ne ben veit (J) Ke home nel sent ne l'en veit (S) | [786] Si en istera
hors o. u q. (S1S) | [787ff] See S1 no. 63 below. | [791ff] See S1 no. 64 below. In J
790–1 are not separated. | [791] Si volet aver autre e. (S1)) 791–802 are found in MS B.
L. Sloane 962 (s.xv) f. 61r | [792] Gardez dunc ki ben seit feit (J) Si gardet ben ke dunt
seit feit (S1) | [797] MS *bon*. Uncore vus dirray autre f. (J) | [810] Bon saner e ben r. (J)

BEIVRE A PLAIE GARIR

Un beivre vous vodrai elire
812 Ke vaut a plaie, ce os bien dire,
Kar bons mires l'ont dit plusors
Ke entre mil ne n'a nul meillor:
Pernés plein poigne de la parele,
816 Une herbe que est bone et bele
Kaunt la plaie purge et nettie
Si que ordure n'i remaint mie.   f.10va
La salle pernés et le chin
820 Ke le defent de palasin,
Et la violette et la flour
Ki assuage la chalour,
Et vetoigne qui est contre fevre
824 Ki a home jovene trop greve,
Launcelee que crest el faunc
Por ce que ele restreint le saunc,
Et plantein que crest es chemins
828 Ke revaut encontre venims.
Et si metés la pelosette,
Ele cure plaie et tient nette.
L'ere terrestre et egremoigne,
832 Ces .ii. i metés sauns assoigne.
Totes ces herbes me pernés,
Triblés les bien, puis les quirés
En bone cervoise ou en vin,
836 Si le boive a seir et au matin.
Miel i metés por adoucir,
Se le poés donc le plus lonc tenir.

AUTRE

Jo di, si vous vient talent,
840 Fere poés bon oignement   f.10vb
Et de meimes de ice jus
Des herbes dont j'a[i] dit desus,
Fors soul taunt que remuerés,
844 La pelosette en osterés.

[811ff] See S1 no. 65 below. J has red rubric *Bone boivre a plaie*. | [813] Ce afichent m. p.
(J) Ce sevent m. p. (S1) | [817] neie (J) nie (S1) | [819] De sauge pernez le tim (J) De
sauge me pernet et le tim (S1) | [820] MS *le p.*; garrist (J) | [822] dolur (JS1) | [823]
ke tout f. (JS1) | [824] Ki en plaie sout estre rievre (JS1) | [828] Ki sout enchacer les v.
(J) | [830] E ovre la p. (J) | [831–4] E egrimoine, ces herbes touz les pernet / trinlet
ben, pus le quiset / en bone serveise ou en vin / si beive al seir e al matin. (Sl. no. 65) |
[831–2] L'escrite umcore testimoine / mettez i cre terestre [sic, see also 855, 949, 969] e
egrimoine (J) | [838–9] not separated in J. | [839ff] See S1 no. 66 below. J has only
lines 839, 840 and 850. |

Si cele herbe mise estoit,
La plaie vous aoveroit.
Metés i mel et oile et cire
848　　E siu de moton fetes frire.
Issi faites vostre oignement,
La plaie garras erraument.

A PLAIE SORSANEE

A plaie que est sursané
852　　Et qui n'est mie bien mundee,
Si fer ou fust ou rien i ait
Que ne seit mie bien fors trait:
L'erre terrestre me pernés
856　　Et pelosette ovec metés,
Cheüe pernés et vetoine
Et morele sauns nul essoigne.
Vetoigne la plaie ov[r]era
860　　Et le venim en ostera
Et fust et fer getera hors
Ke point remaindra en le cors,
Si os ja issir l'estuet,
864　　Kar autrement estre ne puet.
L'autre beivre beive ensement
Et longuement dont dis devant.

f.11ra

A PLAIE OVRIR

Ki veut tenir la plaie overte
868　　Por la dolor k'en a sofferte,
De l'oef devés batre l'aubun
Et oile o tot que tot seit un,
Et blaunc sel maigre bien [ars en] aistre,
872　　De ce si faites vostre emplastre.

POR SANER PLAIE

Emplastre por plaie saner
Et por garder de sorsaner:
Cire et oile me pernés,
876　　Limeure d'araim querés,
Et si la fisike ne ment,
L'en i mettra de l'orpiment,

---

[846] vus aneyt (J) | [851] J has red rubric A *sursaneure*. | [853] fere u ruil (J) |
[857] E la cegue (J) | [870] seit commun (J) | [871] E bel siel ki seit ars en l'astre (J)
| [873] J has red rubric *Emplastre*. | [877] Umcore cum ieo l'entent (J) | [878] Co-
vient mettre (J) |

Kar l'orpiment et la limeure
880   Manjuent de la plaie l'ordure,
L'oile assowage et la cire,
Ce os jo por verité dire.   f.11rb
Et quant sont bien mellé ensemble,
884   Plaies garisent, ce me semble.

AUTRE

Autre dirai bele et nette
Por traire espine ou seite:
Por faire ceste medicine
888   Covient il de noir espine,
Pernés la moisse et l'entrerus,
Bien vous dirai quei en frés plus.
En cerveise egre les quirés
892   Ou en fort vin, si le avés.
L'enplastre metés tot desure,
Ice l'entraira sauns demure.

AUTRE

Pernés racines de rosel,
896   Raés les et lavés les mult bel,
O tot ice pur miel batés
Et sor la dolor l'emplastrés.

POR OS FREINT

Si il est houme qui ait os frait
900   Emplastre covient ki il ait:
De segle pernés la ferrine,
Bien covient a la medicine.
De la flour les .ii. pars pernés,   f.11va
904   De vin chaut la tierce part avrés,
L'aubun de l'oef o tot mellés,
L'emplastre sor le mal metés.
Aprés ce ke vous averés ce fait,
908   Un beivre covient ke il ait.
Pernés consoude et confire
Et omonde ovec deit quire,
Ou cru ou quit le covient beivre
912   Si tost veut saunté receivre.

[880] En plaie ne remainent ordure (J) | **[883]** ensemble sunt justez (J) | **[884]** g. ben assez (J) | **[884–5]** not separated in J. | **[886]** Por cancre e. e s. (J) | **[889]** MS *les tendrons*, cf. 447, la musse e letteruse (J) | **[892]** U en forte aisil le lavez (J) | **[894–5]** not separated in J. | **[899]** MS *fraint*; frainte (J) |

Glossary on pp.403–12

A PLAIE OVRIR

A plaie ovrir et saner
Et de rancle et venim oster,
La mort char tot ostera
916   Et bien et bel le sanera:
Des ebles pressés fors le(i) jus
E d'aluine autretaunt ou plus,
De neire ronce les tendrons,
920   De l'ortie les couperons.
Le jus de ache ovec seit mis
Et aubun de l'oef, ce m'est avis,
Un poi de fiente de geline,
924   Et de segle aiés ferine.   f.11vb
Ensemble les faites boillir
Ke ensemble voilent tenir.
Desor un drap tost l'emplastrés
928   Et sor la plaie le metés.
Se ce desecchist, se metés
Jus d'ache, bien le arousés.
Ki cest sagement(es) fra
932   Entrait bon et verrai avra.

A FAIRE OIGNEMENT

Aprendre vous voil ensement
A faire .i. bon oignement,
Por plaie garir et saner
936   Ne covient meilur demander:
Pernés l'anguille grosse et grasse
Dont en ces vivers ad grant masse.
Decoupés le, si le quisés
940   [. . .]
La grasse de l'owe o de geline
Colés a ceste medicine.
Et si pernés del gras moton
944   Del blaunc siu d'entre lé roignon.
Et le bel siu de cerf pernés,
Oint de fresceng ovec metés.   f.12ra
Puis triblés rue, aloint et sauge
948   En .i. morter ou en .i. auge,
La lancelee, ere terrestre,
Od les autres triblés doivent estre.
Ces herbes dont ai dit desus

[918] MS E *liuus*; E d'alusne atant e nent plus (J) | [924] J adds two lines: Desur le fu tut ceo mettez / e tut iceo cire querez. | [928–9] om. (J) | [938] Dunt en marreis (J) | [940] E la gres tut cuilliez (J) | [946] fres cenge (J) | [949] E la cheinlange cre terestre (J) |

952   Triblés et si premés le jus.
        Ensemble faites tot boillir
        Et la grasse desor quillir,
        Tot freit coilir et puis eschaufer
956   Et parmi .i. net drap coler.
        Poudre de encens od tot mellés,
        En vos boistes le metés.

        [AUTRE]

        Une autre manere d'entrait
960   Vous dirai et coment ert fait:
        De segle ferrine pernés
        Et aloine mult bien triblés
        Et miel od tot i soit ajoint
964   Et .ii. fois le remués le jor.
        [. . .]

        BEIVRE A PLAIÉ

        Un beivre a plaié vus dirai
        Si com en l'escrit trové l'ai:
        Pernés viole et egremoine   f.12rb
968   Et tanesie et vetoine,
        Yere terrestre, bugle et plauntain,
        Le jus bevés, si serés sain.

        POR PLAIÉ GARIR

        Le livre nous dit et comaunde
972   Ke il se deit garder de viaunde,
        De tot egrun, de lait, de fruit.
        Si il femme haunte, ce le destrust.
        Char de chastris manjust poudree
976   Auques et de sel assaudree.
        Grasse geline, feisauns, partris
        Manjust, mult tost sera garis.
        Et si s'en gart de corocer,
980   Plaié seut por ce empirer.

[959ff] See S1 No. 67 below. J has red rubric *Entrait*. | [963ff] J has Oillie de olive e bon veuz oint / e mel od tut i seit aiont / deus fiez le remuez le jor / pur eswager si grant dolor; S1 has Od oyle de olive e bon veil unt / e mel a tut i ceeit ajoynt / deuz fethe le remuet le jur / pur asuager la grant dolur. It is therefore likely that two lines are missing from the MS, but as there is some uncertainty I have not included them in the line numbering, as I have when an incomplete couplet suggests a single missing line. | [965ff] See S1 no. 68 below. | [966] om. (S1) | [971ff] See S1 no. 69 below. J has red rubric *Autre medicine*. | [972] MS g. ce me semble. | [973] Herbes furmage e l. e f. (S1J) | [976] Ou ke il seit sale e fumee (S1J) | [980] Sa plaie puroit comparer (J) Sa plaie purra le meuz saner (S1) |

Ou seit por graunt ou por petit,
Le saunc del cors li bout et frit,
En chalor, en ire et en fu
984   Le saunc est tot commeu.
La plaie rougist, si li dout,
Emfler, ranclier aprés seut.
Sages est qui garder se poet
988   Quaunt veit que fere li estuet.   f.12va

POR PLAIÉ GARIR

Pelosete donés a beivre
Par quei volés aparceivre
Se li naufré devra garir
992   Ou de cele plaie morir.
Si il retient, tost garir poet,
Si il vomist, morir l'estoet.

ENTRAIT

Entrait a plaié vous dirai
996   Et a confire vous aprenderai:
Ache pernés, si le triblés,
Aprés flour de forment querés.
Un tortelet enpestricés
1000   Od miel et puis si le quisés.
Al fu nel metés mie quire,
Mes au fu manier come cire
Devrés en autre plusor feis.
1004   En miel remoillierés vos deis.
Taunt le devés manier issi
Que il seit auques emplastri.
Si cru le metés sor la plaie,
1008   Dolor n'i avra que il n'entraie.

A PLAIE SANER   f.12vb

A plaie que ne veut saner
Estue[t] la morte char oster:
A ce pernés hastive[me]nt
1012   Mult bon encens et arrement,
Trestot em poudre le batés
Et sor la plaie le metés.

[989ff] See S1 no. 71 below. | [995] J has red rubric *Entrait a plaie.* | [996] fere (J) |
[997–1004], [1007–8] See MS B. L. Sloane 962 (s.xv) f. 61r. | [1005] si maner (J) |
[1006] Ki le puis ben amoiller (J) | [1009ff] See S1 no. 59 below. J has red rubric *A la
plaie ki ne veut saner.* |

A PLAIE TOST GARIR

A plaie tost garir faites saim de lart
1016 Et ferrine de segle et miel et vin de autre part,
Gardés qui de chescun seit mis owelement;
Quant ert quit, sor la plaie metés cest oignement.

ESPERMENT

Si vous volés prover si home plaié vivera,
1020 Pimpernele triblé od ewe bevra.
Si il deit morir, par la plaie en istra,
Si il nen ist par la plaie, donc garir porra.

POR TOUZ PLAIES GARIR

Por totes plaies me pernés arrement,
1024 Escorce de tremble, siu et sel owelement,   f.13ra
Lart ausi en .i. nuef pot tot ovec arderés,
Sor la plaie de la poudre por garir i mettrés.

A CANCRE SANER

A cauncre saner covient force:
1028 De nuef arbres pernés l'escorce:
L'escorce de l'ere et del fraine,
De neire espine et de cheine,
De hous, de tremble, de pomer,
1032 De pruner et de bolacer,
De tous ces nuef faites coillir
Et en douce ewe lé faites boillir.
Taunt seient boili et tant quit,
1036 Ce nous aprent nostre escrit,
Si com melles escorchié sont,
Si com plusors houmes en ce font.
Puis getés les escorces hors.
1040 L'ewe soit requite lors
Et taunt longuement quire deit
Que l'ewe bien espesse seit.
Miel purgié donc o tot metés,
1044 Puis issi tot reboillés.
Quaunt ert espés, si l'entraiés,
L'emplastre sor le mal metés.   f.13rb

[1015–18] Written out as prose. Om. (J) | [1019–22] Written out as prose. Om. (J) Cf.
S1 no. 75 below | [1023–6] Written out as prose. Om. (J) | [1027] J has red rubric
Autre medicine. | [1029] Le corce de oser (J) | [1031] De holis (J) | [1037] S. c. les
escorces s. (J) | [1038] Sunt p. genz en ke i funt (J) | [1040] ne seit requisse (J) |

Glossary on pp.403–12

AUTRE

A cancre oscire ou ke ele nesse,
1048   Que felonesse est et engresse:
Donc me pernés enneire
Flor de segle, pu[d]re de veire.

AUTRE

Ou pernés caus vive et sablon,
1052   Lé pertuis emplés environ,
Ce garist bien cancre afestri
Et festre par soi autresi.

AUTRE

Pernés le corn de .i. bovet
1056   De .ii. ans aukes jovenet,
Et pernés racine de ortie,
Laiterole ne obliés mie.
De fou devés prendre l'escorce
1060   Ou legierement ou a force,
Poumes de chaine et limaison
Qui de escale fait maison.
Et de tot ce emplastre frés
1064   Et sor les pertuis le metrés.

BEYVRE POR LA CANCRE

Un beivre li freés o tot
Ke a cancre et a festre vaut mult:
Centoire, sanicle et avance,
1068   Bugle et vetoigne qui l'avaunce,   f.13va
Ouquelesconsce et pelosette
Et tanesie et kauketrappe,
O tot metés le limeure
1072   De corn de vif boef et bure.

POR CANCRE GARIR

La foille pernés del navet
Et gleire de oef novel et net,
Desor le cancre l'emplastrés,

[1047] J has red rubric *Autre medicine*. | [1050–1] Not separated in J. | [1051] savun (J) | [1055] J has red rubric *Autre medicine*. | [1055] P. de lart del bovette (J) | [1058] La tuel (J) | [1059] De sauz (J) | [1080] Home le saut saut [sic] rater par force (J) | [1062] Prendre devez od sa m. (J) | [1064–65] Not separated in J. | [1067] cenicle (J) | [1069] Mes l'escunse (J) |

Glossary on pp.403–12

1076   Le maus esteindra, ce est verités.

AUTRE

Ou pernés poudre de arrement,
O vieus oint seit triblé fortment,
Cele emplastre metés desore,
1080   Si l'averés gari en peu d'eure.

AUTRE

Arrement o miel o vin
Faites boilir en .i. bacin,
Iceste chose mult i vaut
1084   Ki sor le mal le mettra chaut.
Ou les poumes dé bois querés
En la brese puis les quirés,
Dous jors ou .iii. i seront liés,
1088   Sor le mal chaut aparellés.

AUTRE   f.13vb

Si vous volés faire autre medicine,
Pernés crue char de geline,
Tot issi chaut le metés,
1092   La plaie aprés bien lavés.
D'ewe de pluie laverons,
Par fisike issi l'enseignons,
Et si cel ewe nen avés,
1096   L'ewe de tan pure pernés
Et mainte fiez i a valu
Sotil poudre de tan batu.

POR FESTRE ET CANCRE

A festre et a cancre pernés
1100   Un oef et l'aubun fors getés,
Puis metés ens saugemme o sel,
L'un et l'autre par owel,
O argille ben l'estopés
1104   Et en bres[e] le metés.
Kaunt tot seit ars, si le devés moudre

[1076] ennuiera ce verrez (J) | [1080–81] Not separated in J. | [1081] U la ment (J)
| [1087] nuiz (J) | [1093ff] De l'ewe lavez idunke / ki troverez dedenz le trunc / de pluie
ki ens ert chaez / lavez la pleie e fetes nez (J) | [1098] La p. ki est (J) | [1099] J has red
rubric A cancre e a festre. | [1103] Od aisil (J) |

Ou batre, taunt ke tot s'espoudre
Mult deliés et mult sotil.
1108   Ovec cele poudre gentil,
Si vous volez fere a dreiture,
De l'araime pernez la limure,   f.14ra
Ens deit estre la tierce part
1112   Si vous le faites bien par art.
Ceste poudre, ce dit l'escrit,
Ke la cancre et la goute oscist.

AUTRE

Uncore dirai autre medicine:
1116   Vous prendrez les oes de geline,
Ostez l'aubun et metez issi
Et si le metez tot ouni,
Et spis de segle et orpiment,
1120   Poudre de veire et d'arrement.
La poudre ert corosive mult,
Cancre et festre garist de tot,
Si est bien en autre (autre) arsee
1124   Et puis par .i. linge drap passee.

AUTRE

Por cancre oscir dirai el:
Pernez crotes de lievre et sel,
La sieue de la maison
1128   Ignelement mis et par raison,
O gleire de oef le destemprés
Et sor le mal le metez.

AUTRE

A goute festre devez prendre
1132   Le jus premt fors de lavendre.   f.14rb
En cel jus estoupes moiliez
Et sor la plaie les metés.
De lentilles pernez del jus,
1136   De pain(e) autretant ou plus,
Et pur orge devez puis prendre

[1110] De l'a. ki chet la l. (J) | [1115] has red rubric *Autre medicine.* | [1118] E cel e
siu tut uni (J) | [1119] Espie de s. e arrement (J) | [1120] e orpiment (J) | [1123-4]
om. (J) | [1125] J has red rubric *Pur cancre occire.* | [1126] de chever (J) | [1128]
Ouelement (J) | [1131] J has red rubric A *gute festre.* | [1135] J precedes with red rubric
Autre medicine, and reads De wantileye | [1136] De la paene (J) |

Glossary on pp.403-12

En .i. nuef pot ardir en cendre.
Od le jus devez ce pestrir
1140   Et metre au mal por tost garir.

AUTRE

Une autre oncore dire voil:
Pernez le jus de chievrefoil,
Treis fois le jor au mal metez,
1144   Le pastel sor lierez.
Treis moeus de oes puis pernez
Et l'aubon fors engetez.
Et puis metez ignelement
1148   Mel et sel et arrement,
Et grain de segle et nele
Et semence de camvre bele,
De .i. viel tacon .i. grant piece,
1152   Poivre i metés od verdegrece.
En .i. pot tot ce ardez
Et cele poudre bien gardez,   f.14va
Kar goute festre garist bien
1156   Et cancre sor tote autre rien.

POR CONUSTRE LES MAUS

Ore seroit mult bon a savoir
A conustre ces maus por voir,
La quele est festre et la quele non,
1160   La quele est cancre par raison.
Une esprove vous aprendrai,
Icele que bien esprové ai.
Le freis formage me pernez
1164   Et de net miel l'endaubez,
Sor le mal liés de primsoir,
L'endemain poez bien voir,
Si ce formage est entamé,
1168   Donkes i a le cancre esté.
Et si il remaint tot entiers,
Donc n'est li maus uncore festriers.

AUTRE

Si aucun musart dit tel controve,

[1141] J has red rubric *Autre medicine*. | [1142] de cerfoil (J) | [1147] ouelement (J)
 | [1157] J has red rubric *Medicine espruvé*. | [1162] cum apris l'ay (J) | [1164] O miel
luignez sil mettez (J) | [1165] Si vus le liez primes al seir (J) | [1166] L'e. pur veir (J) |
[1169-70] om. (J) | [1171] Plusurs diunt ki ce est controve (J) |

1172 Por ce dirai .i. autre esprove:
   Pernez l'anguille et l'emplastrés
   Ou grosses roches i metés.
   Sor lin ou caunvre seient mis   f.14vb
1176 Net et bien lavé et tot vifs,
   Sor la plaie seient lié.
   Si l'endemain seient mangé,
   Donc poez bien saver de fi
1180 Que goute festre est, ce vous di.

AUTRE

   De autre chose garde pernez
   Kaunt vous les plaies esgardez.
   Le cancre manjue le quir,
1184 Si fait la plaie aneircir.
   Mes festre le fait autrement,
   La plaie fait parfondement,
   Joste les os, joste les ners
1188 Et les jointes crose en travers.
   La festre est mult fort a garir,
   Kar n'i puet om preu avenir.
   Ce poez mult bien prover,
1192 Kar tente i puet om boter.
   A cancre poés emplastre metre,
   Jus et poudre, ce dist la lettre,
   Si poés la cancre amortir
1196 Et aprés la plaie garir.
   Entre cancre et festre a deseivre,   f.15ra
   Kar por la festre covient beivre
   Ke le mal puist amortir
1200 Et la plaie dedens garir
   Et qui en puist geter l'ordure
   Et fors metre la porreture.

POR TAILER

   Quaunt vous trovés croes lé pertuis,
1204 Tentes metés, poudres et jus.
   Tailez en long le bel braon
   E deliés come lard(r)on,
   De vos jus d'erbes l'arousés,
1208 De vos poudres le poudrés,

[1173–80] om. (J) | [1172/81] Not separated in J. | [1181] Si vus del mal garde pren-
drez (J) | [1182] E si vus le pleies gardez (J) | [1188] jountes entur vers (J) | [1195]
anentir (J) | [1197] le festre de cancre deceivre (J) | [1199–1200] om. (J) | [1202–
3] Not separated in J. | [1206] Lunge e delez un lardun (J) |

En cel crois le botez parfunt
Issi [ke] cirurgians le font.
Si la tente ne l'ateint taunt
1212   Ke del mal viengne devaunt,
Donc face la plaie effondrer
Là endreit ou quide trover
Le liu ou li mal est aers,
1216   Mes gard braon, veines et ners,
Ce li defent bien a tocher.
Si il ne poet sauvement ovrer,   f.15rb
Effundrer le deit par dreiture
1220   Et geter hors la porreture,
Puis garira hastivement,
Ce os dire verraiment.

POR PISSER

Houme qui a mal en la vessie
1224   Si ke estaler ne puisse mie,
De l'ewe prenge la favee,
Ovec seit mente triblee.
Od vin blaunc destremprez
1228   Ou a chaude ewe le bevez.

AUTRE

Une autre: pernez comin
Et grumil, bevez a fort vin.

AUTRE

Uncore vous voil enseigner
1232   A ceus ki ne poent pisser:
De cerises pernez les pieres
– Qui sage est mult les tient cheres –
En .i. morter bien les triblez,
1236   De benoite ewe les arousez.
Ki en Deus ferme creance a
Tot certain seit, bien garira.

[1209] El tuez e batez einz parfunde (J) | [1210] Si garra ben meuz de mond (J) |
[1211] E sil ne poet atendre tant (J) | [1212] De si kal mal ki est avant (J) | [1214] La
tendrait u la q. t. (J) | [1216] brauns (J) | [1217] a etifirer (!) (J) | [1223ff] See T
281ff; S no. 80 below. J has red rubric *Pur estaler.* | [1228–9] Not separated in TJ. |
[1229] Uncore p. (TSJ) | [1230] Sil beivet od plein hanap de vin (TJ) E bevez plain
hanap de vin (S) | [1231ff] J precedes with 1291–6. See T 295ff and S no. 79 below. |
[1234] Hom les deit tenir mut cheres (TSJ) | [1236] ja i usez (T) i ajustez (S) | [1237]
ferme om. (TSJ) avera (TSJ) | [1238] Sachez ke de cel mal garra (S) Tut en sur seit ki
garra (J) |

Glossary on pp.403–12

AUTRE   f.15va

Plusors medicines valent
1240   A ceus ki le sanc estalent:
        Warance rouge me pernez,
        En .i. morter bien le batez.
        Boillez en cerveise ou en vin
1244   [. . .]
        Si la racine de peresil
        Metés ovec, tost ert gari.

POR PIERE EN LA VESSIE

        Kicunques a piere en la vessie
1248   – Trop est forte cele maladie –
        Kaunt il estale, maintenant
        Desure vait com paile flotaunt.
        Le penil enfle et dout
1252   Et ne puet pissir quaunt il vout,
        Cruel mal i a et rievre,
        Ausi fait trembler com fevre.
        Le manger pert et si languist,
1256   Mains dort assez ki il ne vousist.
        A ce me pernez le grumil,
        Le rouge ortie et peresil,
        Semence de fenoil et blaunc peivre,
1260   De ce li fetes vous une beivre.
        Tot ce deit estre en vin boilli,   f.15vb
        Mes une poudre metez i.
        Le pel de lievre si pernez,
1264   En .i. nuef pot puis l'ardez,
        Ensemble od vin le fetes boillir,
        En baign le bevez por garir.

AUTRE

        Une autre vous dirai mult fine:
1268   Del ravle pernez la racine,
        Od .i. coutel bien le parés,

[1239ff] J has red rubric *Ki sanc estalent.* See T 303ff and S no. 81 below. | [1241] La wderove de le bois (T) La woderove du boys (S) La wouderove de cel bois (J) | [1242] Poez cuillir a vostre chois (TSJ) | [1243] Bevez en chaut ço est la fin (TSJ) | [1244] En bone cerveise u en vin (TSJ) | [1245–6] om. (TSJ) | [1247ff] J has red rubric *Ki ad peres en la vessie.* See T 309ff and S no. 76. | [1253] Fort m. (TSJ) enrevre (T) revre (S) encevre (J) | [1256] Ne pot dormir e si vomist (TSJ) | [1259] blaunc om. (TS) | [1260] De ceo lui fres vus un b. (TSJ) | [1265] od vin om. (TS) | [1266] Qui l'usera sil pot garir (TSJ) | [1266–7] Not separated in J. See T329ff and S No. 77 below | [1267] Uncore v. d. (TSJ) | [1268] De raiz (TSJ) |

Glossary on pp.403–12

En roeles le decoupez
Taunt ke il i ait cinkaunte nuef.
1272 En .i. hanap tot blaunc et nuef
Metez les ens et miel assés
Et de ce vous dejunerés
Par .ix. jors, si com jo vous dirai
1276 Et (l)oures vous deviserai:
Le premer jor .ix. mangerez,
L'endemain .viii., ce est assez,
Puis .vii., puis .vi., puis .v., puis .iv.,
1280 Issi le devés vous abatre
Et chescun jor amenuiser
Et si en decressaunt manger.
Al neveime jor serés gari   f.16ra
1284 Kaun[t] ce avrez fait et acompli.

POR LA PIERE

Si aucun a el conduit gravele ou piere,
De mirre face poudre et de la goume d'ere,
Il deit en blaunc vin et en clier destemprer
1288 Et par jor cel beivre deit il en baing user.
Au tiers jor deit l'urine parmi .i. drap coler,
Si il i a piere ou gravele en la drap, l'en porra trover.

KI NE POET TENIR SA URINE

Ki son estal ne poet tenir,
1292 Ce veit om a meint houme avenir:
Ungles de porc a ce pernés,
En le fu a poudre les ardés.
La poudre metez en sa viaunde,
1296 Ce dist fisike et comaunde.

POR DOLOR DES RAINS

Souffre en poudre moudrés
E pois en jus de rue le destemprés
Et sel et mel ensemble [triblez]

[1271] MS = *kaunte nuef* with a bar through kaunte, and trente written above in a later hand. TSJ have cinquante. | [1272] om. (J) | [1276] Si cum jo le d. (T) E si com jeo d. (S) E sicum jeo vus d. (J) | [1278] ben le purrez (T) bien le poez (S) s'en porez (J) | [1282] user (J) | [1285–90] Written out as prose. Om. (TSJ) | [1291ff] See T289ff and S no. 82 below. | [1291] A meint home issi avent (TSJ) [1292] Que sun estal pas ne retent (TSJ) | [1296] Co volt f. (TS) Ce voet cil ki si le comande (J) | [1297] The rubric is written in the ink of the text as if forming part of the receipt proper, with the first letter of Por as a red initial. The receipt is omitted in TSJ. |

1300   [Et puis] sor les rains lierés.

     A l'houme qui a fevre ague   f.16rb
     C'est li retors quant om sue.
     Si deit jus de alisaundre beivre,
1304   Par taunt porra bien aparceivre
     Si il sue bien, si deit garir,
     Si non, si li covient soffrir.
     Ki donkes averoit ewe rose
1308   Ce lui seroit mult bone chose
     Laver ses temples et son front,
     Ses mains, se[s] jointes com eles sunt,
     Por les humors del cors hoster
1312   Et por lé miels destorber
     Et a fere suor issir
     Ki ains ne pout hors venir.

     Puis pregne foilles de pescher,
1316   De pruner, sau sec et ciricer,
     En ewe lé fetes boillir
     Et puis les piés dedens tenir.
     Et tele emplastre li revaudra
1320   Od la graunt chalor ke il a
     Pernés flour d'orge bien passee,
     Plantaine, jubarbe et sarree,
     Et canellie ensement   f.16va
1324   Et la morele ignelement.
     La flour od le jus pestrissés,
     Sor .i. drap linge le couchés,
     A destre part le devés metre
1328   Sor la foie, ce dist la lettre.

     POR FIEVRE TERSAINE

     Bien sai ke la fevre tersaine
     Mult malement plusors gens maine:
     Bevez .iii. plauntes de plauntain
1332   Devant l'accés, si serez sain,
     Treis au matin et .iii. au seir,
     Nuef jors si volez saunté aveir.

[1301ff] J has red rebric A *fevre ague*. See T535ff and S no.170 below | [1306] fort li est le s.(TS) | [1310] Les pouz (TJ) Les poins (S) | [1311] Pur la savur k'om deit o. (TSJ) | [1312] E les pores desestuper (TS) E ses pores destuper (J) | [1315ff] om. (T) J has red rubric *Uncore* | [1316] Perer pomer e ceriser (S) Perer pruner e c. (J) | [1319ff] See S no.171 below. J has red rubric *Autre medicine*. | [1320] Pur la g. (S) | [1321] Pernez plantein b. p. (S) | [1322] E jubarbe e favee (S) la fauce (J) | [1324] oelement (S) | [1325] destemprez (S) | [1329ff] See S no.173 and S1 no. 57 below. J has red rubric A *fevre terciene* | [1329–30] om. (S1) | [1330] demeine (SJ) |

POR COTIDIANE

La cotidiane fevre
1336   Cele est mal et enrevre:
Pernez .i. oef que seit mol quit,
Del blaunc versez hors .i. petit,
Une femme i viegne avaunt
1340   Ke norisse .i. masle enfaunt,
Treis goutes de let i degot,
Li fevereus le deit humer de tot,
Mes cil taunt coiement le face
1344   Ke li fevereus n'oie nel sace.   f.16vb

POR FEVRE QUARTAINE

Ore vous dirai de la quartaine,
Haschee i a et mult grant paine:
Vous covendra fere un beivre,
1348   Pernez quatre vint greins de peivre,
Triblez la rue et la sanguine,
Od vin le beive la mescine.
Pernez plein poin de launcelee
1352   Et de egremoine une poinee
Et sel pernez a une fois
Taunt solement a vos .iii. dois,
Ensemblement mult bien les t[riblez]
1356   Et od mult bon vin les destemprez.
Puis le bevez devaunt l'accesse
Par si ke la fievre vous lesse.

POR FEVRE AGUE

Aprés recordez fevre ague
1360   Ke il la caleur aukes remue:
Si li doint om centoyre a beivre
Ki le mal decache et deseivre.
Le jus de senesçon bevera,   f.17ra
1364   Ja puis, ce di, ne recharra
K'i[l] lui dora puis le retor.
De consoude bevera la flor,

[1335] See S no.174 and S1 no. 58 below. J has red rubric A fevre cotidiene. | [1335–6] om. (S1) | [1336] MS = malevre; revre (J) | [1337] MS = mal quit | [1343] cointement (SS1J) | [1344] li malade (SS1J)) mot ne sace (S) ne le sace (S1) | [1345] J has red rubric A fevre quartaine. The receipt is not found in SS1. | [1346] haschet (J) | [1348] utante grainnis (J) | [1349] la rue saugine (J) | [1359] J has red rubric Pur fevre ague. See S no.172 below. | [1359] Puis le record de f. a. (S) Apres le retur de f. a. (J) | [1360] MS = a coleur | [1361] doine fumtere (S) home fumeter (J) | [1363] Ou qui le s. (S) Ki la s. (J) | [1364] Ja en le mal n. r. (S) ce di om. (J) | [1366] cosuede (J) |

Puis le suor, s'il boit aprés,
1368   De cel ne recharra més.
O la semence de parele
Bien garist malle et femele.

POR FORSENÉ

Maint houme est ke en peu de tens
1372   Pert sa memorie et son sens.
Si il n'ait hastif confort,
Mieus li seroit ke il fust mort.
Solsecle et averoine pernez,
1376   La sauge pas ne obliez,
Ces herbes li donez a beivre,
Si porra bien saunté receivre.
Ki veut memorie recovrer,
1380   Mult li covient bien dieter.
Les herbes ke jo ai dit desus
Cinc jors beive ou aukes plus,
Li bon maistre deit encerchier
1384   Ke il devra user et manger.
Les herbes beive o bon vin voir   f.17rb
Ains ke il manjust, matin e soir.

POR ESROURE MEDICINE

Ore vous dirai ke ai loé
1388   A ceus ki sont esroé:
En vin facent boillir savine
Et miel metés en la medicine
O feves, ce dit nostre escrit,
1392   Chaut les mangés en brese quit.

AUTRE

Une autre truis, ce me semble:
Les tendrons pernez de tremble
Et pernez d'eble la racine,
1396   En vin quisez ceste medicine.

[1371ff] See S no.179 below. J has red rubric *Ki pert sa memorie*. | [1373–4] om. (S) | [1373] A ceus covient h. c. (J) | [1374] Mult meuz veint kil fussent mort (J) | [1375] solsequie (J) | [1378–9] Separated in J by red rubric *Autre medicine*. | [1379] v. sa sancte r. (J) | [1383–4] om. (S) | [1383] Et le chous face apareiler (J) | [1384] Ceo ki devera le jors manger (J) | [1385] Quire deivent en b. vin (SJ) vin u viner (J) | [1386] mangera (S) | [1387] See S no. 72 below. J has red rubric *Autre medicine*. | [1388] enroe (J) | [1392] Ail m. (SJ) | [1393] See S no. 73 below. J has red rubric *Autre medicine*. | [1394] l'entrerus (S) l'entrus (J) trembel (J) |

User le deit matin et seir
Ki tost vodra saunté aveir.

AUTRE

Ou de mente le jus bevez
1400   Kaunt quit en cerveise l'averez.
Mangez lait quit, kar ce vaut mult,
Et miel et frés formage o tot.
Un oef mol quit prendre devez,
1404   Oile et peivre dedens metés,
La nuit quaun[t] vous coucherez   f.17va
Humez le tot, puis reposez.

AUTRE

Jus d'ache et mel devez boillir
1408   Et puis en vostre bouche tenir,
Issi en la bouche maime
Devez fere gargarime.

AUTRE

Pernez racine de rais,
1412   Racine d'aune, ce m'est avis,
Pas de cheval i ajostés
Et marobre n'i obliez.
En vin les fetes bien boillir
1416   Et laissés dedens gisir
Par .iii. jors et .iii. nuis temprer
Et puis ses poez bien user.
Houme ki si fere le vodra
1420   La vois mult li esclarcira.

AUTRE

Ki seit esroé sodeinement
Por chaut, por fumee ou por vent,
Les poriaus face bien tribler,
1424   Prendre le jus et bien coler.
Si il veut ki sa vois esclaire,
Il deit gargarime faire.

[1398–9] Not separated in J. | [1402–3] Separated in J by red rubric *Autre medicine*. |
[1406–7] Not separated in J. | [1410–11] Not separated in J. | [1411] de la raiz (J) |
[1412] Racine de aune e de latriz (J) | [1413–4] om. (J) | [1421ff] See S no.196
below. J has red rubric *Autre medicine*. | [1421] roe (J) |

POR ESCHAUFEMENT DE FOIE   f.17vb

　　　　　Seignurs, d'echaufement de foie
1428　　　Vous dirai que jo vous loeroi:
　　　　　Del fenoil premés hors le jus,
　　　　　Del peresil autretaunt ou plus
　　　　　Et de lettuis owelement
1432　　　Et de fumitere ensement.
　　　　　Le jus de ces quatre pernés
　　　　　Et a lent fu le boillerés,
　　　　　Parmi .i. drap bien le colés
1436　　　Et cizre od miel ovec metés
　　　　　Les queus seient mis owelement
　　　　　Ovec cest jus par essient.
　　　　　Od chaude ewe le destemprés
1440　　　Et quatre fois ou .iii. l'usé[s],
　　　　　De jor et de nuit sauns dotaunce,
　　　　　De mal vous fra deliverance.
　　　　　Ou vous pernés cicoree,
1444　　　Lavandre n'i seit obliee,
　　　　　Licoriz, goume arabike,
　　　　　De ce fait beivre mult riche,
　　　　　Por chalor hors del cors oster,
1448　　　Ne sai meillor enseigner.   f.18ra.

POR FI AL QUER

　　　　　Corn de cerf en fu ardez
　　　　　Et puis en poudre le molez,
　　　　　Mult bien le fetes bulleter
1452　　　Et parmi .i. drap bien passer.
　　　　　Quaunt la poudre ert bele et delié
　　　　　Et blaunche come neif negié,
　　　　　Le metés en vostre aumonere.
1456　　　Vous le devés aver mult chere,
　　　　　Kar a multes enfermetez
　　　　　Vaudra, si vous a droit l'usez.
　　　　　Au premerain morsel le jor
1460　　　Pernez la poudre de la flor,
　　　　　Come sel le poez desevrer,

[1427] J has red rubric *Pur eschaufisun.* See S no. 45 below. | [1427] Pur eschaufeisun del feie (J) | [1428] jeo en loie (J) | [1431] tut ensement (SJ) | [1432] oelement (SJ) | [1436] E le cler jus de ceo pernez (SJ) | [1437] A ceo mettez u sucre u mell (SJ) | [1438] Par tut gardez ke soit owel (SJ) | [1439] Od ewe clere [teve, J] le devez [deit, J] temprer (SJ). J now breaks off (f. 99rb) | [1440] | E puis le devez ausi user (S) | [1441–8] om. (S) | [1449ff] See T431ff and S no. 66 below. J has red rubric *Pur meneisun.* | [1449] Perche de c. (TSJ) | [1450] batez (TSJ) | [1460] Vostre pudre metez desure (T) | [1461] Cume sel la pudrez desure (T) Ausi come seel poudrez desure (S) Cum cele

Puis le mangez sauns demorer.
Ce vaut por fi et por corchon
1464   Et si vaut contre meneison,
Et si vaut a maus plusors,
A femme qui ens nori dolors.

AUTRE

Autre medicine truis issi
1468   Que mult vaut contre le fi:
Dedens meson fowez la tere
Et faites une fosse fere   f.18rb
Treis piés lonc et .ii. lee
1472   Et .ii. piés de parfondee.
Et puis i face fere un feu
De sec ligne de seu,
Tiules metés por eschaufer,
1476   Pieres si les poés trover.
Kaunt bien seront chaut, le fu ostés
Et la brese(s) sus rastellés.
La tiule remaine a delivre,
1480   Celidoine i metés deseure,
A l'us percié com une selette
Seit mis sor la fosselette
Ou li malades deit ser
1484   Et tot le chalor recoiller.
Bien deit estre de dras covert,
Desus seit li cul overt.
Illekes se deit (s)il tenir
1488   Taunt com il plus porra soffrir.
Deus jors ou .iii. face il issi,
Hastivement sera gari.
Mais ains qu(i)'il se voile estuver,
1492   Se li covient il defumer.   f.18va
Primes seit secché le seu
Et poudré seit de tan batu.
Aprés ice .i. oef pernez,
1496   Le blaunc de l'escale pernez,
Le poudre seit el moel mise,
Ensemble pestri en tele guise,
Et ce deit il primes manger

poudre seit mis desure (J) | [1462] en poi de ure (T) sanz demure (SJ) | [1463] cursun
(J) | [1465–6] om. (SJ) | [1467] J has red rubric *Autre medicine*. | [1471] Pecez de
lunge e deus de le (J) | [1474] seke buche e de sui (J) | [1475] Tuille (J) | [1476]
Kaillous ki ce ne poet trover (J) | [1479] La pere r. cel oure (J) | [1480] La celadoine
m. d. (J) | [1481] Un aiez percie cum une sete (J) | [1484] recivre (J) | [1486] |
Fors d. de cel overte (J) | [1492] Sil deit ben diuner (J) | [1496] versez (J) |

1500 Ou volentiers ou a daunger.
   Puis deit entendre et aparceivre
   Ke plein hanap li covient beivre
   De celidoine bien triblee
1504 Et ke seit devaunt bien colee.
   Od bone cerveise ou od vin
   S'en beive plein .i. mazelin.
   Puis li seit a son oés tot prest
1508 Une herbe ke a a non panifest.
   Quite en brese et si chaudette
   Seit mis en une paellette,
   Si chaut le deit au mal tenir
1512 Cum plus chaut le porra soffrir.
   Pernez del sel une poinee
   Et de flour de segle bien delié,   f.18vb
   En .i. noef pot seient taunt quit
1516 Ke poudre seit, ce dit l'escrit.
   La poudre manjust od le pain
   Si il desire estre mult tost sain.

   AUTRE

   Uncore vous dirai avaunt
1520 Que devez fere a fi sanaunt:
   Si vous sentez ke il vous doile,
   Si bevez la bone quintefoile
   Et od let de chievre l'usez,
1524 Juns et saul bien le bevez.
   Ou vous triblez la moleine
   Ke a tel mal est bone et saine,
   Od cerveise le destemprés
1528 Et .iii. jors gesir le lerrés.
   Puis si le deit par .ix. jors beivre
   Ki sa saunté vodra receivre.

   AUTRE

   Uncore vous dirai avaunt
1532 Ke vaut contre le fi seinaunt:
   Mirfoil, mentastre, launcelee,
   Chascune seit mult bien triblee,
   I covient ke i[l] beive aprés
1536 Si sa saunté desire prés.   f.19ra

[1501] Ensemble oi cest aceivre (J) | [1502] Li covient une hanape b. (J) | [1504] Apres beu anisee (J) | [1508] painfest (J) | [1510] drapelet (J) | [1512-13] Separated in J by red rubric *Autre medicine.* | [1519] J has red rubric *Autre medicine.* | [1522] cinfoil (J) | [1532] MS = *feinaunt* |

Sor le moron miel metez vel
Et poudre arse que seit de sel.

POR SANC ESTANCHER

Kicunque vodra autre aider
1540 Kaunt del niés le verra seiner
Pervenke li doint a tenir
En sa bouche si il le veut garir.
1542a Taunt com en sa bouche l'avera
1542b Quatre goutes de saunc ne segnera.

AUTRE

Si vous volez autre fere,
1544 Betoine et seel devez quere,
Tribler le bien et mettre aprés
Al niés celui ke seine adés.
Il larra tauntost le seigner,
1548 De ce ne vous covient doter.

AUTRE

Ki quintefoille li dorra
Et od vin le destempera
Et son front lavera de aisil,
1552 Tost garira de cel peril.

AUTRE

Celes escales me pernés
Dont les poucins enclos veés,
El niés les metés, si garra   f.19rb
1556 Et tauntost estaunchera.

AUTRE

Pernez la racine d'ortie
Et feutre veus n'obliez mie,
Od fort aisil bien le mellés,
1560 Es pauperes le lierés.

[1537] Sur moroide mettre mele (J) | [1539] Home ki veut (J) | [1540] Kan i vait del (J) | [1541] Parvent (J) | [1542a/b] Portant cum iloec le avera / Une gute ne seignera (J) | [1547–8] om. (J) | [1549] dirray (J) | [1550] distemperay (J) | [1554] esclos (J) | [1556] Kar assez tost enchangera (J) | [1558] f. ars (J) | [1560] E le poceres ben liez (J) |

Glossary on pp.403–12

POR SAINIER DE VEINE

Si il i a home ou femme ke corusé seit
De chose ke il oit ou veit,
Ou por chaut ou por freit,
1564   Ke de son sen estrangié seit,
Si issi est ki son chief li doile
Aukes plus ke il ne voile
Et les oreilles li tounent
1568   Si cum le cervel li estounent,
Avis li est ki il n'oie point,
De bon marciaton seit oint.
Si se face bien covrir
1572   Ki suer poet et bien garir.
Mais si d'autre part veut torner
Ke le bras comence a enfler,
Ou par travail ou par forfait
1576   Ou par manger ke mal li fait,   f.19va
Gruel d'aveine donc prendrez,
En ewe mult bien le quirez,
Ou le wimauve seit ens quite,
1580   Kar le livre issi l'endite.
Sor .i. bel drap l'emplastrerez
Et sor le bras le lierez.

AUTRE

L'achon triblez, ce dist l'escrit,
1584   Et puis si seit en saim frit,
Si chaut seit a rauncle mis,
Si assera, jo le vous plevis.

AUTRE

Ou vous pernez flour de forment
1588   Et le jus d'ache ensement,
Siu de moton metez o tot,
Si l'oscira trestot de bot.

[1561ff] See T347ff. J has red rubric *Pur le brace emflé*. | [1561] Home ki en seigne gruce
(J) T347ff is garbled. | [1562] De acun rien dunc se corouce (J) | [1563] Ki ait oy u veu
(J) | [1564] Pur quei i seit irascu (J) J now adds U seit pur chaud u pur vent / kil seit
estume ensemnt. | [1565] E seit ce ke le chief (TJ) | [1566] D'asez plus ke li plest u
voille (TJ) | [1568] MS *estoupent* Ke la cervele li estunent (TJ) | [1570] mareicon (T)
marciatorie (J) | [1572] om. (J) | [1575] surfeit (T) surfet (J) | [1576] U p. m. u par
aultre feit (J) u par fet (J) | [1582–3] Not separated in J. | [1583] Le ache (TJ) |
[1587] See T375ff. J has red rubric *Autre medicine*. | [1589] o tut metez (TJ) | [1590]
Ensemble mut ben le quisez (TJ) TJ now add A l'emfle seit mis e lié / si [en, J] avera tost
[sempres sa, J] sancté / u feves mulues pernez / en ewe u en vin [les, J] quisez. T concludes with

AUTRE

Flur d'orge od semence de lin
1592   Quisiez en aisil ou en vin
Ou en cerveise que viele seit
Quise taunt com quire deit.
L'emplastre chaude metez i,
1596   Si assera tot, jo vous afi.

AUTRE

Flour de forment o miel pestri
Rauncle oscist tot autresi.   f.19vb

POR DELIVRER DE MORT ENFANT .

A femme ke travaile taunt
1600   Por delivrer de mort enfaunt:
Pernez tost ache et verde rue
Et seit bien triblé et batue.
Et peivre blaunc mul[t] bel et net
1604   Et la semence de cholet
E le bibues tot bien triblez,
Od vin destemprer le devez.
Le mente mult bien me frotés
1608   Et a son ventre le liez.
De cerf querez une coroie,
Delivres ert si ses flauncs lie.

AUTRE

Boive ditan, boive sarree,
1612   D'ewe beneite destempree.
Et si me pernez .xiii. grains
De coriaundre ou onze au mains,
Puis les liez en .i. cince.
1616   Gardez ke ele seit de linge
Et seit a senestre quisse
Ataché ke ne li misse,

1589–90, whilst J modifies these lines to Seu de mutun od tut mettez / ce ocist rancle bien le
sachez. | [1591ff] See T385ff. | [1597f] See T391f. In J there is no division between
1596–7. | [1599ff] See T449ff. J has red rubric *Femme ki travail de enfant.* | [1599] t. de
enfant (J) | [1605] E l'artimese (T) E l'artemese (J) | [1606] destempré lui dunez (T)
| [1606–7] Separated in TJ. J has red rubric *Autre medicine.* | [1609] De sel (T) Seil (J)
| [1610] De ce seigne tute veie (T) De ceo seit ceinte tut veie (J) | [1611ff] See T461ff.
In J there is no division between 1610–11. | [1611] sanee (J) | [1613] treis g. (J) |
[1614] coliandre (J) | [1616] Mult net e bel seit de drap linge (TJ) | [1618] Mult suef
ataché e mise (TJ) |

Glossary on pp.403–12

Et la femme gard bien qu'ele l'ost
1620   Kaunt li enfés ert né tauntost.   f.20ra

POR AMEGRIER

A meschine ke est trop grasse
Dont om poet trover une masse:
Prendre devez le bel maroil,
1624   Peresil, ache et fenoil,
En vin deivent mult bien boillir,
Miel i metés por adoucir.
Et quaunt ce sera quit assez
1628   Le beivre puis mult bien colez.
Tot jun l'usez par matin,
Ce vous amaigr[ir]a enfin
Et vous tendra en vigor
1632   Et dorra mult bele color.
Si vous cest beivre usez sovent,
Le cors averez mult bel et gent.

POR LAIT DE NORICE

Kaunt lait a la norice faut,
1636   Un beivre face que mult vaut:
Pregne fenoil, pregne letue,
Pernez vervaine et pernez rue,
La bele flour de l'aube espine
1640   Mettre devez a la meschine,
Si ele use cest beivre et fait,
Mult graunt plenté avra de lait.   f.20rb

POR DORMIR

A home ki dormir ne poet
1644   Emplastre fere li estuet:
Pregne mente et canellié,
L'une et l'autre seit bien triblé,
Et kaunt mult bien triblé seront,
1648   Metés as temples et au front.
Le front, les temples emplastrés

[1619] Mes si gardein gard ben (T) k'il ost (TJ) | [1620] Apres l'enfant en haste e tost (TJ) | [1621ff] See T393ff and S no.182 below. J has red rubric *Pur damiseles saner*. | [1623] devez eble e m. (S) 1623–4 are found in MS B. L. Sloane 962 f.131r | [1626] endulcer (S) enducir (J) | [1628] b. nettement bien (S) | [1629–30] Found in MS B. L. Sloane 962 f.131r | [1630] enmegra (TJ) enmegrira (S) | [1633–4] Found in MS B. L. Sloane 962 f.131r | [1635ff] See T407ff, S no. 89 and S1 no. 55 below. J has red rubric *Pur let a norise*. | [1638] Prenge euruke [euruge, J] prenge rue (TJ) Prenge euruque [eruke, S1] prenge letue (SS1) | [1640] MS = *et la m.*; medicine (J) | [1643ff] See T415ff. J has red rubric *Pur ben dormir*. |

A l'oure ke dormir vodrés.
Mes letues avaunt mangez
1652 Ou viande apareillés
Od semence de pavot,
De dormir prendra tot son escot.

AUTRE

Fiente de columbe et miel et cire
1656 Vaut as mameles, ce os dire.
Ki l'emplastre mettra deseure
Emfle et dolor tout en poi d'eure.

POR CLIER OI[R]

Ki dolors as oreiles a dunt il n'oit pas clier
1660 Poudre de neir soffoigne deit od aisil meller,
Et miel bien purgé ne deit il oblier,
Ke il n'i mette as oreilles dount il orra plus clier.

A FAIRE CILECTRE   f.20va

Si vous volez fere cilectre,
1664 Donkes vous covendra mettre
Gome de ere et orpiment
Et bon aisil, com jo l'entent.
Oes de formies assés i ait,
1668 De ce si est cilectre fait.
Tot là ou il tochera,
Sachés ke la pel en charra.

A FAIRE CRESPE CHEVELURE

A faire crespe chevelure
1672 Et longue faire par nature:
Pernez mai les foilles de fou,
Quisez les bien et neient pou.
Le chief en lavez mult sovent,
1676 Aprés fetes cest oignement:
Jus de mirfoil en oile frit,
Si vous en oignés par delit.

[1651] cuvent manger (TJ) ǀ [1652] v. autre apareller (TJ) ǀ [1653] Od oillette de popi (TJ) ǀ [1654] Si dormira tut en suffi (T) Si endormira vus afi (J) ǀ [1655ff] See T427ff with the rubric A mameles emflees. J has red rubric As mameles. ǀ [1656] oi dire (TJ) ǀ [1659ff] Not in TJ ǀ [1663ff] See S no.189 below. J has red rubric Ki voet fere letire. ǀ [1663] siletire (J) ǀ [1665] de cre (J) ǀ [1668] la letire (J) ǀ [1670] crestra (J) ǀ [1671] J has red rubric A crespe chevelure. ǀ [1672] E lung cru solum nature (J) ǀ [1673] P. la juneler del f. (J) ǀ

Glossary on pp.403–12

A TEINE GARIR

  A cele gent ki sont teignus
1680 Raez tot hor[s] teigne et cheveus
  Od fiel de tor et od aisil
  . . .
  Celidoine i met cil,
1684 Tost garira de cel peril.
  Aprés me pernez siu de tor,
  Kar i vaut a cel mal fin or.   f.20vb
  La troche arse de (de) ail pelé
1688 Od le sel arse seit mellé,
  Oile o tot ce mis seit,
  Donc garira, si garir deit.
  A lius placheus ou li peil faut
1692 Bien vous dirai que mult vaut:
  Pernez mosche[s] et ces metés
  En .i. nuef pot et les ardez.
  Od ce metez jus de cerfoil
1696 Et nois petites de cel bruil
  En poudre arses mult sotillement,
  Miel et oile tot ensemble.

A FAIRE NEIR CHEVELURE

  Autre dirai al mien espeir,
1700 Si vous volez aver le chief neir:
  De vigne fraunche pernez sarment,
  Leissive faites ensement,
  Sovent de icele vous lavez,
1704 Bruns et tot neirs cheveus avrez.

POR FAIRE CHEVELURE ROUS

  K[i] veut aver les cheveus rous
  Ce voil enseigner a vous:
  La fraunche vingne devez prendre,   f.21ra
1708 Laissive faire de la cendre,
  Metez i safran et bresil,
  Si serés rous come gopil.

[1679ff] See S no. 37 (prose) below. J has red rubric *A ceus ki sunt teignus*. | [1680] Reez le chef ce dium nus (J) | [1681] O felt e o aisile (J) | [1682] Garist mult ben de cet peril(J) | [1683–4] om. (J) | [1687] La trese de le aile pelé (J) | [1688] MS = Od le *troche arse*; O seit bon melé (J) | [1690–91] Separated in J by red rubric *As places u le peile defaut.* | [1693] e si ardez (J) | [1694] et sil metet (J) | [1698] J adds Ki de cest l'em oindra o tut / Le peill i crestrait tut de but | [1699] J has red rubric *Autre medicine.* | [1701] De fr. vif (J) | [1705–10] Not in J. |

POR AVER LONG CHEVEUS

Femme ke ni a cheveus longs,
1712 Si ce avient por les sirons
Ke la desus es cheveus pendent,
Ki lé manjuent et ses fendent,
Un pain de segle mult i vaut
1716 Kaunt om le trait del for si chaut.
Le pain tot si chaut fendez
Et les cheveus dedens metez.

A tous ceus ke ont manjue
1720 Et com bren ont la char nue
Et soeffrent el chief le moleste
Et g[r]ateison graunt en la teste:
Pernez la semence d'ortie,
1724 Triblez le od vin graunt partie,
Le chief en faites bien laver
Et od le savon bien froter.
Puis pernez le jus de kerson
1728 Od grasse d'owe ou de capon,   f.21rb
De ce si faites oignement
Et le chief en oignez sovent.

LAVEMENT A DAME

. Dirai vous une laveure,
1732 Esteint, ke a cheveus bien dure:
Pernés .i. pot ou ait pertuis
Ou .ii. ou .iii. ou aukes plus,
Cendres de cheine metez i
1736 Et espis d'orge autresi.
De l'estreim d'orge une litiere
Et puis la cendre que ele apere,
Puis l'estreim et puis la cendre
1740 De lit en lit devez estendre.
Que vous en dirai jo plus?
Ewe coraunt versez desus,
Leissive en faites, s'en lavez,
1744 Icest tains vous dura assez
. . .

[1711ff] J has red rubric *Pur ciruns.* | [1711] Cheveus ne poent crestre longes (J) |
[1712] Ce est pur voz cironis (J) | [1718–19] Separated in J by red rubric *Pur la grate e le manjue.* | [1719] Pur le grate et le mangue (J) | [1720] Encumbrement a la char nue (J) | [1721] la moleste (J) | [1722] Dunc gratet en la t. (J) | [1731ff] J has red rubric *Bone laveure.* | [1731] Ore v. dirray une bone l. (J) | [1734] U treis ou quatre (J) | [1740] entendre (J) | [1742] Chaud ewe (J) | [1744] E si taint (J)

Appendix

RECEIPTS IN MS ST JOHN'S COLLEGE D.4
not found as part of the 'Physique rimee'[23] in
MSS Trinity College 0.1.20 and 0.8.27:

St John's	Trinity 0.1.20
[f.84rb] 1. *A jaune cheveleure:*[24]	*Por jaune cheveus avoir* [f.239v]
Un bon consail dirra[i] a ceus	
Ki desirent [. . .] cheveuz.	k. d. avoir jaune c.
Les trus des cholez facent prender,	
Secher e arder puis en cender,	
De ice fere une bone lessive	De ce face om b. l.
De ewe de funtaine vive,	Et de e.
E prender la flur de geneste,	
Garder le poeiz, si le vus plest,	
L'an outre en utre tut enter,	tot plenier
Ki bonement le veut secher.	
En la lessive le bullez	quisez
Einceis ke vostre chef muillez,	Eins
[f.84va] Laver poez par resun	
O assez petit de savun.	O mult tres petit de savun

[f.85vb] 2. *Pur oster lé tecches del vis:*	*Por tecches en le vis* [f.236r]
Quele ki seit, dame u pucele,	La quele
[Ki] coveit aver face bele,	Ki desire
Ne s[a]i bele femme en pais	F. ne sai en nul p.
Pur quei ki [e]lle ait tecches en le vis	
Ki forment ne li mesavenge.	
[. . .] Por quele chose qui avigne	
Si tecche ait ke en vis asperge,	
Si face quire gumme de (c)ere	prendre
E fel de tor, si triblez ensemble.	
Le liu deit froter, se me semble,	
Endrait le tecche ben froter	Totes les t. doit f.
E tut le vis ben laver.	mult b.
Aprés ceo tut a recurer	E enaprés par dreiture
Dait aver autre laver.	D. a. a. laveure
Foïr dait o une beche	
La racine de la liuvesche,	
Laver le deit e fer net,	
[f.86ra] E quire en un pocenet.	bel p.
Mut deit quire, e ceo grant masse,	Ki soit degasté del jor g. m.
Tant cum cel ewe en seit grasse.	
De drait gresse seit oille,	De cele g. s. doldee [sic]
De ceo se leve autrefie.	Et del plus clier abevree

3. *Bone laveure*   *Por faire clier vis* [f.236v]
   Al mais de mai al tens (de) noel
   Prenge le pain de cucuel,
   Lave mult ben, la face net,   fetes le n.
   Sil par[e] ben od une knivet.   coutelet
   U il met puis en un morter   Puis le metez
   E tut le face depescer.
   Kant ceo serra forment pesé,   pilé
   Si sait parmi un drap culé.
   En une noef pot puis le mettez
   E de net ewe le quisez.   arosez
   Issi seit dekes le novim jor,
   Mes le ewe en(s) hostét chescun jor,
   Autre mettez mult clere e bele
   De rive u de fontainele.   De rivere
   Al darraim jor seit ceo osté,
   Parmi un drap seit ben culé,
   Seccher le lessez atant,
   Pudre devendra maintenant
   Plus blanche ki flur buleté,
   Kar se semble naif gelé.   Si semblera
   Ce fet cler vis e bel e net,
   Mes apre est, mult ceo vus promet.   Si om lait de anesse avec met

4. *Autre medicine*   *Autre*
   Aprés iceo, vus promet,   [f.237r]
   Vus aprenderay de fer un siwet.
   Suef fet quir e bele e plain   Qui fait la face b. et p.
   E mut bon culur e sain.   Le vis et la colur sain
   A veile dame (e) a vis frunci
   Fra le vis bele, plain e oni;   P. et o. le fra et delie
   A la meschine, a la pucele,
   Fet la face aver cler e bele,
   E le vis tant ben culuré
   Cum est la rose en tens de esté.
   Home deit fuïr o un beche
[f.86rb]   La racine de la luvesche
   E de la viemauve ensement
   E de fenoile tut ouelement.   ignellement
   La face nettement laver
   E de un cutel mut ben parer.
   Puis seit tut detrenché menu
   E mis a builler sus la feu,   sor / A douce ewe doivent
   A petit feu mut a leisir,   boillir / A petit fu tot a leyssir
   E quant ceo serra quit assez,
   Cele gresse ewe me pernez.
   Avez dunc prest seu de mutun   Aiez
   E seu de cerf, oint de chapun,
   E oint de grasse geline   [f.237v]

Notes on pp.366–67

Revaut a ceste medicine.   Que mult valent
E pur fer la bosine   Por meuz f.
I revaut le oint de la cigoine.   Mete om siu de c.
Le seu deit estre mult blaunchet   blaunche
E tut ben fet e bel e net.   Auques novele clier et fraunche
De tal seim fres puis me pernez   Novel s.
E o les autres mettez.
Puis me pernez trestuz iceo,   Quant ke ai avant nomee en-
    semble met

Sis mettez quire en vostre bro.   Si les metez q. en le bruet
Lessez ben quir e(n) ben bullir
E puis pessez ben freider.
Quant tut ceo refreidé serra,
Cuillez ki desus flot[er]a.
De tel puis [. . .] en un vescel   Batez le p.
E si le cuillez ben e bel.
Puis ki vus averez fet issi,
Vos pudres bones mettez [i],
Muge, girofre e franc encens,
Ceo i covent, si cum jeo pens.
De une verge seit mu
E ben pestri e ben batu.
En veire home pusse mettre   En v. le doit om puis m.
Pur estuer, ceo dit la lettre.   Por meuz garder [f.238r]
Ceo surmet ert de grant valur   [corr. suwet?] Cel siu en est
E mut gentil fleirur,   la flaur
Ce fet le vis net e bele.
Si vus volez aver ruvencele,   rovençel

[f.86va]   Fere le say bel e gentil.   le sa
Vus devez reer le brasil
Pleine culure al men avis,   P. quiller
E de ewe cuillierez sis,
Ov blanc alum deit puis bullir,
Une petit puis refreichir [sic]   Un petitet p. refroidyr
E deit puis estre mis   A l'un des deis d. e. m.
Ou colur deit estre al vis.   c. sera en le v.

5.   *Laveure a dame e a damoysele*:   *Por face lentilluse e froissie*
    [Face] lente(le)iluse e frunsé
    Covient consil e bon aie.   Avroit mester de b. a.
    Anceis ki li die ceo mahagne,   Mainte bele face est m.
    Si prenge savun de Espaigne   Por ce en ai jo eu grant paine
    E voile la face ben quire   [corr. En oile?]
    O vif argent, ce dist le mire,
    Riches dames a Munpele[r]s   [see below p.215]
    E[n] ont le vis beles e cleris.

6.   *Autre medicine*:
    Un oef de geline pernez,

L'aubun del moel deseverez,
L'aubun remetez arer,
Ensemble fetes bullir
Une petit mut a leisire
Ki seit solum mesure,
Ci ad mut bone laveure.

7.   *Pur garder sei de chanir:*   *Por chanir* [f.239r]
Home se deit queintement tenir   Sagement se doit contenir
Ki se veut garder de chanir.
Face lessive, si sen seit.   leve
[. . .]   Bon est qui bien le set fere
Ore vus dirray coment ceo vaut.   ce vait [f.239v]
Lu viemauve par buillir o let   Le wimauve b. l'en fait
En ewe de funtaine vive
Dunt serra(y) fet la lessive,
Ce est de racines de trus,   Cendres de r.
Ki mut par vaut, ce dium nus.   Tele leissive v. a estrous
En le baigne de ewe vus laver   En baigign v. en devez l.
E devez ben cest us garder.   Cest us vous d. trop b. g.

[f.87va] 8.   *Ki parol en dormant:* [25]
Un maveys use on li aquant
Ki solaient parler en dormant.
A lur couls devent athacher
Une croiz entailé de meller
Ou crest sus sulement itant.
[. . .]
E averoine sachez pur veir
[f.87vb]   Od eiscil deven[t] beivre a seir.

9.   *Pur l'aleine pulente:* [26]
Cil ki ont l'aleine pulente
Si beivent puliol e mente,
Si face sa buche escurer,
Cum dis avant, e ben laver.
Si li ert nule dent purrie,
De ceo vent cel pulentie.
Mun consail est ki il en ost
En haste e mut tost.
Bones especes deit user
Pur cel orde fleirur oster,
Clowes de girofre e noiz mugat,
Ki cel mal odur abat.

10.   *Ki perde sa parole:*
Si home pur mal perde sa parole,
Pernez puliol e viole,
Triblez, e a beivre donez,

En le oriele le versez.
La parole recovera
Ki cointement celi durra.

11.   *Ki (en) senglute*:
      Home ke est en mal sanglute,
      La vie li est mut en doute.
      Pernez vin e rue e peivre,
      Entre liu li donez a beivre.
      U pernez ache u comin,
      Buillez en iscel veu vin,
      Castoreum e calament
      Li donez a beivre ensement.
      U si(l) esturnuer porrait,
      Si garra, si vivre deit.

12.   *Pur la jaunez*: [27]
      A la jauneice si me pernez
      Yvoire e rerobe [?] devez,   [corr. recopé]
      Od duz leit seit destempré,
      Al(a) malad[e] seit doné.
      Les gelines as jaunes pez
      A manger li apareilez,
      Savur de sage u de comin
[f.88ra]   Od le safrun ou o le blanc vin.

13.   *Autre medecine*:
      Un uncore vus dirray,
      Verray esprové le ay.
      Li marogerin me pernez,   [corr. maroge chenin?]
      En un morter ben le triblez.
      Ki le fet privement le face,
      Si ki le malade nel sace.
      Le urine pernez al malade,
      Le beivre en ert uaytuse e fade.
      Le herbe de ceo en destemperez,
      A beivre puis le donez.

14.   *Pur ventrail*:
      Encontre le deding de ventrail
      Vus dirray le men consail.
      Iceo avient a mult de genz
      Ki funt un tuiz asés pulenz.
      Vetoine en vin mult ben bullez
      E mel a ceo beivre mettez.
      Plain hanap chaud beivra
      La nuit quant i[l] se cochera.
      La ceintorie buille[z] en vin,
      Bevez a seir e al matin.

Notes on pp.366–67

15. *Por la tusse*:
    Home ki de la tusse veut garrir
    Bone cerveise deit buller
    En vessel de arreim.
    Home ki veut estre sein
    De chesn prenge fugerole
    E la luvesche e la viole
    E puliol ovec si mette
    E jubarbe ki mut seit nette.
    Ensemble seit ben bulli
    E pus cuilli e ben refreidi.
    Seir e matin le deit user,
    Tel beivre fet ben a garder.

16. *Autre medicine*:
    Tel tusse ki del quer v(e)ient
    E al quer e al pomun tient:
    Prendre devét une drap linge

[f.88rb]
    E tailler en longe un c(e)ince
    E par treis feiz lessez gesir
    E li[e] de mede e vin juster.
    Puis entraiez issi muilee
    E seit o vent ben esseuié.
    Aprés pernez de peivre tant
    Bien a deus deners pesant.
    E mettre ki ben priser seit
    Le peis de treis deners teniét[?].
    De blanc encens tut autretant
    E sufre un dener peisant.
    De tut iceo pudre i facez,
    O cire vi[r]gine le mangez.
    E drap ling limignun
    E la cire poet [?] envirun.
    O cire e od linge tail
    Devez fere une chandeile.
    Home ki veut entre
    Un pain de segle deit pus prendre
    Od un carrez parte seit
    E un corn partie ester deit.
    Kant la chandeil ert alumee
    E al pertus del pain seit buté,
    E l[e] cornet seit par desus
    Butié encontre le pertus.
    Li malade ert desus acis,
    Le cornet a sa buche mis.
    La chalur cov(e)ient survenir
    Tant cum il purra suffrer,
    Ost e remette mut feiz,
    Sufre si sent, ceo est draiz.

De manger li dirray la cure,
Mangue cru let e mel e bure.

17. *A la seck tusse*:
    De l'estreit piz e secche tus
    Prenge un lardun, ce dium nus,
    Tenu e teillie en tele manere,
    Met sur un chaud pere.
    Sur ceo met comin ovoc,
    Sun corn parceié si ert iloc,

[f.88va]   Issi se redeit estuver,
    Si li vaudra ben suer.

18. *Autre medicine*:
    Desus a mun dist quer puis
    Ore parlerumus de une autre t(r)us,
    Par nuil, par chaude u par freit,
    Par poi achesun venir deit.
    A ceo pernez maroin chenin,
    Ache, persil e cumin,
    A une sesun ajustez
    [. . .]
    E les cims de la bruere.   [corr. ciuns]
    Bulli serrunt en tele manere:
    En une pot quisent, ce est la fin,
    En bone serveise u en vin.
    Les herbes engete e si prenge
    Saim de bele frescenge
    E mel o tut, car ceo (ke) est dreit
    E puis seit bulliante feiz.
    E quant del feu serra osté,
    Si reserra autre feiz cuillé.
    E aprés ce beivre deit,
    A vespre chaude, al matin freit.

19. *Autre medecine*:
    Ore vus dirray autre manere
    Ki a fere est assez legere.
    E marol chenin me pernez,
    En bersile la quisez
    E uncore vus covient aver plus
    U licorice u le jus.
    Quant ensemble serunt builliz,
    Ceste beivre tout la tus del piz.

20. *Pur gute caïve*:
    Hom ki ad gute kaïve,
    Si voliez k'il garrisse(z) u vive,
    Tost le [. . .] al tor pernez,

En une noef pot les tuz ardez,
La poudre a beivre le donez,
S'il cr[e]aunce ait, si est savez.

[f.88vb] 21. *Autre medecine*:
Uncore vus dirray autre medicine:
De luvesche pernez la racine,
Treis moz escrivez desus:
Jesu + Christus + dominus.
Tant cum avera al col pendu
Ne cherra mes, ben est seu.
S'il eit en Deu ferme creance,
Toz jors garri est sanz dotance.

22. *Autre medecine*:
Pur ceo mal vus dirra[i] aprés.
Face sei li home ben confés
E deus chandeiles eit de cire,
Si fra un messe dire.
Tel messe deit estre deite
En le noun de Saint Espirite.
E[n] les chandeiles dont vus avez dit
Serrunt les nouns dé jors escrit.
A l'autier deit les home offrir
E le malades deit choisir
Une en bone fay e pure,
E prendra la par aveinture.
A cel jor s'ill truverat,
A[l] devant le cors Deu vouerat
Par sun mal e par sa maladie
Jammés jor de sa vie
Por tant cum il sun nun tendra,
E meintenant garri sera.
A cel jor ne mangera,
Si pain nun, e ewe bevera.

23. *A home ki seit amuÿ*:
A l'home ki seit amuy
A(a)loin od ewe doint a luy.
Od cutel overez lé denz
E le beivre versez dedenz.
U gazere u sage u pionie
Li doint home tost sanz esoignie,
Por iveresce done a beivre
Vetoine ki mut maus desevre.

24. *Encontre venim*:
[f.89ra] Encontre venin bevez centorie
E vetoine en bone memorie

Notes on pp.366–67

E rue e sang autresi
Ainz ke mangez, bon est issi.
Ache e aloine, fenoil e raiz
Bevez, si tost garriz.

25. *Por pointure des ee[s]:*
A la pointure des ees pernez
Foile de mauve, si triblez,
Sur la pointur[e] la mettez
E par meismes garri serrez.

26. *Pur morsur[e] de chien:* [28]
Si vus de chin aiez morsure,
Pernez ruge ortie a dreiture,
La morele, beu lard crue,
Ensemble seit ben batue,
E[n] bure quisé(n)t bel e gent,
Si garra par cest oignement.

27. *De chien aragé:* [29]
Un chien aragé, s'il vus mord,
Le plei vus devendra mut fort.
Mut fort sause detemprez
E la plei de cest lavez.
Aprés ce pernez la plantaine
E de egremoine plaine la maine,
Ensemblement ben les(c) triblez.
Aubun de l'oef e mel i mettez
U veuz oint o la plantaine,
Cest oignement vus fra tost saine.

28. *Pur morsure de yraine:* [30]
Ce n'est mie ben k'issi remaine,
Por la morsure de l'yraine,
Ke ne vus die la medicine
Ki mult par est verray e fine.
Muches grant masse purch[a]cez
E de ceo la morsure oignez.
Puis pernez fuilles de raiz,
En vin sein[t] mult buillez.
Quant quit serrunt, ben lé triblez
E sur le pley lé mettez,
[f.89rb]   La plei overte tendra
E l[e] venime enchacera.
De foilis me(s) pernez
E od mel les estampez.
Sur la plei puis lé mettez,
Si deliverement sanez.

Notes on pp.366–67

29. *Pur gute:* [31]
La gute voil a mult orb noil [?]
E grant dolur fete al col,
Es espaules ensement,
Si ouelent angusement.　　　　　　[corr. duelent]
Od mel primes vus oignez,
De feves la ferine pernez
E foiles de cre ensement　　　　　　[corr. de ere]
E de mel fetes oignement.

30. *Autre medicine:*
Uncore vus dirray iceo plus.
De artemese premez le jus,
Od oile e cire le mellez,
Oignez vus e ben garrez.
Rue en fort aisil quisez,[32]
Si chaud sur la dolur mettez.
U savine u verveine pernez,[33]
En vin flur de feves mettez.
Bon oint de ver metez o tut,
Ce garra la dolur de bot.

31. *Pur la gute as reins:* [34]
Home ki ad la gute as rains,
S'il vout garrir e estre sains,
De ortie preng[e] la racine
E cento[r]ie ki est la fine,
E odlescunse mettez o tut.
Ces treis herbes bevez de but,
Ventuser deit u garser
Pur quay i puis estere.
E s'il umcore se sent feble,
Deus feiz u treis se beine en eble.

32. *As genuiz emflez:* [35]
Si acun ait le genuiz emflez,
La rue e[n] beau(l) mes me quisez,　　　[corr. mel]
[f.89va]　　L'emplastre a genuil seit lié,
Tost recevera sa santé
Une medicine dirray bele:[36]
Pernez vie(z)mauve e parel[e],
Cel ki en ewe crestre sout,
Le lu emplastrez u ceo dout.

33. *Autre medicine:*
Uñ autre vus fray ben cert
Ki fu le medicine sein Cutebert,
Ce ki angeles li aprist,

Ki creance ait, ben garist.
. . . now follows T 1–6, succeeded by 7–12

34. *Encontre morsure de serpent:* [37]
Cil ki serra de serpent mors
Hastivement prenge lors
Une forte curray de cerf,
De deus parz seit lié le nerf,
En quel lu ceo seit,
De deus parz seit lié estrait.
Une geline seit tost prise,
Plumé a la morsure mise,
[Ha]stiment e sanz demur
Le fundement tenez desur.
Quant l'em vera(y) k'ele seit emflé,
Si seit cele geline osté.
Un autre seit maintenant quise
Ki ensement soit remise.
Issi seit fet cum iceo le divise
Deskes cel enflure seit asise.
[f.89vb]   Dragance beive e matefelon
E morel par resun.

35. *Pur blesure en l'oile:*
Li home ki est blescé le oile,
Ce face ki dire voile,
Ce ki l'escrit nus teymoine.
Prenge del jus de egrimoine,
O ce prenge l'aubun de l'oef
En une drap linge viez u noef,
Si fetes cotun, si moillez
E sur le oil suef cuchez.
Si ceo nient avez, pernez lin,
L'emplastre le garrist enfin.

[f.98vb] 36. *Pur seigner:*
Ore voil aprender e enseigner
Coment li home se det seigner.
Par tut covien[t] sen e resune
Ki voet overer solum nature.
Li fleumatic e li sanguin
Ne se seignent mie matin,
Mes entre tierci hur de jor.
E june seignent, ce dit le autur.
Colirien a midi
Se deit seigner, ce vus di.
E ki est malencolien
A nun put se seigner ben,
Car sulum les hures del jors

Soleient regner le quatre humors.
E pur les homur menuser
Si deit li home suvent seigner.
Home se deit seigner sagement
E garder se deit ensement.
De tut surfait se deit garder
E quant ke est trop deit eschuer.
E puis manger cele viande
Cum sa nature li demande.
Dunc li covient aver bon pain,
Le blanc levé li est plus sain.
Les oefs moles poet il user
Pur [l]e chef e conforter.
Mirsaus de char de porc en fine,
Pucin, perdriz, fesant, geline,
E sain char est de chapun
E char poudré de mutun.
Petit u nent manjut de fruit
Si ceo n'est une pome par deduit.
Swef vin blanc lors beivera,
Une bone serveise k'il ad.
A manger lerra s'il est sage
E auz e chous e let e furmage.
E[n] dormir e (l)en veiller
Iceo ki afert a commover,
Le travail e le curuce[r]
E trop penser e veiller.
Quei vus en dirra[i] mes?
Deus jors u treis aprés se gard en pes.
En pais seit e en oscurté
K'il seit aukes recoveré.
E pur la veine resaner
Home se deit sur tut rien garder.

COSMETIC RECEIPTS IN MS TRINITY COLLEGE 0.1.20 ONLY

[f.238r]

Por face lentilluse et froissie
  Face lentilluse et froisie
Avroit mester de bon aie,
Mainte bele face est mahaigne,
Por ce en ai jo eu grant paine
De trover .i. verai espeirement
Ke valer peust apertement.
De feves me metés ferrine
Et des cherveles la racine,

Metez i poudre de orpiment
Et oes de formies ensement:
[f.238v] Tot ce soit ensemble triblé.
Et fetes fere oile de blé
Od let de anesse owelement,
Si destemprés vostre oignement.
Pain levé en ewe teve mis,
De ce soit eins lavé le vis.
Aprés, quant est bien assués,
Vostre face oignez, lent ne seez,
Si seron sans fronches et sans lentilles,   [corr. sera]
Kar ce vaut a meres et as files.
Et si avec est mis vif argent,
Plus clier en ert le vis et gent.
Enpoudre om les cheveus esteins
E en salive, ce est la fins,
Et issi esteint om vif argent,
Ce ne sevent pas tote gent.

Lavement a dame par corteysie
Dame et pucele al cors gentil
Que doute hounte e peril,
De cele doit hom pieté avoir,
Que n'est trop coveitos de avoir.
Mainte femme i a de haut quer
Que ne(l) metroit a nul fuer
Sor sa face nul oignement.
[f.239r] Celes voil enseigner brefment
Un lavement par corteysie.
Et de la racine une partie
De luvasche me pernez
Et de fenoil et bien les lavez,
Minciez les bien menuement.
De saugemme et de orpiment,
Et de roses, poudre freez,
Et mastic i ajosterez.
De un oef metez le moel
Et .i. petit de puliol,
Et si i metez blanc encens
En un noef pot par grant sens,
Les fetes bien ensemble boillir
Mult longuement tot par leysir.
Aprés, jus del fu le metez,
De un petit vostre vis lavez.
Ce fetes chescun jor au seir et au matin,
Blanc vis averez et clier et sein.

Chapter Five

AN ANGLO-IRISH RECEIPT COLLECTION

MS London, British Library, Additional 15236 is a collection of botanical, medical and prognostic texts copied, for the most part, around 1300.[1] It was acquired by the British Museum on June 18, 1844 as lot 265 at the sale of books belonging to the interesting collector Benjamin Heywood Bright. The medico-botanical texts are noteworthy for a number of Irish glosses which they contain (see below).[2] Traces of ownership are found on f.153v (Johannes Deane, in a 17th C. hand; Henricus Howler, in a 16th C. hand beside the date 1598) and on ff.13v and 188v (William Eden). On f.57r a hand has written 'proved on my selfe 1614' beside a receipt *Ad delendum morfeam sive lepram cutis*.

The MS has been cut down and now measures approx. 148 x 108 mm. The quires have been mounted separately. Of the fifteen which make up the MS the first four (ff.2–52) seem to have been written slightly earlier than the rest of the contents. The most important texts for present purposes are:

1. ff.2r–13v an alphabetically arranged botanical glossary or list of *synonyma herbarum* giving Latin names with French and English equivalents,[3] the whole written in a neat, elegant hand of c.1300. The glossary proper (ff.2r–9r), another copy of which is found on ff.172v–87v, is followed by two lists of herbs under the headings 'calida et sicca' (ff.9r–10v) and 'frigida et sicca' (ff.10v–11v) and by a miscellaneous glossary of plant names.

2. ff.14r–24v a second, similarly organised botanical glossary (ff.14r–22r), followed by lists of herbs under the headings 'calidum et siccum' (ff.22v–23r), 'calidum et humidum' (f.23v), 'frigidum et humidum' (f.24r) and 'frigidum et siccum' (f.24r/v). This is the work of a second scribe, also of c.1300.

3. ff.172v–187v another copy of the opening glossary which here furnishes the qualities of each plant e.g. 'Absinthium amarum: calidum primo gradu, siccum in secundo gradu'. The indication of these properties is always underlined in red. There are letters in the margin (badly cropped) indicating the Latin *synonyma* and alternating red and blue initials for each alphabetical section. Folios 182v and 183r are so badly rubbed as to be illegible. At the bottom of f.184v are found six verses on the *scabiosa* (Walther, *Initia* 6449) which are also found in MS Oxford, Bodleian Library, Digby 86 f.201v.

4. ff.29r–78r a collection of medical receipts, beginning with a charm. Folios 29–39 are part of an original gathering of 12 folios (there is a leaf missing after f.32) numbered in a medieval hand from 1 to 12 (5 = the missing f.32*). Folios 28 and 40 are a bifolium from another quire and have a series of puzzles and receipts in a later, fourteenth-century hand which is also responsible for the addition of recipes and similar material on ff.14v, 15r, 15v (in French), 16r, 24v, 30v, 31r, 32r, 33v, 36v, 37r, 39v, 41r, 46v, 48r, 54r, 55r, 55v, 56r, 61v, 62r, 63v, 71r, 72r, 76r, 78r, 79r, 80r, 86v, 90v and all the contents of f.91r/v. The first group of receipts contains a large number of grotesque heads in the margins (ff.29r–33r), whilst the second group has no such illustrations and is written, in a variety of hands of the early fourteenth

century, on ff.41r–71r which are numbered in a medieval hand from 13 to 50 (foliated as far as f.64r = 36 and paginated thereafter). Folios 71v–78r (med. pag. 51–63) are occupied by an index to the collection, *Incipit tabula de medicinis supra scriptis et etiam infra scriptis*.[4] The internal folio references which it provides are accurate and include the receipts which follow, in a variety of fourteenth-century hands, on ff.78v–90v (med. pag. 64–88).

The exact provenance of the MS is not known. The scribe does not seem entirely at home with the Irish glosses and may simply have copied them *tant bien que mal* from an exemplar produced in Ireland. These glosses occur in both the glossaries and the receipts. Those appearing in the glossaries, which I have already annotated elsewhere (see note 1), are distributed as follows:

[ff.2v/3r] ciclamen, panis porcinus, malum tere idem, anglice eorþenote, hibernice colranys (also f.5v); [f.8r] sigillum sancte Marie, herba est quedam, hibernice mas tork; sangguinaria, bursa pastoris, g. sanguinarie vel oumener, hibernice lus ne galdan (and again f.11v, MS reading both times *ius*); [f.11v] tapsus barbastus, g. moleyne, a. feltwrt, hibernice kinnil mury; [f.12r] lapacium rotundum forte vocatur anglice vel hibernice pobel; [f.15r] buglosa anglice wodeburne .s. bugle, hibernice glaskil; [f.17r] filago, mouser, lethlas; [f.17v] herba munda, anglice spurge, hibernice gid coru?; ypia minor, gracedeu que dicitur hibernice lus mide; [f.18v] melotum, hibernice sanrothirath; morsus demonis, hibernice lethan corhygh; [f.19v] paranetum, hibernice aneoit, dile; pigula, lingua avis, anglice stitchwort, hibernice ur agus crin.[5]

At the bottom of f.49r the scribe has written a brief account of measures as follows:

Nota quod unus denarius cum quadrante faciunt unum scrupulum et sic scrupulum debet scribi ɔ. Item duo denarii cum obulo faciunt unam dragmam et dragma debet sic scribi .ȝ. Item octo dragme faciunt unam unciam et uncia debet sic scribi Ƭ. Item sexdecim uncie, et secundum aliquos quatuordecim uncie, faciunt unam libram. Item octo libre faciunt unam lagenam vini vel servicie vel alterius liquoris qualiscumque sit.

In printing the receipts below I have numbered those composing the first gathering (ff.29–39), which may originally have been independent from the rest, separately from the bulk of the collection (the numbering of which is accompanied by an asterisk in the glossary). The unrubricated charm and the first remedy (*Pur fundure*), the ingredients of which are listed over two columns, are indicated in the glossary by C. and O. respectively. The standard format of receipt collections begins on f.30r and I have commenced the numbering of the receipts from this point.

[f.71v] *INCIPIT TABULA DE MEDICINIS SUPRA SCRIPTIS ET ETIAM INFRA SCRIPTIS*[5]

Absinthium: Nota de multis virtutibus medicinalibus absinthii .46. (f.69r)

Albedo: Contra albuginem occulorum .3. (f.31r) .8. (f.35r) .31. (f.59r) plura de hiis infra *occulus*

Antrax .i. feloun: Contra antracem per laminam plumbi .3. (f.31v) et idem valet pro fistulis, vulneribus et aliis morbis contagiosis

Pro antrace interficiendo: .31. (f.59r) .87. (f.90r)

Item pro omne genere antracis si surrexerit infra corpus nec extra apparuerit .5. (f.32* missing) .17. (f.45r)

Item pro antrace cum fuerit ostensus vel non ostensus .17. (f.45r)

Item pro antrace ammovendo de uno loco ad alium ubicumque extra apparuerit .5. (f.32* missing) .31. (f.59v)

Item pro antrace rubei coloris .i. rouge feloun .6. (f.33v)

Item ad sanandum antracem cum antrax fuerit interfectus .32. (ff.59v–60r) et idem etiam valet pro omni genere plagarum dummodo plage non sint nimis profunde et idem etiam valet pro omnibus pistulis sanandis .i. bylis

Apostema: Contra apostemata .8. (f.35r) .10. (f.37r) .15. (?)

Item experimentum ad sciendum utrum homo habet apostema vel non

Item contra apostemata laterum et tumorem et dolorem eorundem .9. (f.36v) .32. (f.60v)

Appium: Nota de commendacione appii quoad diversa medicamenta .46. (f.69r)

Annisum: Nota de multis virtutibus annisi medicinalibus .46. (f.69r)

[f.72r] Argentum vivum: Nota de mirabili affectu eiusdem .41. (?)

Aures: Contra dolorem aurium et vermes .10. (f.37v) .12. (f.39v) .46. (?)

Auditus: Contra difficultatem auditus .3. (f.31r) .11. (f.38v) .12. (f.39v) .18. (f.46v) .46. (?)

Arena: .i. gravel. Respice infra urina ubi scribitur

Anus: Contra anum exeuntem una etiam cum bottouns .76. (f.84v)

Arsura: Contra arsuram .50. (f.71r)

Brook: Contra predictam infirmitatem .67. (f.80r) .88. (f.90v)

Bottouns: Contra bottouns exeuntes sive fluxerint sanguine sive non .85. (f.89r) 87 (f.90r) .15. (?) .47. (?)

Casus: Pro malis casuris .i. lithir fallingys .14. (f.42r) .16. (?) .85. (f. 89r)

Cancer: Contra cancrum: .1. (f.29r) .2. (f.30r) .3. (31r) .5. (f.32* missing) .8. (f.35r) .26. (f.54r) .33. (f.61r) .82. (f.87v) .83. (f.88r)

Carmina: Carmen pur festyr, kaunkyr, goute corable, rancle, et tot maner de goute .i. (f.29r)

Item carmina plumbi pro antrace, fistula, vulneribus et aliis morbis .3. (f. 31v)

Item carmen contra dolorem dencium .23. (f.51v) .33. (f.61v)

Item carmen contra albedinem occulorum .27. (f.55r)

Item carmina contra febres .14. (f.42v) .18. (f.46r) .19. (f.47v) .26. (f.54v)

Capud: Contra dolorem capitis intollerabilem .9. (f.36v) .5. (f.32* missing) .11. (f.38v) .13. (f.41v) .16. (f.44v) .18. (f.46v)

Capilli: ad nutriendum capillos .10. (f.37v)

Item ut capilli nascantur .12. (f.39r)

Morbus caducus: Contra hoc .2. (f.30v) .20. (f.48r) .84. (f.88v)

Calculus: Infra lapis

[f.72v] Cibus: Cuiusmodi cibaria debent sumi in quatuor temporibus anni .s. in vere, estate, autumpno, et in hyeme necnon et de qualitatibus et de incepcionibus et terminacionibus eorumdem .48. (f.70r)

Coitus: Que sunt illa que coitum provocant et confortant .21. (f.49v)

Concepcio: Ut mulier non concipiat .12. (f.39v) .41. (f.66v)

Item ut mulier concipiat .18. (f.46v) .26. (f.54r) .43. (f.67v)

Constipacio: Contra constipacionem .3. (f.31v) .14. (f.42v) .19. (f.47r) .26. (f.54v) .31. (f.59v) .41. (f.66v) .68. (f.80v)

Item contra eandem passionem infra electuaria

Item combustio: Supra arsura

Dentes: Contra dolorem dentium .5. (f.32* missing) .9. (f.36v) .23. (f.51v) .33. (f.61v)

Dormicio: Ut homo dormiat .10. (f.37v) .13. (f.41v) .36. (f.64r)

Entracta: Ad faciendum entractum quod gratia Dei vocatur .34. (f.62r) .71. (f.82r)

Epar: Contra calefactionem epatis .7. (f.34v) .13. (f.41v) .35. (f.63r)

Ebrius: Ne ebrius fiat aliquis .12. (f.39r)

[f.73r] Contra ebriosos: .9. (f.36v)

Item si vis aliquem inebriare .12. (f.39r)

Electuaria: Electuarium laxativum maxime cum fleuma dominatur in corpore et ad purgacionem fleumatis .19. (f.47r)

Item electuarium laxativum ad purgationem colere .20. (f.48v)

Item electuarium laxativum .20. (f.48r)

Item electuarium confortativum sive restauracio .20. (f.48r)

Item electuarium optimum qui vocatur diapigamon; valet enim contra omnes malos humores ex quibus diutine infirmitates proveniunt, valet enim contra debilitatem stomachi et viscositatem et omnem guttam et parelesim expellit, renum et inferiorum partium dolores mitigat, naturam perditam restaurat et semen coagulat .20. (f.48v)

Item electuarium quod vocatur diasaturion ad reddendum hominem potentem in opere venereo .21. (f.49r) .22. (f.50v)

Item potio pro eodem .22. (f.50v)

Item electuarium ad reddendum hominem inpotentem in opere venerio pro perpetuo .23. (f.51r)

Item electuarium ad reddendum hominem inpotentem in opere venereo ad tempus .23. (f.51r)

Emoroidas: Contra istam passionem .14. (f.42r) .47. (f.69v) .85. (f.89r) .87. (f.90r)

Experimenta: Experimentum ad sciendum si homo evadet de fluxu ventris vel non .3. (f. 31v)

Item experimentum ad sciendum an infirmus vivet vel morietur .11. (f.38r) .18. (f.46v)

[f.73v] *Ferrum*: Ad extrahendum ferrum de ossibus .6. (f.33v) .64. (f.78v)

Item ad extrahendum ferrum sive fuerit in stomacho sive fuerit in [in]testinis hominis .42. (f.67r)

Febres: Pro febre acuta .6. (f.33v)

Item contra febres tertianas .36. (f.64r)

Item contra febres .10. (f.37r) .14. (f.42v) .18. (f.46r) .19. (f.47v) .26. (f.54v) .79. (f.86r)

Item contra febrem tertianam et etiam cotidianam .28. (f.56v)

Fetor: Contra oris fetorem .9. (f.36r)

Fistula: Contra fistulam .1. (f.29r) .8. (f.35r) .82. (f.87v) .14. (f.42r)

Fluxus: Ad fluxum ventris restringendum .6. (f.33r) .10. (f.37v) .33. (f.61v) .83. (f.88r)

Item contra fluxum ventris .30. (f.58v) .41. (f.66v) .33. (f.61v)

Item de eodem supra experimentum

Item pro fluxu continuo matricis .15. (f.43v)

Item contra fluxum sanguinis, infra sanguis

Fleobotomia: Quando facienda est fleobotomia .47. (f.69v)

Fetus: Ut mulier pariat quemcumque fetum .12. (f.39r)

Ferrum: Ad portandum ferrum ignitum .12. (f.39r)

Festir: Pro omni genere de festir .14. (f.42r) .1. (f.29r) .8. (f.35r) .82. (f.87v)

Notes on pp.368–72

Foundur: Contra fundacionem que provenit ex subitanea **[f.74r]** potatione post laborem .1. (f.29r) .7. (f.34r)

Frenesis: Contra frenesim .9. (f.36v) .47. (f.69v)

Furtum: Ad inveniendum furtum .25. (f.53r)

Fumeterre: Nota de XII virtutibus fumiterre .45. (f.68v)

Fantasmata: Contra fantasmata .35. (f.63v)

Gutta: Contra guttam currentem .1. (f.29r) .16. (f.44v)

Item contra guttam et paralisim .2. (f.30r)

Item contra guttam .13. (f.41r) .10. (f.37r) .68. (f.80v) .74. (f.83v)

Item contra guttam frigidam in capite vel alibi emplastrum .10. (f.37r)

Item pro omni genere guttarum .13. (f.41r)

Item contra guttam frigidam et etiam currentem .31. (f.59r)

Item contra guttam que non est frigida nec calida et que movet se de loco .32. (f.60v)

Item contra guttam que aliquando est frigida aliquando calida .33. (f.61r)

[f.74v] Herba sancti Johannis: Nota pulcrum miraculum eiusdem herbe quoad punctum temporis in quo Christus natus est .33. (f.61r)

Inflacio: Contra omne genus inflacionis et rankyl .1. (f.29r) .10. (f.37v) .16. (f.44v)

Item contra inflacionem colli .12. (f.39r)

Item contra inflacionem brachii de fleobotomia .9. (f.36r)

Ilyaca passio .i. jaundys: Contra hoc .40. (f.66r) .83. (f.88r)

Item inpedigines .i. . . . .⁶ Contra hoc .8. (f.35r)

Lapis sive calculus ad lapidem frangendum .88. (f.90v) .10. (f.37v) .37. (f.64v) .34. (f.62v) .45. (f.68v) .47. (f.69v)

Lepra: Experimentum ad probandum an homo sit leprosus natura vel a causa et si sit a causa, de cura eiusdem .38. (f.65r)

Item lepra cutis .29. (f.57r) .45. (f.68v)

Loquela ad eos qui non possunt loqui pre infirmitate .2. (f.30v) .11. (f.38r) .19. (f.47v)

Libido: Ad extinguendum libidinem in meretricibus .31. (f.59r)

Livor: Contra livoris dolorem que provenit ex percussione .46. (f.69r)

Latera: Contra tumorem et dolorem laterum et apostemata eorundem .9. (f.36v) .32. (f.60v)

[f.75r] *Manus:* Contra crepaturas manuum .36. (f.64r)

Matrix: Pro mola matricis precipitatione et suffocatione eiusdem et ad provocandum menstruum .21. (f.49v) .29. (f.57v) .30. (f.58v) .47. (f.69v) .76. (f.84v)

Item pro subito assensu matricis .i. aþie þe verliche rakynggys offe þe modyr to womanhus hert .42. (f.67r) .83. (f.88r)

Item ad purgandum matricem et ut mulier concipiat .43. (f.67v)

Menstruum: Si mulier nimis cito vel nimis tarde habuerit flores suos qualiter est reducendum suum statum naturalem et ad tempus debitum .43. (f.67v)

Item ad restringendum menstruum et etiam fluxum matricis continuum .15. (f.43v)

Item menstruum supra, matrix

Minucio: supra, fleobotomia

Morsus: Pro morsu canis et etiam lythyr prichynggys de ferro acu vel de spina .16. (f.44r) .47. (f.69v)

Mors: De .vii. signis mortiferis in homine infirmo .31. (f.59v)

Morbus caducus: Contra predictum morbum .2. (f.30v) .20. (f.48r) .84. (f.88v)

Morfea .i. mool sive lepra cutis ad hoc delendum .29. (f.57r)

Mulier: Pro illa infirmitate que est in mulieribus et est quasi quid vinum discurrens huc illuc intra corpus mulieris .4. (f.32v)

Item pro quadam infirmitate que est in muliere et cum quid gibbosum et durum in se nec movetur per corpus sed semper in uno loco continue sistit .15. (f.43r)

Item ad mulierem que non potest per se post partum libere purgari .10. (f.37r) .75. (f.84r)

Item ut mulier pariat quodcumque fetum .12. (f.39r) .13. (f.41r)

Item ut mulier liberetur a partu suaviter et sine periculo .75. (f.84r)

[f.75v] Ut mulier statim pariat .13. (f.41r)

Item ut mulier (non) concipiat .18. (f.46v) .26. (f.54r) .43. (f.67v)

Item mamilla: Contra infirmitatem gravem mamillarum .67. (f.80r)

Mus: Contra mures et vermes ne corrodant pannos .46. (f.69r)

Occulus: Pro rubedine et lippitudine occulorum .2. (f.30v) .5. (f.32* missing) .6. (f.33r)

Item pro occulis percussis .6. (f.33r)

Item pro occulis egris contra noctem .6. (f.33r)

Item pro occulis continue lacrimantibus ex excessu caloris .32. (f.60r)

Item contra omnes infirmitates occulorum .11. (f.38r) .31. (f.59r) .46. (f.69r)

Item pro albugine occulorum et pur la tey .6. (f.33r) .8. (f.35r)

Item carmen pro eiusdem .27. (f.55r)

Item collirium electum .i. confectio herbarum et aliarum rerum pro occulis et clarificatione visus .3. (f.31r) .5. (f.32* missing) .10. (?) .12. (f.39r)

Item ad auferendum sanguinem de occulo .9. (f.36v)

Visus ad confortandum visum .11. (f.38v)

Item ad clarificandum visum .46. (f.69r)

Opilacio: Contra opilaciones epatis .45. (f.68v)

Pannus: Ut pannus videatur ardere et non ardebit .12. (f.39r)

Palpebra: Contra rubedinem palpebrarum .6. (corr. .7. = f.30v) .5. (f.32* missing)

[f.76r] *Partus:* supra, mulier

Paralisis: Contra paralisim .4. (f.30r) .8. (f.35r) .33. (f.61r)

Pectus: Contra stricturam pectoris .6. (f.33v)

Item ad dilatandum pectus .35. (f. 63v)

Item ad pectus dolens et ad pectus purgandum .9. (f.36r)

Pedes: Contra pedes inflatos vel dolentes ex itinere .10. (f.37r)

Item contra frigus pedum .10. (f.37r)

Pistule .i. bylys; Pro pistulis sanandis .32. (f.60r) .45. (f.68v)

Pili: Ad deponendum pilos in quocumque loco corporis fuerint nec unquam excres . . . et ad sanandum eundem locum .24. (?) .28. (f.55r) .69. (f.81r)

Item ad faciendum ut pili crescant seu nascantur .12. (f.39r)

Item ad nutriendum pilos .10. (f.37v)

Item ne pili crescant .50. (f.71r)

Plaga: Pro omni genere plagarum .3. (f.31r) .14. (f.45v)

Item ad sanandum plagas .30. (f.58r) .31. (f.59r) .32. (f.60r) .44. (f.68r)

Item pro plagis curandis pocio .2. (f.30v)

Item ad faciendum sanativum quod vocatur poysoun pro plagis curandis .24. (f.52r)

Item contra dolorem livoris que provenit ex percussione .46. (f.69r)

Porrus: De effectibus bonis et malis porri .30. (f.58r)

Pulmo .i. longyn: Contra malum pulmonis .30. (f.58r?) .40. (?)

Punctura: Contra puncturas graves de acu vel spina .16. (?)

Purgacio: Supra, mulier

Pruritus: Contra hoc .45. (f.63v)[7]

[f.76v] *Raucitas* sive raucedo: Contra hoc et etiam tussim et malum pulmonis .30. (f.58v) .40. (f.66r)

Renes: Contra dolorem renum .14. (f.45r) .18. (f.46r) .47. (f.69v)

Sanguis: Ad constringendum sanguinem de vena infissa vel de naribus vel de vulnere .9. (f.36r) .14. (f.45v) .18. (f.46r) .19. (f.47v) .34. (f.62v)

Item si ex naribus vis producere sanguinem .12. (f. 39r)

Sausfleme: Ad hoc delendum .31. (f.59v)

Scabies: Ad deponendum scabiem in facie et eandem scabiem sanandam .24. (f.55r) .28. (f.55v) .35. (f.63r)

Item ad delendum scabies manuum et etiam tetrys .29. (f.57r)

Item ad delendum scabies existentes in capitibus et in servicibus juvenum .29. (f.57r)

Item contra scabiem et pruritum .45. (?)

Serpens: Si serpens os hominis intraverit .35. (f.63v)

Spina: Ad extrahendum spinam .2. (f.30v) .6. (f.33v) .42. (f.67r) .64. (f.78v)

Sompnum: Supra, dormicio

Stranguria: Hoc est quando homo non potest facere urinam, contra hoc .9. (f.36r)

Sterilitas: Supra, concepcio

Item ad probandum sterilitatem in viro et muliere .30. (f.58v)

Stomachus: Contra stomachum frigidum .6. (f.33v) .74. (f.83v) .76. (f.84v) .18. (f.46r)

Item ad confortandum stomachum et ad provocandum appetitum .45. (f.66v)

[f.77r] Item contra stomachum obstructum .18. (f.46r)

Item contra dolorem stomachi .19. (f.47r)

Item contra dolorem stomachi et cordis arsuram .30. (f.58v)

Item contra frigidum stomachum et obstructum ex nimia repletione et ad purgandum stomachum et ventrem constipatum de malis humoribus .32. (f.60r) .41. (f.66v)

Surditas: Supra, auditus

Splen: Ad mundificationem et confortationem splenis .45. (f.67r) .46. (f.69r)

Singultus: Contra singultum que provenit ex plenitudine .46. (f.69r)

Tetris: Ad delendum omne genus tetris .29. (f.57r)

Testiculi: Contra testiculos inflatos .28. (f.56v)

Timpora: Contra dolorem timporum .13. (f.41v) .16. (f.44r)

Torsiones: Contra torsiones ventris et stomachi .9. (f.36v)

Tumor: Contra tumorem brachii de fleobotomia .9. (f.36v), plura de hiis supra, inflatio

Tussis: Contra tussim .5. (f.32* missing) .7. (f.34v) .11. (f.38r) .18. (f.46v) .30. (f.58v) .40. (f.66r?)

Tret: Ad faciendum tret diversimode .34. (f.62r) .71. (f.82r)

Tristicia: Contra tristiciam .47. (f.69v)

[f.77v] *Vermis:* Contra vermem .11. (f.69v)

Item contra vermes et mures ne corrodant pannos .46. (f.69r)

Item ad extrahendum vermem .2. (f.30v)

Item contra vermem generatam in matrice mulieris .4. (?)

Item si vermis os hominis intraverit .35. (f.63r?)

Venenum: Contra venenum .34. (f.62v)

Visus: Supra, occulus
Urina: Contra difficultatem urinandi .8. (f.35v) .9. (f.36r) .10. (f.37r) .11. (f.38r) .47. (f.69v)
Item cum homo non poterit urinam suam retinere .9. (f.36r) .36. (f.64r)
Item qui sanguinem mingunt .36. (f.64r)
Item quicum urina[m] simul mingunt et arenam .i. gravel .34. (f.62v)
Wrechyng: Contra hoc, supra, inflacio
Virga: Contra arsuram virge .28. (f.56v)
Vomitus: Ad provocandum vomitum .11. (f.38v) .35. (f.63r)
Item ad restringendum vomitum .11. (f.38v) .18. (f.46v) .35. (f.63r) .46. (f.84v)
Vox: Ad clarificandum vocem .36. (f.64r)
Uva .i. strichyl: Ad uvam pendentem .36. (f.64r) .37. (f.64v)
Vulnus: An homo evadet de vulnere vel non .35. (f.63r)
Item de hiis consimilibus, supra, experimenta
Item contra vulnera stillancia .46. (f.69r)
Venter: Contra dolorem ventris .47. (f.69v)
Ventositas: Contra ventositates .46. (f.69r)
Ydropisis: Contra ydroposim [sic] qui accidit ex fundacione .1. (f.29v) .7. (f.34r)
[f.78r] Item contra ydropisym antequam infirmitas sit radicata seu confirmata in corpore et precipue antequam venter sit inflatus .72. (f.82v) .73. (f.83r)
Item contra ydropisim .45. (f.68v)[8]

[f.29r]
Veez ci la charme seinte Susanne ke Gabriel l'aungle li aporta de part Nostre Seignor pur charmer les crestiens de vers, de festre, de goute corable, de rauncle, de caunkre, et pur toute manere de goute.[9] Fetes chaunter primerement une messe del Seint Espirit au matyn et seit li malades present et pus li fetis charmer: In nomine Patris et Filii et Spiritus Sancti, Amen. Ausi verraiment cume Deus est, ausi verrey-ment cum kaunt ke il dit bien dit, ausi verreiment cum kaunt ke il fit ben fit, ausi verreiment cum de la seinte pucele char prist, ausi verreiment cum en la seinte croiz se mist, ausi verreiment cum cink plaes suffrit pur touz pecheours de mort reindre, ausi verreiment cum en la seinte croiz fu estendu, ausi verraiment cum entre deus larruns fu pendu, ausi verreiment cum en la destre fu de une launce feru, ausi verreiment cum sa seinte teste fu d'espines corouné, ausi verreiment cum ses meins et ses pez furent des clous fichez, ausi verreiment cum en la seinte sepulcre sun cors reposa, ausi verreiment cum au tierz jour de mort sei resuscita, ausi verre-iment cum en enfern ala, ausi verreiment cum les portes d'enfer brusa, ausi verrei-ment cum le maufé lya, ausi verreiment cum lé seinz sus amena, ausi verreiment cum il a ciel munta, [f.29v] ausi verreiment cum a la dextre sun pere reposa, ausi verreiment cum a le jour de juyse vendra, ausi verreiment cum chescun home en char et en saunc en age de trent aunz levera, ausi verreiment cum Nostre Seignur touz a sun pleisyr jugera, ausi verreiment cum ce est veir et veir serra, ausi verreim-ent Deu, Pere et Filz et Seint Espirit, verrai Roy, simples, douz, deboneir, humles, pitous, et plein de misericorde, pur celes seintes angoisses ke Vous sufrites en la seinte croiz garricez cesti .N. de cele maladie. Diez au malade ke il ne deporte nule manere de viaunde. Diez ceste charme a la secré de la messe.

0. *Pur fundure* seu contra ydropisim qui accidit ex fundacione:[10] Persil-rote, fenoil-rote, radich-rote .m. .i.; violette, dayse, strowberywise, bugle, scabiose, musere, hertistunge, cetrac, pollitricum, adiantos .m. .ii.; wallewrt-rote, fumetere, corticis sambuce .m. semis. Terantur et coquantur in aqua usque ad consumpcionem tercie partis et postea clarificetur et addatis si velitis de zuccura vel liquiricio et bibat inde paciens unam mediocrem quantitatem mane et sero. Istud veraciter est probatum.

1. [f.30r] *Pocio pro plagis curandis*: Accipe semen vel summitates canabi, summitates veprium rubeorum, summitates oleris rubei, summitates urtice rubee, tenesye, avence, herbe Johan, herbam Roberti, herbam Walteri, sanicle, plantaginem, consolidam minorem, pentafilon .i. quintefoil, millefolium, linguam avis .i. bridistunge vel stichewrt, bugle et ad pondus omnium istarum herbarum waranciam .i. madir. Deinde terantur omnia in mortario mundo ad modum minutissime salse et fiant inde pile et desiccentur ad solem et dentur vulnerato mane et vespere, in vino vel cervisia defecata vel aqua, et ponatur super vulnus folium caule rubee et lavetur vulnus tepida aqua semel vel bis in die.

2. *Ad cancrum*: Flewrt,[11] herbe Robert, heyhove simul terantur et fiat emplastrum et superponatur loco et sanabitur paciens domino mediante.

3. *Pur gute et paralisi*: Pernez oint de jars .i. gandirsmere et de chat madle et de cire virge le peis de .iii. souz et une bone poyne de cressuns et autaunt de sauge et treis oyngnouns et oint de porc sengler une livere et mellez touz ensemble et le triblés ben et metez toute dedens le jars et le rostez trében et requilez le seym ke en istera. Si le gardez bien [f.30v] e kaunt bosoyne serra, en oignez la gute au fu.

4. *Pur goute*: Egremoyne, weybrede, musere, scabiose, carsin, warmot, pimpirnel .i. flewrt, heyhove, alisaundre, wodethunge, spinacle, herbe Jon, bremilcrop, red-cowilcrop. De hiis et butiro de mayo fit optimum unguentum pro gutta.

5. *Pro rubedine oculorum*: Conteratur albumen ovi cum lana alba et munda et sume de succo plantaginis duas partes et tertiam partem de albumine ovi simul mixtas et inde pone in oculis antequam vadas cubitum.

6. *Ad extrahendum spinam vel vermem*: Recipe egremoyn, columbinam et pinguedinem apri et ex hiis fac emplastrum et appone loco.

7. *Contra morbum caducum*: Accipe semen columbine et detur infirmo ad bibendum, vel ponatur in pane vel potu suo. Probatum [est]. Detur etiam semen columbine infirmo carenti loquela et loquetur.

8. *Contra rubedinem palpebrarum*: Accipe succum pomorum silvestrium et pone in pelvi bene mundata et sit ibi per novem dies naturales et omni die bene fricetur liquor(um) cum cote in pelvi et post .ix. dies pones in vase eneo et omni nocte[12] [f.31r] inunge palpebras quando vadis cubitum.

9. *Contra cancrum experimentum optimum et leve*: Primo pure confiteatur paciens. Deinde sumat herbam Roberti et bene terat eam in mundo mortario et apponat morbido loco et sanabitur mediante domino Jhesu Christo.

10. *Collirium electum* pro occulis et pro albedine occulorum:[13] Pernez une poigne

de eufrase et autaunt de rue et la tierce part de fenoil russe, si triblez ben ensemble et colez parmi un drap linge. Et fetes seym de porc en un vessel de areme et veez ke cel oint seit de porc madle, ou pernez oint de cok ou de gelyne, si colez parmi un draplette, cum est avaunt dit, et metez en une paele, si le quisét nettement. Et pus pernez le jus des treis herbes[14] avaunt dites, si les boillés ensemble et movez ben au funz, si primez parmi un draplette et pus lessét refreydir. Si metez en un boist, si l'estuez par tut le an et de ceo metez as euz quant vus irez cocher.

11. Bevez chescun jour rue et le mangez jun et vus fra bone vue.

12. *Pur dur oye*: Triblez mente e pernez le jus et metez teve as orailles.[15]

13. [f.31v] Si vous volez saver si home que est en fluxe pusse eschaper u nun, donez li treis feiz en treis jors le peis de un dener de semence de cressun du jardyn .i. tuncars a manger et pus li donez a beivre vyn u cerveise estale. Et si il estaunche, si garra, et si nun, il murra. Et si il estaunche, li donez a beivre jus de planteyne et jus de ache .i. merche et mellez en cel jus un pou de ferine de feves et fetes li pacient beivre cel jus au seir chaude et au matyn freide.

14. *Si home ne se pusse delivrer*: Si home ne pusse sei deliverer[16] a chaumbre, prenge semence de lyn et le face ben quire en eawe et pus ochte l'eawe et mange[17] la semence et serra soluble.[18]

15. *Pro antrace, fistula, vulneribus et aliis morbis contagiosis*:[19] Accipias laminam plumbi ita longam et latam sicut vulnus. Postea in quolibet angulo fac unam crucem et unam in medio et dum facis ipsas cruces dicatis omnia ista: 'Domine Jhesu Christus, qui passus es pro nobis in cruce, da sanitatem huic famulo tuo .N. "Vulnera quinque Dei sint medicina sui / Sit medicina sui pia crux et passio Christi".'[20] Postquam hoc perfeceris cave ne predicta lamina tangat terram quia, si fecerit, perdet virtutem suam. Et sciendum quod ad quamlibet crucem dicere [f.32r] debes: 'Domine Jhesu Christe', ut prius cum ceteris. Postea ponendo dictam laminam super morbum dicere debes istud carmen cum tribus benedictionibus: 'Dame seinte Marie, mere au Sauveour, pur les cink joyes ke vous aviez de vostre cher filz, kaunt vous le conceutes, saunz humayne compaignie et l'enfauntastes virgine saunt peyne, et vous le veites du mort relever a vie e par sa vertu demeyne au ciel mounter et kaunt il vos corona sur toutes autres creatures; jeo vous en pri ke vous priez vostre cher filz pur les cink plaes ke il sufri en la croiz, ke il garrisse ce mal'. E a checune feiz ke vous[21] dites ceste charme, donez la beneiçun 'In nomine Patris et Filii et Spiritus Sancti, amen. Sicut plage domini nostri Jhesu Christi non putruerunt nec ranclerunt nec vermes fecerunt, ita plaga ista non putrescat nec ranclescat nec vermem faciat, sed ad sanitatem perfectam perveniat'.[22] Gardez ben ke la plate ne seit remué avaunt treis jours. E pus pernez la ruge cholette et quisez bien en eawe ové toute la racine et l'escorz et debrusez ové vos meins et metez point de fer et quisét taunt ke la meité [de] l'eawe seit retret et pus lavét la plate sovent et le mal et recuchez la plate autre feiz et pus dites cest oreysun: 'Domine Jhesu Criste, qui precioso sanguine tuo nos peccatores in cruce redemisti, mittere[23] [f.32v] digneris benedictionem tuam super plumbum istud, ut quicquid infirmitatis ex eo tactum fuerit per virtutem sanctissime passionis tue accipiat sanitatem per Christum dominum nostrum, amen'.

16. *Postea dicat istam orationem:*[24] 'Ausi verreiment cum Nostre Sire Jhesu Crist fu mis en la croiz en le mount Calvarie, et ausi verreiment cum il sufrit cink plaes pur nous, et ausi verreiment cum ses plaes ne festrerent ne ranclerent, ausi verreiment ne pussent lé plaes cesti .N. rauncler ne festrer. E ausi verraiment cum il se resuscita au tierz jour de mor en vie, ausi verraiment pussent ces plaes aver saunté et garrisoun, amen. In nomine Patris, et Filii et Spiritus Sancti, amen'. Pur garrir[25] festre, verme et cankre et toute manere de plaey overte, fetes cum jeo ay dit et saunté avera li pacient par la grace Deu.

17. *Pro illa infirmitate que est in mulieribus et est quasi vivum quid discurrens huc illuc intra corpus mulieris:* Recipe de madir manipulos duos, ribbewrt .m. .i., mugwrt .m. .i., warmot .m. .i., wodesur .m. .ii. et bene terantur in mortario et postea coquantur in vino rubeo vel in cervisia forti, et defecata, si vinum non inveniatur, usque ad medietatem et fiat inde pocio. Postea detur mulieri circa horam primam jejuno stomaco ad bibendum nec post ad bonum tempus . . .[26]

18. *Pro oculis percussis:* Accipe consolidam minorem / .i. briswort[27] / et albumen ovi et simul tere et sume de succo et oculis infunde et sanabitur.

19. *Pro oculis egris contra noctem:*[28] Capias eufrasiam et tere bene. Postea sume pinguedinem auce vel galline vel porci masculi et frixentur bene in patella. Postea cole per pannum lineum et pone in pixide et unge inde oculos. U pernez greyn de centirgalle et metez chescun[29] jour en l'eoil un greyn u deus u treis. *Prescripta medicina valet contra albuginem occulorum.*[30]

20. *Pur blanc de eus e*[31] la teye: Pernez fel du levre et mel owele mesure et mellez ben ensemble et de ceo metez dedenz l'oyl. Ou pernez le jus de chous et eysil owele mesure et metez dedenz un pot de areme et le coverez ben dedens la terre .ix. jurz et de ceo metez en l'oyl, si garra.

21. *Contra rubedinem et lippitudinem oculorum:* Sume calaminam et pinguedinem caponis et simul frige et inde unge palpebras.

22. *Ad idem:* Accipe pulverem cimini et cum succo rute confice et bombace intincta pone super oculos.

23. *Ad fluxum restringendum:* Sume capillos porri et mundentur bene et coquantur in aqua usque ad medietatem. [f.33v] Interim coquantur 4. vel 5. ova in vino vel aqua quousque durescant. Postea volvantur sub prunis usque ad fracturam testarum. Deinde comedat vitella ovorum et bibat moderate de aqua cocta et sic abstineat usque in crastinum.

24. Pur freid estomak: Pernez centoire et quisez ové mel et mangét au matyn.

25. Pur dolur de denz: Pernez pelusel / .i. mouser, vel capillos Veneris .i. maydynher[32] / et triblét ben et metez entre les denz malades et tenez lungement et pus lessez curre de la bouche la glette en un bacyn et verrés le verme, s'il i ad point.

26. Pur estrer fer de l'os: Pernét egremoygne e la gresse du porc madle[33] et metez a la playe.

27. Pur ruge felun: Pernez launcelé et conseude la petite et solsiecle owelement et

ataunt de morele cum des treis et seient bien triblez ensemble et seient mis sur le mal.

28. Ad stricturam pectoris: Accipe unctum porcinum recens quando extrahitur de porco et mundatum penitus a carne frustatim in panno lineo ponatur et iuxta ignem extorqueatur pinguedo. Postea admisceatur tercia vel quarta pars de cera virginea in patella super ignem tepidum et inde unges pectus pelle super-posita.

29. Pur la fevre ague: Pernez bugle et burnette et les braez ben et les temprés en eawe et donét au[34] [f.34r] pacient a beivre, e garra.

30. Contra fundacionem que provenit ex potacione subita post laborem: Fiat siru-pus ex hiis herbis[35] .s. radicis: petrosilli, feniculi radicis, mugwrt-rote, matefelun-rote, de qualibet manipulum usum: corticis ebuli, mediam corticem sambuci, manipulos duos; violete, hertistunge, strouberywyse, mousere, herbe Jon, bugle, sanicle, maydenhere, cetrac, adiantos, de qualibet manipulum .i.; liquiricie libra semis. Postea coquantur in aqua usque ad consumpcionem ter-cie partis aque. Postea clarificetur et bibat inde paciens mane et sero. *Expertum est certe.*

31. [f.34v] *Contra calefactionem epatis*: Recipe fenyl-rote, persil-rote, violette, dayse, weybrede, hertistunge, musere, liverwrt, centorie, linary, bugle, sanicle, strowberywyse, warmot, cetrac, maydenhere, adiantos,[36] de qualibet .m. .i.; de alleluia .m. 3., liquirice libram semis, et fiat syrupus sic: simul terantur et co-quantur in sexterio aque usque ad consumpcionem tercie partis et deinde clari-ficetur cum albumine ovorum et postea coletur per pannum lineum et utatur paciens mane et sero.

32. *Contra tussim*: Recipe de peniwrt .m. .i. et .m. 2. de watercars et simul terantur et extrahatur succus cum panno lineo et coquatur cum butiro proportionabili toti succo. Et modicum ante finem[37] decoctionis mittantur 3. manipuli de alle-luia. Postea simul coquantur ad tempus et ammoveatur.

33. *Contra tussim et tisim:*[38] Recipe mugwrt-rote, matefelum-rote, hertistunge, herbe Jon, musere, bugle, de qualibet .m. .i.; alleluia .m. 3.; licorice quarterium unum. Terantur simul et fiant ex eis .xv. [pile] quarum quelibet [f.35r] se ha-beat ad quantitatem ovi. Et prima nocte ponatur una pila in bursa linea et co-quatur in ciphato vini cum dimidio vel in forti cervisia usque ad consumpcionem tercie partis et utatur pocio et reservetur bursa cum pila et su-matur eadem mane et eodem modo coquatur et post decoctionem exprimatur succus pile et similiter utatur pocio tepida sicut contra noctem. Postea proicia-tur pila. Sic fiat singulis pilis.

34. Ad albedinem frangendum: Recipe mel, vinum et urinam pueri masculi virginis et succum feniculi et edere terrestris qui .s. succus se habeat in dupla propor-cione respectu mellis et aliorum et commisceantur in vase mundo et perma-neat usque ad descensum impuri et de puriore lineantur oculi.

35. *Contra*[39] *fistulam, cancrum et apostema*: Recipe burnettam maiorem et south-rinwde. Simul terantur cum sangui[n]e porcina recenti et fiat emplastrum.

36. *Contra impediginem*: Accipe dok-rote et rue et simul terantur et exprimatur succus et obtemperetur cum vino albo et inde inungatur locus.

37. *Unguentum calidum contra paralisim specialiter*: Recipe duas libras de salvia, unam de lavendula, et unam de primula veris, unam de narsturcio ortensi, unam de avencia, unam de foliis lauri .i. lorer et origani .i. puliol real, unam de centaurea [f.35v] .i. cristisladdir, unam de bissopwrt, unam de gasir, unam de sinapio, unam de urtica rubea, unam de narsturcio aquatico, unam de ebulo .i. wallewrt, unam de puliol muntayne, unam de peretro .i. peletre, unam ambrosii, unam de ache, unam de feniculo, unam de petrosillo, unam de rafano .i. radich, unam de menta et parum de savina. Iste herbe colligantur circa festum Johannis Baptista et, collecte, bene terantur et cum fuerint bene trite, appone ad libram herbe dimidia libra uncti porcini et iterum bene terantur simul et cum fuerint bene trite, fiant de illis pilule et sic ponantur in vase eneo et superponatur multum de viridi herba et sic jaceant per novem dies. Tunc iterum pistentur et bene coquantur in vino rubeo. His factis fortiter primantur per canabum fortem et non nimis spissum, aqua rejecta. Quo facto commisceatur hoc unguentum cum unctis cati, apri, anseris, altilium et cum medullis cervi et bulliantur iterum ad debitam mensuram et commisceantur huic unguento pulveres zinziberis, incensi, euforbii, gariofili et similium ac cum gummis et refrigerentur. Et ungatur infirmus circa locum percussum et spina dorsi donec sudet et sanabitur domino concedente.

38. *Ad difficultatem urinandi*: Succus millefolii potatus cum aceto prodest.

39. *Ad ventrem solvendum emplastrum*: Mel cum semine lini [f.36r] coctum mediocriter et super umbilicum positum ducit ad cellam quantum sibi placet.

40. *Ad constringendum sanguinem de vena infissa et vulnere*: Accipe far[i]nam de ligno quod vermes terunt, et melius si sit de quercu, et pone super et manu tua plagam obstrue pulverem inponendo et altera pulverem sparge super assidue, ut fluminis impetus medicinam reiciat et quamvis nimius sit fluxus cessabit. Probatum est.

41. *Ad tumorem brachii de fleobotomia*: Mel et lac caprinum equaliter misce et farinam de frumento adde ut nec satis molle nec satis durum et cataplasmetur et salvus erit.

42. *Contra difficultatem urinandi*: [40] Fiat emplastrum. Recipe cinerem radicum et foliorum ebuli .i. wallewrt et ipsum diu bullire facias in aqua vel vino. Deinde calidus quam tolerari potest in aliquo sacculo super pectim imponas et statim paciens reddet urinam.

43. *Contra oris fetorem*: Nota quod teste Avicenna fetor oris potest curari si paciens per annum integrum jejunus masticet siler montanum vel semen petrosilli macedonici.

44. *Aliud ad idem*: Frequens comestio apii removet oris fetorem.

45. *Ad pectus dolens*: Marubium cum pulegio in olla nova [f.36v] cum sale modico coquet[ur] et jejuno da bibere.

46. *Item ad pectus purgandum*: Utere pulvere butti.

47. *Ad dolorem dencium*: Scoriam tremuli cum aceto tritam in ore tene.

48. *Ad fluxum sanguinis de naribus*: Radix urtice super tegulam calidam usta et pulverizata. Fluxum sanguinis de naribus intus missa stringit.

49. *Item*: Combure in testa ovi sanguinem inde fluentem. Postea pulverem illum suffra in naribus per canalem. Probatum est.

50. *Ad torsionem ventris et stomachi*: Apii seminis et feniculi seminis, piperis similiter, tenuissimum facies pulverem ex quo in aqua calida potabis tria coccleariata.

51. *Item*: Testarum ovi cinis in calida potetur aqua.

52. *Ad latris tumorem et dolorem*: Marubium .i. horhunne, serpillum et sal modicum coquet[ur] et desuper pone.

53. *Contra ebriosos et venenum*: Si aliquis ebriosus fuerit, cerfolium [41] comedat et liberabitur, et si jejunus comederit, non inebriabitur nec intoxicabitur. [42]

54. *Contra frenesim et capitis dolorem intolerabilem*: Teratur lactuca, succus eius exprimatur in quo tepido pannus lineus humectetur et contra timpora ponatur.

55. *Ad auferendum sanguinem de oculo qui ibi induratur*: Accipe (accipe) farinam frumenti et pulverem cimini et distempera cum succo rute et fac inde parvulos panes [43] [f.37r] ita quod eosdem poteris separare per medietatem et eos coque super tegulam calidam coopertos et cum cocti fuerint, finde per medium et primum pone unam medietatem super oculum et postea aliam et sic fac sepius in die et infra duos dies liberabitur.

56. *Ad mulierem que non potest post partum libere purgari*: Succum de foliis porrorum vel boraginis cum oleo misceat et bibat.

57. *Qui mingere non possunt*: Semen lactuce cum vino veteri bibant.

58. *Ad pedes inflatos vel dolentes ex itinere*: Allium cum sepo pistentur et ad ignem bene ungantur.

59. *Item*: Multum valet contra frigus pedum.

60. *Optimum emplastrum ad guttam frigidam in capite vel alibi*: [44] Sumantur pise albe et adequentur et pistentur. Sumatur stercus columbe et in vino bono bulliatur et ita calidum sicut potest sustineri addatur.

61. *Ad destruendum guttas et apostemata*: Fiat potio de hiis herbis: capiatur una libra de fumetere, alia libra de musere, tertia libra de spinacle, et terantur bene et postmodum ponantur in vino albo et sint ibi per novem dies. Deinde bibatur modicum jejuno stomacho.

62. *Contra febres*: Fac balneum cum edere terrestri .i. heyhove bene cocta et cum fuerit in balneo, pone super capud tuum herbam calidam et cave ne aqua tangat brachia tua et ibidem minuetur in duobus brachiis. Probatum est. [45]

63. [f.37v] *Ad capillos nutriendos vel confirmandos*: Lini semen combure et oleo commisce et unge capud tuum.

64. *Ad dolorem aurium*: Butirum et mel et vinum congregatum bene commisceantur et tepefacta mitte in aures et dolor, quamvis inveteratus sit, tolletur.

65. *Ad dolorem oculorum summa medicina est*: Sume fel arietis et fel galli et fel anguillarum, sucum rute cum modico de melle in vase ereo pones et inde unge oculos tuos et proderit.

66. *Ad oculos clarificandos*: Sume succum radicum feniculi cum melle et clarificabit oculos.

67. *Ad fluxum ventris*: Caseum recentem et mel et vitella ovorum assatorum duorum et equaliter coque parum et fac quasi electuarium et da comedere. Probatum est.

68. *Ut homo dormiat*: Sume fel leporis et da bibere et dormiet.

69. *Ad inflacionem*: Sume acetum et album ovi, grossiorem farinam avene et simul commisce et superpone.

70. *Item ad idem*: Sume narsturcia rubea aquatica et tere furfur frumenti, succum lini, lac vacce, sepum ovis mascule, coque omnia simul quousque fuerit spissum et pone super infirmitatem.

71. *Ad lapidem frangendum*: Accipe radicem porri cum gromille et coque bene in veteri cervisia vel dulci [f.38r] vel vino et da pacienti bibere. Probatum est.

72. *Si vis scire an infirmus vivet vel morietur*: Accipe artemesiam et sub capite infirmi pone ipso nesciente et si dormierit vivet, si non, morietur. Probatum est.

73. *Ad eos qui non possunt loqui pre infirmitate*: Aloyn .i. warmot distempera cum aqua et da pacienti bibere. Pro[batum est].

74. *Contra omnes infirmitates oculorum*: Coque bene rubeam testudinem cum aqua et collige pinguedinem et inde unga [46] oculos sero. Probatum est.

75. *Ad eos qui non possunt [47] bene urinare*: Tepefac urinam caprinam cum vino et da bibere.

76. *Contra tussim*: Accipe sinapium et bene tere et distempera cum aqua tepida et cole per pannum. Postea fac ebullire et da pacienti bibere calidum jejuno stomacho. Probatum est.

77. *Item ad idem*: Recipe mugwrt-rote, matefelun-rote, hertistunge, herbe Jon, rathele, bugle, de qualibet *manipulum unum*, wodesur .m. .iii., licorice .m. .ii.. Simul terantur et postquam fuerint trite fiant .xv. pilule et contra noctem sumatur una pilula et ponatur in bursa linea et bene coquatur in vino vel cervisia forti et bibatur illud. Et mane coquatur illa eadem pila et iterum bibatur et sic fiat de aliis.

78. [f.38v] *Contra dolorem capitis*: Recipe alisaundir-rote, persil-rote, fenil-rote, columbine-rote vel semen betonie, rue, ysop, eufrase, simul terantur et coquantur in dulcidrio, anglice wrt, et fiat inde cervisia et bibatur omni die et lavetur capud aqua decoctionis camamille et feniculi.

79. *Ad visum confortandum*: Fiat secundum tenorem istorum versuum: 'Feniculus, vervena, rosa, celidonia, ruta: / Ex istis fit aqua, que lumina reddit acuta'.[48]

80. *Contra surditatem aurium*: Recipe warmot et ova formicarum et simul terantur et exprimatur succus earum et misceatur cum pinguedine anguille aque recentis et ponatur inde in auribus tepidum.

81. *Ad vomitum provocandum*: Recipe summitatem matefelun et coquatur in aqua et bibatur tepida.

82. *Item ad idem restringendum vel sedandum*: Recipe radicem predicte herbe et coquatur in vino vel forti cervisia et bibatur.

83. *Contra vermem*: Fac formellum de lacte dulci et postea scinde per medium uno tractu et lini illam partem fissam cum melle et sic pone super vulnus et in crastino invenies vestigium vermis. Sequenti nocte sume pedelyun et tere et pone super vulnus. Tamen inter herbam et cutem pone pellem tenuem et in pelle fac foramen parvum ex opposito vulneris, ut vermis **[f.39r]** inde gustet et sic sanabitur.

84. *Ad clarificandum oculos*: Omnium piscium adeps liquefacta, cum sale et melle admixta, claritatem oculorum facit.[49]

85. *Ut mulier pariat quemcumque fetum*: Da ei ysopum in aqua calida et pariet.

86. *Contra guttam inossatam*: Pix et hedera simul coquantur, capud radatur, et in panno lineo super capud involvatur.

87. *Ut pili nascantur*: Sume anguillam nigram et combure in olla et fac pulverem, misce cum melle et confert.

88. *Ad ferrum ignitum portandum*: Frica manum cum herba waldeca [50] fortiter et non nocebit.

89. *Ut pannus videatur ardere et non ardebit*: Argentum vivum cum modico aceto coquatur tam diu donec coaguletur sicut unguentum. Postea superponatur panno et non ardebit.

90. *Ad tumorem vel inflacionem colli*: Stercus columbarum, sulphur, semen lini, unctum, lolium coquantur simul et fiat emplastrum et sanabitur.

91. *Si ex naribus vis producere sanguinem*: succum marubii .i. horehunne pone in naribus et sanguis sequetur.

92. *Si vis aliquem inebriare*: Rute pulverem sume et in vas quod volueris mitte et cum ipso de ipso vase non bibas.

93. *Ne ebrius fiat*: Betonicam ante sumat quam cibum aliquem.

94. *Item*: Ovum crudum sorbe et medullam trunci **[f.39v]** caule comede jejunus.

95. *Contra dolorem aurium*: Lignum fraxini viride pone in igne et liquorem qui de summitate eius stillat collige et inpone. Dolorem sedat et auditum emendat.

96. *Contra vermes aurium*: Stilletur succus absinthii et interficies vermes.

97. Item: Fel caprinum cum lacte mulieris temperatum et cum melle et modica mirra. Summa est medicina.

98. Item: Fel caprinum mixtum cum succo pori auri infusum dolorem tollit et auditum restituit.

99. Item: Succus cepe cum lacte mulieris injectus mire dolorem placat.

100. Item: Medullam recentem vituli tritam infunde auribus et, quamvis dolor fuerit acerrimus, mirifice sanabit.

101. *Ad idem*: Butirum et mel tritum et vinum tepefactum mitte in aures et, quamvis dolor sit inveteratus, sanabitur.

102. *Contra surditatem aurium*: Fel bovinum mixtum cum urina capre tepida auribus instilla.

103. Item: Fel leporis, lac mulieris et mel bonum bene commisce et tepefac et in aure stilla et multum valet.

104. *Ut mulier non concipiat*: Coagulum leporis post partum datum potui non sinit ultra concipere.[51]

1. **[f.41r]**[52] *Pro omni genere guttarum*: Fiat oleum de subscriptis herbis: Recipe yeke[sters] sive wodeþong, heneban, ramnus, ysop, camamyl in equali proporcione et bene terantur et cum fuerint bene trite, misceantur omnes herbe simul bene et permittatur sic in vase mundo stare per .ix. dies. Hiis diebus transactis, capiatur vinum et oleum in equali proporcione et superfundatur quousque herbe trite fuerint cum licore spissitudinis gruelli. Deinde ponatur totum in aliquo vase terreo perforato et apto pro eodem alio vase terreo supposito et sepeliatur in terra, tali videlicet loco ubi sol poterit obumbrare et bene cooperiatur de terra et sic permittatur stare per alios .ix. dies. Et hiis transactis de terra eripiatur et quicquid defluxum fuerit de vase perforato in vase supposito, illud diligenter custodiatur et guttarum loca bene ungantur et sine hesitatione aliqua sanabuntur omnes qui dictam paciuntur infirmitatem qualitercumque fuerit fortis gutta sive frigida sive calida. *Sepius probatum est.*

2. *Item pro mulieribus in partu laborantibus*: Scribatur in cedula subscriptum carmen modo videlicet subscripto et scripta cedula firmetur dicta cedula cum aliqua ligatura ad ventrem mulieris modicum .s. ultra membrum ipsas litteras scriptas videlicet ad ventrem et dicant astantes quelibet mulier secretius Pater Noster et Ave Maria et sine dubio liberabitur sine periculo.[53] **[f.41v]** Omnimodo tamen cavendum est ne dicta cedula ponatur ad mulierem nisi cum in partu laboraverit: + In + nomine + Patris + et + Filii + et + Spiritus + Sancti + amen + Maria + Christum + genuit + matrix + eius + non + doluit + ipsum + enim + genuit + qui + nos + suo sanguine + redemit + iam + redit + et + virgo + redeunt + saturnia + regna + iam + nova + progenies + celo + dimittitur + alto + nate + mee + vires + mea + magna + potencia + solus + talia + prestabat + memorans + fixusque + manebat + agyos + athanatos + ymas + eleyson + Ave Maria, gratia plena, dominus tecum, benedicta tu in mulieribus et benedictus fructus ventris tui Jhesu, amen.[54]

3. Item contra guttas calidas, item contra dolorem capitis ex calore, item contra dolorem capitis in accutis febribus, item ad provocandum sompnum in eis, item contra calefactionem epatis, item contra dolorem timporum procedentem ex calore: Recipe populeon; herbarum quedam confectio est et invenitur cum spicers. Quod quidem populion fit hoc modo: recipe violarie, plantaginis, umbilici Veneris .i. peniwort, jusquiami, barbe Jovis, morelle minoris que portat nigros fructus, ana .i. de qualibet manipulum unum, occulorum populi .i. bourjuns de pepeler ad quantitatem omnium, butirum in bona quantitate terantur simul et postquam fuerint bene trite, fiant masse parve et te [f.42r] neatur sic per tres septimanas et postea sumatur una lagena vini et proiciantur predicte masse in illo vino et decoquantur usque ad consumpcionem vini. Deinde coletur et usui reservetur.

4. Item pro malis casuris, anglice .i. lithyr fallingys

5. Item pro guttis frigidis: Fiat unguentum sive confectio de subscriptis gummis: baucon, marciaton, oleum laurinum.

6. Item balneum vero pro predictis: Fiat de subscriptis herbis, walwort, alizaundir, hockys, heyhove.

7. Item pur oynnement fer a sauver hom de emoroydys: Pernez feltewort, yarou, vrtidegres .i. brounewort maior, morel, southirnewode, et fronkencens, oynt de pork ou de berbis et muel be beuf, anglice couhismarch, et ponét ben ensemble et pus festis boyller ensemble houtir le fu et si colét parmi un drap et unnez ben le male et garra. Pro[batum est] . . .[55]

8. Item alia medicina pro eadem infirmitate: Recipe mouser et bene teratur cum butiro recenti eodem die [f.42v] facto in quo sal nunquam erat positum et cataplasma .i. fiat emplastrum et superponatur et paciens isto emplastro utatur quousque fuerit sanus effectus et sine dubio salvabitur. Pro[batum est].

9. Item contra constipacionem: Pernez linory, polipodi, racine de gladyne, violet, livyrwort, persoyl, fynoyl, si quisét ben en wort anglice et donét a malad a bevyr, si garra.

10. Item ad idem emplastrum optimum: Coquantur bene et diu helryn-rindis et deponatur exterior pars corticis; betyn-rotis in equali proporcione sumantur. Item hokkys quantum de duabus aliis et fac emplastrum et ponatur super ventrem et super spinam dorsi ita quod nullo modo tangant latera dorsi propter calefactionem eppatis et sanabitur. Probatum est. Si vero paciens post deliberacionem torsiones habuerit in ventre, iterum emplastrum sibi apponatur et utatur ad prandium broués videlicet in brodio bovino et pullis galinarum et colys.

11. Item pro febribus cuiuscumque fuerint nature: Primo dicat qui dicturus est subscriptum carmen + In nomine Patris et Filii et Spiritus Sancti, amen. Deinde dicant ambo quilibet per se secretius Pater Noster. Postea faciat crucem in fronte iterum dicendo + In nomine Patris etc. Deinde dicat carmen et ante quodlibet verbum carminis fiat crux cum police in fronte prout hic signatur dicendo + Christus + vincit + Christus + regnat + Christus + imperat + [f.43r] Christus te sanet +. Pater Noster ab ambobus videlicet silenter et quilibet per se. Deinde dicatur + Christus natus est + Christus passus est + Christus tercia die resurrexit a mortuis + sanet te Pater per potenciam suam +

sanet te Filius per passionem suam + sanet te Spiritus Sanctus per bonitatem suam + sanet te Trinitas Sancta per gloriosam omnipotentiam suam a febribus cuiuscumque fuerint nature et ab omni alia infirmitate, amen. + In nomine Patris etc. Pater Noster et Credo ab ambobus dicatur et quilibet per se et silenter. Eligat insuper febriscitans quo die sanari voluerit et eligat semper nomine Trinitatis tertium diem et sanabitur domino concedente. Probatum est.

12. *Item medicina pro quadam infirmitate que est in muliere, que etiam infirmitas provenit ex corrupto sanguine in matrice et ibidem congludinatur et cum quid durum in se ad modum unius glebe nec per corpus movetur, sed in uno loco semper sistit:*[56] Fiat pacienti balneum una cum bonis herbis et balneat se mulier binis vicibus in die, mane videlicet et sero, et sedeat in balneo modicum ultra nates et non ultra ullo modo [. . .] Medio vero tempore terentur herbe subscripte bene videlicet ribwort, weybred, attirloue, non autem attirlobery, quia attirloue dicitur ipsa herba seu folia, attirlouebery dicitur ipse fructus. Istis autem tritis **[f.43v]** ponatur in parvo sacculo lineo ordinato et facto ad longitudinem et latitudinem tocius menbri mulieris. Postea ponatur super eandem ita quod emplastrum cooperiat totum membrum et ibidem stet usque ad aliam balneacionem et sic semper balneando et cataplasmando quousque sana fuerit effecta. Probatum est.

13. *Item pro fluxu continuo matricis:* [57] Recipe subscriptas herbas videlicet weybred, yarou, streberiwyse, lus crey (hibernicum nomen est); [58] equaliter de omnibus terantur bene et cum fuerint bene trite, capiatis furfur in bona quantitate et simul commisceas et ponatis herbas tritas una cum furfure sic mixtas in diversis parvis sacculis, galice en diverse peti pouchis pointe a la maner de un actoun. Postea coquantur omnes sacculi parvi in vino albo, si potest habere, vel rubeo, (in aceto, quod melius est)[59] et cum fuerint cocti, galice mettez un pouche apré une autir ausi chaute cum ele pust suffrire sur tote sa membre et sur la greynnour parti de sun quiis et sic semper utatur mulier talibus sacculis parvis calidis cum talibus herbis et cum furfure, ut dictum est, quousque sana fuerit effecta.

14. *Item pro eodem fiat insuper sibi pocio talis:* [60] Recipe omnes herbas prenominatas una cum istis herbis subscriptis videlicet bursam pastoris anglice porswort, sourdokys, rubeas rosas, senekyl, equaliter de omnibus, liquiriciam in **[f.44r]** bona quantitate; terantur omnes herbe. Teratur liquiricia etiam et postea coquantur modicum in bono vino rubeo [61] et post decoctionem stet sic in pace per noctem vel saltem per dimidium diem. Deinde colatur pocio per bonum pannum et bibat paciens cum pocio fuerit clara unum bonum tractum antequam vadat cubitum et nullo modo commedat vel bibat aliquid postea et sit pocio sua illo tempore calida. Similiter mane bibat bonum tractum jejuno stomaco ante horam prime et sit pocio sua illo tempore frigida et per magnum spacium temporis postea non commedat aliquid vel bibat. Similiter non commedat carnes bovinas nec congruum nec anguillas nec lang nec ray. Non bibat novam serviciam nec acetosum lac .i. sour milk. Vinum est potus optimus pro ea. Si paciens sit ita fortis quod poterit sibi minuere, minuat sibi omni mense binis vicibus de duobus brachiis, una vice de uno brachio, alia vice de alio et qualibet vice modicum valde. Omnia predicta faciat quousque sana fuerit effecta.

15. *Item pro morsu canis* and lithir prikkyngys de ferro vel de aliis: Recipe rutam anglice ru et teratur cum melle et fac emplastrum et superpone et sine dubio sanabitur. Pro[batum est].

16. *Contra dolorem timporum* non tamen provenientem ex calore: Primo minuat sibi paciens de vena capitali modicum vel sit inter duas scapulas anglice yhornid. Deinde terentur [f.44v] herbe videlicet pervenk, stichewort, quantum de aliis duabus. Hiis vero tritis comisceatis cum hiis albumen ovi, sanguinem hominis, una cum farina fabarum et fiat emplastrum de predictis et ponatur super tinpora etiam a medietate frontis usque ad auriculam et sanabitur domino concedente. Probatum est.

17. *Item contra dolorem capitis intollerabilem ratione cuius doloris* inflantur oculi una cum facie. Aliquando inflatur unus occulus tamen. Minuat sibi paciens de vena timporis modicum et hoc post commestionem et statim sonabitur. *Probatum est.*

18. *Item pro omni genere inflacionum anglice* for al maner swolling and wreching optimum emplastrum: Recipe lac caprinum vel lac bovinum vel lac ovinum [62] et similam avenaticam, anglice grittis, et sepum ovinum et fac simul bullire quousque fuerit spissum. Deinde de istis fac emplastrum tuum sicut vobis videbitur et superpone et sanabitur.

19. *Item pro eodem:* Capias anglice þe rede mosse of þe mor cum aqua propria quantum possibile est et fac diu (diu) valde bullire et ita calidum sicut pati poterit. Superponatur et sine dubio sanabitur. Ista sepius sunt probata.

20. *Item pro gutta currente:* Bibat paciens omni die hora prima jejuno stomaco succum herbarum videlicet mouser, matfeloun, yarou, houndefenyl tem[f.45r]peratarum cum vino vel servicia bona defecata. Pro[batum est].

21. *Item pro antrace* .i. feloun cum fuerit ostensus vel non ostensus in corpore et precipue cum fuerit ostensus per modum parve vesice albe in pede; talis enim antrax est mirabiliter periculosus nisi citius occuratur et statim. Infra enim duos dies illa albedo convertetur in nigredinem et ascendet usque ad capud et ex tunc vix aut nul lum est remedium cum fuerit illa parva vesica sic semel denigrata; provenit enim iste antrax ex sanguine. Cum igitur fuerit ostensus vel non, ut prius dictum est, primo minuat sibi paciens simul de duobus brachiis multum etiam usque ad swownyng anglice. Postea bibat succum herbarum videlicet mouser, matfeloun, temperatarum cum aqua et jejuno stomaco hora prima bibat nec per magnum tempus postea aliquid commedat vel bibat et faciat paciens abstinenciam per tres vel duos dies et sanabitur. Probatum [est].

22. De emplastro vero pro huismodi antrace ostenso: Fiat ut dictum est supra hoc et infra.

23. *Item pur mal de reyns:* Pernez la racine de gletener graunt, anglice mucheclit, et triblez la gletener bene et verseez servoyse eyns et beveez sele a seyre chaut et a matine freyde.

24. [f.45v] *Item ad constringendum sanguinem de vena infissa et vulnere et fluxum sanguinis de naribus:* Capiatur pannus laneus et intingatur in eodem sanguine con-

tinue quousque pannus omnino fuerit madefactus et plenus sanguine. Deinde comburatur et panno conbusto pulverizetur. Hoc facto pone super et manu tua plagam obstrue pulverem inponendo et altera manu pulverem sparge super assidue ut fluminis impetus medicina reiciat et quamvis nimius sit fluxus, cessabit.

25. Idem etiam facit sanguis collectus in testis ovorum conbustus et pulverizatus. Isti etiam pulveres fluxum sanguinis de naribus intus missi stringunt sufflando videlicet pulverem in naribus per canalem. Probata sunt ista.

26. *Item pro omni genere plagarum nisi sint mortifere*: Recipe pannum azorii coloris, anglice blu cloth, et scindatis per particulas ad longitudinem et latitudinem vulneris et intingatis unam particulam illarum in vino rubeo bene quousque videlicet illa particula fuerit omnino madefacta et super plagam pone. Deinde, si vobis videbitur expedire, ammoveatur paniculus ille binis vicibus in die eundem paniculum videlicet de novo in vino intingendo, ut prius et denuo superponendo. Unus autem paniculus satis bene ministrabit per duos dies. Ista medicina optime et pulcre de mundo vulnera sanat. De eodem et melius infra 30 [=f. 58r].

27. [**f.46r**] *Ad omnes febres* colige tria folia salvie dicens ad primum 'In nomine Patris quesivi te', ad secundum 'In nomine Filii inveni te', ad tercium 'In nomine Spiritus Sancti colligo te'. In primo scribatur 'Christus vincit', in secundo 'angelus nunciat', in tercio 'Johannes predicat'.[63] Postea distemperentur cum aqua munda et a quadam virgine detur febricitanti.

28. *Item ad idem*: Sume tres oblatas quarum in una scribatur 'Pater est Alpha et Omega', in secunda 'Filius est vita', in tercia 'Spiritus Sanctus est remedium'. Tunc detur egroto jejuno stomaco primo die prima oblata, secundo die secunda, et tertio die tertia et antequam commedat aliquam illarum omni die dicat Pater Noster et Credo. In prescriptis etiam scribatur 'Increatus Pater, increatus Filius, increatus Spiritus Sanctus'.

29. *Ad stomacum obstructum*: Recipe et tere simul ciminum, absincium .i. warmot, morel .i. attirlouebery, apium .i. merche, panem acidum bene assatum et sepius in aceto tinctum et simul trita pone et sue simul in sacculo lineo et deinde coque totum in aceto et appone super orificium stomachi ita calidum sicut potest pati. Sic fiat per 3. dies, si necessitas id deposcat.

30. *Item ad constringendum sanguinem de vena infissa*: Scribatur in fronte hominis 'Veronica' et salvetur.

31. Item ad renum dolorem: Betonice succus ovo pleno mellis coclear unum et postea in calice mitte et vinum superfunde et bibe.

32. [**f.46v**] *Pro auditu*: Accipe succum ebule .i. walwort qui dedat auditum ei qui longo tempore fuerat surdus et tepidum mitte in aures.

33. *Contra vomitum*: Fac emplastrum de barba Jovis et de farina ordei et pone super orificium stomachi vel accipe ciminum et pone in sacculo et postea coque bene in aqua et pone super orificium stomachi.

34. *Contra tussim pocio*: Lingua cervina .i. hertistong, violaria .i. violet, radices ar-

tamesie .i. mogwort-rotis, capillus Veneris .i. maydynher, centaurea .i. centory, solsequium .i. roddis, liquiricia: ista terantur in mortario et coquantur in aqua et detur egroto ad bibendum.

35. Si vir vel mulier steriles sint: Accipe ova de nido corvi nono die ante kalendas Apprilis et coque in aqua munda ita ut bulliant et postea remitte ova in nidum proprium et dimitte ibi demum veniet corvus et inventis ovis excoctis ibit et afferet petram et ponet eam in medio ovorum suorum et reviviscent, quam petram sume et lava cum aqua benedicta et da bibere viro et mulieri et postea generabunt. Pullos vero accipe et incide colla eorum et fac pulverem et misce pulverem cum succo celidonie et da bibere animalibus et omni morbo carebunt.

36. *Propter dolorem capitis:* Celidonia cocta in butiro et cola per pannum et ponatur in pixide et inde ungatur capud. Postea lavetur capud cum aqua decoctionis celidonie, rute, feniculi et eufrase albe.

37. Si vis scire utrum infirmus evadet vel non: Combure testudinem .i. snayl et da ei pulverem in cibo vel in potu: si evomuerit, non evadet.[64] **[f.47r]**

38. *Pocio ad stomachi dolorem:* Anetum, apium, ciminum cum aqua (aqua) calida bibe.

39. *Pocio optima contra constipacionem:* Recipe endive manipulum semis, violet manipulum unum, borage manipulum unum, maydynher manipulum semis, petrosillini .i. persel-rotis manipulum semis, lyvyrwort manipulum unum, siccorie / .i. roddis[65] / manipulum semis, maratrum .i. fenyl-rotis manipulum semis, bugyl manipulum semis, polipody manipulum semis, liquiricie libram semis, linory manipulum unum. Hiis habitis vel aliquibus istarum, si omnes inveniri non poterunt, primo pistentur, deinde coquantur in aqua in estate, in dulcidrio in yeme et hoc usque ad terciam partem; quibus coctis, sic simul stare permittatis in aliquo vase ligneo et mundo tota nocte, in crastino vero per pannum coletur et postea clarificetur et utatur mane jejuno stomaco et sero modicum ante cubitum et utatur isto potu omni tempore frigido. Ad omnes predictas herbas sufficiunt tamen due lagene cum debeant coqui sive in aqua sive in dulcidruo .i. wort.[66]

40. Item electuarium optimum pro eodem maxime cum fleuma dominatur in corpore, quod quidem specialiter ordinatur ad purgationem fleumatis: Recipe turbith dragmam .i., esule dragmam .i., lignum aloes dragmas .ii., dyagredii dragmam .i., hermodactuli dragmas .ii., sandali albi et rubei ana dragmas .ii., **[f.47v]** rosarum, dragaganti ana dragmas .ii. et fiat pulvis.

41. *Item contra fluxum sanguinis* per menstrua:[67] Plantago, barba Jovis, absinthium, arthemesia, edera, menta, lingua cervina et ordeum coquantur et coctura detur ad bibendum. Contra idem etiam valet cer(vi)folium bibitum crudum vel coctum.

42. *Item contra sermonem subtractum:* Succum salgie in ore potatur vel absinthium in aqua vel succus separum vel savina vel folia pini arboris cum pipere simul temperata.

43. *Ad restringendum sanguinem tam in presencia quam in absencia cuiuscumque pacientis fluxum sanguinis dummodo nomen eiusdem habeatur:* [68] In nomine Patris et Filii et Spiritus Sancti, amen. Longinus miles latus domini nostri Jhesu Christi perforavit, in continuo exivit sanguis et aqua. In nomine Patris cessat sanguis .N., in nomine Filii restat sanguis .N., in nomine Spiritus Sancti non exeat gutta sanguinis .N. Et dicatur Pater Noster et Ave. Probatum est.

44. *Item alia medicina:* Scribatur super membrum ubi fluit sanguis istud verbum tetragramaton cum cruce in principio et in fine.

45. *Item pro febribus:* Scribatur in sedula subscripta verba per modum infra scriptum et ligetur sedula super manum dextram et dicat paciens .3. Pater Noster cum totidem salutacionibus virginis gloriose et simbolo cum maxima devotione quolibet die mane jejuno stomacho per tres dies. Tertio vero die removeatur sedula et comburatur et cineres in aqua currentes proiciantur + + + hympnus + artus + arus + tremens + eloy + ventus + affricat + angelus + nunciat + Christe [f.48r] + liberet + Amen + + + Probatum est.

46. *Contra morbum caducum:* Collige herbam pilocellam .i. lathyve vel mouser, quod idem est, cum oratione dominica ita ut cum dixerit 'sed libera nos a malo' eradicat eam in nomine resurrectionis dominice. Deinde tantum quantum cum vino per novem dies sufficere possit distemperetur. Postea tres missas de resurrectione cantare facias quas tu diligenter audias et pocio distemperata iuxta altare sit posita per omnes missas, quibus expletis paciens per quadraginta dies cum oratione dominica in nomine resurrectionis bibat. Per hoc experimentum Judeus multos vidit Rome liberatos. Item ponatur titulus circa collum. Hic est titulus: 'Triumphalis Jhesu Nazarenus rex Judeorum'.

47. *Item alia medicina pro eodem:* Deglutiat paciens apem alveariam, anglice a be off hyve, vivam, aculeo primo ab eadem abstracto. Sepius est probatum. . . .[69]

48. [f.49v] . . . *Pro mola matricis* et suffocatione matricis et precipitatione matricis et menstruum provocandum: [70] [f.50r] Recipe mentastrum .i. horsmyntis, mentam [71] rubeam, nepte, salgiam ana uncias .ii.. Item radices feniculi, petrosellini, ache, scolopendria .i. hertistong, endivie, scarioli .i. hyndhal, lactuce, ysope, marol .i. horbound ana uncias .iii. Item violet, epatik .i. livyrwort, absincium, enule campane .i. horsel, mater herbarum .i. mogwort ana unciam .i. et semis. Item rubei tinctoris .i. madir [72] uncie .ii. Item anys quarterium unum. Item liquiricie libra .i. et semis. Terantur minutatim et coquantur in quatuor lagenis albi vini vel rubei, si vinum album inveniri non poterit, vel in dulcidrio, si vinum haberi non poterit, [73] usque ad tertiam partem ad quarum etiam coctionem vini apponatur ad minus una lagena aque et clarificetur et utatur binis vicibus in die mane videlicet tepidum et in sero frigidum. Post cuius sumpcionem in sero non sumatur cibus vel potus et utatur paciens ista pocione per duos vel tres dies ante descrescenciam lune usque ad finem lunacionis, quod si paciens multum debilitatur per emissionem menstrui seu sanguinis ratione dicti potus supersedeat de assumpcione dicti potus [74] et utatur sepe vino bene calido tam in prandio quam in cena quam etiam aliis temporibus etiam si voluerit jejuno stomacho ad cuius etiam assumpcionem apponatur unum coclear de aceto, si haberi potest, et cessabit fluxus. Istud etiam vinum taliter sumptum per se in instanti prestat juvamen contra suffocacionem et precipitationem matricis que

fit aliquando per se. Ista pocio de dictis herbis sit facta, [f.50v] destruit totaliter molam matricis et eius suffocationem et precipitationem et menstruum
provocat, si ea ut dictum est utatur. De hoc etiam infra 76 [=f. 84v].

49. *Ad confortandum et provocandum coitum pocio*, correspondens electuario quod
vocatur diapigamon et electuario quod vocatur diasaturion que quidem electuaria fiunt pro eodem. Recipe salgiam manipulum unum, mentam rubeam .m.
.i., puliol real .m. .i., tyme .m. .i., puliol montan .m. .i., ysopum .m. .i., camamyl .m. .i. Item semen levistici unciam .i., semen carwey unciam .i., semen
dauci unciam .i., semen saxifragii unciam .i., semen urtice unciam .i. Terantur
omnia minutatim et coquantur in duabus lagenis vini rubei usque ad tres potel-
los et sic stare permittatur in aliquo vase ligneo per diem naturalem. Deinde
per pannum colatur, quo facto, pulveres subscriptarum specierum in panno
lineo inclusi apponantur, videlicet zinziberi, galange, macis, clovys, cinamomi,
nucis Indie, pistacis, piperis longi, ana dragmas .ii. Primo igitur capiatur de
electuario, deinde sumatur de pocione ad quantitatem .vii. vel .viii. coclea-
rum, mane videlicet jejuno stomacho et sero ante cubitum. Nec comedat alico
modo at bibat post sumpcionem in sero et multo melius operabitur si a cenis
vel saltim a superfluitate cenarum abstinuerit. Post sumpcionem vero in mane
laboret aliqualiter etiam si poterit usque ad sudorem . . .[75]

50. [f.51r] . . . *Ad hoc autem ut aliquis non sit totaliter impotens* [f.51v] nisi tamen
ad tempus videlicet pro uno anno vel dimidio. Subtrahatur tamen terra in qua
habitantur formice de predicto electuario. Notandum quod ova formicarum ad
hoc ut de eis fiat pulvis primo debent desiccari in aliquo vase ultra ignem, quibus desiccatis redigantur in pulverem. Deinde liquefiatur camphora que est
quedam gumma, qua liquefacta, imponatur pulvis ovorum formicarum et
totum simul in pulverem redigantur. Formice vero debent cum cribro colligi
quia terra per cribrum expulsa, hoc est ysiftyte anglice, remanebunt formice et
debent poni in alico vase concavo et obturato vel vesica ad hoc apto, et sic
custodiri quousque fuerint mortue, quibus mortuis, terrantur, quibus tritis,
omnes pulveres una cum terra in qua habitantur formice simul misceantur et
fiat electuarium et utatur ut supra dictum est. Notandum etiam hic quod
capud hominis quem vis reddere impotentem simpliciter vel ad tempus debet
in pergameno vel in aliqua alia re protrahi in omnibus quam est possibile iuxta
formam suam, videlicet si sit calvus vel lenis vel longos crines habens,[76] si
habet occulos nigranos vel grossos vel protensos vel parvos et eodem modo
quoad nasum. Fiat tunc tale capud et hoc facto predicta effigies debet poni in
predicto electuario seu involvi vel in pulveribus includi seu una cum pulveribus poni, si videlicet debeat uti pulveribus illis in potagio vel aliquo alio liquore liquido.

51. *Contra omnem dolorem dencium*: 'In nomine Patris + et Filii + et Spiritus Sanctus + amen + Christus vincit + Christus regnat + Christus imperat + Christus
hunc [f.52r] famulum tuum .N. ab omni malo et dolore dencium quocumque
defentat + Conjuro vos vermes et alium dolorem dencium quemcumque per
Patrem et Filium et Spiritum Sanctum + et per adonay + agios + emanuel ++
alpha et omega ++ et omnes sanctos et sanctas Dei, ut non noceatis alicui hoc
breve portanti nec potestatem habeatis nocendi per virtutem domini nostri
Jhesu Christi et beate Marie virginis et omnium sanctorum Dei sed pocius ad

nichilum redacti ipsum .N. dimittite in pace et sanum et incolumen ab omni malo et omnimodo dolore dencium pristine sanitati restaurari permittite. + In nomine Patris + et Filii + et Spiritus Sancti + Amen +++' Prescriptum carmen per prescriptum modum scriptum portet paciens circa collum et sanabitur.

52. *Pur fere poysoun*: Pernez bugyl, senekyl, pigyl, verveyne, betoyne, pimpirnol, herbe Water, herbe Johan, herbe Robert, herbe ive, flur of brome, spinakyl, wodsour, percepere, filago, turmentille, quintefoyl, burnet, croysry, fymter, hyndehale, pulleol montayne, plantayne, clavyr .i. samrok vel trifolium portans florem rubeum, non autem trifolium portans florem album, mouser, milefoyl, valerian, eskeban, egremoyn, madefeloun, nepte, scabios, streberiwyse, sauge, ragwort, ribwort, wodbynd .i. wethwynd, [f.52v] dayce, primrol, cropleswort, dittoundir, tansey, sperge .i. pé de colum, horshunde, solsekyl, horpyn, violet, columbyn, wildnetil, le tendrun de warence .i. madir, le tendrun de caumbre .i. hennpe, le tendrun de rounce .i. bremmyl, le tendrun de urtye .i. netyl, le tendrun de ruge cholet, groundyswyly, hevyrferne .i. polipody, wodrove, fillis, conferry, herbe coppi, dauke, dente de lyoun, lavandir, suthirnwodde, puleol real, avance: *summa omnium herbarum* 66. Item de istis omnibus herbis sit equalis proporcio. Item de butiro de maii ad pondus omnium istorum. Primo igitur bene et minuatim terantur herbe, deinde liquefiatur butirum, quo liquefacto per aliqualem morulam quousque videlicet fex descendit ad fundum, et tunc per pannum coletur et sic fiat duobus vel tribus vicibus. Postmodum omnes herbe trite in predicto butiro liquefacto ponantur et bene simul misceantur et sic stare permittatur ad omne minus per novem dies. Verumptamen omni die semel ad minus simul admisceantur bene cum sacro ewangelio Johannis dicendo. Hiis completis ad ignem ponatur et iuxta proporcionem materie vinum apponatur album, si haberi poterit, sin autem rubeum. Ista igitur simul bene et diu coquantur et [. . .][77] quo liquore ad medietatem bullito seu cocto de igne deponatur et per pannum bonum et fortem fortiter coletur et sic stare permittatur per diem adminus naturalem. Deinde quod coagulatum fuerit colligatur et usui reservetur. Hic etiam sciendum est quod ad unam petram de butiro maii requiritur adminus una lagena vini. Istud coli [f. 53r] rium valet ad omne genus plagarum et utatur mane et sero ad mensuram unius fabe in aliquo liquore ut puta vino vel servicia defecata et folium super vulnus ponatur tamen et sic convalescet. Exibit plagam eo modo quo bibit quod si non sit spes convalescentie, non exibit. Item predictum colirium valet ad plagam prius etiam male sanatam, quia, si utatur modo predicto, scrutabitur corpus nec cessabit quousque pervenerit ad locum illum male sanatum et locum plage seu ipsam plagam de novo apperiet et ipsam de novo et integraliter sanabit.

Istud est carmen quo sciri potest furtum . . .[78]

53. [f.54r] . . . *Contra cancrum experimentum infallibile*: Accipe farinam de siligine .i. ry-mele et farinam de vermibus, anglice wrmele, eque porcionis et decoque eas in melle, quibus decoctis pone super folium caulis mane et sero, et postea super livorem in omni renovacione lavetis plagam cum urina hominis et in qualibet locione dicatur continue Pater Noster et Ave Maria et evitet anguillas, carnes bovinas, panem et serviciam de siligine, lac dulce et sanabitur. Probatum est sepius.

54. **[f.54v]** . . .[79] *Contra constipacionem seu materiam congelatam et ad purgandum omnes malos humores et nocivos et superfluos in utroque sexu existentes, sine enim aliqua violentia mirabiliter purgat et ventrem solvit nec in aliquo nocet, si semel omni mense sumatur:* Recipe de zucura uncias .vi., de turbit uncias tres,[80] de gingibero unciam unam cum dimidia. Fiat pulvis et sumatur post matutinas vel in aurora tamen una vice unum coclear cum aliquo liquore, ut puta vino vel scero .i. wey, vel pireta .i. puree, et caveat a carne noctis precedentis, ut stomacus aliqualiter vacuus inveniatur.

55. **[f.55r]** *Contra albedinem occulorum:* Ponatur in vola manus modicum de terra, deinde expuetur super dictam terram et incipiatur illa signando signo crucis dicendo 'In nomine Patris et Filii et Spiritus Sancti, amen'. Deinde de duobus predictis fiat lutum et in faciendo lutum dicat continue et repetat carmen subscriptum adminus ter nomine Sancte Trinitatis: 'Expuit Jhesu in terram et fecit lutum ex puto et linivit lutum super occulos ceci et dixit ei "Vade lava in natatorio siloe quod interpretatur missus". Abiit ergo et lavit et vidit et credidit Deo. In nomine Patris et Filii et Spiritus Sancti, amen'. Facto vero luto per modum prescriptum signetur signo crucis palpebra occuli exterius silicet lutum imponendo per modum crucis cum ventriculis digitorum, pollicis videlicet et indicis, in dicto luto madefactis dicendo 'In nomine Patris et Filii et Spiritus Sancti, amen', sic ter faciendo in honorem Trinitatis, lutum qualibet vite imponendo. Ista medicina fiat per .3. dies continuos et binis vicibus in die mane videlicet et vespere et sine dubio macula destruetur. Sepissime probatum est. Vitet paciens per .9. dies carnes bovinas recentes, caseum, lac dulce, pisas, anguillas, ova, porros, alleum, sepas, novam serviciam, et breviter omne genus prandii guttosum, anglice goutouse.

56. *Ad depondendum pilos in quocumque loco corporis fuerint. Et etiam ad deponendum scabiem in facie et scabiem sanandam. Primo utamini unguento corosivo, secundo unguento sanativo, que quidem unguenta fiunt modo subscripto. Unguentum corosivum*[81] **[f.55v]** fit sic. Fiat lexivium super cineribus fraxinis ita forte sicut fieri poterit. Isto lexivo facto et purificato capiatis calcem non extinctum et cineres fraxinos duplicem videlicet proporcionem de calce respectu alterius et simul misceantur. Deinde ponatur per modum spissi emplastri super stramina avenatica vel super herbas ad hoc aptas vel ponatur in sacculo lineo ad hoc apto si vobis videatur vase bono et mundo supposito. Postea calefacias lexivium et ita calidum sicut fieri poterit. Effundatur circulariter et lente super predictum emplastrum seu mixturam et ita fiat novies lexivium .s. semper calefaciendo et super vinum et idem plastrum seu mixturam effundendo. His factis capiatis calcem non extinctum purum .i. similam eius et parum de sulphure bene pulverizato et parum de alym pulverizato et simul misceantur et ista cum lexivio prenotatio ignia apponantur et bulneantur simul bene. Quibis bullitis de igne deponatur et sic stare per .3. dies permittas. Transactis tribus diebus effundatur totum lexivium in aliquo vase mundo et residuam partem .s. feces eiusdem soli vel vento exponatis et sic stare et seccare permittas quousque in pulverem omnino redigantur. Medio vero tempore capiatis butirum et sepum cervinum in dupla proporcione respectu butiri et coquantur bene in predicto lexivio. Quibus coctis de igne deponatur et sic stare permittas quousque fuerit omnino frigidum. Deinde colligatur quicquid fuerit coagulatum. Demum vero coagulacio capiatur et igni[82] **[f.56r]** apponatur et liquefiat. Quo bene liquefacto de igne

deponatur et sumatur de pulvere illo seccato, sic soli et vento exposito, et cum una manu continue pulvis[83] id infundatur rei liquefacte et cum alia manu continue cum spatula moveatur quousque totum fuerit omnino frigidum et spissum. Non tamen infundatur pulvus rei liquefacte nimis spisso modo aut tenuo, sed modo mediocri. Quam cito igitur totum fuerit infrigdatum in pixide ponatur et usui reservetur. Istud est et dicitur unguentum corosivum eo quod statim corodit etiam usque ad nudam et puram et vivam carnem.[84]

57. *Unguentum vero sanativum fit hoc modo dicte infirmitatis*: Recipe hyndehale, merche, de qualibet equaliter, folia solsequii .i. roddis in quarta proporcione respectu unius predictorum, ragydwort eodem modo, weybreed eodem modo, glassyn kylle[85] eodem modo, bremmylcroppis eodem modo, ribwort eodem modo; iste herbe bene terentur. Quibus minutatim et bene tritis fiant pilule et ponantur postea pillule super undam terram sub aliquo lecto et sint ibi per sex dies quousque videlicet fuerint effecte cane, anglice yhorydde. Deinde sumantur et in patella ponantur et cum butiro equi ponderis cum omnibus predictis herbis bene purificato coquantur et illis coctis totum per pannum colatur et sic stare permittas quousque totum fuerit frigidum et coagulatum. Demum vero tota coagulacio colligatur et in pixide [f.56v] ponatur et usui reservetur. Istud unguentum dicitur sanativum eo quod mirabiliter et cito sanat. Cum igitur uti volueris dictis unguentis pro scabie, primo sumatur modicum super digitum de unguento corosivo et ungatur tenue locus infirmitatis et statim corodet scabiem etiam usque ad crudam carnem. Hoc facto statim sumatur unguentum prescriptum sanativum et spisso modo ungatur dictus locus infirmitatis et citius quam credi poterit sanabitur. Cum etiam volueris pilos corporis deponere, fiat cum predictis unguentis prout dictum est de scabie et nunquam iterato crescent.

58. *Contra arsuram virge*: Contra arsuram virge virilis ex muliere recipe farinam fabarum et commisceatur cum melle et aceto et coquatur et fiat emplastrum et superponatur.

59. *Ad idem*: Item ad idem. Recipe folia salicis et decoquantur in aqua et in illa aqua fovietur.

60. *Item ad testiculos inflatos*: Recipe alteam .i. wymawe et rutam cum auxugia et simul tere et superpone et sanabuntur.

61. *Contra febrem tercianam et etiam cotidianam medicina infallibilis*: Recipe semen levistici et teratur bene et temperetur cum aceto bono (bono) et puro. Deinde per pannum colatur et faciat micas .i. miis in dicto succo seu liquore et de hoc commedat quam voluerit hora prima et vespertina et nullo alio cibo vel potu aliquo modo utatur paciens per tres dies. Et si paciens multum sitierit predictis diebus, commedat paciens de micis positis in predicto liquore et sine hesitatione liberabitur[86] [f.57r] de infirmitate. Tertio vero die minuat sibi paciens. Hoc tamen habet intelligi: si in principio infirmitatis sue fecerit predictam medicinam, si vero per magnum tempus stetit in infirmitate, non minuat sibi paciens, quia per hoc forte nimis debilitaretur.

62. *Item ad delendum morfeam sive lepram cutis, anglice mool þat is oppe þe velle of manis body*:[87] Recipe sulphur et minutatim frangatur. Deinde recipe glaream

ovi et ex hoc fiat aqua et commisceantur simul in aliquali spissitudine et ungatur locus ubi sistit morfea mane et cum ieris cubitum et infra tres dies delebitur
illa macula corporis et si multociens ungeris dictum locum sive dictam maculam, tanto citius delebitur macula annotata.

63. *Item ad delendum omne genus tetrys humani corporis*: Recipe sepum cervinum,
vel sepum ovinum si sepum cervinum non poterit haberi, et ru in dupla proporcione quoad pondus. Deinde teratur ru bene et minutatim. Quo facto liquefiatur sepum, quo liquefacto predicta herba trita inponatur et bene simul
frixentur. Deinde bene per pannum et fortiter colatur et quod coagulatum
fuerit colligatur et in pixide ponatur et usui reservetur. Et cum uti volueris
dicto unguento facto pro dicta infirmitate, ungatur locus infirmitatis prope
ignem, eo quod dictum unguentum est de natura sui durum.

64. *Item ad delendum scabies manuum et tetris* [88] et ad reducendum manus ad pristi-
num statum infra paucos dies, medicina infallibilis: [f.57v] Recipe lymyk /
senekyl [89] /, wodeþong sive yekesters, quod idem est, equaliter de tribus. Item
vertgrys, item sepum ovinum [90] quam de herbis in pondere. Pulverizetur
vertgrys, terantur bene herbe, liquefiatur sepum ovinum. Quo liquefacto inponatur vertgrys eo modo quo fit in factura viridis cere. Deinde omnia herbe trite
et sepum ovinum simul commisceantur et bene super ignem frixentur. Et postea per pannum fortiter colatur et quod coagulatum fuerit coligatur et in pixide ponatur et usui reservetur. Et cum uti volueris dicto unguento, ungantur
manus prope ignem eo quod dictum unguentum de sui natura est durum et
sine dubio sanabitur.

65. *Item ad delendum scabies existentes in capitibus et in cervicibus juvenum medicina
experta*: Recipe sirpos qui sunt in genere suo duri et graciles et crescunt commu-
niter in dura terra et prope moras prout crescunt sirpi marini prope mare. Con-
burantur sirpi illi duri et graciles. Quibus conbustis, commisceatur cinis
illorum sirporum cum lacte mulieris parturiantis et nutrientis infantem masculum. Hiis factis ungantur capita et colla juvenum qui paciuntur infirmitatem
et sine dubio sanabuntur.

66. *Item contra suffocacionem matricis*: Recipe manipulum unum de lorel, item manipulum unum de violet, terantur bene. Quibus tritis, ponatur in uno potello
vini et utatur paciens isto potu binis vicibus in die, mane videlicet et sero, post
cuius sumpcionem in sero non sumatur cibus vel potus.
[f.58r] *Nota de virtutibus et viciis porri . . .* [91]

67. *Ad sanandum plagas*: Accipe oleum olive et vinum sed minus de vino quam de
oleo et incorporentur simul et ad ignem calefacientur. Deinde ponatur de
dicta confectione in vulnere cum penna et in crastino lavetur vulnus cum
vino albo, si poterit haberi, vel [f.58v] rubeo et bene mundetur et iterum linietur vulnus sicut prius et sic facies quousque fuerit sanum. Probatum est sepius.
Experimentum rysystokys [sic].

68. *Item ad raucedinem et contra tussim et malum pulmonis*: Accipe de auripimento
et pipere et croco de unoquoque quam denarium pensat et tribula fortiter et
postea misce mel cum vino et inpone pulverem et permitte multum bullire et

exinde jejunus bibe. Tussim sanat, pulmonem curat, et vocem restaurat amissam.

69. *Item contra raucedinem*: Recipe radices petrosilli, folia de violet, horhound, ana. Predicte bene coquentur in dulcidrio. Deinde sero de predicto liquore bibatur et valebit.

70. *Item ad provocandum menstruum*: Semen lini coctum cum lacte in cibo vel in potu datum mulieri quando vadit dormitum. Statim provocat menstruum.

71. *Item contra dolorem stomachi et cordis arsuram*: Menta trita coquatur in pasta triticea sub cineribus et cum extractum fuerit ab igne perforetur multis parvis foraminibus et inponatur parum aceti et stomacho superponatur. Probatum est.

72. *Item ad sterilitatem probandam*: Inpleantur duo vasa de granis ordei et urinentur vir et mulier in dictis vasis, quilibet videlicet in suum vas. Deinde ponantur dicta vasa in aliquo loco frigido per .vii. dies et cuius grana post non germinaverit, eius culpa est.

73. *Item contra fluxum ventris*: Ungatur umbilicus egroti et regio, .i. spina dorsi tota,[92] eius communi oleo. Postea super aspergatur pulvis cornu cervi conbusti.

74. [f.59r] *Item ad plagam sanandum*: Tere centrum galli et pone super plagam et cito sanabitur. Probatum est et si caro inflatur, pone id recens quousque sanetur.

75. *Item ad extinguendum libidinem in meretricibus*: Da eis bibere betonicam et nimpheam cum aceto. Probatum est.

76. *Item ad idem*: De herba nimphea .3. uncie date in diversis cibis mulieri meretrici, a luxuria cessat, vel bibat betonicam et solsequium et cessabit luxuria.

77. *Item ad antracem interficiendum*: Recipe succum de heyreve et de burnete et similam ordei et de illis fac emplastrum et pone super antracem et interficietur.

78. *Item contra guttam frigidam*: Recipe croppis offe þe red netyl et heyreve in equali proporcione et sal et urinam veterem hominis: terantur omnia simul bene et exprimatur succus per pannum fortiter et cum illo succo ungat se paciens ad ignem locum infirmitatis et sanabitur. Probatum est.

79. *Contra albuginem occulorum .i. wyte et lippitudinem occulorum .i. bleriyne[s] et galyrsoul:* [93] Recipe eufras manipulos duos, ribwort manipulum unum, ben-levis .m. unum, celidoniam unum manipulum.[94] Terantur bene herbe simul, quibus tritis colatur tritura fortiter per pannum. Hoc facto sumatur pinguedo caponis .i. chappounys-gres et etiam barchys-greys, equaliter de ambobis,[95] si poterit haberi, ad pondus dictarum herbarum. Liquifiatur predicta pinguedo, quo liquefacto simul conmisceantur usque succus herbarum et pinguedo et super ignem ponatur et bulliat modicum et inpone de copros ad quantitatem unius fabe pulverizato [f.59v] et ad quantitatem durarum fabarum de attramento pulverizato. Hiis factis et conpletis de igne deponatur et colatur per pannum et quod coagulatum fuerit usui reservetur . . .[96]

80. *Contra constipacionem*: Recipe flores violarum et boraginis et epitimi, liquoricium, annisum, semen maratri .i. feniculi, croci .i. safran, ana dragmas .ii. Item

sene ad pondus omnium aliorum fiat pulvis et utatur jejuno stomacho cum cervisia vel sero in aurora sumpto. Probatum.

81. *Ad delendum sausfleeme*: Fiat in urinali aqua de floribus fabarum et ungatur facies sepius cum illa aqua et delebitur illa infirmitas.

82. *Ad antracem de loco ammovendum si sit supra hanelitum vel quocumque loco alio*: Sume de radicibus pede leonis et edere terrestris, tere et pone in testa nucis maioris et pone super locum ubi volueris quod descendat antrax et sine dubio trahet ad se antracem. *Ut igitur interficiatur antrax*, sume succum de heyrive, gallice glavelye, et de burnete .i. moderwort et fac succum ex eis et sume de simila ordei et fac pastum et fac inde emplastrum super antracem et interficietur. [f.60r] Interfecto igitur antrace, recipe malvam minorem .i. lityl hook[97] et butirum ita quod tres partes sint de malva et quarta de butiro. Terantur simul in mortario diu et bene et hoc facto ponas emplastrum super morbum binis vicibus in die, si oporteat, et sanabitur. Et notandum quod istud genus emplastri sive ista medicina non solum valet pro omnibus antracibus sanandis, verumpeciam pro omnibus pistulis .i. bilis et pro omni genere plagarum dummodo non sint nimis profunde valet et ultra modum ista medicina suaviter et celleriter sanat.[98]

83. *Item pro frigido stomacho et obstructo ex nimia repletione* et ad purgandum stomacum et ventrem de malis humoribus: Recipe warmot, reed may, reed mynt, reed netlys, sage, halfwodde, fymeter. Terantur modicum et ponantur in vino vel servicia defecata et stet sic per diem naturalem. Postea sumat paciens omni die jejuno stomacho unum bonum tractum post cuius sumpcionem vadat spaciatum et moveat bene corpus suum ambulando et sic faciat per .9. dies continuos et totum stomachum et ventrem purgabit et appetitum provocabit.

84. *Item optima medicina pro occulis lacrimantibus ex excessu caloris*: Recipe sex coclearia de aqua rosacea et sex coclearia de aqua facta ex albuminibus ovorum coctorum et conmisce ambas aquas simul et accipe [f.60v] unam dragmam de caudi [pulli] et unam dragmam de vitreolo viridi .i. copros et pone simul in predicta mixtura aquarum donec liquefiant et ponatur una gutta predicte medicine in occulo in principio noctis .s. quando paciens vadit ad lectum suum et alia gutta post (post) primum sompnum vel circa mediam noctem et optime sanat. Fit autem aqua de albuminibus ovorum per modum istum: accipe .xii. ova et coque illa donec fuerint omnino dura et tunc separa albumina a vitellis et tere albumina in uno disco cum manubrio cultelli et cum fuerint bene trita, ponatur discus cum albuminibus in aliquo foramine humido in pariete remoto omnino a sole et stet ibi per tantum tempus quam poteris dicere exequias mortuorum cum .ix. lectionibus et tunc exprime succum eius per pannum lineum fortiter et habebis aquam clarum. Deinde pone discum secundo in eodem loco per tantum tempus et secundo exprime ut prius et secunda aqua est f[r]igidior et melior.

85. *Contra apostema laterum* et eorum dolorem: Ita quod homo non potest nec audet ponere sub lateribus manum suam, teratur bene red may .i. huundefenyl et temperetur cum aqua benedicta et exprimatur per pannum lineum et bibatur omni die per novem dies continuos jejuno stomacho et sanabitur et salvabitur.

86. *Item pur gout que n'est freyd* ne chaud que se remue de lu en lu: Pernez saunk d'un aignel et jubarbe et boyllez ensemble. Pus pernees **[f.61r]** gres de chever ou oyl de olive et les friez tut ensemble et quant ce serra fet, mettez en un boist et là ou vous sentez la gout, liez pardesus et pardesuz. Pus festes garcer un pou et pus mettez a la gout un enplastre de cele boyste et la gout s'en irra dedens trei jours.

87. *Item pur gout freyde et chaude*: Pernés herbe Johan et medefeloun, si lé triblez et mellés en cervoyse et donez a beivre au pacient, si mettez la drache sur le mal . . .⁹⁹

88. *Item contra cancrum*: Accipe burnetam maiorem, southrinwode et herbam Roberti in bona quantitate et simul terantur cum uncto porcino et lavetur infirmitas cum aqua decoctionis centauree et unguentum ponatur super linum et infirmitati superponatur et bis lavetur in die, mane .s. et vespere, et similiter bis superponatur unguentum.

89. *Item contra paralisim*: Accipe salgiam, hindehale, watircars, primerole, piper, avencia, wythewynde, **[f.61v]** butirum de maii, equa porcio istarum colligatur et bene terantur et lique butirum, quo liquefacto stet ad tempus in pace antequam herbe inponantur et quod butirum sit multum super herbas in coctione et coquatur usque ad spissitudinem et cum frigidum fuerit, reservetur unguentum hoc in pixide et inungatur infirmus.

90. *Item contra fluxum ventris*: Recipe lac caprinum et farinam furmenticeam et simul coque et post decoctionem bonam pone in disco et tere unam vel duas tortas panis frumenticii bene assatas et commedat ita calide sicut potest et bibat vinum calidum quando indiget, sed curetis quod istud non fiat in principio infirmitatis, sed post bonum tempus et hoc semel mane et secundo ad vesperas, et nisi post hoc fuerit emendatus, est in periculo.

91. *Item contra dolorem dencium*:¹⁰⁰ In nomine Patris et Filii et Spiritus Sancti, amen. Apud Alexandriam passa est beata Apollonia, virgo et martir, cuius primo persecutores omnes dentes ab ore illius excusserunt. Unde per merita et intercessiones ipsius deprecemur dominum nostrum Jhesum Christum, ut omnis dolor a dentibus huius famuli vel famule .N. excutiatur, ita ut nullam passionem doloris in dentibus paciatur, sed per virtutem Dei et domini nostri Jhesu Christi fiat sanus, amen. Scribatur ista medicina in scedula et teneat eam paciens inter dentes et sanabitur mediante domino nostro Jhesu Christo. Probatum est.¹⁰¹

92. **[f.62r]** *Item ad faciendum entractum quod Gracia Dei vocatur*: ¹⁰² Pur fer bon entret pernez deus poignes de pimpirnole et deus de betoyng et deus de verveyne et .ii. de puliol reale et une poigne de merche et .i. de rathele et .i. de violet et .i. de bugle et .i. de conseude la petite ¹⁰³ et une de mouser et une de bugyl savage et .i. de celidone et .iii. poygnes de wodesour. Pus lé triblés bien et pus pernez un quarter de cire virgine et un quarter de roysine et un quarter de mastik et un quarter de franc encens et les triblés bien si qu'il seint ben menu et de storacia calamit un dragme et pernez un quarter de turbentine et un pou de oyle de olive et dymy dragme de la vine, si vous le poez aver. Pus pernez un novel pot et pernez un poteau de vin, si mettez les herbes en le pot et le vyn

ensement et les festis bolyr jekys a la tiers part. Pus les outhez et colez parmy un drap et quant ce serra colé, pernez un autre noveau pot et mettés cel vine dedens. Pus mettez la cire et l'oyl et la rosine et storax calamite et les lessez ben boyller et movez tutdis et quant ce serra ben boyllé, les otte[z] de fu. Et pus pernez le mastik et le ensens et mettez dedens et le turbentine et la baume encement [104] [f.62v] et tut feez lé movez et quant ce serrunt ben mellé, remettez au fu et lessez rechaufer. Pus otthez du fu et colez parmi un drap et mettez en un vessel; ce est la suverein entret que seit.

93. *Contra calculum, pur la gravel:* Pernez un levre vif et mettez en un noveau pot, si le ardés tut enter et fetis poudir et donez a malade a manger en soun potage et li donez greyn de elisaundre a manger et pissera mult et gettera mult de la gravele. Si il seyt pleyne de gravele, fetis li manger purnelys dé boys .i. slou et il li frount deliverer de la gravel. Quaunt aust vendra, pernez purneles dé boys et fetis ben boyller, pus les triblés au meuz que vous poez, pus le mettez en un pot ové mel et li donez a manger checun jour en l'iver jun un quiller et il garra.

94. *Item contra venenum pocio,* pur poysoun: Pernez let du chevere et semence de caumbre et boillez ensemble, ce est le meillour bei[v]r[e] que seit pur poysoun.

95. Item pur estauncher flux du saunk: Pernez cink foillis de pervenk et machez sauns transgluter; ou pernez un feve et fendez et mettés sur la veine; ou pernez vers .s. anguiltwychis et triblez et mettez sur la playe; vel accipe bothum et inde fac cinerem et pone super plagam.

96. [f.63r] *Item ad vomitum reprimendum:* Fac emplastrum de barba Jovis et de farina ordei et pone super orificium stomachi et sumas ciminum et pone in sacculo lineo et bene coque in aqua et pone super orificium eius. Item recipe pugillum seminis aneti et quinque grana piperis et modicum mellis et tere simul et distempera cum vino et calide bibatur vel coquatur radix matefeloun in vino vel forti cervisia et bibatur.

97. *Item ad vomitum provocandum:* Recipe teste [105] ovi plenitudinem vini et tantumdem mellis et tantum terciam partem de succo ebuli et misce et bibe.

98. *Item contra scabiem pocio:* Recipe warmot, centoyre, fumtere, mugwort-rote, matefeloun-rote, hertistong, hokkys, mouser, dayse, herbe Jon, livyrwort, bugil, senicle, scabiose, ex hiis fiat pocio et ungatur paciens unguento facto ex hiis quatuor herbis videlicet mercuriali, luvache, fenil et celidoyn.

99. *Item contra calefactionem epatis emplastrum:* Recipe weybred, attirlouebery. Simul terantur et ponantur in bursa linea super dextrum latus.

100. Item si volueris scire an homo evadet de vulnere vel non, des sibi ad bibendum secundo vel tertio die aut amplius post vulneracionem villis, cerfoyle gallice, quam si evomuerit, morietur, si non, salvabitur dummodo bene custodiatur.

101. [f.63v] *Item ad dilatandum pectus* electuarium: Sume pulegium montanum et confice in pulverem et bulliatur mel et zucura addatur et eiciet illud quod est putridum.

102. Item si serpens vel vermis nocivus in os hominis introierit, attramentum cum vino mixtum bene spissum bibat. Probatum est . . .[106]

103. [f.64r] . . . Item ad crepaturas manuum: Ablue manus in spuma mellis et aqua frigida. Probatum est.

104. Item contra febres tercianas: Collige tres plantas de plantagine dicendo orationem dominicam in colligendo et admisce quam duobus digitis levare poteris de sale et contere fortiter et da bibere pacienti anti accessionem et post et sanabitur.

105. Item ad eos qui non possunt continere urinam, sed mingunt sub se dormientes: Coque cortices liliorum in aqua et cum bene cocti fuerint, fac emplastrum et appone renibus.

106. Item ad eos qui sanguinem mingunt, hec potio valet: Accipe appium, feniculum, anetum, petrocillum, gromyl, ana et simul terantur et ponantur in olla nova et coquantur in vino vel in servicia defecata vel in dulcidrio, ut quidam dicunt, donec medietas excoquatur et per pannum lineum colatur et inde bibat paciens jejunus vel quando surrexerit a sompno.

107. Item ad clarificandum vocem: Furfur ordei coque in aqua et bibe.

108. Item ad provocandum sompnum: Distempera apium .i. merche cum tenui albumine ovi et unge inde capud et timpora.

109. Item ad uvam pendentem .i. strichil et distillantem: Recipe centauree folia cum vino trita, bibat jejunus; vel allium cum sale tritum pone in cocleari et tange uvam pendentem.

110. [f.64v] Item ad idem: Recipe hundefenyl et medwort ana, terantur cum sepo porcino veteri et super verticem capitis .i. mold bene calide ponatur et salvabitur.

111. Item ad calculum frangendum: Recipe radicem mactarum [corr. malvarum?], radicem urticarum, radicem .i. poukspere vel semen carwey, linguam servinam, corticem radicum malvarum, radicem petrocilli, semen feniculi, semen macedonici .i. elisaundir, semen vel folia edere ana .m. .i. Maior pars tamen sit de tribus primis. Terantur herbe et coquatur super clarum et lentum ignem in tribus potellis vini albi, si haberi potest, usque ad unam lagenam. Deinde coletur et clarificetur cum modico melle, bibatur inde mane et sero tepide, commedatur semen feniculi ante prandium et post. Caveatur a lacte, a salsis etiam piscibus et carnibus etiam salsis et caseo et a viscosis cibariis et potibus et a nimia sessione. Item appone saxifragium, si habes, et herbam grani solis .i. gromyl, et si volueris loco mellis ponatur liquiricia vel zucura, quando etiam bibit limpha vinum cum illa aqua. Experimentum optimum et probatum.

112. Item ad idem: Recipe saxifragium et bona quantitate et aliqualiter teratur et ponatur in vino vel in forti cervisia defecata nullo autem modo yma et cum manu vel baculo moveantur simul bene. Deinde obturetur bene os olle cum straminibus avenaticis et sic stare permittas per duos dies naturales. Tertio vero die et ex tunc cum uti vo[f.65r]lueris predicto potu non ammoveatur

obturatio, sed permittas licorem in effundendo transire per illa stramina in cipho et bibat quam et quotiens et quando voluerit omni die. Insuper cum voluntas urinandi eum arripuerit, capiantur folia illius herbe que vocatur walwort vel radices eiusdem cum foliis caruerit, et extrahatur truncus quod est in medio radicis .i. spir et deleatur et residua pars bene teratur. Coquantur folia vel predicti radices bene in aqua, quibus decoctis balneetur virga cum tota bursa bene. Postea apponatur predicta decoctio super totam virgam et bursam ad modum emplastri ita calide sicut potest pati et sic stet per aliquod spacium temporis. Deinde faciat urinam predictis existentibus circa virgam et bursam et emittet urinam cum modica aut nulla pena. Facta vero urina deponantur omnia si voluerit et sic faciat paciens quociens voluntatem habuerit urinandi et cum potus fuerit consumptus, de novo fiat alius potus et sic faciendo continue tam bibendo quam virgam et bursam balneando et cataplasmando quociens necesse fuerit, sine dubio liberabitur a calculo et salvabitur. Istud est experimentum efficacissimum et probatissimum.

113. *Item experimentum ad probandum utrum homo sit leprosus a natura*, hoc est si infirmitas traxit originem a parentibus vel si homo sit leprosus a casu, hoc est a causa accidentali, cum videlicet malus potus vel cibus venenosus sumebatur vel potabatur **[f.65v]** vel cum homo abutebatur muliere prius cognita a leproso, et si isto modo, hoc est a casu, de remedio sanativo eiusdem. Nota igitur tale est experimentum. Sumatur ovum galine eodem die vel die precedenti natum et ponatur ovum in disco multum concavo et minuat sibi paciens ita quod sanguis eius fluat super ovum in predicto disco existens et ad tantam quantitatem minuat sibi paciens quousque videlicet totum ovum sit coopertum sanguine. Deinde ponatur predictus discus com ovo et sanguine in aliquo securi loco et mundo ita quod ex tunc nullo modo moveatur discus nec ovum in sanguine existens, set stare permittatur a tempore minutionis, hoc est a mane usque ad horam vesperarum. Post horam vero vesperarum extrahatur ovum de sanguine et deponatur eius testa, quod si repereris in deposicione teste eius albumen aliqualiter durum fetens et corruptum vitellum autem totum inmaculatum, vel si adhuc vitellus pro aliqua sui parte tantum sit maculatus seu viciatur tendens ad corruptionem et fetens residua parte vitelli remanente integra, talis omnino est leprosus a natura, set a casu, hoc est a causa accidentali, et poterit curare. Quod si vitellus totus una cum albumine ovi sit aliqualiter durus, corruptus et fetens, talis homo traxit infirmitatem a parentibus et sic habet infirmitatem a natura nec aliquomodo poterit curari. *Cum igitur infirmitas* processerit a casu, hoc est a causa accidentali, talis est sibi cura adhibenda. Recipe salgeam, urticam, mentam, warmot, hundefenyl, de qualibet **[f.66r]** libram unam. Item unum quarterium de radiche. Terantur omnia bene, quibus bene tritis ponantur in tribus potellis vini rubei et simul bene misceantur. Hoc facto obturetur bene os olle. In crastino vero eodem tempore quo ponebantur herbe in vino iterato simul bene cum baculo misceantur et iterato os olle bene obturetur et eodem modo tertio die fiat. Transactis vero tribus diebus utatur paciens predicto poto per .xii. dies continue ita quod infra tres dies semper bibat unam quartam adminus et binis vicibus bibat in die, mane videlicet jejuno stomacho et cum iverit cubitum, et si pluries in die biberit, magis prodest. Et pro certo infra predictos duodecim dies curabitur prout expertum est.

114. *Item contra jaundis*: Recipe endive, maydynher ana, coquantur in aqua usque ad medietatem cum liquiricia aliqualiter prius trita in mortario vel post decoctionem ponatur zucura et sic stare permittas per diem naturalem. In crastino vero capiatur quod purum est et clarificetur et facta clarificatione in olla usui reservetur et tunc zucura addatur si liquiricia prius non fuerat apposita. Utatur igitur paciens de predicto potu ad quantitatem unius magni salsarii alternis diebus jejuno stomacho et tunc utando apponatur qualibet vice ad quantitatem unius fabe de reubarbe pulverizato et sanabitur infra paucos dies.

115. [f.66v] [107] *Contra raucitatem*: Recipe horsmynt, herb Jon ana, coquantur in vino vel in servicia defecata modicum et utatur predicto potu ita calida sicut potest cum iverit cubitum et statim coopereat bene capud suum et facto bono sudore in capite sanabitur . . . [108]

116. *Item contra malum stomachum et repletum et precipue contra constipacionem*: Recipe nuces avellanas in bona quantitate et coque eas nuces cum tota testa bene diu in aqua ac si coquentur carnes, quibus decoctis colantur per pannum, quibus colatis statim frixentur cum sepo porcino salso vel recenti et multo melius est si in predicto sepo coquantur. Quibus coctis seu frixis extrahantur et teste nucum frangantur et de curnellis calidis calide commedat paciens unum bonum pastum et sine dubio reddit eum solubilem et . . . et ad cellam quam voluerit et ventrem purgabit et stomachum et appetitum provocabit.

117. *Item contra fluxum ventris et nedynggys quod est magna pena*: Recipe herbam que vocatur mousgras vel horwey, quod idem est, in bona quantitate et teratur bene. Qua trita temperetur cum cervisia defecata et extrahatur succus totus per pannum mundum. Deinde fiat potagium .i. hymmerolys modo consueto et ponatur in [f.67r] potagio de [?] illo succo . . . et hoc facto detur potagium pacienti post cuius sumpcionem binis vicibus vel amplius, si oporteat, vel minus, si oporteat. Sine dubio cito post cessabit fluxus et nedynggys nec sinit ultra ad cameras privatas accedere qui secundum modum alias consuetum.

118. Item hic medicina de veretro scervi, respice infra.

119. *Item ad extrahendum* sive ad expellendum ferrum sive fuerit in stomacho sive fuerit in [in]testinis hominis. Recipe salgeam et fiat pulvis de salgea et utatur paciens omni die jejuno stomacho et cum iverit cubitum illo pulvere in cervisia defecata vel vino et infallibiliter ferrum per sua posteriora finaliter emittet seu expellet.

120. *Item pro subbito assensu matricis*, hoc est aþye þe verliche rakynggys off þe modyr to wommanhis hert:[109] Recipe cropleswort vel brounwort, quod idem est, et tere bene et temperetur cum vino vel servicia defecata et exprimatur succus et bibat ad quantitatem unius salsarii et hoc fiat tociens quotiens arripuerit sibi passio et non ante. Et si volueris, cum predicta herba fuerit bene trita, ponatur tota tritura in predicto licore et sic stare permittatur quousque liquor attraxerit ad se totam fortitudinem herbe et obturatur bene os olle et utatur modo quo prius [f.67v] dictum [?] quod liquor transeat per illa . . . et effusione liquoris.[110]

121. *Item pro matrice quando videlicet mulier non habet* flores suos temporibus debitis, sed magis temporibus indebitis: aliquando enim mulier habet menstruum aut nimis cito, et hoc fit propter nimiam habundantiam menstrui, aut mulier habet menstruum nimis tarde, et hoc fit propter nimiam carentiam menstrui. Ad reparandum igitur omnia ista et ad reducendum menstruum ad tempus suum debitum et ad purgandum ipsem matricem et ut mulier concipiat, talis est medicina. Tertio die quo mulier habet flores suos vel si mulier non habet flores suos nisi tamen per duos dies, secundo igitur die quo mulier habet flores suos, capiantur folia illius herbe que vocatur wallewort vel capiatur radix eius cum foliis caruerit et bene terantur et temperetur cum aqua et per pannum exprimatur et sumatur eius succus ad quantitatem unius salsarii et propositum in omnibus predictis optimebit. Sed sciendum est quod post predictam sumpcionem statim magnam penam sustinebit eructuando, spuendo, evomendo et proiciendo tam inferius quam etiam superius, quod si tamen mulier fuerit ita dure complexionis quod post eius sumpcionem non evomit nec proicit sursum vel deorsum, tunc secundo cum ipsa habuerit flores suos sumat potum de predicta herba predicto modo factum et incontinenti sumat aliquod liquidum [f. 68r] ut purum potagium vel brodium calidum vel aquam calidam et ita statim provocabit ad predicta facienda et si tanta virtus in eius fuerit natura, concipiet nisi defectus viri fuerit in hac parte vel nisi ipsa in etate nimia processit vel per maleficia vel per alias causas accidentales a concepcione inpedita fuerit . . .[111] tamen mulierem ad debitum statum quo alia supraposita rediit. Post etiam sumpcionem predicti potus cesset mulier a sumpcione cibi quousque illa passio fuerit totaliter scedata.

122. *Pulvis pro plagis sanandis:* Recipe bremmylcrop, reed-coulcrop, hempcrop, reed-netilcrop, fenylcrop, tansy, ana; maddyrcrop ad quantitatem omnium aliorum. Terantur bene et minutatim et simul bene misceantur in tritura. Quibus tritis fiant pile parve et seccantur extra solem et ventum et pluries in die volvantur et revolvantur in manu . . .[112] caniciem quibus ad plenum et perfecte seccatis usui reserventur. Cum igitur uti volueris, fiat pulvis de eisdem sic videlicet terantur pile in uno mortario ereo quot volueris, quibus bene tritis cribretur munde et utatur paciens. Sit . . .[113] cum modico liquore ad quantitatem trium cocleariorum mane jejuno stomacho et sero ante cubitum. Post cuius sumpcionem in sero non sumatur cibus vel potus nec diu etiam in mane post sumpcionem eiusdem et folium [f.68v] olleris rubei morbo seu plage apponatur. Probatum est sep(s)ius verum.

123. *Item aliter et levius et melius pro plagis* sanandis et aliorum etiam morborum foraminibus in corpore existentibus et tamen etiam valet pro eiusdem negotiis quam omnes alie herbe suprascripte et etiam maioris est efficacie prout expertum est sepius per illum medicum de Lechlyn. Recipe pimpirnol, bugyl, senekyl ana . . .[114] Terantur bene et fiant pile et fiat pulvis eodem modo per omnia sicut de suprascriptis herbis et eodem modo utatur . . .[115]

124. [f.71r] *Item contra arsuram sive conbustionem cura: Recipe fimum* seu stercus aucarum et sepum ovinum sic videlicet quod duplex proporcio sit de fimo seu stercore aucarum et cum sepo predicto bene frixentur et frixura colatur per pannum et in illo unguento colato intingantur panniculi diversi facti iuxta

quantitatem combustionis et apponantur quotiens opus fuerit quousque sanus fuerit effectus. Ista medicina cito sanat et optime prout sepius est probatum.

125. Item ut pili evulsi non crescant, cum lacte canis locum inungere debes.

126. Item ut pili non crescant; Pernés lé graundes formies .i. emotis et ostez lé testes et de cele oyngnour oyngnez la ou vus voderés.

127. Ad idem: Pernez les eofs des formies et destemprez mult bien od aysel, si enoygnez.[116]

128. [f.78v] *Ad extrahendum seu expellendum ferrum de corpore*: Recipe archam angelicam .i. blyndenetil, agrymoniam .i. egyrmoyn, ditonia .i. dyttaundyr, peluseta .i. mouser, salgeam ana. Iste quatuor erbe terantur in mortario et de istis accipias succum et coquas dictum succum cum duplicata parte puri mellis quousque sit tam condensum sive spissum sicut salsa de zyngibero. Et detur ad potandum pacienti omni die jejuno stomacho ad quantitatem unius coclearii pleni cum alio parvo liquore, vino videlicet vel servicia defecata vel cum sero et pro certo per spacium temporis eiciet ferrum omnimodum fixum in corpore. Probatum est.

129. *Electuarium quod vocatur dyasaturion:*[117] Dyasaturion dicitur a saturionibus qui ibi recipiuntur vel a saturis quos fama pronos in Venerem devulgavit. Valet enim contra debilitatem renum. Debilitas autem renum quandoque fit ex calore, quandoque fit ex frig[id]itate, quandoque ex viscoso humore. Quando autem fit ex calore, non detur quia magis augmentaretur dolor caloris. Et debilitas quando fit ex frigiditate detur cum vino tepido. Quando autem fit ex viscoso humore detur cum vino decoctionis feniculi et petro. Libidinem exitat. Coitus etiam debilitatur ex defectu spumum, aliquando etiam ex defectu humorum, aliquando ex frigiditate, aliquando ex calore. Quando autem debilitatur ex calore, non detur, quando autem ex frigiditate debilitatur, detur cum vino mediocriter limphato. Quidem autem dant cum vino decoctionis stinccorum, sed male fa[f.79r]ciunt[118] quia sic ignem igni addentes dum putant excitare libidinem ipsam extingunt. Accepturis diaforon probatum est electuarium. Utatur bono cibo et generante humores multos et postquam acceperit sumat dactilis vel ficus vel penideon vel amigdalas.

130. *Item*: Saturiones calidi et humidi sunt in tertio gradu, excitant libidinem quia grossos humores resolvunt et ventositates. Unde virgam tendunt et inflant. Herba est cuius radix in vere colligitur et competit usui medicine et per annum servari potest.

131. *Item*: Baucie calide et humide sunt sanguinis et spermatis generative, alio nomine dicitur pastinata. Radix competit medicine et ponitur hic ad excitandum coitum quia sperma et sanguinem generat et ventositates et excitat libidinem et ideo ponenda est in medicina.

132. *Item*: Eruce .i. skyrwyttys calide et sicce sunt in tertio gradu. Herba est cuius semen ita appellatur et semen ponitur in hac medicina propter causam dictam, quia grossos humores generat et resolvit in ventositates. Semen per tres annos servari potest. Herba ipsa cocta cum carne irci et commesta dyasaturion est rusticorum.

133. Item stinccorum viriduum .i. recentium. Stincti enim calidi sunt et sicci. Pisces sunt qui in transmarinis partibus et in istis regionibus in fontibus scilicet inveniuntur. Transmarini autem meliores sunt et maioris efficacie. Illi maiores sunt et grossiores, alii vero minores et graciliores. Circa caudam maioris sunt virtutis propter causam assignatam positam hic. [f.79v] Si sint recentes, debent inponi siu autem inponentur secci. Saliuntur duos et seccuntur et per tres annos possunt servari.

134. Item: Semen bu[l]bi .i. cepule sive semen separum, quod idem est, calidum et humidum est. Ponitur hic ad exitandam libidinem quia grossas generat humores et resolvit in ventositates; in vere colligitur, per annum servari potest.

135. Item: Lingua avia .i. semen fraxini calidum et siccum est et est herba que lingue avis similis est; propter predictam causam ponitur hic. Per annum servari potest, quanto recentior tanto melior. Contra siccitatem pectoris detur decoctio eius et diadragantum.

136. Item: In aqua quidam ita conficiunt saturiones et baucias crudas .i. pestirnepis et ea que non possunt pulverizari conterunt et distemperant cum melle qui postea addunt pulveres specierum sed sic confectus cito corrumpitur. Melius autem conficitur sic: saturiones et baucias in melle in quo cocta sunt conficiantur. Deinde amigdale et penideon per se constricte addantur, ad ultimum pulveres specierum ponantur; per annum servari potest.

137. *Item de eodem .s. de diasaturionum radicibus*: Saturiacis enim grece, erectio virge dicitur latine. Proprie datur illis qui renum debilitatem paciuntur. Libidinem mirabiliter provocat ex aliqua occasione perdita, sine mora restaurat. Recipe saturionum testiculos viriduum, bauc[i]e, nucis indice, pistacee, setacum, pinnearum emundatarum ana dragmas .xii., anisi, eruce, seminis lingue avis ana dragmas .v., cinamomi, caudarum stinccorum, seminis bullii ana dragmas .13. et musci grana .vii. Confice sic; sit ibi tantum mellis de[f.80r]spumata quod sufficiat. Ponantur saturionum testiculi et baucie, setacul unamquamque per se bene tritum et per se similiter in melle mittantur et cum spatina unde conmisceantur et bulliant et cum aliquantulum bullierint ab igne deponantur et pulvis supradictarum specierum ibi conmisceatur. Ad ultimum vero mustus cum aqua rosacea apponatur et sic usui reservetur. Detur in sero cum condito vel vino dulci coclearium unum.

138. *Pro gravi infirmitate mamillarum quas mulieres acerime sepius paciuntur in mamillis suis et similiter pro brook*: Cum igitur predicte infirmitates inceperint crescere, recipe ru[tam] et teratur bene cum puro et mundo melle et superponatur. Quod si per duo vel tria emplastra talia cessaverit dolor et caro sive cutis dealbescat, signum est quod paciens est in convalescendo et tunc utatur predicto emplastro paciens quousque sanus fuerit effectus. *Quod si non cessaverit dolor* propter predictum emplastrum, sed augmentatur et inflatur caro et rubescit, vel si ad tantum devenit infirmitas quod caro etiam iam putrefacta est et etiam caro peciatim cadit de mamilla et sic insunt foramina, recipe subscriptas herbas, videlicet sourdokkys crescentes in campis que sunt macillentiores aliis crescentibus in ortis vel pratis, smal-hokkys, roddis, warmot, weybred; ana terantur bene et [119] [f.80v] minutatim valde. Deinde apponatur predictis herbis pura pinguedo lactis .i. [c]reeme et bene insimul

conmisceantur et superponatur binis vicibus in die, mane videlicet et in sero, et sine dubio per ista emplastra apposita infirmitati, quotiens opus fuerit, sanabitur. Pro[batum] est.

139. *Item contra guttam sive passionem inflativam que accidit in iunctur(i)a humeri ita quod homo non potest levare aliquam manum ad capud vel etiam manum ex opposito directe extendere pre gravamine passionis:*[120] Recipe warmot et teratur minutatim valde. Hoc facto ponatur dicta tritura sive emplastrum super totam iuncturam binis vicibus in die, si oportuerit, et scedabit passionem. Quod si predicta passio non solum tenet pacientem in iunctura humeri, sed etiam passio descendit per brachium, tunc ponatur dicta tritura non solum super ipsam iuncturam, sed etiam super ipsam iuncturam et totum brachium et totam manum usque videlicet ad ultimas iuncturas omnium digitorum et sic fiat quotiens opus fuerit et sine dubio sanabitur paciens [dei] adiutorio mediante, prout sepius expertum est.

140. *Item contra constipacionem:* Recipe .14. vel .16. vel plura grana, si vobis videatur, de seminibus ipsius gladyn et terantur bene in uno disco. Postea sumatur unum ovum molliter assatum et loco salis inponatur dictus pulvis et sic bene misceantur et hoc facto absorbeat quicquid est in ovo. Ponatur etiam .16. vel .17. grana de predictis seminibus in eodem vase et terantur bene et addantur duo coclearia de servicia deffecata [f.81r] et misceantur bene simul et sumatur statim post sumpcionem ovi integraliter uno sorbunculo. Ista medicina poterit dari pacienti ante prandium et etiam post, sed postquam data fuerit, paciens non commedat aliquid quousque paciens fuerit purgatus. Habebit enim paciens post eius sumpcionem cellerem et optimam purgationem inferius et binis vicibus ad maius vomitum superius. Ista medicina est valde suavis et sine periculo. Quidam vero dant succum radicis eiusdem cum alio liquore simul bene mixto. Aliquando autem dant cum potagio, sed istud est aliqualiter periculosum eo quod nimis violenter laxat. Eo igitur laxato et purgato sumat paciens aliquod confortativum.

141. *Item ad deponendum pilos ubicumque fuerint in corpore:* Recipe de cineribus infrascriptis quantum volueris, proportionaliter tamen, prout hic in exemplo ponitur et fiat unguentum corrosivum et sic recipe de calce vivo non extincto .ii. libras. Item de cineribus fabarum .i. de stipitibus fabarum combustis .i. de ben-helme combustis .ii. libras. Item de de cineribus fraxinis unam libram. Item de cineribus de wyche-hasil unam libram. Item de cineribus vrticarum unam libram. Item de woodeactyn duas libras. Istis igitur habentis et simul bene mixtis fiat cum istis lexivium et sic ponantur omnes cineres bene simul mixtos in una patella cum aqua et coquantur aliqualiter .i. habeat tres vel quatuor walmys et de principio usque [f.81v] ad finem decoctionis cum spatula moveatur. Deinde deponatur de igne et colatur per pannum vel transeat per cribrum ad hoc aptum posito modicum de feno vel de straminibus prius in cribro. Postmodum capiatur illa aqua colata et calefiatur bene et sumantur de cineribus novis et in eadem quantitate simul bene mixtis ut prius et ponantur in parvo cribro posito modicum de feno vel de straminibus sub illis cineribus et alio vase subposito cribro in quo fundendus est liquor et infundatur sepius illa aqua bene calefacta seu lexivium quousque tota virtus illorum cinerum sit extracta per tales infusiones. Facto igitur isto lexivio sic per .v. vel .vii. tales

infusiones, proicia(n)tur quicquid est in cribro et ponantur tunc nova stramina vel fenum in cribro et postmodum cineres de wodacsyn et calcem vivum
ponantur super illud fenum et ex tunc fiat eodem modo cum isto lexivio lexivium calefaciendo et super predictos cineres et calcem infundendo prout per
omnia fiebat de aqua et in fine quicquid remanserit de isto lexivio per pannum coletur. Hiis omnibus completis et cetera ut su . . .[121] Vel si volueris
cum primo deposueris de igne, infundatur illa aqua super illos cineres in cribro contentos. Hiis omnibus completis ad unam quartam predicti liquoris sumatur una uncia de calce vivo et sumatur una uncia de orpiment et illud
quod est grossum .i. ballis vel cnappis est melius quam illud quod est subtilis
.s. pulvis eiusdem et illi [122] cnappis frangantur bene et in pulverem redigantur
et simul cum predicto calce misceantur. Et si vis quod predicta confectio sit
ultra modum corrosiva, addantur de resalgar dragme due, item de salpetyr
dragme due, item de alym dragme due, et redigantur in pulverem et simul
misceantur ut prius et coquantur simul movendo continue cum spatula quousque videris quod penna inposita poteris levi tactu manus eam excoriare seu
depilare. Deinde ponatur predicta confectio in vaso terreo (sed melius cus-
toditur in vase ereo), eo quod vas terreum perforabit. Cum igitur uti volueris
predicta confectione, cale[f.82r]fiatur una pars illius confectionis semper in
utendo et sumatur una pecia parva de panno laneo, ad quantitatem videlicet
loci illius cuius loci crines deponere seu depilare volueris, et illa pecia humectetur in predicta confectione et calida sicut potest pati ponatur super locum.
Et iaceat ibidem illa pecia per unam horam vel . . .[123] et non ultra, quia si ibidem ultra moram traxerit, corrodet cutem etiam usque ad carnem vivam.
Pecia igitur deposita de loco levi tactu digiti deponas et deponere poteris
crines. Quibus igitur depositis ad hoc ne crines iterato crescant ibidem, sumatur de sanguine vespertilionis et cum penna intincta in illo sanguine linietur
bene et spisse locus predictus . . .[124] Vel sumatur de eddyrgomme vel de lacrima eddere – quasi fere idem est in genere, nisi quod eddyrgomme fit artifi-
ciose de predicta arbore, lacrima vero eddere est ipsum gomme fluens ab ipsa
arbore – et liquefiatur modicum de butiro vel sumatur modicum de oleo olive
et in eodem oleo vel butiro liquefacto. Liquefiatur sive resolvatur predictum
gomme et cum penna vel cum digito intincto linietur ut prius predictus
locus. Quod si crines iterato crescerint, fiat iterato cum supradicta confectione, ut supra dictum est.[125] De isto unguento corrosivo et etiam sanativo
habetur supra 27,[126] sed hic habetur melius.

142. *Item ad faciendum entret commune pro parvis vulneribus et fistulis et pistulis .i.*
bylys sanandis: Sumantur due uncie de cera virginea vel de alia cera. Item de
rosyn sive coode quatuor uncie. Item de oleo olive vel de auxu[f.82v]gia porcina .i. wyt saym vel de butiro una uncia et simul liquefiantur. Quo liquefacto de igne deponatur et inponatur modicum de turbentyn et moveatur
continue quousque totum turbentyn fuerit liquefactum. Deinde effundatur in
una scutella .i. plateyn non multum concava et cum fuerit coagulatum scin-
datur per parvas pecias. Istut [en]tret sanat antraces cum fuerint interfecti et
etiam parvas plagas et pistulas .i. bylys. Poterit etiam fieri sine turbentyn licet
non fuerit tante virtutis sicut cum turbentyn.

143. *Item contra ydropisym antequam infirmitas sit radicata seu confirmata in corpore et*
antequam venter precipue sit inflatus: Recipe de succo de spurge unum disca-

tum vel duos et recipe mel purum ita quod tertia pars semper sit de melle et due partes sint de predicto succo. Conmisceantur simul bene. Quibus conmixtis ponatur ad ignem et coquatur semper quousque videlicet perveneris ad portionem quam posuistis de melle et habita illa portione deponatur de igne et in vase mundo ad utendum prout inferius dicam custodiatur. Hiis omnibus peractis, sumatur unus discatus vel sumantur duo discati de succo feniculi et ultra ignem cum albumine ovorum clarificetur et cum fuerit clarificatum, ponatur in vase mundo et usui reservetur. Cum igitur uti volueris, sumatur de prima confectione unum bonum coclear et de ista secunda confectione .v. vel .vi. coclearia quousque videlicet videris quod sit satis tenuis ad bibendum et utatur [f.83r] mane jejuno stomacho et hoc semel vel bis in ebdomada. Quod si pro tempore anni non poteris habere succum feniculi, capias radices feniculi et mundentur et extrahantur stipites qui sunt in medio et cum aqua coquantur quoadusque tota virtus radicum sit per coctionem extracta. Et utatur cum prima confectione ut prius et sanabitur dummodo ista fiant in principio infirmitatis et antequam venter infletur.

144. *Item ad idem*: Capias .3. ova et effundas totum albumen eorum et remaneant vitelli in testis suis. Et postea inple ova loco albuminis cum succo illius herbe qui vocatur walwort anglice et conmisce simul succum cum vitello in testa sua bene et pone intus modicum de sale valde et calefacias ova aliqualiter ad ignem et absorbeat ea. Et utatur sic tribus ovis vel duobus, ad minus unum, omni die per novem dies et ulterius, si oportuerit, jejuno stomacho et necessitas infirmitatis deposcat et sine dubio sanabitur Domino mediante, nisi infirmitas fuerit in corpore radicata prout prius dixi. Nec est cura si pedes inflati fuerint. Dum tamen inflatio non ascendat ad ventrem, et ad inflacionem pedum, una cum predictis medicinis vel cum predicta medicina sumantur subscripte herbe videlicet goutfan, walwort, hokkys, heyhove, chikynmet et cum istis subfumigentur pedes et melius est cum syndyr vel cum lapidibus quam cum coctione herbarum in aqua. Et ista omnia fiant quousque fuerit effectus sanus.

145. [f.83v] *Item contra guttam frigidam sive stantem sive currentem summa medicina et infallibilis*: Recipe unam libram de salgea et de succo senecii sive cardui benedicti, anglice groundyswyly, unam libram. Teratur salgea minutatim cum toto predicto succo senecii. Postea accipe de oleo olive ad pondus succi senecii vel salgee et conmisceantur omnia bene simul, quibus simul bene mixtis, sic stare permitte per .9. dies. Omni die tamen materiam semel bene cum spatula movendo decimo vero die igitur exponatur et cum fuerit ad plenum bene calefactum sive frixatum, coletur per pannum lineum et cum fuerit infrigdatum, colligatur quod est coagulatum et in pixide usui reservetur. Cum igitur operari volueris, ungatur locus infirmitatis ad ignem semel vel pluries in die prout opus fuerit et infirmitas exigit quousque sanus fuerit effectus, et sine dubio sanabitur de infirmitate. Set hic sciendum est quod ad unam libram de oleo olive debent sumi due uncie de cera boni ponderis et cera debet liquefieri antequam. Predicta confectio debeat igni exponi et cera ad plenum liquefacta. Debet tunc predicta confectio imponi in eadem patella cum cera et cum omnia fuerint bene simul frixata, coletur et fiat ut supradictum est.

146. *Item contra frigidum stomachum et ad calefaciendum stomachum et ad provocandum appetitum: Recipe salgeam, urticam,* mentam, et cetera. Omnia recipiantur et fiant in modo et quantitate prout dictum est de cura leprosi .39. [=f.65v] et sanabitur.

147. **[f.84r]** *Item ad mulierem que non potest per se post partum ad plenum purgari vel si post partum torsiones graves ultra modum habuerit in ventre:* Recipe unciam .i. de turmentille, item uncias .ii. de ysopo, item dragma .i. de ruta .i. ru. Teratur turmentille et fiat ex inde pulvus si radices non fuerint recentes. Et facto pulvere terantur predicte herbe. Quibus tritis misceantur simul pulvus cum herbis et ponantur in uno potello vini albi vel rubei vel servicie defficate, si vinum nullo modo poterit haberi, et coquatur usque ad tertiam partem .i. tertia pars eiusdem liquoris sit consumpta in coctione et hoc facto coletur fortiter per pannum et utatur paciens sepius isto potu et hoc semper tepide .i. wlakke et liberabitur et sanabitur. Istud sum expertus. Quod si turmentille .i. radices eiusdem fuerint recentes, hoc est noviter de terra extracta, teratur primo turmentille aliqualiter. Deinde inponantur herbe et terantur omnia simul et fiat cum vino vel servicia prout iam dictum est.

148. Item ut mulier liberetur a partu suaviter et sine periculo. Fiat sic: cum mulier fuerit vicina partui per duas vel tres vel quatuor septimanas ante partum utatur balneo facto cum hiis herbis .s. fenyl, smal-hokkys, holyhokkys, chikkynmette, heyhoue. Et sedeat in balneo usque ad umbilicum .i. navyl super pulvinar factum de furfure frumenticeo. Et balneato corpore statim post balneum corpore siccato ungat se ad ignem cum istis unguentis prius simul bene mixtis videlicet maciaton, deauté, oleo laurino. Et ungat se videlicet ab umbilico et infra et circa vulvam **[f.84v]** et infra crura usque ad genua et spina dorsi videlicet ab opposito umbilici et infra et renes et ab uno hyppebon usque ad aliud hyppebon. Et hiis factis paretur pannus lineus ad modum blodebende ad latitudinem illius uncture et in illo panno firmetur lana et superponatur totum locum uncture que est a retro et firmetur pannus in anteriori parte et sit ibi pannus ille de balneatione in balneationem. Et de unctione ad unctionem sit firmatus et cum denuo debeat reponi, primo calefiatur bene pannus ille ad ignem semper et eidem loco superponatur et omni ebdomada ista fiant balneando videlicet et ungendo tribus vicibus in ebdomada et una etiam et eadem aqua facta pro uno balneo poterit sibi ministrare pro tota ebdomada de novo semper calefaciendo eandem aquam.

149. *Item contra frigidum stomachum et infrigdatum et vomitum reprimendum:* Recipe zynziberum unciam .i., galangam unciam .i., sucuram uncias .iii. Fiat pulvis et utatur paciens isto pulvere in vino simul calefacto ita quod frigiditas vini tamen sit expulsa et sic bibatur. Item ad unum ciphatum vini sufficit ponere dimidium coclear de predicto pulvere ad omne maius.

150. *Item contra anum exeuntem:*[127] Recipe urticas, weybred, waterca[r]s. Ana terantur[128] et purgetur de sale et fiat una pila de predictis et ponatur pila ad anum et sedeat super pilam illam vel pilas quotiens opus fuerit et pro certo reintrabit et curabitur.

151. *Item mulier que non habet flores suos sive menstrua nec habuit per multa tempora nec habere potuit ad provocandum igitur menstruum,* cura: Recipe neptam, sal-

geam, calamynt, pulliol real, ysopum, mentastrum .i. horsmyntis, verveyn, mogwort, [f.85r] askeban, herba Johannis .i. herbe Jon, maddyr ana manipulum unum. Terantur herbe. Quibus tritis ad unam libram herbarum tritarum addatur unum quarterium de anys et unum quarterium de liquiricia et unam lagenam vini et unam quartam aque et pistentur bene et minutatim tam anys quam liquiricia. Et postea cum herbis tritis simul bene misceantur et igni exponantur et coquantur usque ad tertiam partem. Et hoc facto sic stare permitte usque in crastinum. Deinde coletur et clarificetur et usui in vase mundo reservetur. Et isto potu utatur paciens prout dictum est supra .22. [=f.50v] [129] et dicetur etiam infra.

152. *Sciendum est* etiam quod ad istum potum sibi debet fieri una subfumigatio .i. unum stu cum hiis herbis:[130] recipe camamyl et calamynt, mentam rubeam et mentam [131] albam, mentastrum,[132] ana manipulum unum. Item de code dimidiam libram. Pistentur herbe bene, pistetur etiam coode et simul cum herbis tritis misceantur et omnia in sacculo ponantur et os sacculi bene ligetur vel suatur et omnia coqua[n]tur in duabus lagenis aque. Quibus coctis ponatur in uno potto sub sedili et sedeat mulier nate discooperto super sedile et ordinetur sic pottus et sedile cum pannis coopertis quod totus fumus exiens de potto quam est possibile ascendat totaliter ad nates et ad claustrum pudoris. Cum igitur corpus mulieris sic sedendo per aliquod tempus fuerit bene calefactum, bibat tunc sedendo unum tractum de predicto potu mane videlicet tepidum et in sero frigidum et post sumpcionem potus sedeat mulier super sedile per tantum tempus per quantum sedebat ante sumpcionem potus antedicti. Et sic faciat omni die binis vicibus, mane videlicet et in scero, post cuius sumpcionem in scero nullus cibus vel potus exinde [f.85v] illa nocte sumatur. Quod predicte herbe pistentur et in sacculo ponantur et sic coquantur. Hoc fit ad cautelam ne alii percipiant que conveniunt ad subfumigationem. Et sciendum est quod illa eadem aqua cum predictis herbis cocta poterit sibi ministrare per .v. vel .vi. dies sine renovacione aliarum herbarum, observato etiam modo in omnibus prius dicto.[133]

153. *Item ad* hoc fiat sibi emplastrum sic, videlicet recipe malvam agrestis .i. smalhokkys libram unam ad minus. Item unum quarterium de cimino. Teratur ciminum bene per se et hokkys per se. Quibus tritis misceantur simul bene et ponatur totum in sacculo formato ad modum totius umbilici cum suis ligaturis ita quod saculus extendat se a navyl usque ad os claustri pudoris et de uno hyppebon ad aliud hyppebon in latitudine et punctetur sacculus et hiis factis frixetur sacculus in sepo porcino .i. wyt seym vel wyt gres vel in oleo olive vel in butiro et ligetur calidum cum illis ligaturis super umbilicum seu ventrem et sit ibi continue nisi cum debeat ire ad lectum mariti sui vel cum debeat uti predicto stu seu predicta subfumigatione. Et cum predictus sacculus inceperit desiccari, illa pars sacculi que ponetur ad umbilicum seu ventrem calefiatur tantum ad ignem et ungatur cum istis unguentis modicum simul bene mixtis videlicet maciaton, oleo laurino, deauté et demum ventri superponatur et sic fiat quotiens opus fuerit. Et una cum hoc ponat infra corpus suum .i. in claustro pudoris radicem altee recentem .i. rot of þe wymaw vel radicem accori .i. gladyn ad longitudinem .vi. pollicorum intinctam prius in oleo communi vel unctam cum predictis unguentis et sit ibi etiam continue nisi in casibus prius dictis de emplastro et in dies renovetur radix, hoc

est omni die capiatur nova radix recens[134] altee vel accori et sit preparata et [f.86r] intromissa et sine dubio menstruum provocabit. Demum vero per tres vel quatuor dies ante tempus quo solebat habere flores suos lavet bene pedes suos et tibias et crura sua cum aqua calida in qua herbe bone sint cocte videlicet feniculum, heyove, lovage, chikynmet, walwort. Et statim post minuatur de vena que est sub cavilla pedis .i. ancle et si sanguis non exierit bene de vena, ponat pedem in aqua calida ad quantitatem lagene et extrahatur sic sanguis in tantum quousque aqua fuerit effecta ad modum vini in colore. Sequenti vero die de reliquo pede et[iam] extrahatur sanguis secundum virtutem eius, quoniam in omni egritudine respiciendum est ad virtutem pacientis[135] et maxime timendum est ne nimis debilitetur et sciendum est pro certo quod si ista fecerit medicinam in dies continue, curabitur et flores suos habebit.

154. Item pro eadem infirmitate respice supra .21. [=f.50r], melius hic.

155. Item contra febres: Recipe febrifugam .i. fethirvoy et commedat jejuno stomacho de predicta herba þre croppis cum sale per unum vel duos dies vel tres continuos et pro certo liberabitur. Et est sciendum quod primo die post primam commestionem habebit unam gravem accessionem et non plures et si habuerit hoc, raro invenitur et raro videtur. Cum igitur sanus fuerit effectus, si postmodum casu aliquo in eandem infirmitatem reinciderit, fac ut primo dictum est et curabitur et etiam tociens quociens reinciderit . . .[136]

156. [f.87v] Item contra vermem, fistulam .i. festyr et contra cancrum et maxime contra vermem: Recipe herbam que vocatur violet et tere minutatim. Qua trita ponatur per modum emplastri super morbum. Postea recipe mel et pone super paniculum lineum vel super linum aliqualiter spisse et ponatur super dictum emplastrum de violet. Quibus positis et super morbum ligatis, usque ad fatigationem moveat se paciens. Dicta enim medicina mirabiliter acerbe pacientem infestabit et ideo quanto magis movet se paciens tanto minus gravabit eum medicina et tanto magis et melius operabitur premissa medicina. In crastino vero eadem hora renovetur medicina et fiat per omnia, ut prius dictum est, et sic fiat per .iii. dies continuos. Quarto vero die, si perceperitis aliquo modo aliquem motum ad modum vermiculi repentis, anglice 'any stiryng as a crepinde worme', addatur adhuc morbo predicta medicina et fiat motus corporis prout prius dictum est. Quarto vero die vel quinto recipe herbam que vocatur brounwort et teratur minutatim et per modum emplastri super morbum ponatur binis vicibus in die, mane videlicet et in sero, et sic fiat per alios .iii. dies continuos. Septimo vero die vel octavo sumatur herba que vocatur ragwort et in mortario minutatim pistetur. Qua pistata stilletur et inpleantur omnia foramina illius morbi cum succo illius herbe. Quibus inpletis ponatur super morbum dicta herba bene trita cum toto suo succo integro et in sero renovetur predicta medicina eodem modo et sic fiat omni die quousque sanus fuerit effectus. Et lavetur in omni renovacione cum urina veteri propria vel aliena. Ego ipse loquebar cum homine qui dictam infirmitatem cum multis foraminibus in tibia paciebatur [f.88r] per .xv. annos, ut dixit, nec unquam per quamcumque aliam medicinam poterat curari nisi per medicinam solummodo antedictam.

157. Item contra cancrum: Recipe radices flagris .i. seggys illorum videlicet qui crescunt in dura terra et sicca maxime et temperantur minutatim et apponantur morbo mane et sero et in omni renovacione lavetur seu mundetur infirmitas per penam cum propria urina et salvabitur.

158. Item contra assensum matricis .i. rakynggys: Recipe rybwort et commedat duo vel tria folia ex illis et statim sentiet allevacionem. Deinde recipe predictam herbam et herbam que vocatur seynte Mary wort ana et simul terantur et extrahatur succus et bibatur et non solum cessabit rakynggys, sed etiam eam ex toto purgabit.

159. Item contra illiacam passionem .i. jaundiz: Recipe selvegren et modicum aceti purissimi. Teratur selvegren et extrahatur succus eius et addatur unum coclear bonum de predicto aceto ad .4. vel .v. coclearia succi selvegren et bene simul misceantur et in predicto liquore sit panniculus lineus bene madefactus et ponatur panniculus predictus super epar sic videlicet quod nullo modo tangat stomachum et cum panniculus fuerit siccatus apponatur alius panniculus bene madefactus et tociens sic quotiens opus fuerit et salvabitur.

160. Item contra constipacionem: Recipe ysopum .i. ysop et teratur minutatim. Qua trita temperetur cum lacte acido spisso et per pannum coletur et bibatur mane jejuno stomacho et cum iverit cubitum et sic totiens quotiens opus fuerit et liberabitur. Probatum est.

161. Item contra fluxum ventris: Recipe tormentillam totam herbam .s. cum suis radicibus et terantur modicum in mortario et coquantur in lacte [f.88v] dulci bovino et hoc facto eiciantur herbe cum suis radicibus et cum illo lacte fiant pultes .i. potagium sive gruellum vel pappe cum pura simila siliginis et utatur paciens isto potagio ita calide sicut potest, mane videlicet jejuno stomacho et in sero cum iverit cubitum, et sic hoc tociens quociens opus fuerit et salvabitur.

162. Item contra epilenciam .i. morbum caducum:[137] Recipe .i. fiant .xii. candele de cera iuxta numerum .xii. apostolorum et in qualibet candela nomen unius apostoli scribatur ita quod .xii. candele nomina .xii. apostolorum comprehendant. Hoc ordinato et facto, audiat paciens missam de feria quarta de jejunio videlicet quatuor temporum ante festum beati Michaelis et illa missa celebrata statim audiat paciens aliam missam .s. de Spiritu Sancto. Et dicto offertorio offerat tunc paciens omnes candelas accensas simul in manu sacerdotis quibus oblatis extrahat de manu sacerdotis de illis (de illis) .xii. candelis (candelis) accensis unam casualiter non deliberando quam illarum vult extrahere et illa candela sit extracta. Vigiliam illius apostoli cuius nomen est in illa candela scriptum omnibus diebus vite sue jejunet in pane et aqua, nisi gravis infirmitas obsistat in hac parte, et per annum integrum abstineat a coitu. Et notandum quod a principio prime misse usque ad oblationem secunde misse paciens debet semper tenere omnes candelas accensas simul in manu sua et sit prius mundo confessus et contritus de peccatis suis commissis et pro certo salvabitur si sit bone fidei. Hec igitur sunt nomina apostolorum duodecim: Petrus, Andreas, Johannes Ewangelista, Jacobus maior, Thomas, Jacobus Alphey, mi[f.89r]nor Johannis, Bartholomeus, Matheus, Simon cananeus, Tadeus, Mathias. Isti .xii. apostoli conposuerunt simbolum sacrosanc-

te matris ecclesie. Tadeus qui postea Judas dictus est prout in passionario habetur, festum eius una cum Simone simul celebratur prout festum Johannis et Jacobi apostolorum uno et eodem die ab ecclesia sollempnizatur.

163. Item propter casum ab equo propter quem casum corpus vel aliqua membra corporis sunt concussa .i. ystoneyd:[138] Fiat potio de subscriptis herbis: recipe askeban, ysop, briswort, confory ana et coquantur cum liquiricio in dulcidruo vel in servicia defecata vel in vino et bibatur omni die jejuno stomacho. Item locio: coquantur in aqua merche, hokkys, chikynmet, heyhoue, una cum bona furfuris quantitate. Quibus coctis lavetur bene locus lesus. Deinde ponantur herbe cocte super unum manutergium amplum et ita calide sicut potest sustinere. Iaceant ille partes corporis lesi super predictas herbas. Herbis vero infrigdatis, ponatur emplastrum super predicta loca lesa bono modo calide quod quidem emplastrum fieri debet de subscriptis herbis. Recipe merche, lymyk, ana et terantur bene in mortario et frixentur cum sepo ovino vel cum butiro et melius si cum utroque fiat et calide apponatur vel ungantur loca lesa cum marciaton, dauton, oleo laurino simul mixtis.

164. Contra bottouns exeuntes sive etiam currentes sanguine sive etiam non currentes, precipue tamen contra bottouns sanguine fluentes et vocantur alio nomine etiam emoroide. Sunt enim ibi quinque vene descendentes a vertice capitis usque ad locum illum et cum tres ex illis exierint et sanguine fluxerint, cum difficultate [f.89v] curatur paciens et si ultra tres exierint et sanguine fluxerint, ex tunc secundum medicos est incurabilis. Cura: recipe semen jusquiami .i. heneban vel folia eiusdem herbe, si semen aliquo modo non poterit haberi, et fiat pulvis de semine et recipe sepum ovinum et liquefiatur sepum et liquefacto sepo inponatur pulvis jusquiami in bona quantitate. Et hoc facto ponatur una pars illius confectionis super panniculum laneum et ita calide sicut potest bono modo pati apponatur loco .i. super botouns sive venas sic exeuntes et desuper sedeat. Et cum frigdatum fuerit, iterum calefiatur panniculus cum confectione et apponatur loco et sic fiat tribus vel quatuor vicibus in die vel pluries, si oporteat, et quarto magis diutius cederit super predictam medicinam tanto magis et melius operabitur ipsa medicina et sic faciat per tres vel quatuor dies continuos. Quibus diebus transactis recipe ceram virgineam et tus .i. stor et ciminum. Hiis habitis fiat pulvis de cimino et incorporetur pulvis cimini in bona quantitate cere virginee et turi prius liquefactis et cum predicta confectio fuerit coagulata et bene incorporata per manuum attractionem et palpacionem capiatur una pars illius et ita calide sicut potest bono modo pati apponatur illa pars sive porcio sic ad ignem calefacta loco et sepius in die hoc fiat et desuper sedeat, prout per omnia dictum est ante de alia confectione et hoc faciat singulis diebus quousque sanus fuerit effectus. Istud est experimentum infallibile prout didici ab illo qui dictam infirmitatem paciebatur nec aliqua medicina poterat curari nisi solummodo ista medicina et ex tunc illam infirmitatem nunquam habuit.

165. [f.90r] *Item contra bottouns exeuntes et sanguine fluentes*: Recipe yarou, feltwort, radices wymau, weybrede, sepum porcinum vel wyt sayme, sepum ovinum fere ad quantitatem herbarum. Terantur herbe et liquefiatur sepum ovinum. Quo liquifacto commisceantur simul bene in mortario herbe et sepum. Deinde exponatur igni et simul bene frixentur. Deinde per pannum

fortiter coletur et usui reservetur. Et cum paciens debeat uti illa medicina, faciat per omnia, prout dictum est in precedenti medicina, et de sepo ovino et pulvere jusquiami videlicet ponatur una pars et cetera.

166. Item contra bottouns exeuntes sed non sanguine fluentes: Recipe predictas herbas in precedenti medicina proximo scriptas et sepum porcinum vel wyt sayme. Terantur simul et frixentur et ita calide sicut potest pati apponatur loco et sedeat super et cetera. Fiant prout dictum est supra in prima medicina videlicet et cum infrigdatum fuerit et cetera.

167. Item contra antracem .i. feloun quamvis in capite apparuerit sive extra fregerit etiam nimis turpiter ubicumque in capite ultra anelitum nec est spes aliquo modo vite sed mortis. Recipe betoyn, maddyr, roddis, bugyl, halfe-wodde ana. Terantur herbe et coquantur in servicia defecata aliqualiter. Quibus coctis ponatur tota decoctio simul cum herbis in una olla et obturetur os olle cum straminibus avenaticis et transeat liquor per stramina illa cum voluerit bibere et sepe et sepissime bibat nec bibat alium potum quousque fuerit ab infirmitate liberatus, et si fuerit aliqua spes convalescentie per istum potum, ad vitam convalescet. Probatum.

168. **[f.90v]** *Contra calculum*: Recipe fructus edere arboree qui crescit circa quercum et perisper ana et coquantur in vino albo, vel rubeo si vinum album non poterit haberi, ita quod ad unam lagenam vini sumatur de utroque una libra et coquatur lagena usque ad unam quartam et sumat mane jejuno stomacho tria coclearia et eodem modo cum paciens iverit cubitum et post hoc non sumat cibum neque potum.

169. *Item pro antrace interficiendo et sanando* experta medicina: Recipe weybrede, wylde sage ana. Terantur simul bene et superponatur et pro certo non solum senciet allevacionem doloris sed interfectionem et nil aliud ponatur ad antracem etiam post interfectionem nisi tamen ista medicina et pro certo morbum sanabit.

170. *Item contra brok*: Recipe mussourounys, .i. poukisthes qui crescit super sterquilinium .i. miskyn, et deponatur pellis exterior et teratur cum pane acido frumenticeo et temperetur cum cervisia defecata, sed melius est cum aceto, et fiat emplastrum et calefiatur et tepide ponatur super morbum. Ista medicina maturescet morbum et franget apostema et ipsum morbum sanabit post cuius fracturam et magnum fluxum eiusdem appetitum paciens habuerit et bene commederit et corpus inceperit fortificari. Evadet si e converso: morietur.

171. *Item ad delendum wertis manuum in aliis etiam partibus corporis*: Laventur manus cum sanguine vulpino .i. foxsisblode et permittatur sanguis stare super manus quousque sanguis totaliter fuerit exsiccatus et quanto diutius steterit sanguis super manus tanto efficacius operibatur medicina et continuet sic quousque manus fuerint effecte sane.[139]

Chapter Six

THE COLLECTION OF MEDICAL RECEIPTS IN MS LONDON B. L. SLOANE 146

MS London, British Library, Sloane 146 is a small volume of 107 folios, measuring approx. 140 x 90 mm. Its contents are wholly medical and botanical. The first three folios have been damaged (f.1r is badly rubbed) and the whole volume cut down, though the prickings are clearly visible on the outer edge of the page. The contents of the MS may be described as follows:

1. ff.1r–68r: a major collection of medical receipts utilizing Latin, Anglo-Norman, and Middle English, largely the work of a single scribe writing towards the end of the 13th C. There are no red rubrics (marginal rubrics in the ink of the text occur from f.57r on) apart from an initial one which is so badly rubbed as to be almost totally effaced. The receipts are simply separated by alternating red and blue paragraph marks with initial letters occasionally being splashed with red. On ff.18v and 21r red scrollwork has been used as a line filler. There are some coloured initials, invariably blue save that an initial on f.6v is red decorated with blue and a similarly executed paragraph mark is found on f.7r. There is remarkably little annotation. Various haplographies have been made good by scribal insertions in the margins (e.g. ff.5v, 7r, 14v, 18v, 20r, 29r, 46r, 53r, 60v). A capital is omitted on f.17v, only the guide letter remaining. On f.4r there is expunction by subscript points and red barring. A sixteenth-century hand has annotated ff.12v–13v. Sporadic use is made of the *de* monogram [1] and where the crossed tironian sign 7 is not used, the conjunction is invariably written out as *e*. The collection of receipts represents an interesting mixture of verses, 'derhymed' verse, and prose pieces, some of which are familiar from the 'Lettre d'Hippocrate',[2] whilst others are unattested elsewhere. The absence of an index and of rubrics would make the collection difficult to use and may account for the absence of the kind of annotation which is normally indicative of use. On f.68r/v a later hand has added a receipt 'Contra scabiem' and two fourteenth-century hands have added, respectively, a receipt and a list of the virtues of the herb fennel. On f.69r there are four receipts in a small hand of c.1300. The third of these is in French and runs 'Pur lé denz malades: Yesu Crit e sa duce mere sainte Marie e sainte Ipolanie [i.e. Apollonia] me doint pes en mes denz e en ma buche, amen. Ter repetatur et ter dicatur Pater noster et Ave Maria'. A larger hand has entered three receipts in French in the lower half of f.69r which are now scarcely legible: '[C]harme bone pur estancher sanc ... [P]ur festre ... [P]ur goute festre ...'

2. ff.69v–72v: an interesting botanical glossary in a hand of the second half of the 13th C. which begins (ff.69v, 70r) with trilingual entries (*gallice* and *anglice* appearing in red), but continues as a Latin-English vocabulary which greatly resembles the Durham plant glossary.[3] Folios 73r–74v are then occupied by a list of plant names, in the same hand as the glossary, accompanied by single Latin verses (occasionally several verses) on their virtues, e.g.

edera terestris: ferventis febris frigus letale recedit

viola: nomen habens a vi virtute resisto dolori
agrimonia: in potu sapor est plaga inquiro retentas

A few vernacular equivalents have been provided on f. 73r, namely: pentafolon: fiflef; salvia: sauge; allium: garlek; celidonia: cheleþeine; [4] petrosilium: persil; ruta: rue; marrubium: horhune.

3. ff.74v–75r: three medical receipts in Latin, in the same hand as the preceding notes on herbs. On f.75r one of the receipts begins 'Collirium magistri Mauri ad omnia vicia oculorum, ad albuginem et pruritum, ad cicatricem et ad lacrimas. Et est tante efficacie quod visum amissum infra .xl. dies restaurat . . .'

4. f.75r/v: a passage on the humours inc. 'Corpus humanum est ex .iiii. humoribus scilicet ex sanguine et colera rubea et ex colera nigra et fleumate . . .' [5] of the type frequently found preceding collections of receipts such as the 'Lettre d'Hippocrate'.

5. ff.75v–79v: a medical treatise on oils inc. 'Humana natura non minus indiget oleis ad sui preservationem quam aquis quorum [sic] quedam sunt calida, quedam frigida . . .' [6] The same treatise is found in MS B. L. Add. 28555 f.37ra/va where it is one of a series of short treatises on waters, oils and sirups, clysters, suppositories, pessaries, siringa, which occupy ff.36rb–39rb and are attributed to Roger Baron.[7]

6. ff.79v–86v: another collection of medical receipts in Latin and the vernacular, many of the latter corresponding to items of the 'Lettre d'Hippocrate' (see notes). There are red rubrics. Latin and vernacular terms rub shoulders, sometimes within a single rubric (e.g. f.81v *Contra le felun medicina*) and occasionally within a receipt (e.g. f.80r 'betonie, agrimonie, benedicte, idem quod senecion, anglice grundeswilie, cerfoile anglice ville, trifolium, pimpernellum, eufrasie . . .'). See text below.

7. ff.87r, 88v–89r: fragments of a treatise with sections on *turtur* (same passage on f.63v), *serpentaria, lingua canis, jusquiamus, basilica*.

8. ff.87v–88v: treatise introduced by a red rubric *Regula optima ad fleobotimationem faciendam.*

9. ff.89v–91v: various medical receipts. On f.89v is found Walther, *Initia* 20125 and on f.90r *Carmen ad oves pro varulis*. On f.90v are found Walther, *Proverbia* 12971 (3 verses), a receipt 'Diayris electuarium', and the following verses on weights; 'Grana quater quinque scrupuli pro pondere pone, / in dragmam surgit, scrupulus ter multiplicatur. / Dat scripulus nummum nummos tres dragma sed octo / uncia dat dragmas, duodena sed uncia libram' (Walther, *Initia* 7292). On f.91r/v is a receipt 'Emplastrum dyastiricos'.

10. ff.92r–98r: short treatise on herbs inc. 'Herbe generaliter dividuntur aut enim silvestres in siccis et altis locis nascentes aut domestice in ortis vel locis orientes aquosis et humidis . . .' [8]

11. f.98r–v: a short treatise introduced by the red rubric *Experimentum urinarum* inc. 'Urina pura et supra nebula natans quasi caligo . . .' [9]

12. ff.99r–106v: a new series of medical receipts (see below) in a larger, angular hand with a few red rubrics (mostly badly rubbed).

13. ff.106v–107v: more receipts, mostly in French, in a new hand (see below).

14. f.107v two Latin receipts *Ad dolorem dentium*, in a later hand and now scarcely legible,[10] followed by two lines of a French receipt 'Pernez semence . . .' which is accompanied by a marginal rubric in red *Pur emflure*.

The impressive collection of medical receipts in MS Sloane 146 covers a great variety of conditions, as can be seen from the following table in which the totals include both Latin and French receipts whilst the numbers on the left refer to the vernacular receipts printed below:

1–9 a miscellany of long receipts, including plasters and ointments

10–19   20 receipts concerning varieties of gout
20–35   21 receipts concerning pains in the head
36–37   6 receipts dealing with varieties of scabies
–   30+ Latin receipts concerning diseases of the eye
38   16 receipts dealing with dental problems
39   15 receipts dealing with conditions of the ear
–   4 receipts concerning 'fetor oris'
40   7 cosmetic receipts for facial complexion
41   15 receipts concerning treatment of the hair
42–44   17 receipts dealing with coughs and constriction of the chest
45–52   10 receipts dealing with the spleen and liver
53–56   8 receipts concerning stomach complaints incl. vomiting
–   8 receipts concerning catarrh and 'uvula cadens'
57   6 receipts dealing with quinsy
58   4 receipts concerned with poisonous draughts
59–63   14 receipts concerning constipation
–   3 receipts concerning tormina
64   3 receipts dealing with worms
65–71   13 receipts concerning dysentery
72   1 receipt for diarrhoea
73   2 receipts for stomach pains
74–75   3 receipts dealing with haemorrhoids
76–78   6 receipts concerning the stone
79–82   10 receipts concerning urinary disorders
83–85   8 receipts dealing with diseases of the genitals
–   5 receipts concerning the fig (ficus)
86–89   22 receipts concerning mamillary conditions
–   8 receipts concerning the menses
90–92   11 receipts concerning problems of childbirth
94–96   12 receipts dealing with jaundice
97–102 10 receipts dealing with 'anthrax/felun'
103–13 24 receipts concerning fistula
114–20 13 receipts concerning cancers
121–26 9 receipts concerning wounds
127–29 3 receipts for fractures
132–34/39 8 receipts concerning ailments of the feet and knees
135–37/40 5 receipts concerning 'rancle'
–   7 receipts dealing with scabies
143–45 13 dealing with impostumes (their maturing and piercing)
–   4 receipts concerning warts
146–47 11 receipts dealing with skin complaints
148–49 5 receipts concerning burns
150–51 5 receipts concerning bites from a rabid dog
152   7 receipts concerning snakebites
153   3 receipts dealing with bites from the spider
154   3 receipts concerned with bee and wasp stings
155–56 11 receipts on styptics especially against nosebleed
157   7 receipts dealing with lice, mites etc.
–   4 receipts concerning vomiting
–   2 receipts dealing with stomach upsets
–   2 receipts dealing with the nails
–   3 receipts dealing with 'noli me tangere'
158–59 4 receipts dealing with loss of the voice

Notes on pp.373–78

161–63 4 receipts concerning soporifics
164–66 4 receipts dealing with loss of appetite
167   1 receipt concerning talking in one's sleep
168–69 5 receipts concerning the dropsy
   –   16 receipts concerning the palsy
170–76 20 receipts concerning fevers
177   2 receipts dealing with 'reuma'
178   1 receipt concerning 'glandre'
179   1 receipt concerning dementia incl. memory loss
180   1 receipt for growing fatter
181   2 receipts for slimming

From this point (f.59v) the collection lacks any system of organisation and consists of miscellaneous individual receipts.[11] Nevertheless it can be seen that the assembly of approx. 530 receipts arranged according to the various complaints represents a considerable labour and deserves to be recorded.

At various points in the collection there are references to instances of cures attached to named individuals: f. 20v 'magister Helyas vidit famulum avunculi sui curatum de squinantia sic'; f.33r 'magister T. vidit quendam curatum de antrace solo succo iacee nigre'; f.34r 'Experimentum magistri Ricardi contra fistulam et cancrum ubicumque fuerit preterquam in trachea arteria'; f.40v 'Secundum magistrum Ricardum contra tumorem pedum et tibiarum'; f.47v 'sic enim curatus fuit frater N. de Credetoun in terra sancta'; f.52v 'Nota quod succus marubii frequenter potatus optimus est in ydropisis calida secundum magistrum Johannem de Roseto'; f.53v 'oximel magistri Thomae Comin contra paralesim'.

The language of the receipts is heavily influenced by the vernacular which is latinized in forms like *feverolam* (f.21v, cf. *faverole*), *stuppis madidis* (f.22v, cf. *estoupes moillez*), *rotula raphani* (f.28r, cf. *roele de raiz*), *lesca* (cf. *alesche*), *stufa* (cf. *etuve*), *rubea parella* (cf. *ruge parele*), *wastellum* (cf. *gastel*) etc. Surprisingly little use is made of English, though some English words appear as glosses to plant names (see notes).

1. [f.1r] Pernez demie livre [12] . . . de peys resine, un quarterun de cire, un quarterun de franc encens, un quarterun de dragant, un quarterun de gomme arabich, un quarterun de aloe epatic, un quarterun . . . un quarterun de fenegrec, un quarterun de comin . . . pois, un unce de sarcocolle . . . peys resine . . . gumme arabich. Puis . . . franc encens . . . sarcocolle, puis dragant, puis . . . puis comin . . . au derain. E puis le colez parmi un drap en eawe froide. E puis . . . e puis le metez en eawe chaude e le lavez bien la dedenz. E puis le tenez au feu e puis le metez en sauf.

2. Pur fere precius entret e precius oignement a plaie e a totes dolurs pur . . . er lungement: Pernez sauge, bugle, pigle, consoude, agrimoine, pimpernole, plantaine, ache, quintfoil, cerfoil, coperun de runce, confirie, verveine, lovesche, cerfoil, lancelé, pervenke, avence, frasere, smerewort, [f.1v] osmunde, foille de poret. Ces herbes seient pris oelement, puis seient triblez en un morter e friz en bure de may, et seient bien quis ensemble. E dunc porrez preendre le jus parmi un drap. E le jus seit remis en la paele. E pernez franc encens e peiz e dragant e gumme arabich e cyre virgine e seient menuement triblez e mis en cel jus. E boillez bien ensemble, e quant serra refreidi, metez en boistes. Ices herbes seient

quilli en may. Totes plaies, totes dolurs, totes rancles e totes choses nomez bien garist sanz dute. Esprové chose est.

3. Pur fere bon entret a plaie e a brusure e a rancle: Pernez peiz e seu de motun e cyre virgine e franc encens. Primes metez peiz en la paele, si fetes merer bien. Puis metez le seu de motun, puis pernez la cyre virgine, si metez tuz treis ensemble. Puis au derain metez le franc encens bien molu en poudre si bien chaut deske a comencement au boillir e sovent movez les ensemble de un fusselet.

4. Pur fere bon e noble entret (e) [contre] plaie e contre felun e tutes maneres de apostemes: Pernez peiz e cyre virgine [f.2r] e code e franc encens e mastich e gumme arabich e comin. E sei[en]t menuement triblé en pudre e seient tuz ensemble mis en une paele e friz ov siu de motun u od siu de sesun, ke puis i a. . .t, e od bure de may. Esprové chose est.

5. Ceo est la recette de entret ke mult vaut contre brusure de corps e cheyure e baterie e pur ameurir tuz apostemes: Pernez quatre unces de fenugrech e une poyne de comin e treis quarteruns de franc encens. E fetes les batre en un morter a menue pudre. E puis pernez une livre de cyre virgine e dous livres de poys reysin e une demie livre de bure de may e un quarterun de blanc saym de pork e demi livre de oyle de olive e treis quarteruns de siu de sesun. E puis le fetes fondrer en une paele, si ke les gummes seient bien defites. E puis pernez les poudres avant nomees, si les boillez ensemble e puis les fetes preendre parmi un drap e facez bien mover deskes il seit refreidi.

6. Pur totes maneres de boces e pur emflure e pur plaie e autres mals saner bon entret:[13] Pernez trois poignez de aloyne e autretant [f.2v] de ache e autretant de centorye e une poigne de l'escorce del neyr espine e une de pomer dé bois e une bone partie de corn de cerf e une poigne de la racine de feugerole. Totes cestes choses boillez en eysil tant ke les .viii. parties seient quites e la .ix. partie remeine. A l'une meité pernez .iii. unces de mastik e une unce de encens e un unce de peis resin e deus unces de peis neir. Si fetes tut mult delié pudre. Sil medlez al jus devant dit. Si metez treis unces de cyre virgine. Pus si medlez bien ensemble. E cest entret est apelé apostolicon.

7. A fere bon oignement pur freide gute: Pernez lavendre e sauge e primerole e cressuns de fontayne e avence e ambrosie e planteine e launcelee e milfoil e quintefoille, herbe Johan, pelueite, moleyne, ache, la menue consoude, celidone, le coperun de la runce tendre, le coperun de l'aube espine, la foille de lorer, foille de egremoyne, medewrt, osmunde, coperun de seu, pigle, sanicle, bugle, rouge cholet, thaneseie, la foille de chevrefoille, herbe Water, tormentine, yere terrestre, trifoille, sparge, creppe malve, fenoil, lovasche: totes ces herbes a ouele [f.3r] mesure, fors ke de foille de lorer eit autretant cum des autres quatre herbes.[14] Ices herbes seient tuz batuz ensemble. Puis mellez totes ces herbes od blanc saim freis. Cil fetes boiller a un boillun sanz plus. Puis sil metez en un beau vessel. Si lessez ester .iiii. jurs. Al quint jur pernez beau saim e cyre seit le quart encuntre tote la gresse devant dite ceste. E pernez franc encens e matik e kode, peis resine, galbanum, oppoponac, almoniac: de totes ces gummes avant dites ouelement, fors ke de franc encens demie livre, de peis resine demie livre, de kode de Nortweie une livre. Ices choses seient tutes fundues ensemblement od le saim devant dit. Pus si pernez les herbes destempré, si les fetes quire ensem-

blement od les gummes a leisir e a petit feu. Pus les fetes preendre parmi un drap e mettre en boistes ou en autre vessel a garder. Ki vodra aguser cest oignement, si mette arubre e castor[ie?].

8. Oignement mult chaut encontre freide goute: Pernez sauge, lavendre, prim-erole, aloigne, naveldrote, ruge ortie, foille de lorer, gazere, avence, savine, rue, lovache, [f.3v] herbe Johan, mente, calamente, thime, oel peis de chescun; flur de geneite al peis de tuz les autres herbes; e quisez les herbes en un poi de vin e bure de may bien pure. E metez demie livre de oile de olyve e de noiz a tut. Quant les herbes sunt bien quites, que il eient un bon boillun, e si escume vent, si seit ostee. E de l'hure que il sunt mis a quire tote feez movez lé belement e puis colez lé parmi un drap. E quant il serrunt refreidiz e le fundiz osté, si il i point al funz, mettez les autrefez en une bele paele sur le feu e cyre virgine, solum ceo que il i a plus u meins, e franc encens triblé en poudre en meime la manere. E si il i ert poudre de gingivre od tut, si vaudra mult le meuz. E quant il serra quit un boillun e refreidi, metez le en sauf vessail e si durra en bone vertue plusurs a(i)nz.

9. Chaut oignement contre parlesye: Pernez sauge, lavendre, primerole, aloyne, na-veldrote, ruge ortie, foille de lorer, gazere, avence, oelement par peis de ches-cun. E si par aventure foille de lorer ne seit trové, pernez oille de lorer, que ne seit pas quit od les [f.4r] herbes, mes mis au derain od les especes. Puis si pernez ices herbes e triblez en un morter net. Puis si prendrez bon vin al peis de tuz ces herbes. E puis pernez bure de may meré e bien pure al peis del vin e de tuz les herbes e mettez ensemble a quire en une paele e quisez le od mesurable feu bien longement deske l'em quide ke le vin seit gasté. E puis prendre les parmi un poke de kanevaz e quant il serra refreidi, si il i a point de fundriz, ostez le, e puis pesez le par ame. Si il i a quatre livres, mettez poudre de gingevre treis unces e de baie de lorer bien triblé en poudre deus unces e atant de cyre virgine cum un oef de geline e tant de franc encens triblé en poudre. E remetez sur le feu entem-pree a prendre un boillun. E puis ostez le e movez belement quant il serra refrei-di, que l'em puisse suffrir le dei. Metez une unce e demi de castorie bien batuz, kar il ne suffreit pur la chalur de estre boilli. E puis movez le, que le castor[ie] seit medlee e puis quant il est refreidi, metez le en boistes que sunt encyrés e il serra le plus sauf pur lungement estuer. . . .

10. [f.4v] . . . [f.5r] . . .[15] Oignement encontre chaude goute emflé: Pernez jubarbe, morele, herbe yve, mathefelun, violette, plantayne, e friez les en bure de may bien pure. E puis fetes le preendre parmi un drap e puis mettre le en sauf liu.

11. Ad idem: Cuillez une bone partie de neirs lymachuns en les prees en tens de may. E puis les mettez sur une bele table e trenchez chescun d'un cotel en tra-vers le do(r)s un pou. E puis les poudrez bien de sel e les mettez ensemble en une poke de bon kanevaz e les pendez sus e mettez un vessel desuz e recevez ceo ke desgustera e de ceo oignez la chaude goute. . . .[16]

12. Pur goute enossé: Pernez [f.5v] lesches de pain de segle, si tostez bien al feu. Pus les plungez en fort ai[sy]lle et mel, si liez sur la goute par .iii. jurs. Pus per-nez jus de eble e vin par ouel peis e flur de segle. Puis le quisez bien deske il seit espés. Si metez desure en un drap.

13. Autre: Emplez .ii. ruges oignons [17] de peivre e les envolupez en un drap e pus estupez moillez, si quisez en breses e puis les triblez od oille. Si metez sur la goute l'emplastre. . . .[18]

14. Pur goute des espaules: Oignez vous primes de miel. Pus pernez farine de feves e foille de iere e miel e medlez ensemble. Si vous oignez de ceo.

15. [f.6r] Ad idem: Pernez rue, si boillez en eysil e mettez si chaut cum vus poez suffrir sur la dolur.

16. Pur goute es rayns: Pernez rascine de ortye e centoyre e triblez ensemble e bevez le jus. E mult vaut a ceo ventoser e jarcer. Si ceo ne vaut, baigne sei .iii. foiz ou .iiii. en eble.

17. Uncore pur goute es espaules: Pernez savine e verveyne e flur de feves e quisez en fort vin. Pus medlez a ceo oint de veir. E de ceo oignez la dolur.

18. Autre:[19]

>   Meinte foiz iceo avient
>   K'en aukun liu goute vous tient.
>   Querez un herbe en sa saison
>   Ke calketrappe ad a nun.
>   Triblez le bien e le jus pernez
>   E od blanc vin le destemprét
>   Ou od cervoise ke vin vaut,
>   Un maselin plein en beive chaut.
>   Pus prengne de segle farine,
>   Pestré soit od la mescine
>   Ou od jus de eblee soit pestri.
>   Pus freez ceo ke jeo vus di:
>   Deus turtels fere devez
>   E en la brese les quisez.
>   Quant serrunt quit, sil treez hors,
>   La croste desus hostez lors.
>   E le turtel al mal metez,
>   Tut issi chaut bien le tenez.
>   E quant cel turtel freit serra,
>   L'autre turtel si soit mis la.
>   Autrefoiz [f.6v] une pece aprés,
>   Si ne poez aver relés,
>   Querez ke eiez oint de tessun,
>   Ou de butor u de leun.
>   Si la goute oignez de cel oint,
>   La goute n'i remeindra point.
>   E ki vodra santé receivre,
>   Si devera polipodie beivre,
>   Betoyne en cervoise ou en vin,
>   E jun le bevez par matin.

19.

>   Ore vus aprendrum ensement [20]
>   A fere mult bon oignement.
>   Veil oint de veer e(n) bure e mel
>   E siu de buk, pus cyre e sel.
>   La ruge ortie e la sarree,

Cerfoil ewe[21] i seit gettee.
Le kersun ewage pernez
E od les autres la triblez.
Puis seient quit e bien colez,
Ceo vaut a meint enfermetez.

20.[22] Encontre dolur de la teste e des oils, oignement esprové: Pernez la flur de eglenter bone partie e la flur de rose e la flur de malve e la flur de gwymalve e de crespe malve e la semence de persil e de fenil oele partie; la flur de trifoil, la flur de chevrefoil, un poy de ysope vert, un poy de lavendre, un poy de cama- mille, ambroyse, reynette, eufrasye, la flur de consoude la grande, thyme, herbe Johan, une partie de puliol real e de l'autre pu[f.7r]liol. E quant avez ces herbes quilli od les flurs avant només, fetes les tribler bien en un morter. E puis i mettez bure une bone partie. Si mellez bien ensemble e lessez puis reposer en un vessail bien .xv. jurs, u meins si vus volez. E quant vus le volez purer, metét le outre le feu en un pot de terre ou en une paele. Si versez dedenz ewe rose bone partie, si vus le poez aver. Si le boillez bien ensemble une pose. E quant vus verrez qu'il soit assez, retreez aucune chose vostre feu, si ke vus le tiegnez en sa chaline d(r)eskes vus le eez bien prent parmi une pouke ke [est] fet de kanevaz. Si lessez ester dekes[23] il soit bien refreidi. E pus pernez le sus un autre jur, si ostez le fundriz, si metez derechief ultre le feu e le fetes boillir un poi. Si ostez l'escume e gardez que vus eez prest vostre cyre virgine bien fundue e bien escumé. E versez dedenz, si le mettez aval. E pernez vostre poudre de franc encens bien molu, si esparpelez desus e tutes fiez le fetes mover tresque il soit refreidi. E de cest oignement devez oindre les temples e les narilles un poi dedenz, e ceo si sovent cum vus avrez[24] mestier.

21. A la dolur de chef [f.7v] que longement dure: Pernez une poigne de rue e un autre de iere terestre e autretaunt de foilles de lorer e .ix. bays de lorer e quisez tut en vin u en ewe. E de ceo oignez le chief deske vus seez gari.

22. Item: Triblez bien ensemble feil de lievre e mel, tant de l'un cum de l'autre. Si oignez les temples.

23. Item: Destemprez ensemble averoygne e sauge e iere (de) terestre en ewe. Si donez le malade[25] a beivre.

24. Item: Triblez mel e rue e eysil ensemble, si fetes emplastre e metez sur le chef.

25. Item: Quisez les foilles de egremoyne od mel e metez cum emplastre sur le chef.

26. Item: Quisez celidoyne bien ov bure, si le colez parmi un drap e oygnez le chef. E puis quisez selidoyne en ewe e de cel ewe lavez le chef.

27. Item: Quisez en ewe camamille, betoyne e de cel jus lavez le chef e l'emplastre metez desure.

28. Item: Destemprez la foille de ere terestre od oleo[26] e od eysil e oygnez les narilles.

29. Item: Triblez les foilles de ere e de eysil e od le blanc de un oef e de ceo oignez le frunt.

30. Item: Pernez jus de fe[f.8r]nuil e de ru(i)e e de lovasche, peivre, od mel e od vin destempré e beyve jun.

31. Item: Fenuil, aloygne, quit en eysil, e de ceo lavez le chef e oygnez le frunt sovent.

32. Item: Triblez savine(z) od oleo [27] de ro[se] e de ceo oygnez le chef. . . . [28]

33. Item: Quisez puliol en eysil, si mettez as narilles que l'en sente le odur. E fetes une corune de cel puliol quit, si en corunez le chef.

34. Contra vertiginem capitis: Quisez en ewe pyoyne, cyremontayne, primerole, labrum veneris .i. vouthþistel seed [29] e un poy de cedewal. E seit menu [f.8v] batu e pus quit. E beive la [sic] matin e le seir teve une bone quantité.

35. Item: Pernez rue e ere terestre e triblez bien ensemble e pernez le jus. Pus mellez a ceo le aubon de l'eof. Pus de ceo fetes emplastre sur un drap lunge e quant la teste serra rese, mettez cel emplastre desure.

36. Item: Pur mangue de la teste: Triblez semence de ortie e mellez en vin e lavez le chef e frotez bien de savon. Pus pernez jus de kerson et mellez od grece de owe ou de chapun. E de ceo oignez sovent la teste.

37. Al teignus: Fetes le chef rere. Pus si le oignez de fel de tor e de eysil mellé bien ensemble. Pus pernez seu de tor e la tresse arse de aus e seit bien mellé od seel ars e od oylle. E de ceo oynez le chief. . . .

[f.9r] . . . [f.9v] . . . [f.10r] . . . [f.10v] . . . [f.11r] . . . [f.11v] . . . [f.12r] . . . [f.12v] . . . [f.13r] . . . [f.13v] . . . [30]

38.[31] Item: Pernez de orge e sel e mel ouelement e mellez od eysil. E de ceo frotez les dens. . . .

[f.14r] . . . [f.14v] . . . [32]

39.[33] Item: Veraie medicine pur maladie des orailles ou tut surt u survenue: Pernez en yver la racine de primerole u en esté les foilles e fetes jus de cel. E versez en les orailles e il orra bien aprés. . . .

40. [f.15r] . . . [f.15v] . . . [34] Pur femme pale fere colur aver: Face laver sun vis de ewe chaude e od savun, si la lest sechir. Pus si metez la roventele od la salive là ou ele vodra colur aver. E ceo durra par .iiii. jurs. . . . [35]

41. La ou chevelure [f.16r] faut: Pernez grant partie des ees ke funt le mel e ardez les en un pot novel. E mellez a ceo jus de cerfoil e noiz petites arses en poudre. E a ceo metez mel e oile e en facez oignement. E oignez la ou peil faut. . . .

42. [f.16v] . . . [f.17r] . . . [36] A la dolor del piz e encontre tuz les mals del quer: Triblez bien maroyl e ysope. Sil quisez bien en cervoise estale u en blanc vin. Sil bevez au seir. . . .

43. [f.17v] . . . [37] Pur la touse e destresse del piz: Bevez ysope, esclaré, centorie, maroil, puliol real, puliol montaine, verveine.

44. Pur la touse: Boilez bone cervoise en un vessel de quivre. Pus pernez feugere de chesne e violette e luvesche e puliol e jubarbe e seient ensemble boilliz en cele

cervoise. Pus le colez parmi un net drap e use ceo a beivre al matin freit e al seir chaut. . . .[38]

45. [P]ur eschaufesun del foie:[39]
> Bien vus dirray
> Que jeo l'orroie.
> De fenoil pernez hors le jus,
> De persil autant u plus,
> De letue tut ensement,
> De fumetere oelement.
> Le jus de ces quatre pernez
> E a lent feu bien les boillez.
> Parmi un drap pus bien les colez
> E le cler jus de ceo [f.18r] pernez.
> A ceo mettez u sucre u mel,
> Par tut gardez ke soit owel.
> Od ewe clere le devez temprer
> E puis le devez ausi user.

46. Autre: Pernez violette, frasere, cerlange, endivie, cycoree, coupere / .i. livre-wort[40] / medene(c)her, roses, la rasine de fenoil e de percil e liquoriz e lé quisez en ewe. E si il ne soit mie le chaut mal, metez un poi de ysope.

47. Medecine pur l'esplen: Pernez de centonicle, calamente, ermoyse, averoyne, rue, de chescune une poigne; semence de fenoil, persil, anis, de chescun un unce; licoriz .ii. unces; de mel .ii. livres. Quisez les herbes e les semences brisez en deus galuns de ewe treske la tierce partie seit gasté. E pernez de ceo un petit hanap plein, teve au matin e au vespre.

48. Autre: Pernez la racine de gledene e autretant de la racine de wymalve. Si lé debrisez bien menu. Si lé boillez bien en bure freis, si que la tierce partie seit gasté. E puis seit prent parmi un canevaz. E de cel oignement oignez le esplen .ii. fiez le jur u treis.

49. Ou en autre manere:[41] Friez la chose en bure e fetes emplastre. Si le metez teve sur le mal .ii. fiez le jur [f.18v] e coverez le de un tenve quir.

50. Autre: Pernez .i. livre de oylle de olyve e .i. de bon vinegre e boillez le deske le vinegre seit degasté. E oignez l'esplen sovent.

51. Autre: Pernez les racines de fenoil e de persil ouele porcion e kneþistel a la quantité de ces deus racines avant diz e de l'escorce de frene a la quantité des racines avant nomez[42] (nomez) e pur enducir le metez liquoriz suffisaument e donez vostre pacient a beivre, al matin freit, al vespre chaut.

52. Autre: Face sei seigner de kevil del pee dedenz e si se seit de chauz humurs, face sei seigner de le main senestre entre le petit dei e l'autre. . . .

53. [f.19r] . . . Encontre ceo ke home vomist e ne pot retenir sa viande: Pernez les deus parties del jus de fenoil e la tierce de mel e quisez deske il seit (seit) mult bien espés. E de ceo usez al seir e al matin. Si vus vaudra mult a l'esplen e al pomun e ostera la glette e la vomite del quer.

54. Ad idem: Pernez puliol real e maroil e peivre e quisez ben en ewe e metez du mel bone partie. Si le fetes beivre de ceo sovent. . . .[44]

55. A fere vomite: Pernez .v. eschales de oefs pleins de jus de ieble e .iii. de beau saim de porc freis e .l. greins de peivre e une bone ra[f.19v]cine ou deus de gingivre. Triblez en menu pudre. Puis quisez tut ceo ensemble e le usez bien chaut.

56. Autre legiere: Pernez l'entrures[45] de seu e le raez del seu de un cotel. Si vus volez vomer, raez le en contremont. Si vus volez aver bone solucion, raez le en valant e le bevez od ewe chaude. . . .

57. [f.20r] . . .[46] Pur esquinancie e pur aposteme: Triblez bien la brune ameroke en vin u en bone cervoyse u en ewe. Si donez al malade a beivre, si garra bien tost. . . .

58. [f.20v] . . . [f.21r] . . .[47] A garir home que est enpoysuné: Quisez lait de chevre jeske a la tierce partie od la semence de chanvette e le bevez .iii. jurs en jun. Suz ciel n'i ad si bone medecine for triacle. . . .

59. [f.21v] . . .[48] Ad idem: Pernez laureole e les baees de lorer e claree e quisez tut ensemble en ewe e donez le malade a beivre.

60. Ad idem: Pernez la semence de lin e la quisez bien en ewe. E pus pernez la semence, si la friez bien [en] seim de porc, si le donez a manger. . . .[49]

61. Ad idem:
> Ore vus dirrai [a] droiture
> Ke revaut mult a costiveure.
> Aloigne en cervoise boillez,
> Cervoise forte, egre e vieuz.
> Si mette od tut e mel e bure.
> De eble pernez a droiture,
> En un morter ceo bien triblez,
> Le jus pernez e bien colez.
> Treis escales d'eofs pleins de jus,
> Une de saim e [f.22r] nient plus.
> Quant bien iert quit e escumé,
> Beive le, si avera santé.
> Pernez cler lard, si l'entaillez,[50]
> Un long lardun ja n'i faillez.
> De mel l'oignez bel e gent,
> Pus soit poudré d'arrement.
> Tut environ bien le pudrez
> E el fundement le metez
> E iloques le lessez tant,
> Ke ceo remett[r]e avient.

62. Item: Pernez grundeswilie, fenoil, karewy, ache, saxifrage, de chescune une poigne. E quisez tutes ces choses en .ii. galuns de ewe, si que la terce part seit quit einz. E moillez un linge drap duble en l'ewe chaude si quite e metez sovent sur le ventre al costivé. Quant il (il) est mult sek, le moillez autre foiz en la avant dit ewe chaude e seles avera.

63. Autre: Pernez d'eble la racine e destemprez en un hanape de mek de vache e beive le malade deske il soit soluble. . . .

64. [f.22v] . . .[51] Pur verms as enfanz:
> Ore voil aprendre as enfanz

Pur verms dunt il nurisent tanz.
Pernez kersun, si me triblez,
E l'enplastre a l'umblil metez.
Milfoil bevez, quant ceo iert fet,
Ke seit destempré od duz let.
E la norice le receive
E od ceo la centoyre beive.
Les verms s'en istrunt finement
E l'enfant garra sanement.
. . .

65. **[f.23r]** . . .[52] Ad idem: Pernez un pot novel de terre, si emplez le de flur de furment. Si le metez en un furn, si quisez le tant cum le pain. Si covrez le pot de une tuile. Pus le pernez hors del pot **[f.23v]**, si le braez en un morter, si le destemprez od let de chevre u de vache. Si en fetes papelotes. Si donez al malade a manger. E cel estanche menesun. . . .[53]

66. Ad idem:

Perche de cerf en feu ardét
E pus en poudre tut batez.
Mult le fetes bien boleter
Ou parmi un drap bien passer.
La pudre iert bele e deliee
E blanche come neif que est negee.
Metez en vostre aumenere,
Vus la devez avoir mult chiere,
Kar en plusurs enfermetez
Vaudra, si vus a droit l'usez.
Al premer morsel le jur
Vostre pudre metez desur.
Ausi come seel poudrez desure
E puis mangez sanz demure.
Ceo valt pur fi e pur cursun
E si valt mult a menesun.

67. Autre:

L'arestebeof en champ querrez,
Triblez bien e la quisez.
Puis la versez en une gate,
Ses pees i mette li malade.
Par tant que dedens les tendra,
Talent de ceo ne li prendra.

68.

Uncore vus dyrrai un autre bele:
Il deit beivre la pelusele
Od let u od ruge vin fort.
Ceo garist meint ho**[f.24r]**me de mort.

69. Autre:

Pernez la grace venesun
E le sanc de gras motun
E seit od la grece bien fet.
Si garra bien – mar s'en esmait!

70. Item:

> Pernez le frés formage
> Bel e bien fait que soit de vache,
> En eysil le facez boillir:
> Si en mangue que volt garir.

71. Item: Pernez trestuz les os de la teste del luz, si les ardez e en fetes de ceo pudre e metez de ceo dedens un oef,[54] si le donez a manger. . . .[55]

72. Si vus volez saver si home que ad forte menesun puisse garir un nun: Donez li a manger un dener pesant de la semence de kersuns de cortil par .iii. jurs, ceo fet asaver le premer jur un dener pesant, e beive aprés un tret de vin teve. Si le face il par .iii. jurs e nent plus. E si ceo lui vaut, si garra; si nun, murra.

73. Contre dolur del ventre: Boillez betoyne en vin bien e a ceo mellez mel e bevez de ceo bone partie quant vus irrez cocher, ou beive al matin centorie boillé en vin. . . .

74. [f.24v] . . .[56] Pur emeraudes abatre ke emflent pur destresce de menesun: Pernez de la mie de gastel e autretant des moeaus des eofs durs e les destemprés od le jus de plantaine e metez sur le mal. E bevez chescun jur jun le jus de milfoil deske vus seez gari. . . .[57]

75. Al fundement que ist hors e ne poet entrer: Triblez mult bien l'amaroke e donez al malade le jus a(l) beivre. E fetes emplastre de ceo meimes. Si metez al mal. . . .

76. [f.25r] . . .[58] Item ad idem:

> Ky ad pere en la vescye,
> Ceo est mult forte maladie.
> Quant il estale, meintenant
> Desus vait come lait flotant.
> Le penil luy emfle e dout,
> Ne peot pisser quant il vout.
> Fort mal i ad e mult est [f.25v] revre,
> Car trembler fet home cum fevre.
> Le manger pert e si languist,
> Ne peot dormir e si vomist.
> A ceo me pernez le gromil,
> La ruge ortie e persil,
> Semence de fenoil e peivre,
> E de ceo lui frez un beivre.
> Tut ceo deit estre en vin boilli,
> Mes une poudre metez i.
> La pel de levre me pernez,
> En un neof [pot] tut l'ardez.
> Ensemble le metez boillir:
> Ky le usera si peot garrir.

77.

> Unquore vus dirrai une fine:
> De raiz pernez la racine,
> Od un cotel bien la parez,
> En roeles le decoupez
> Tant que il i eit .lix.

En un hanap blanc e tut neof
Metez les ens e mel assez,
E de ceo vus desjunez
Par .ix. jurs, cum jeo vus dirray
E si cum jeo deviserai.
Al premer jur .ix. mangez,
L'endemayn .viii. bien le poez,
Puis .vii., pus .vi., pus .v., pus .iiii.,
Issi les devez vus abatre,
Chescun jur amenuser
E si en descreissant user.
Al .ix. jur serrez gari
Quant tut ceo averez acumpli.

78.[59] Ad idem: Donez al malade a beivre la tere des niz des arundes od ewe chaude. . . .

79. **[f.26r]** . . .[60] Ad idem:

Des cerises pernez les peres,
Hom les deit tenir mult chieres.
En un morter bien les triblez,
En ewe beneite i ajustez.
Ky en Deu creance avera,
Sachez ke de cel mal garra.

80. Ad idem:

Home que ad mal en la vessie
Ke estaler ne puisse mie,
De l'ewe prenge la favee
[f.26v] E seit od la mente triblee.
Od vin blanc la destemprez
E od chaud ewe la bevez.
Uncore pernez le comin
E bevez plain hanap de vin.

81. A cels que pissent sanc:

Plusurs medecines valent
A cels que le sanc estalent.
La woderove du boys
Poez coillir a vostre chois.
Bevez en chaut, ceo est la fin,
En bone cervoise u en vin.
. . .[61]

82. Ky ne peot tenir sun estal:

A meint home issi avint
Ke sun estal pas ne retient.
Ungle de **[f.27r]** porc a ceo pernez,
En feu tut en pudre ardez.
Le pudre metez en sa viande,
Ceo vout fisike e comande.
. . .[62]

83. Item: Si la verge seit eschaudé a femme, prenge fiente de owe, si le frie en bure de may ou en freche bure e puis le face colir parmi un drap. Puis oignez le liu

de une penne e il garra pur veir. Ou leve sun membre de sa premere date aprés que il avera fet sa folie e doute n'avera. . . .[63]

84. Pur tuz vices del menbre: Pernez milfoille, parele, chenlange [f.27v], si triblez od seu de motun. Si le eschaufez en une paele, si le metez en un linge drap e le metez environ le menbre tedve. Si garra tost. . . .[64]

85. Ad idem: Pernez rose, violette, flurs de chevrefoil, meydeneher, honisoccle, anete, mauve, wilde tesel, e fetes un emplastre e metez i. . . .

86. [f.28r] . . . [f.28v] . . . [f.29r] . . .[65] Item: Si femme ad maladie as mameles, donez lui treys jurs a beyvre en ewe benette[66] treys verms que l'em apele en engleis angeltwaches. Si garra.

87.
> Chenulé bien triblé od vin
> Socurt a la mamele en fin.

88. Pur mameles enflez: Quisez wymalve en ewe e pus triblez le od seim freiz de porc e de ceo fetes emplastre e metez i. . . .

89. [f.29v] . . .[67]
> Quant let a norice faut,
> Un beivre face que mult vaut.
> Prenge fenoil e la rue,
> Prenge euruque, prenge letue.
> La bele flur de l'aube espine
> Mettre devez a la mescine.
> Ki cest beivre use e fet,
> Mult grant plenté avera de leet. . . .

90. [f.30r] . . .[68] Pur femme ke travaille de enfant e prestre ou clerc i seit: Lise cest bref .iii. fez desus sa teste e pus le mette la femme en sun sein e le tienge desuz sun umblil [f.30v] encontre sun ventre e tost enfantera e sun enfant ne morra ne cele ne perira. '+ In nomine Patris et Filii et Spiritus Sancti, Amen. + Anna peperit Mariam, Elizabet peperit Johannem Baptistam, Maria peperit dominum nostrum Jhesum Christum sine sorde et absque dolore. In nomine illius precibus et meritis sancte Marie virginis et Sancti Johannis Baptiste exi, infans, sive sis masculus sive femina, de utero matris tue absque morte tui et illius, Amen.' Pater Noster .iii., Ave Maria .iii.

91. Autre: Donez li a beivre ditayne ou donez li a beivre ysope od ewe chaude e enfantera sanz peril, mes ke i seit mort ou porri dedenz luy.

91a. Pur dolur de enfanter: Quisez ortie en vin, si le donez a beivre.

92. Femme que est malmise a enfanter: Roses en vin beive le matin e le seir jeske ele seit garie. . . .

93. [f.31r] . . .[69] A femme que a dolur [f.31v] fet sa urine: Cervoille e alisandre e persil e luvesche e fenoil e ache e burnette e grumil quisez ensemble en vin blanc e bevez le matin e le seir jeske vus seez garie. . . .

94. [f.32r] . . .[70] Autre: Pernez la rascure de yvoyre e triblez le oveke la racine de parele e od farine de furment bien boletté e od un poi de safran. E puis si fetes

de ceo petites pelotes e quant li malades les deverat user, quisez .iii. sur le carbun e le donez a manger. Issi le facez .ix. jurs e chescun jur .iii. jun.

95. Pur jauniz dedens u dehors: Pernez savine e pioyne, luvesche, ache, rue, celidoine, plain poin de sauge, andra, origanum, ysope, ouelement. Si les triblez
ensemble e quisez en estale cervoise de furment. Si le bevez al matin freit e al
seir chaud, e ceo fetes tote la quinseyne.

96. Pur le feie malade e pur jauniz: Bevez recoupé sovent, si garrez. Esprové chose
est. . . .

97. [f.32v] . . .⁷¹ Ad idem: Pernez la morele, si le lessez boillir en sa grece demeine e metez sur le felun ausi chaut cum il purra suffrir. E pernez avence,
valeriane e centorie e les boillez en ewe deske a la meité. Si le donez a beivre.

98. Ad idem: Bevez mathefelun. Pus ardez l'eschale de un oef e mellez cele
poudre od [f.33r] cel herbe. Pus pernez ache e persil e boillez ensemble en
vin u en bone cervoise. E ceo bevez al soir e al matin.

99. Quant felun est depescé: Pernez jus de lancelé e de menue ache e mel e le
aubun de l'oef e flur de furment. Si metez sur le mal.

100. Pur le felun: Fetes emplastre del moel de l'oef e de seel e quant il iert depescé,
fetes emplastre de jus de ache e de herbe Robert e de mel e de flur de furment
u de orge deske le mal seit mort. E pus le sanez od oinement cum autre plaie.

101. Pur totes maneres des feluns: Pernez la racine u le grein de argentille u de
l'ame(s)ruske u des tutes treis. Si li donez a beivre. . . .

102. [f.33v] . . .⁷² Pur tuer felun: Nim merch ⁊ wiflef ⁊ bruswort ⁊ spirgras ⁊ ribbewort ⁊ weibrode ⁊ þe vouueþistel ⁊ mathefelun ⁊ confirie ⁊ atterloþeberien
ant soech am in watre. ⁊ do þerto þree croppes of þe rede caul ⁊ þroe of⁷³ þe
rede brer. ⁊ num mest of þe merch ⁊ nim buttre of may ⁊ schepes-smere ⁊ recheles ⁊ huni ⁊ swines-smere ⁊ clene whetene flur. ⁊ 3ef þe salve bith
muchel, num two ayren ⁊ 3ef habith lutel, nim on ey. . . .

103. [f.34r] . . . [f.34v] . . . [f.35r] . . .⁷⁴ Ad idem: Pernez le pudre de franc encens e vinegre fort e medlez ensemble, que il seit ausi espés cum un coliz.
Puis moillez une nette cinse en sele bature e metez sur le mal, matin e tard. E
pernez .ii. poignez de [f.35v] egremoine e quisez en .ii. galuns de eawe, si que
la tierce partie seit quit einz. E beive le malade matin e tard.

104. Autre: Pernez la racine de hermodacle bien lavez e secchez e batuz en pudre e
metez le en mel bien boilli e escumé e metez cest emplastre bien espés al mal,
matin e tard. E quant vus hostez l'emplastre, metez i de memes icel pudre
avant nomé.

105. Autre: Parboillez bolaces un poy, si que vus puissez oster nettement la pel que
nient ne remayne. E pernez dunc nettement tute la sustance des bolaces e
pus friez cele sustance en mel que il seit si espés cum past. E metez sur le mal
cum en liu d'emplastre .ii. feez le jur, al matin e al seir. E avant que vus facét
ces choses, lavez le od date u od vinegre.

106. Pur festre chancré: ⁷⁵ Pernez flur de segle e le pestrez en mel si que le past seit

dur. E pus en fetes petiz turtels e metez as pertuz. E quant il sunt bien moillez, metez autres.

107. Quant festre comence: Pernez farine de orge e le jus de wilde tesle e fetes un emplastre e metez i.

108. Pur festre; Pernez warence, avence, semence u la foille de chanvre, ruge cholet, herbe Robert, herbe Water, egremoine, ambrosie, le [f.36r] tend-run [76] de runce, seient boillé en vin e diz jurs ne bevez nul autre chose. E si ceo ne valt, pernez franc encens e triblez le e metez le desur la plaie .iii. jurs. E autre .iii. jurs pernez vinegre e jus de plantaine autant e franc encens e fetes emplastre e metez desure.

109. Encuntre goute e festre beivre esprové: Pernez bugle, sanicle, herbe Johan, herbe Robert, herbe Water, mel, avence, sparge, pelusette, plantaine, phil-ago, paritarie, de totes ces herbes oele partie. Si les fetes tribler e quire en bon vin u en bone cervoise deske a la meité. Si lui donez al matin e al seir teve. E de memes cel beivre lavez les plaies chescun jur e quant vus verrez que la maladie seit bien esmundé de la quiture, dunc purrez estoper les plaies od la pudre de mastik. Meis toteveis usera sun beivre deske il seit sein.

110. Autre pur goute festre: Pernez avence, herbe Robert, sparge, paritarie, si fetes tribler en un morter e preendre le jus parmi un drap sanz autre liquor for le pur jus tut creu e donez lui a beivre. E perne[z] la drache de ces herbes, si liez sur le mal e issi fetes chescun jur. Mes toteveis quant vus ostez la drache (es-mundez la drache) esmundez les plaies de une [f.36v] penne nettement. E pus metez autre, car chescun jur sun beivre deit estre renovelé e la drache mis sur la plaie. Cest est bon a povere gent.

111. Pur festre medecine verraie: Pernez crowesope, moleine, avence, planteine, herbe Robert. Totes ses herbes quisez en ewe u en vin e donez al malade a beivre e metez la drache sur le mal.

112. Item: Pernez avence, cerlange, egremoine, ambrosie. Bien triblez e quisez en bon vin u en cerveise clere e bevez sovent e metez ces herbes issi quites [77] sur le mal.

113. Autre: Pernez avence, herbe Robert, sparge, chanvette,[78] warance, saxefrage, peluette, de chescun oele partie. E si vus avez une livre de tuz les herbes, metez a tut un galun d'eawe e quisez le od petit fu. E quant la terce partie seit wasté, metez le jus e bevez le al seir e al matin. . . .

114. [f.37r] . . . [79][f.37v] Autre: Pernez le oef que est failli desuz la geline quant ele cuve, si le depescez e moillez dedenz les estoupes des linz e metez sur le cancre e tost le oscira.

115. Item: Pernez mel e feil de chevre e triblez bien ensemble e oignez le cancre, si le sanerat.

116. Medecine esprové pur cancre: Pernez orevale e plantaine e braiez le bien od sel. Si metez a la plaie. Ou pernez freidele e metez al cancre, si garra.

117. Autre: Orpiement, sel ars, vive chauz, corn de tor, os de hume, de chescun

oelement pudre, e metez a la plaie. Puis fetes emplastre de ache e de celidoine e de mel e de flur de segle e metez desus l'autre.

118. Autre: Pernez arrement e corn de cerf e neire feves e trace de ail. Si ardez
chescun par sei. Si pernez des pudres de chescun oel, sil medlez ensemble.
Pus sil metez al mal jeske il seit afundré.

119. Autre: Pernez menu pudre de tan un unce e le pudre de tartaro .i. fece vini
demi unce e medlez le ensemble e metez de cest pudre sur le mal.

120. Pur tuer cancre: Nim boef of[80] þre ʒer old ant a cherne ⁊ scolen of garlec ⁊
grund yvi ⁊ ribwort ⁊ tan dust ⁊ huni ⁊ a schelle [f.38r] ful of salt ⁊ do hit in
to þe fur þat þe schelle beo ibarnt ⁊ do þe salt to þe beof. . . .

121. [f. 38v] . . .[81] A garrir totes maneres des plaies par beivre: Pernez la racine de
warence e le croup de cholet vermail e le croup de ortie vermail e le croup de
taneseye e le croup de chanvre e le croup de runce vermail et ambroise,
avence, bugle, sanicle, e veez que ceo seit fait el moys de may. Pus peisez les
en une balance que chescun seit oel. Pus veez que la warance peise contre tuz
les autres. Pus les triblez mult menu en un morter mult net. E pus si en fetes
menuz pelotes de ces herbes al grandur de une noiz. E pus les metez sur un
bord a secchir, que vent ne solail n'i avienge. E a celui qui est plaié durrez
une pelote al matin e un autre al seir od vin u od [f.39r] cervoise. Si serra lié
a la plaie une foille de cholet vermail sanz plus. E veez que la plaie seit chescun jur lavee de la date le pacient. E la foille de cholet seit chescun jur renovelé, si garra bien e tost. . . .[82]

122. Pur tolir anguisse de fresche plaie: Pernez aloigne e linoys oel porciun. Si les
fetes bien tribler e quire en gresse de porc madle. Si metez a la plaie, si chaut
cum il le poet suffrir.

123. Pur oster anguisse de plaie: Pernez mel bien boilli e escumez e flur de furment
e vin. Si fetes une bone bature, si les fetes bien boillir, si metez a la plaie
chaut.

124. Pur overir plaie que est sursané: Pernez de savun e de vive chauz e mellez ensemble e metez desure e liez le ferm. L'endemain triblez aloigne od oint de
porc, si metez desure [f.39v] deske ele seit chei. E si la plaie est parfunde,
metez une tente de verte grece. E pus si metez entrete, si garra bien.

125. Pur trere menuz os hors de plaie: Ardez les lung verms de terre, si metez mel a
cele poudre, si metez sure, si garra.

126. Autre: Metez sur le mal fente de chievre pestrie od vin, si garraz bien.

127. A garir os brisé: Pernez le jus de ache e le moel de l'oef e farine de furment e
bure pur. Si fetes meller ces choses ensemble e estendez un drap ke voit deus
feez entur le menbre depescé. Si metez l'enplastre desus e envolupez entur la
blessure. E pus moillez un drap en le blanc de l'oef par desus. Pus si metez un
feutre ke se joigne outre tut cest. Pus si le enplentez mult mainement, ne trop
ferm ne trop lache. A chief de .vii. jurs seit l'emplastre renovelé en memes la
manere.

128. Autre: Pernez .ii. parties de farine de segle e la terce partie de vive chauz e

mellez od l'aubun de l'oef e fetes emplastre, si metez sur le mal. E si beive chescun jur le jus de consoude, confirie, osmunde, si garra.

129. A home debrusee: Pernez bugle, confirie, sanicle, lavendre, taneseie, osmunde, consoude, avence, betoyne. Si les quisét en bone cervoise e usez le beivre.

130. [f.40r] Pur nerfs coupeez:
> A home que ad coupé les nerfs
> De la tere pernez les gros verms,
> Les facez laver e esquaser
> E pus a la plaie lier.
>
> [Por os plaié]
> Si os seit remis en la playe
> E n'i eit home ke l'entraye
> Ou fer u fust que dedenz seit
> Ke home nel sent ne l'en veit,
> De ditayne deit beyvre le jus
> E le pastel lier desus.
> La viole en eawe quite,
> C'est un herbe bone e eslite.
> Sus les pez metez le pastel,
> Sin istra hors os u quarel.
> . . .

131. [f.40v] . . .[83] Item: Triblez cerfoil .i. tunfille e donez al pacient a beivre. E si il retient, il garra; e si il le vomit, il murra. . . .

132. [f.41r] . . . [f.41v] . . .[84] As genoilz enflez: Quisez rue en mel e fetes de ceo emplastre e metez a tot.

133. Autre: Pernez wimalve e parele que crest en ewe e de ceo emplastrez les genuls.

134. Contre enflure des pees par cheminer: Pernez siu e auz e mellez ensemble e de ceo vus oignez.

135. A rancle: Pernez semence de lin e flur de orge e boillez en vin u en eisil. E pus mellez a ceo siu de moton e de ceo oignez le mal e si le garist e felun ausi.

136. Autre: Quisez bien lynois e a ceo mellez let de chevre e feves triblez e siu de moton e oignez de ceo le mal.

137. Pur abatre rancle: Pernez la racine de wimalve, la racine de liz, la racine de eble, le croup de aloigne, lynois, jubarbe, morele la petite, la racine de brionie e menu ache. E pernez de chescun oel porciun e pus si le fetes bien tribler e pus si le fetes frire en gresse de porc madle. E quant il serra bien quit, si le fetes coler parmi un drap a une [f.42r] livre de l'oignement. Metez un demi quarterun de cyre pur endurcir le.

138. Pur brusure e morsure de chien, cheval, e pur rancle: Pernez lemeke e lynois e chikenemete, senesun, aloigne, oel porciun de chescun e fetes le frire en gresse de porc madle u en oille de olyve. Pus si le metez ausi chaud cum il le poet suffrir.

139. Pur enflure des chambes e de peez: Pernez le ruge kersun, sil mincez menu, sil metez en un pot od espesse lie de vin e ové bran de forment e ové siu de moton e quisez ensemble deske il seit bien espés. E pus pernez un drap que puisse coverir l'emflure, si liez ové l'emplastre si que il seit entur l'emflure. Si le lessez estre tote une nuith, si garra.

140. Pur rancle oscire medecine vrai: Pernez la mie de pain de furment od ewe e od gleire de l'oef e triblez tut ensemble e metez desure. . . .

141. **[f.42v]** . . .[85] Pur aswager dolur des nerfs coment qu'il seient blescez: Pernez .ii. poignez des foilles de aube prunere e de violette e de malves e une poigne de aloigne e demie livre de wymalve e de la semence de lin sotilement fet en poudre une partie e seit fet un emplastre de ceo en la manere avant dite, e si n'i ad let prest, seit quit en ewe. Icest emplastre vaut a enswager dolur de chescune plaie e de chescun nerf blescee. Mes quant a la plaie deit om mettre le aubun de l'oef primes sus la plaie e pus le emplastre.

142. Pur aswager emflure e dolur de bras aprés seigné: Pernez .ii. poignez de foille[s] de aube prunere ou treis e bien les triblez a feor de sause e pus seint quit en let duce **[f.43r]** e seit ajusté semence de lin sotilement poudré e farine de forment menu deske il seit espés e un poi de sanc de porc frees e seit bien triblez ensemble e seit mis sur le emflure e a la dolur del braz. . . .

143. **[f.43v]** . . . **[f.44r]** . . . **[f.44v]** . . .[86] Pur haster clous e apostemes crever: Pernez columbine e brusez en eawe e le bevez le matin.

144. Pur apostemes durs fere ameurir: Pernez seneisun e oynt de chapun ou de veir e metez desus e incurira e depescera.

145. Ad idem: Esquassét de cees longs verms de la terre e metez a l'aposteme e le fra depescer. . . .

146. **[f.45r]**[87] A dertes en face ou aillurs: Orpiement, jus de parele, aloen e savun mellez e oignez. . . .

147. **[f.45v]** . . .[88] Pur dertre / .i. tertre / : Pernez arguil, si le fetez arder .ix. foiz, si que il soit ausi chaud come feu e chescune foiz le fetes estendre en vinegre. Pus le fetes braer en un morter de arrem ausi menu com vus poez e si le destemprez od le avant dit vinegre, ke il soit ausi tenve come coliz. Pus le versez ens une bage de canevaz e pendez cele bage sus e si metez desuz la bage un vessel de veire pur receivre le oyle ke degoutera de la **[f.46r]** bage e de cel oyle oignez là ou le dertre est. . . .[89]

148. A home que est ars od feu ou cors ou menbre ou visage: A ceo pernez saim de oes e od une penne de owe moillez de cel saim mult bien le arsun. Aprés ceo pernez wymalve e fetes mult bien[90] boiller, si secche com l'em purra en un pot net. Pus soit batu tant que soit mol e si chaud com l'en purra si le mette sur le arsun e iceste chose renovelez chescun jur tant que l'arsun soit requiree, e ki n'ad la grant malve, prenge la petite.

149. Pur eschaudeures: Quisez eble od tote la racine e pus emplastrez iloec.

150. **[f.46v]** . . .[91] Pur morsure de chien: Perne[z] ruge ortie e morele e lart creu e batez ensemble. Pus quisez ceo en bure e de ceo oignez la ou il est mors.

151. Pur morsure de chien enragé: Fetes bien forte sause de sel e de eawe, si vus n'avez sause de mer, e de ceo lavez mult bien la morsure. Pus pernez plantaine, agrimone e triblez ensemble. Pus mellez a ceo mel e aubun de l'eof e oignez de cel oignement. . . .[f.47r]

152. [f.47v] . . .⁹² Pur morsure de serpent: Fetes lier la plaie de .ii. pars bien estroit tantost de coreies de quir de cerf. E fendez en deus une vive geline u un vif cok e ausi chaud le metez sur la morsure. Pus beive dragante, morele e matefolon [sic]. . . .

153. [f.48r] . . .⁹³ A morsure de yrayne: Pernez grant masse de mosches e esquassez e de ceo oignez la morsure. Pus perne[z] foille de rays e fetes bien boillir e pus triblez e metez a la plaie. E ceo tendra la plaie overte. Pus pernez de cele meimes foilles e mellez od mel e metez sur la plaie. . . .⁹⁴

154. Ad idem: Triblez foille de malve e metez sur la pointure u le fente de vache chaude.

155. [f.48v] . . .⁹⁵ Ad restringendum sanguinem de naribus et undecumque effluat de vena: Scribantur hee litere in fronte pacientis in sanguine proprio: + a + g + l [f.49r] + a, et dicatur istud carmen: 'Nostre Dame sist sur un banc e tient sun cher fiz en sun devant. Veraie mere, verai enfant, verraye veine, tien ton sanc. El non de Jhesu te comant ke goute ne isse des ore en avant'. Et dicat paciens .iii. Pater [Noster] et .iii. Ave Maria cum eo qui carmen dixerit. Ter dicatur carmen. Nunquam deficiet.

156. Contra san[guinis] fluxum post munutionem [sic] . . . pur sanc [estancher]: Ardez une cince e la destemprez od vin egre e estanchera. . . .

157. [f.49v] . . .⁹⁶ Pur cyruns as oils: Pernez un oef chaut quit dur e le quassez menuement. Pus pernez un drap de lin blanc e metez as oils e de sus ceo metez le oef sur les cilles si chaut cum il le peot suffrir. E cels cyruns istront contre le chaut a l'oef. E escouez le drapel e vus les purrez oir croissir – ceo sunt cil cyrons ki manguent la char entur les oils e funt les oils verflez cum veer poez de meinte genz. . . .

158. [f.50r] . . . [f.50v] . . . [f.51r] . . .⁹⁷ A home ke pert la parole par maladie: Triblez puliol e viole e en beive le jus e lui verse on en l'oraille sotilment. Item a home ke pert la parole: Overez lui les dens d'un cotel e li donez aloes a beivre mellé od eawe e od pudre de pioyne.

159. Autre: Pernez un oef quit dur e le pelez, si lui fetes riere la teste entre le col e le haterel e pus li metez le oef eschaudant.

160. A celui que parole en dormant: Porte entur sun col croiz de meller ou eit escrit desus ceste chose: Jesus + Jesus + Jesus +. E beive al seir averoyne destempré od eysil.

161. Oignement pur bien dormir: Pernez la racine de mandrage e la semence de chenulé e de popi, si les triblez bien ensemble tut a pudre. Pus pernez gresse de porc e friez ensemble, si enoignez les temples quel hure que vodra dormir.

162. Autre: Pernez les foilles de popi e de chenulé, si en facét eawe com l'en fet eawe rose e oignez vos jambes e vos temples, si dormierét bien.

163. Autre: De morele bevez le jus e eschaufez l'emplastre, si liez entur le chief, si
     dormierét bien. Autre: Pernez mente e chenulé e le triblez bien od let [f.51v]
     de femme. E pus de ceo emplastrez vostre front e vos temples mult bien
     quant vus vodrez dormir. E mangez letues u metez a vostre viande oille de
     popi. . . .[98]

164. Ad idem: Pernez aloigne, anete, rue, livesche e runce e quisez en bone cer-
     voise e bevez le bien chaud.

165. Ad idem: Bevez le jus de puliol e de aloigne destempré en vin.

166. A doner talent a manger: Pernez centorie, si la quisét bien en cervoise. Pus la
     triblez bien, pus la remetez a quire en mesme la cervoise. Pus lé colez parmi
     un drap, pus metez une partie de mel, si quisez tut ensemble tant que il seit
     espés. Pus le metez en boistes, si donez al malade a manger chescun jur jeun
     .ii. quillerés deske il seit gari.

167. Si home reive e parole quant il dort: Donez li a beivre averoigne destempré
     en vin. . . .

168. [f.52r] . . . [f.52v] . . .[99] Encontre freide ydropesie: Pernez semence de fenil,
     de percil, de anise, karewi, gromil, saxifrage, alisandre, coriandre, livesche,
     mente, ache, gingivre, de chescun le peis de .v. deners, safran le peis de .vii.
     deners, liquoriz un unce. Si fetes pudre, si le usez sovent.

169. Item: Pernez racine de fenoil, percile, mente, avence, puliol, ermoyse, kersun
     de eawe, scabiouse, organie, herbe Johan, aloigne, capillus Veneris, cerlange,
     de chescun demi poigne, polipodie .i. quar[t], anise .i. unce. Seient quites en
     .iii. galuns de berzize ou en bone cervoise. Si les usez sovent. . . .

170. [f.53r] . . . [f.53v] . . . [f.54r] . . . [f.54v] . . . [f.55r] . . . [f.55v] . . .[100]
     A home que ad fevre ague
     C'est le retor quant on en sue.
     Il deit d'alisandre le jus beivre,
     Par tant purra l'on aparceivre,
     S'il sue bien, si deit garir,
     Si nun, fort li est le soffrir.
     Ke donques averoit eawe rose
     Iceo ly cerroit bone chose
     Laver les temples e son front,
     Les poins, les jointes cum il sunt,
     Pur la suur que l'en deit oster
     E lé porez desestoper.
     E face la suur issir
     Ke einz ne pout fors venir.
     Si prenge foille de peccher,
     Perer, pomer e ceriser,
     En eawe les fetes boillir
     E pus ses peez dedenz tenir.

171.
     Un emplastre lui revaldra
     Pur la grant chalur k'il a.
     Pernez plantein bien passé

E jubarbe e favee
E chenulé tut ensement
E morele oelement.
[f.56r] La flur od le jus destemprez,
Sur un drap linge le cochez,
Al destre part le devez mettre
Sur le faie, ceo dit la lettre.

172.

Puis le record de fevre ague
Ke la chalur aukes remue.
Si lui doine fumitere a beivre
Ke le mal chace e deceivre.
Ou qui le senechun bevera,
Ja en le mal ne recherra.
Ky li durra pus le retur
De consoude beive la flur.
Pus la suur, si beit aprés,
Al mal ne recherra il mees,
U la semence de parele,
Bien en garrit madle e femele.

173. A fevre terceine:

Bien sai que la fevre terceine
Malement plusurs demeine.
Bevez .iii. plantes de plantain
Devant l'accés, si serra sain,
Treis al matin e .iii. al seir,
Noef jurs s'il volt santé aveir.

174. A fevre cotidiane:

La cotidiane fevre
Mult est male e enrevre.
Pernez un oef ki seit mol quit,
Del blanc versez hors un petit.
Une femme veigne atant
Ke norisse madle enfant,
Treis goutes de lait i degoute,
Cele lui doint a humer tute.
Mes tant cointement le face
Ke li malade mot ne sace.

175. Charme pur chescune manere de fevre: Ki ke veut estre charmé deit prier la
charme par charité. E celui qui le deit charmer le deit demander quel jur il
veut estre gari. E il respundra 'le tierz jur' e il ne deportera a manger ne a
beivre par enchaison de la maladie. 'Beau Sire, le verrai cors de Vus seit honuré ausi verraiment com Vus estes [f.56v] Pere, Fiz e Seinz Esperiz, treis per-
sones e un Deu. Descendistes en la virgine Marie e pus suffristes mort pur nus
peccheurs e pus resuscitastes de mort en vie denz le tierz jur e descendistes en
enfern e preistes hors Adam par vostre grant valur, par vostre grant duçur,
par vostre grant beauté, par vostre grant humilité. Beau Sire, le verrai cors de
Vus seit honuré. Ausi veraiement donez santé a cest home .N. ou a ceste
femme .N.' E nomez le non e pus aprés covient dire .iii. Pater Noster e .iii.
Ave Maria, ke Deus lui doine santé.

176. Autre: 'Beau Sire Deu, jeo Vus pri e requer ke a tel jur .N. garisez vostre ser-
gant .N. de la fevre k'il ad e k'il mes ne l'eit ausi veraiement com Vus estes
rey pitiuus plain de misericorde, simple, duz e deboneire, sire e seignur de nus
tuz en le honurance de vus e de ma dame seinte Marie e de vostre beneite
croiz e del seint home ki cest charme fist e de tuz vos senz, amen. "Sint medicina tui pia mors et passio Christi, / Sint medicina tui vulnera quinque
Dei" '. Dicat paciens cotidiane quousque liberabitur .iii. Pater Noster e .iii.
Ave Maria. . . .

177. [f.57r] . . . [f.57v] . . . [f.58r] . . .[101] Encontre reume: Pernez ere terestre e un
poi de aloigne e de roses secches e de franc encens e fetes bien boillir en
eawe e receivez la fumee de l'eawe le seir la test covert de un drap. . . .

178. [f.58v] . . .[102] Pur glandre ke flote sà e là: Pernez le wilde nep, si le fetes tut
net e pus le trenchez en la manere de deners e fetes les quire en eawe. E pus
pernez un morter, si le triblez ben od siu de motun e friez les ensemble e
metez sur le glandre ausi chaud cum vus puissez suffrir deskes vus serrez garri.
. . .

[f.59r] . . .[103]

179. [104] A home que pert sun sen:
    Meint home en petit de tens
    Pert la memorie e le sens.
    Solsecle e averoigne pernez
    E la sauge pas ne obliez.
    Ces herbes li donez a beivre,
    Si purra sa santé receivre.
    Ki volt memorie recoverer
    A ceo lui covient dieter.
    Ces herbes dont ai dit desus
    Cinc jurs les beive u aukes plus,
    Quire deivent en bon vin
    Ains que il mangera seir e matin.[105]

180. [106] Pur engrassir: Pernez feniugrez e fetes secchir. Pus le triblez en poudre. A
ceo metez anise e mastik e mellez od bele flur de forment. E tut ceo destemprez od le jus de un herbe que est apelé affodillus e pestrisez ensemble en
guise de pain e le fetes ben levé. E ki a raison tiel pain use, il devendra mult
gras.

181. Pur enmegrir: Quisez bien fenil en eawe e bevez le eawe al seir e al matin.

182. Item:[107]
    Meschine que trop est grase
    Dont l'en poet trover grant masse,
    Prendre devez eble e maroil,
    Percil, ache e fenoil.
    En vin [f.59v] deivent bien boillir,
    Mel i metez pur endulcer.
    E quant ceo serra quit assez,
    Le beivre nettement bien colez.
    A jun le usez par matin,
    Ceo vus enmegrira enfin.

Notes on pp.373–78   *Glossary on pp.428–39*

> E si vus tendra en vigur
> E dorra mult bele colur.
> Si cest beivre usez sovent,
> Le cors averez mult biel e gent.

183. [108] Pur roigne: Triblez la racine de horsselle e de parele e friez les en grece de porc madle.

184. [109] Pur poisun, mal de flanc, e felun e pur totes subites maladies: Pernez espigornele, si le donez a manger u a beivre en jun.

185. [110] Pur mal de flanc: Pernez plaine poigne u plus d'entrerus de fresne e cerlange e la burnette e ceo quisez en vin u en cervoyse e le colez bien e bevez al sier e al matin.

186. [111] Pur verms en ventre: Quisez en eisil u en vin egre milfoille e comin ensemble e de ceo emplastrez le ventre sur le numbil si chaud com vus le poez suffrir e les verms s'en istrunt mors u vifs.

187. [112] Al maladie ke avient al menbre: Triblez primerole e mellez od viel oint frees e metez desus.

188. Autre esprove, tut fust la maladie encancré, e garist gute augere e enossé e meint autre mal: Quisez .xxx. oefs durs. Pus si ostez les aubuns e pernez les moels e les metez en une nette paele e les friez a petit feu. E pernez le oile que en istra e metez a cele maladie.

189. [113] A fere silotre; Pernez [f.60r] gumme de iere e orpiement e formiz esquassez e ceo mellez od eysil e de ceo lavez sovent là ou vus volez ke li peil chece.

190. [114] Encontre le fei eschaufé: Pernez violette, frasere, cerlange, endive, cycoree, coupere .i. livrewort, meideneher, roses, la racine de fenoil e de persil e liquoriz e le quisez en eawe e s'il ne soit mie le chaud mal, metez un poy de ysope. . . .[115]

191. [116] Pur mal des costes: Pernez le jus de jubarbe e farine de orge, si liez al coste. Ou pernez mathefelon e comin e let de femme e farine de segle u de orge e fetes de ceo emplastre, si metez as costez.

192. [117] Pur tecchelure oster del col: Pernez pudre de veire e lessive e lavez le liu sovent bien chaut.

193. [118] Pur la tuse e destresse de piz: Bevez ysope, esclaré, centorie, maroil, puliol real, puliol montain, verveine.

194. [119] A enfans ke trop plurent: Pernez la meule de la bise e oignez les temples.

195. [120] Pur vermes: Pernez la runce que porte les botuns, si la coupez bas a la tere e metez sur le feu e recevez ceo que degoute [f.60v] al chief e oignez les vermes là u il sunt.

196.[121]

> Ki enroés est sudeinement
> Pur chaud, pur fumee, pur vent:
> Les purreals face bien tribler,
> Preendre le jus e bien coler.

S'il volt que sa voiz lui esclaire,
Si en deit gargarisme faire. . . .[122]

197. Ad oculos:[123] Fenoil, verveine, rose, celidoine, rue; de ces poez fere eawe que rendra lumere as oils.

198. [124] Pur enbelir la face de saucefleume: Fetes eawe des flurs de feves com l'en fet eawe rose e lavez la face sovent.

199. [125] Pur grevance de la gorge: Pernez morele e senesçun .i. lashantonwort e arrement e jus de licoriz e quisez e bevez.

200. [126] Pur esclarsir la gorge: Pernez organie e jus de licoriz e quisez ensemble e bevez.

201. [127] Pur crouleure e gute as jambes: Pernez eble e alisandre, primerole, malve, cousloppe e quisez ensemble e lavez sovent les jambes. E pus pernez wymalve e quisez la racine e destemprez od l'eaue des avant dites herbes e fetes emplastre e liez a tut.

202. [128] Pur la kacie: Pernez arrement e mel e le aubun de l'oef [f.61r] e les triblez ensemble par oele quantité e metez l'emplastre sur les oilz. E si rien i eit de sanc u de malveise quiture, tut le entrerra.

203. As oilz ruges e enflez: Pernez fenil [. . .?] e triblez bien ensemble e treez le jus. E pus pernez le blanc de l'oef e medlez bien ensemble e si pernez lin, si moillez e al cochier le metez sur les oilz. . . .[129]

204. [130] Pur cengle: Pernez le sanc de un purcel tut chaud e emplastrez sur le mal e quant ceo iert refreidi, metez autre chaud. . . .

[f.61v] . . .[131]

205. Oignement popilion: Quant le popiler comence a burjoigner, fetes coiller les burjuns .x. livres pesant e fetes les ben tribler od oint de porc freis u bure de may. Pus pernez morele, plantaine, chenulé, violes, letues, les foilles de popi, jubarbe, bardane .i. [f.62r] clote, piloselle .i. musere, foilles de mandrage, coperun de runse, crase geline .i. smerewort, umblil as dames .i. peniwort, tuz les maneres de popi, mercurial, teste de soriz, veir kardun, copere, ana unces .v. Sil fetes tribler od veil oint de porc. Puis fetes pelotes, si lessét gisir .ix. jurs. Puis si pernez trestuz, si les metez en une paele od un galun de eysil. Sil fetes bien boillir que tut seit enbeu einz. Pus si versez en un sac de kanevaz, sil fetes preendre forment hors en un vessel, si le lessez issi(r) estre .iii. jurs. Pus pernez ceo que desus est, sil metez en boistes. Icest oignement est bon a tutes chaudes gutes que sunt e nomeement a agues pur oigdre lur temples e lur umbliz e les plantes e lur pouz. . . .

206. [f.62v] . . .[133] Fetes vus seigner le jur seint Lambert, si n'averez pas la gute chaive cel an ne parletik ne serrez. Meimes le tierz jur u le quart devant einz ceo que le meis se departe ki se fait seigner, il n'avera regard de fevre deske le .xi. jur de averel. Ki le .xi. jur de averil se fait seigner del braz senestre en cel an ne perdera pas sa veue. Ke se fait seigner le .xvii. jur de may del braz destre ne serra tormenté de nule manere de fevre en cel an. Ke en la fin de may le (le) quint u le quart derain jur se fait seigner de l'un braz u de l'autre, nule

fevre n'avera ne la veue ne perdera. Ke se fait seigner le .xvii. jur de marz del bra(r)z destre, il n'avera garde de nule manere de fevre cel an. Ki voldra user chescun jur .iii. foilles de sauge e un grein de pioyv[r]e, il n'avera garde de estre parletik ne de gute chaive tant com il le usera. . . .

[f.63r] . . . [f.63v] . . .[134]

207. [135] A saver si uone femme aime sun barun plus ke nul autre: Pernez un aimant, si metez desuz la teste la femme e si ele vus aime plus ke nul autre, tantost **[f.64r]** vus enbracera, e si ele aime autre plus que vus, ele s'en turnera de vus e dormant cherra hors de lit.

208. [136] Pur faire les chevoilz neirs que sunt chanus: Pernez la verte escorce de nogages, si les destemprez en lescive, ou ardét les en pudre, si en fetes lescive, e lavez les ch[e]voils .iii. feez u quatre. . . .

209. **[f.64v] . . .**[137] Pur enchacer musches:[138] Triblez verveine od eawe beneite e getez parmi la maison d'un wispelon e s'en irrunt.

210. [139] A home afolé par sorcerie u eit mangee cervele de esperver u de chat: Fetes lui manger .ii. ou .iii. huans blancs atirés en guise des gelines rosties. . . .[140]

211. [141] Pur fere voler feu gregeys e depescer le roule: Pernez salpeter le peis de .xvi. deners e carbun de sauz le peis de .iiii. deners maille e suffre le peis de .iii. deners maille. Quant il sunt pesez ouelement chescun **[f. 65r]** par sei, doncs metez les ensemble en un morter, si les braez mult bien. Pus pernez parchemin e pliez entur la corde e fetes issi vostre roule e sufflez le feu hors de ta bouche; + vitam [142] + sanctam + spontaneum + honorem + deo et patrie + liberationem. . . .

[f.65v] . . . [f.66r] . . . [f.66v] . . .[143]

212. [144] Oignement a freide gute: Pernez foille de lorer, savine, les noweus de pomme de pin, armoyse, fetes cestes choses batre en un morter e puis bien frire les en un paele bien lavee e soient friz en bure de maii e puis preiendre le parmi un net drap e receivre cel oignement.

213. Un autre oignement: Pernez le garz de l'owe, si c'est un home, e si c'est un[e] femme, pernez un owe, si le faites plumer e hoster lé entrailes e bien laver. E pus pernez virgine cire le peis de .v. deners e oint de chat sauvage e autretaunt de l'oint de tesson. De cels deus pernez bone partie e dous oignuns e pus les fetes batre en un morter e pus metez tut dedenz l'owe e si la faites costre par tuit ou il i a riens overt. Aprés ceo k'ele est mise sor l'espoi e quant ele est partuit cosue, si la metez al feu rostir e k'ele soit rosté **[f.67r]** tant come riens en voult degoter. E recevez en une bele vessele ceo que en curt de l'owe. Sachez ke c'est le meillur oignement que soit a froide gute. . . .[145]

214. Ceo est la charme a charmer cristiens de vermine e de neof maneres de goute e de goute festre e pur fevres issi ke nule viande ne nul beyvre n[e] lerra:[146] '+ In nomine Patris et Filii et Spiritus Sancti, amen. Ausi verrement come Deus fust e est(re), ausi verrement come ceo ke il fist bien fist, e ausi verrement cum kanke il dist bien dist, e ausi verrement come de la virgine char **[f.67v]**

prist, e ausi verrement cum en la croiz se mist, e ausi verrement cum en sun digne cors cinc playes suffrist, e ausi verrement cum en ambedeu pars de li furent deus leres penduz, e ausi verrement cum ses seins mainz e peez de clouz furent fichiz, e ausi verrement cum sun glorius chef fust des espines coroné, e ausi verrement cum sun seint sanc fust en la croyz espandu par laquele le enemi lié fu e vencu, e ausi cum en la croyz suffri mort humblement par laquele mort avum bapteme communement – ke ceo creit ert sauvé verre-ment – e ausi verrement cum sun seint cors en seinte sepulcre reposa e au tier jour resuscita e cum en enfern descendi e les portes brusa, e ausi verre-ment cum kant li plust au ciel monta e au destre sun pere reposa e cum il au jo(y)ur de juge vendra e checun en char e en sanc relevera e Nostre Sire ses cinc playes mustra e a sun pleysir jugera, ausi verrement cum ceo est veirs, gari seit .N. de goute, de rancle, de cancre, de vermine, e de totes maneres de fevres e de goute. Rancle mort seit, la goute rancle mort seit, le farcine mort seit e morciz de .N.' Puis dites [f.68r] treis Pater Nostres en le nun del Pere e del Fiz e del Seint Espiriz. E puis lessez lire ces quatre evvangelies: 'Rogabat Jhesum quidam Phariseus', 'Cum natus esset Jhesus in Bethleem', 'Recumben-tibus undecim disciplis', 'In principio erat verbum'.[147]

II.

[ff.79v–86v][148]

215. [f.82v] A *sorvenue medicine*: Pernez menu ache e flur de furment e l'aubun de l'of e triblez ensemble e metez sure.

216. Ad *febrem quartanam*: Pernez le jus de la launcelee taunt cum pot entrer en le escale de un of e de [f.83r] ceo humez .ix. jurs [e]n vin. . . .[149]

217. Contra *gutam calidam*: Pernez coypeus ou burjuns de popler la quantité en-cuntre tutes les herbes ke sunt a numer, ceo est a savoir morele, plauntaigne, jubarbe, sanicle, racyne de gletonere .i. clote, stoncrop, violette, herbe yve, mandrage. Cestes herbes seent triblez en seym de porc male ou en bure de may e gardez par .ix. jurs. Pus seint quites en vin egre e pressez parmy un canevaz.

218. Contra *frigidam guttam*: Pernez foile de lorer, savine, lavendre, sauge, rue, baye de ere, primerole la petite e la graunde, eble, herbe Jon, herbe Roberd, lo-vache, avence, alisaundre, wimauve, ceo est a saver pernez foile de lorer e de savine e de lavendre ouelement encuntre tutes les autres herbes, si les triblés en bure de may e gresse de thessun, si aver le porez, ou seym de porc male. Si seint gardez par .ix. jurs. Aprés seint quites en vin e pressez parmy un kane-vaz e a agucer [f.83v] cest oignement metez fens de columb e de castorie, si aver le poez. . . .[150]

219. Ungentum contra *plagas*: [f.84r] Pernez bugle, sanicle, erbe Walter, avence, pimpernele, ambrosie, tendruns de runce, waraunce, tanesy, kanvre, le tend-run del ruge cholet, milfoil, trifoil, quintfoil, matefelun, menu ache, herba munda .i. malva, columbine, orvale, pyluette. Cestes herbes primes seyent tri-

blez en bure de may et reposez par .ix. jurs e aprés quites en vin e al derein purement seit mis virgine cire e oylle de olive.

220. *Pulvis contra cancrum*: Pernez vive kauz ne mie esteinte de ewe e mel, si fetes past de ces deus choses e en fetes pelotes. Si les metez en un test quire al furn oveke payn taunt cum le payn. Pus si le fetes en pudre e pus fetes pudre de vere ben menu e de tan, de chescun ouelement, ceo est asaver del tan e del vere, si metez duble de la premere pudre ki est fet de mel e de vif kauz. Si en-rosez la playe de cele pudre ausi cum beu pudre(r) del seel. Si metez menuz es-tupes sure, si le lessez deskes il se leve nettement par sey. Si metez pus autre deske le malade seit seyn e la nuuef gresse ne oignement n'i tuche. . . .

221. [f.84v] . . .[151] *Pur la destresce del queor*: Pernez cerlaunge e sanicle e maroile, si triblez tut ensemble e le quisez en bure frés, si en usez.

222. *A l'espurgement de tus mals del piz medicine vereie e esprovee*: Quisez pruneles dé boys une partie et triblez ben ensemble en un morter e metez un fort vessel e pernez la serveyse quaunt ele est kolee, si le metez od les pruneles et metez en u[n] nof pot, si fetes en la terre une fosse e metez le pot ens, si le coverez ben e metez la terre sus e seit le pot illoc .ix. jurs e .ix. nuz. E pus pernez un poy en un hanap, si donez a beyvre al malade, le seir chaud e al matin freid. E ceo fetes sovent.

223. [f.85r] *A mal del queor ke fet ke home ne pot manger sa viande mes sunt cuntre queor*: Pernez centorie, si la quisez ben en serveise estale e quaunt ele serra bien quite, triblez la ben e pus la metez en un pot e la quisez ben. E pus si la colez parmi un drap, si la fetez boiler derechef dekes il seit mut espés e le metez pus en une bele boiste, si fetes le malade de ceo manger chescun jur .iii. cuillerés dekes il seit gariz.

224. *Ancuntre ceo ke home vomist e ne pot sa viaunde retenir*: Pernez les dous parties de jus de fenoyl e la terce de mel, si le quisez deskes il seit ben espés, si le beyve le malade al seyr e al matin e li vaudra mut a l'esplen e al pomun. Si li hostera la glette e le vomit.

225. *A home ki per[t] sa parole*: Pernez alun, si destemprez en ewe, si li versez en la buche, si parlera tost.

226. *Pur emflure e dolur del ventre*: Pernez dous kullerees de jus de quintfoil e de sauge, si li donez a humer.

227. *Encuntre costivesun*: Pernez la racine de polipodie ki crest sur la cheine, si raiez l'escorche d'un koutel e pernez les racines, si les fetes quire od char de porc ou od poucinz. E pus si donez le brué a humer e la char a manger, mes metez i comyn ou fenoyl ou anyse pur [f.85v] temprer la ventuosité.

228. *Encuntre menesun*: Pernez la char de motun, si en fetes mosseaus, e pus pernez la mente, si la triblez ben en ewe [. . .?] cel jus e dequisez la char en ewe od mel, si li donez tut a manger.

229. *Item*: Pernez milfoil, sil destemprez ke vus en eez le jus, e pernez flur de for-ment e fetes de la flur e del jus un turtel e quisez e[n] la brese, si mangez le ben chaud.

230. A *la menesun sanglaunte*: Pernez milfoil e plaungtayne e fraser, si eez autretaunt de l'un cum de l'autre, e destemprez ben ensemble. E quaunt vus vodrez, si le destemprez en vin e bevez .iii. foiz le seyr e .iii. foiz le matin, si
garrez.

231. As *feveres quartaynes*: Pernez le jus de artemese, si mellez od ewe teve, si en
oygnez .iii. jurs vostre cors, si garrez.

232. *Home ke ad la menesun, s'il garra ou nun*: Manjusce .iii. jurs le peys de .i. dener
de kersun ke crest en kurtil e beive aprés un tret de vin teve. S'il estaunche,
si garra; si nun, si morra.

233. *Home malade, s'il deit garir ou nun*: Pernez lard e oygne[z] les plauntes des péz e
aprés le gettez al chen. S'il le manjue, garra; si non, il morra.

234. *Encuntre ceo ke home ne pot pissir*: Bevez la terre del ni de arunde od ewe teve.

235. *Bon emplastre pur* [f.86r] *rauncle occire e tuz mauveis mals saner*: Pernez syu de
bof .i. livre e syu de motun .i. livre e de bure fundu .i. livre e .ii. livres de cire,
si le conficez, si entraét la liqur parmi un drap. Pus si pernez plain esquele de
racine de parele ben triblee e une poinee de ache e une de wimauve e une de
aloine. Si le triblez forment, si le quisez en la gresse od feu amiable saunz
flaumbe en une paele de arem ou en nof pot, si le colez parmi un drap, pus si
metez .i. livre de oynt de porc. Si eez aparilee .i. livre de resine blaunche e
demi livre de encens e demi livre de peyz. Fetes tut en pudre, si commovez e
conficez od les autres choses. Cest enplastre est mestre sur totes les autres pur
rauncle.

236. Pur mal de felun est bon le mol de suy u le frut. S'il est triblez e mis sur le mal
.iii. jurs, si est gariz.

237. *Item pur le felun*: Usez le jus de la morele e de cerlaunge e de amarosche e matefelun. Si oynez de la morele le mal.

238. *Encuntre dolur del chef e de gute des oyz*: Pernez vetoine e plauntaigne, ysope e
la racine de gletonere od vin triblé ensemble. Si li donez sovent a beivre, si
garra.

239. *A la tuce occire*: [f.86v] Lavez vostre piz de ewe freide le seyr, si eschaufez les
plauntes des pez e sovent versez l'ewe sur le piz, si bevez vetoine sovent.

240. Item encuntre sarre-piz: Pernez ruwe e averoine e maroil e vin e metez ensemble.[152]

III.

[ff.99r–106v][153]

241. [f.101r] Contra ficum et cancrum et felonem: Pernét tendruns de runces
noveleis e plantaine e chevereflur,[154] solsicle, orpi[ment], menu ache,
popeler. Fetes jus de cete[s] choses e destemperét ov(t) unt de porc male u ov
bure de may e meteis en boites e oinét le malade e lavét la maladye de vin
blanc sovent.

242. A destrure morte char: Fetes pudre de fevis nayris e de drap blu e de escales
de limasun e pernez la gra[f.101v]vele e de la ravre de toneus de vin. En tel
manere osterés vos la morte char. . . .[155]

IV.

[ff.106v–107v]

243. Ki ad perdue la oye par maladie ceo est la medicine a recoverir: Pernez date
de chevre e versez chaud en l'oraile e estopez od leyne nent lavee e lessez
tote nuit. E ceo fetes trei foiz, si garra.

244. A la tusse: Pernez oel peis de orpiment e de peyvre e de saffran. E triblez ben
ensemble e destemprez od mel e od veil vin, si donez a beyvre [en] jun teve.
Ceo sanera la tusse e curat [sic] le estomac e restorra la voiz.

245. Al mal de l'esplen: Pernez betoine e fens de columb e cephalea e oyle rosin e
la breve umbre de le umbre del petit liu e lange de cerf e plusur foiz ajustee
boillez ensemble.[156] Si li donez a beivre e ert garriz.

246. Al mal de la feye: Pernez la coste e rubarbe e fibra lini. Si lui donez a beivre,
si garra.

247. **[f.107r]** Pernez le escorse de freyne quit en vin, si le bevez deskes vus seez
seyn e aloyne quite en vin iceo memes fet. Aloyne e sauge quit en vin bevez
en jun chescun jur une mesure. Ceo sannera le esplen e la feye.

248. A gute podagre: Medlez le mol de l'of od mel e oynez les pez de ceo e pus envolupez de leyne suz trenché, si liez de une bende de linge drap e ceo tout la
dolur e la enflure. . . .[157]

249. Pur enflure ke hume ad en ses gambes ou en ses pez: Pernez la ruge kersun, si
la mincez menument, si le metez en un pot, e de espesse lies de vin e bren de
furment e suy de motun. Si le lessez quire ensemble taunt k'il seit ben espés.
Pus pernez un drap ke pusse coverir la enflure e metez la en[f.107v]plastre
sure e pus sus le mal deskes il seit gari.

250. Pur la dolur des denz: Pernez blaunc encenz e la gleyre de l'of, si le triblez ensemble e metez sur parchemin e metez cel sur la jowe seyne, si lessez estre
tote nuit, si garra.

251. A la voiz amender: Le jus de la mente e dragaunce tenez desuz vostre launge.

252. Pur fere home seyn dedenz le cors: Pernez le jus de eble e ausi gros cum demi
of de seym de porc, si metez en une paele, si fetez ben boillir, pus i metez le
jus dedenz e ke il seit teve e le beyve e li delivra.

Some Sources and Parallels

I give here a list of the receipts in MS Sloane 146 which also appear in the *Lettre d'Hippocrate* (= LH), the *Physique rimee* in MS Cambridge Trinity Coll. 0.1.20 (= PR) and in MS Cambridge Trinity Coll. 0.8.27 (= PRO). In the case of the *Physique rimee* the references are to the line numbers in my edition (ch.4) or to the St John's College, Cambridge MS in the Appendix [= PR(SJ)]

14.	PR(SJ) 29
15.	PR(SJ) 30
16.	PR(SJ) 31
17.	PR(SJ) 30
18.	PR 705 ff
19.	PR 743 ff
21.	LH 8
22.	LH 39
23.	LH ed. Södergård p.10
24.	LH ed. Södergård pp.10/11
25.	LH ed. Södergård p.11
26.	LH ed. Södergård p.11
28.	LH 17
29.	LH 18
30.	LH 19
31.	LH 20
33.	LH 7
35.	PR 97 ff
36.	PR 1923 ff
37.	PR 1679 ff
45.	PR 1427 ff
53.	LH 94
54.	LH 93
55.	PR 427 ff
56.	PR 445 ff
58.	LH 90
61.	PR 491 ff & PRO 471 ff & 489 ff
64.	PR 481 ff & PRO 271 ff
66.	PR 1449 ff
67.	PR 573 ff
68.	PR 583 ff
69.	PR 597 ff
70.	PR 601 ff
71.	PR 611 ff
72.	LH 106
75.	LH 109
76.	PR 1247 ff & PRO 309 ff
77.	PR 1267 ff & PRO 329 ff
78.	LH ed. Södergård p.18

79.	PR 1233 ff
80.	PR 1223 ff
81.	PR 1239 ff
82.	PR 1291 ff
89.	PR 1635 ff & PRO 407 ff
90.	See MS Sloane 3550 (ch.7) no. 36
114.	LH 115
115.	LH 116
130.	PR 773 ff
131.	LH 119
132.	See MS Cambridge, Trinity Coll. 0.2.5 f.116rb & PR(SJ) 32
133.	PR(SJ) 32
140.	LH 124
150.	See Sloane 3550 (ch.7) no. 53 (and note) & PR(SJ) 26
151.	See Sloane 3550 (ch.7) no. 54 (and note) & PR(SJ) 27
152.	PR(SJ) 34
153.	See A. Salmon, 'Remèdes populaires du moyen âge', *Etudes romanes dédiées à Gaston Paris* (Paris, 1891) [pp. 253–66] no. 27 & PR(SJ) 28
155.	See p. 89 no. 34 and note 129
157.	Salmon, 15. Cf. PR 201 ff
160.	PR(SJ) 8
163.	PRO 417 ff
170.	PR 1301ff & PRO 535 ff
171.	PR 1319 ff
172.	PR 1359 ff
173.	PR 1329 ff & Sloane 3550 no. 57
174.	PR 1335 ff & Sloane 3550 no. 58
179.	PR 1371 ff
180.	PRO 249 ff
181.	PRO 263 ff
182.	PR 1621ff & PRO 393 ff
189.	PR 1663 ff
196.	PR 1421ff
202.	LH 28/29
209.	PRO 71 ff
210.	PRO 119 ff

Chapter Seven

PROSE AND VERSE RECEIPTS IN MS LONDON B. L. SLOANE 3550

MS Sloane 3550 in the British Library is an interesting collection of medical texts copied in England c.1300 and containing no fewer than three texts of the popular 'Lettre d'Hippocrate'. Since it appears to be the subject of no printed notice, it is best to begin with a description of its contents and to follow this with a brief discussion of the vernacular receipts which are mingled with Latin in two sections of the volume. Before passing into the collection of the celebrated physician Sir Hans Sloane (1660–1753),[1] the MS appears to have been the property of the notable surgeon and book-collector Charles Bernard.[2] A note on f.1v reads 'Caroli Bernardi chir. Lond. ex dono reverendi Wil. Whitfeld cal. Nov. 1699'.[3] The whole volume offers a valuable picture of medical knowledge and interests in England at the end of the thirteenth century. The principal contents of the MS are as follows:

1. ff.5r–9r [red rubric] *De signis Ypocratis* inc. 'Pervenit ad me quod cum Ypocras morti apropinquaret percepit . . .'[4]

2. f.9v Two sets of verses: (i) 'Al lac glau karapos indigestionem tibi signa[n]t' (8 verses, Walther, *Initia* 723) (ii) [red rubric] *De cognitione colorum urine* inc. 'Pure fontis aque se comparat alba seroque' (19 verses, Walther, *Initia* 14940).

3. ff.10r–21v [Aegidius, *De urinis*] inc. 'Dicitur urina quam fit renibus una'; expl. 'Expliciunt instituta Egidii de iudiciis urinarum'.[5] Heavily glossed.

4. f.22r *Signa salutis in febribus* (2 verses, Walther, *Initia* 20631); *Signa timoris* (4 verses); *Signa mortis* (6 verses); note on humours; *Signa mortis* (7 verses).[6]

5. ff.22v–28r *Incipit summa de urinis* [=*Compendium urinarum* of Walther of Agilon[7]] expl. [in red] *Expliciunt contenta magistri W. Agilun de urinis*. On f. 28v there are further *signa* of maladies detectable by the properties of urines, beginning 'albeus . . . lacteus . . . glaucus . . . karapos (see no. 2 above).

6. ff.29r–32v [red rubric] *De ornatu mulierum* inc. 'Ut mulier suavissima et planissima videatur . . .', expl. [in red] *Explicit liber de ornatu mulierum*.[8]

7. ff.33ra–36rb [red rubric] *De nominibus herbarum* inc. 'Amarusca anglice maythe; 'Fetet amarusca, redolet similis camomilla' . . .', expl. [in red] *Expliciunt nomina herbarum*.[9]

8. ff.36va–37va [red rubric] *Hic ponitur quid pro quo*. A set of drug substitutes.[10]

9. f.37va/vb A passage on weights inc. '[N]unc sciendum est de nominibus ponderum quarum cognitio practice est utilis'.[11]

10. ff.37vb–40v A set of Latin receipts resembling those which compose the 'Lettre d'Hippo-crate' and arranged according to the following red rubrics: *De dolore capitis* (f.38v), *De capillis* (f.39r), *De pediculis* (f.39r), *Contra pullices* (f.39r), *Contra muscas* (f.39r), *De sompno* (f.39v),

De gutta calida (f.39v), *De pilis* (f.40r), *Ut dens cadat* (f.40r), *De capillis* (f.40r), *De lacrimis* (f.40r), *De dolore dentium* (f.40r), *De perforatione dentium* (f.40v), *De fetore oris* (f.40v).

11. ff.41r–76r An alphabetical list of *synonyma* inc. 'Aer idem quod divus', expl. 'Nunc requiem repetam capiunt sinonima metani [MS meta]'.[12]

12. f.76v Miscellaneous verses including Walther, *Initia* 19692 (8 verses), 7108 (2 verses), and 'Esuriens stomachus detur cibus esurienti' (6 verses), together with a receipt by 'Galienus' *Contra antracem.*

13. ff.77ra–84rc [red rubric] *Incipiunt tabule magistri Salerni que sunt .xii. Prima columpna prime tabule agit de emagogie que sic incipiunt*, expl. [in red and blue] *Expliciunt tabule Salerni.*[13] On f.84rd are two medical notes on Diasaturion and Diairis.

14. ff.84v–85r Medical aphorisms with red rubrics *De signo*, *De crisi*,[14] *De afforismo*, *De teorica*, *De practica*, *De dolore*, *De apoplexia*, *De epilensia.*

15. ff.85v–89v [blue rubric] *De urina et quomodo debet iudicari* inc. 'Nota secundum magistrum Walterum Agylem in urina alba et tenui iudica sit . . .'[15]

16. f.89v [red rubric] *Contra fluxum sanguinis* inc. 'Tres boni fratres unum iter ambulabant . . .' A widely attested charm.[16]

17. ff.89v–91v An incomplete copy of the 'Lettre d'Hippocrate',[17] omitting the preface and introductory sections on humours and urines. It begins with *De dolore oculorum.*

18. ff.91v–98v Apparently a continuation of the above, but the Latin and French receipts (see below) are not found in other copies of the 'Lettre'. The Latin and French rubrics in red are as follows: *Probatio egroti*, *De medico*, *Contra instantiam vigilarum*, *Contra ossa fracta*, *De homine qui non potest loqui*, *Pur trer os de play ou fer ou fut*, *Contra tussim*, *De cura . . .*, *Pur suager dolur de play*, *Pur fer atret encontre felun*, *Pur fer ciroine*, *Contra scabiem*, *Contra fluxum sanguinis*, *Contra cancrum*, *Contra tumorem*, *De dolore mamillarum*, *De dolore stomachi*, *Contra lapidem*, *De muliere*, *Contra luxuriam*, *Contra dolorem stomachi*, *Contra febres.*

19. ff.99r.–216r The so-called Gloss of the Four Masters on the *Chirurgia* of Roger and Roland,[18] f.99r [red rubric] *Incipit liber de cirurgia magistri Rogeri* inc. 'Post mundi fabricam eius que decorem . . .',[19] f.100v [red rubric] *Glosa super syrurgiam secundum magistrum Guidonem Arenencium*,[20] f.102r [red rubric] *Divisio libri secundum Rolandum* inc. f.102v 'Incipit cirurgia magistri Rolandi: cirurgia dicitur a ciros . . .',[21] f.154v [red rubric] *Explicit prima particula, incipiunt capitula secunde particule*, f.155r [red rubric] *Liber secundus de vulneribus que fiunt in collo*, f.178v [red rubric] *Incipiunt caputula* [sic] *tertie particule*; [f.179v] [red rubric] *Hic incipit liber tertius de vulneribus homoplatarum*, f.192v [red rubric] *Ecce qualiter vulnus pulmonis curatur a magistro Rolando*, f.215r *Explicit textus*, f.216r [red and blue rubric] *Explicit comentum cirurgie, valete.*

20. f.216v Short treatise inc. 'Li metres ke icete art troverent anumbrent les malurez jurs e le perelurs [sic] ke sunt en le an . . .'

21. f.216v Short passage on flebotomy inc. 'Fleobotomia mentem sincerat . . .'[22]

22. ff.216v–217r [red rubric] *Beda dixit* inc. 'Beatus Beda que sunt dies in quibus si aliquis homo flebotozaverit vel sanguinem minuerit vel sanguis poysonam acciperit et si quos in hiis diebus similiter luestiam flebotozaverit infra .vii. dies morietur . . .' there are some entries in French.

23. ff.217r–219r [red rubric] *Liber Ypocratis missus ad Cesarem quo eum de multis instruxit* inc. 'Ce est le livre ke yo Ipocras envei a tei Sesar ke jo ai od grant cure ajustee ke jo poi . . .'. An abbreviated text of the 'Lettre d'Hippocrate', concluding with Latin receipts on f.219r/v.[23]

24. f.219v Latin verses inc. 'Hec olus urtica tripulus tanasetaque canaps' (Walther, *Initia* 7566).[24]

25. ff.220r–225r [blue rubric] *Ici comense lé medecines ke Ypocras fit* inc. 'Ce est le livre ke yo Ypocras envea[i] a rei Cesar ke jo ai fet od grant cure. . .' A very full version of the 'Lettre d'Hippocrate'. The text ends with a Latin section (f.225r) headed *De splene* followed by

Explicit, but this section is copied from another work, to be found on ff.225v–229v, which is incomplete, but transmits the first two lines of the *De splene* passage under the rubric *Nocent spleni*.

26. ff.225v–229v Treatise 'De conferentibus et nocentibus', variously ascribed in the MSS, inc. 'Conferunt cerebro fedida ut in gravi oppresione cerebri . . .' (the red rubric is effaced).[25]

27. ff.230r–241v [blue rubric] *Ista sunt experimenta Ypocratis que nunquam fallunt quia probata sunt* inc. 'Sicut sunt quatuor tempora ani . . .' Beginning with sections on the seasons and the humours (with cures), the text continues with the red rubric *De conversatione fleobotomie* (f.230v, 'Conversatio fleobotomie et dies caniculares . . .') and *De curatione venarum* (f.231r, 'Curatio venarum que inciduntur si inflatus talis est. . .' with receipts and marginal rubrics). There follows a red rubric *Potio levitima [sic] cui nulla similis est* (f.232v) and then *Ad vocem clarificandam* (f.233v), *Ad eos quibus [cibus] non delectant*. There are frequent marginal rubrics and on f.238v vernacular rubrics (see below). With only one other comparable, but sometimes divergent, copy[26] it is difficult to establish the authentic limits of the text, which in any case ends incomplete.

28. ff.242r–248r [red rubric] *De epilencia* inc. 'Epilencia dicitur egritudo prohibens animata membra ab operationibus . . .'[27] The treatise rapidly becomes a series of receipts with accompanying rubrics such as *De obtalmia* (f.242v), *De rubore oculorum* (f.242v), *De antrace* (f.245r), *De cauterio* (f.246v), *Contra verucas* (f.248v).[28]

29. f.249ra/vb Lists of herbs and spices

Both the collection on ff.92r–98v and the receipts embedded in the miscellany headed 'Experimenta Ypocratis' on ff.230r–241v contain a number of verse receipts written out as prose. Nineteen of these (nos 3, 55–69, 71–73) are derived from the 'Physique rimee' as transmitted in MS Cambridge, Trinity 0.1.20 ff.1ra–21rb (see above pp.142ff.), and four (nos 3, 36, 57 and 58) in MS Sloane 146 (see above pp.264ff.). Another fourteen (nos 20–21, 24, 26, 30, 32–35, 42–43, 75–77) are derived from the 'Novele Cirurgerie', as preserved, for example, in MS Cambridge, Trinity College 0.2.5 (s.xiv) ff.110ra–124vb. Little use seems to have been made of the 'Lettre d'Hippocrate' (though for no. 8 see above p.110 no.10). The scribe regularly writes *t* for *c*.

1. **[f.92r]** Pur goute sang[29] rancle oynement bone ke ben est prové: Pernét de la rouge ortie le coperun, si estampét ben e pernét la urine al(a) malade, si la destemprét, si oynét le leu ou la gote ceyt . . .[30]

2. **[f.93r]** Item pur fere a home dormir:[31] Donét ache a beyvre en chaud euue hu en freit vin et cetera . . .

3. **[f.93v]** *Pur trer os de play ou fer ou fut:*[32] item
        Si os remeine en la playe,[33]
        N'i ad home ke ben trahie,
        U fer u fut ke dedens seit,
        Ke l'en [ne set ne veit]
        . . .

4. **[f.94r]** Pur la touse: Ysope, maroil e la cerlange, plantaine, rophane [sic] en vin boilét e trembét[34] e pus parmi un drap dunt le colét en le pot, si seit remis. Icét dunt vus ore dis od cel e mel u de may bure[35] si poét fere bone cure. Reboylé ceit en cel pot durement ben e parmi un drat [sic] dunt ceit colé mut sagement e sans pose en chaut serveise ou en vin. De set userét par matin e al matin e al seir, de la tose garét pur veyrs.

5. Item: Mel pernét e averoin e maroine [36] e la rue. De cel triblét en fur tres jurs. Userét par matin, la touse e tut le piz delivre.

6. Item: Sovent trovum en escrit / ke mariol en euue quit / pur touse munt vaut a la gent / ke de sel euue huse sovent . . .

7. **[f.94v]** Pur felun: De morele e plantaine le jus bevét, cum emplatre si metét.

8. Pur felun ke fet le chef enfler: Pernét seim de cerf, mel e er(b)e terestre, morele, ferine de orge, si trimblét ensemble e pus raét le chef e metét sur l'emplatre chaut . . .

9. Pur le felun [MS felur] medicine eprové: Primes quant vus vendrét al felun, pernét ache e pé de colun e le mouiuel de l'hef e cel e menue conseude, si batét ensemble, si metét, si garra. Si li donét un beivre de gletinere e de menu consoude e de metafelun e de pé de colun. Le malade ne mange .iii. jurs ou quatre for pan alis e euue hu tisane.

10. Pur le felun: Primes quant vus venét al felun, pernét le mouel de l'oef e doble de cel e melét ensemble e metét al felun.

11. Pur fer oynement en yvens [37] hou quant le vodrét ativement aver.[38] Pernét saym e cire e code e mauve de cortil e roche cholet e friét ensemble. E cet oynement vaut pur suager dolur de playe e autre survenues.

12. Medisine Hubert Gernun.[39]

13. Pur fere atrete ancontra [sic] felun: [40] Pernét avence e bugle e ambroyse, maroyl, rouche [MS roucle] cholet, savine, sauge, mauve de cortil, lancelee, matafelun, plantaine, aloyne, e cire e code e su de motun ou de bef novele. Si confiét ensemble, si metét al felun sur un canevas percé. Si le felun seit depessé, pus si fetes un drap prendre ou lin, si facét une cercle e metét sur le per[f.95r]tus. Pus si pernét un autre canevas, si metét sur cel cercle put ben prendre ors la quiture. Eissi le facét deke ele seit gari, mes atant de pertus cum il i at sur le felun, tans de pertus seint sur le canevas ke plus prés de le felun est.

14. Pur fer ciroyne: [41] Pernez .i. unce de peis e .vii. unce de franc encens e .i. unce de cire e .i. unce de mastix e .i. unce de su de bete sauvage e .i. unce de bure de may e .i. unce de gresse de porc [MS port] e .i. unce de gresse des oyseus sauvage. E boilét tut ycét ansenble e pernét parmi un canevas e metez en boites.

15. *Contra scabiem,* pur roine: Pernét la racine de eble e de parele e de viole e la sanicle e la plantaine e de sparge. Triblét ensemble, si les friét en bure de may, pus li colét parmi un drap, si en oynét.

16. Item: Sufre, veil oynt, vif argent e de la parele la racine e calemente e eisil fort detemperét. La roine sovent oinét.

17. Pur otter la teynne del chef de home: Pernét peis e cire e fetét bullir ensemble. E raét ben le chef e metét l'emplatre en un drap e metét teve sur le chef e ne le ottét mie devant .ix. jurs, si garra pur vers . . .

18. Pur roine: Bevét femeterie en vin e fetét un oynement de doche roche e holioc [42] e bure frés e friét ses herbes dedens e pus pernét parmi un drap. E pus

batét soufre e franc encens e mel oved, si facet un oinem[en]t, si oinét le
malad(i)e, si garra . . .

19. [f.95v] *Contra fluxum sanguinis*, pur sant astancher: Pernét une herbe ke est
apelé sanguinere, si la tenét en votre main, si anstanchera.

20. Pur epurger sant ke remeint en plaie:[43]
Quant sanc en plaie remeint,
Pur espurger la plaie devét sovent
Bevere le jus de calemente;
Engette [sanc] sant nule dote.
. . .

21. Item:
La brioyne ardét en poudre,
Pus menue la facét moudre;
La sant jette tut enfin,
Tele podre bevét en vin
. . .

22. Da aubrey,[44] pur sant astancher de playe e de nes: Le quele ke celu ke seine
seit en present ou non, estanchera de cete charme: 'La virgine mere sur mont
syt e sun virgine afant sur sun devant tint e virginement le lete. Virgine fu la
mere e virgine fu la (f)afant. Ausi verement estanche Deu tun sant'. E num-
mét sun nun. Hicet ceyt dit .iii. fethez, pus anprés trés Pater Noster etc. . . .

23. *Contra cancrum*, [a]ncontre cancre: Pernét le jus de polipodie, si metét desus le
cancre, murra hativement . . .

24. [f.96r] *Contra tumorem*, [p]uur enflure de la verge: [45]
Pur tele enflure e dolur
De ces treis herbes pernét le licur:
De plantaine e de lancelé
E de millefoile, e seint mellé.
De ces treis choses chaufét le jus,
Tant de un come de autre e nent plus.
Ferine de segle en destemprét
E sur la verge la chochez.

25. Item: La primerole seit triblé par sei sur la verge e tut entur, si en gara.

26. Pur aseer rancle de plaie: [46]
Franc ensens e flur de furment,
Jus de eble e de hache ense[me]nt,
Jus de morele metét [i]
E de l'herbe beneite [tut autresi].
En oint de porc tut seint fri(e)t
Cete emplatre est bone eslit [MS e git],
Sur rancle de plaie serra mis
Cete emplatre dunt ore dis [MS dit].
La rancle assét finement
Cele emplatre hativement.

Memes l'emplatre, si vus volét,
Eschafer e metre purét

. . .

27. [f.96v] Item: Pur rancle ocire pernét pain de forment od ewe e gleire de l'of e metét sure.

28. Item: Pernét aloine e tanesie e triblét od mel e metét sure . . .

29. Item: Pur enflure del (le) ventre triblét rue od vin ou en serveise e beive sovent . . .

30. Pur trencheisuns [MS trenchersuns]:[47]
Lart e vetoine bollerét
En let de chevre, pus le mangerét.
Cele dolur acét toute
Cele cure sant nule doute

. . .

31. [f.97r] Pur maladie ke sovent vent a mameles, là ou plusurs pertus sunt:[48] Pernét cire e code e su de motun e mel e facét une entrete. E metet une (a)tente e metét al metre pertuse e liét une cinse desuz e veét ke il eit un pertus sur le cinse contre la(n) tente, e une autre cinse desuz cele cinse sant pertus pur te(ue)nir ens la(n) tente, e garra . . .

32. Pur ossire lumbris: [49]
Si lumbris as en le cors,
Si les volét jeter ors,
Perche de cerf si ardét en pudre,
Pus menument si facét moudre,
Dunc en eisil seit detempré,
A beivre al malede pus doné.
Si n'at eisil, un oef ceit pris
En la poudre; en ço mis,
A humer al malade sera doné,
Si en avera tut sa santé.

33. Item: [50]
La jubarbe triblét od vin,
Munt en beverét par matin,
Ço en ossit tut finement
Les lumbris hastivement.

34. La mente mangét tut autresi,
Lumbris oscit [MS oscis], jo vus afi.

35. En vin detemprét [f.97v] la savine,
Pur meimes cet est bone medesine.
Od vin detemprét arnement,
Ben espés ceit beu sovent

. . .

36. [f.98r] *De muliere*, A femme ke travayle de enfaunter: Liét a sun ventre icét

acrit (acrit): '+ Maria peperit Christum + Anna Mariam + Elizabet Johannem + Celina Remigium + Sator + arepo tenet + opera rotas +' E donét a beivre ditaine, si enfantera sant peryl.[51]

37. Femme ke ad dolur en [en]fanter: Ortie morte e milfoyle quites en vin li donét a beivre.

38. Pur femme ke ne pet enfanter: Donét lu a beivre mente ou ruwe, si enfauntera . . .

39. [f.98v] *Contra febres* . . . pur la fevre: Pernét rue e aloine e peivre e forte serveise e triblét tut ansemble ke seit ben fort. Si li donét a beivre avant ke le mal li prenge, si le facét longement veiller devant; si vomerat ou dormera, si garra.

40. Pur la fevre terteyne: Pernét la recopeye, si la beive, si garra.

41. Pur le fevers: Bevét morele e persil e la scorce de su quit en servese ou en vin, si garrat.

The following receipts are found, mingled with Latin, in the *Experimenta Ypocratis* on ff.230r–241v:

42. [f.231r] Pur plaie:[52]
    A plaie est durement bone atrete
    Ke en tele manere sera fete:
    Pernét viel oint, encens e cire
    E peys e fetes ensemble frire
    En une paele longement
    Ces quatre choses communement.
    Ceste entrete est durement bon,
    Kar plus vaut ke apostolicon.
    A plaie naier [MS raier] e saner
    Munt est bon, sachét pur veir.
    Sur un quir blanc [MS liant] deit etre mis
    E sur la plai chut[53] asis.
    Deuz fet le jur le remuét [MS metet],
    Enchufét [e remetét],
    Deke la plaie seit pur e neste.

43. Entrete pur uverir plaie:[54]
    Ferine de segle [pestrez]
    Od blant de l'of e cuchez [MS cutlerez]
    Sur la plaie, kar tout overa
    Durement ben e sanera.

44. Pur bras ou [MS od] jambe debrusé [f.231v] ou os debrusé:[55] Primes espl[e]ntez le bras, si li donét confir a beivre.

45. Item: De touz seus devét fere emplatre, / de ruge tere de furno hu de astre, / de saim, de lart, vin, mel e sel [MS fel], / ferine de segle, de tuz owel. E eschafét le facét, pus le metét entre les os, si l'esplentez, si beive confire deke il ceit sein.

46. Pur fere a home dormir:[56] Donét ache a beivre en chaut ewe ou en freit vin . . .

47. Pur touse de cheval: [57] Vin vermail e arrement si enchafét en une paelle, si li donét a beivre, si garra

48. [f.233r] Pur menesun, pur la meneisun [58] . . .

49. [f.233v] Pur fere antrete [59] Hubert: Si en pés ou en gaunbe ou ailurs al cors levent meunt burbelettes, fetes une entrete fete de su de motun e de sire e de code e de mel e metét e aseirunt e tut entroyra. [60] De ce garit Robert de Neuport e le suppriur de colun de sa main. Si cete maladie seit durement enrasiné, metét hicete entrete ke plus fort est fete de sire e de mel e de code e de su e de mauve de cortil e de videgrés e metét tut freit ansemble.

50. Pur le stomach ki est astupé: [61] Pernét glaiol e batez ben en un morter, si la destemprét ovec let u ovet meche e pernét flur de furment, si en fetes niuueles, si li donét .vii. (vii), un jur en autre jur, si garra.

51. Pur la meneisun: [62] Beive sanguinere e plantaine e quintefoyle ou milfoile, si enstanchera . . .

52. [f.234r] Contra singultum .i. woxinge: [63] Pernét clou de gilofre e canele e galligal e anise e fetét fer un podre, si li donét a manger un quiler e pus autrefet quant li prent un autre. Si vus ne poét par tant estancher, pernét le jus de mente, si metét le poudre en le quiler sur le jus de mente.

53. Pur morsure de chen aragé: [64]
    Si vus de (de) chen ayét morsure,
    Pernét rouge ortie a dreiture
    E la morele e bel lart creu:
    Ensemble seit batu,
    En bure quisé(n)t bel e gent,
    Si garra par ceit oynement.

54. Pur morsure de chen aragé: [65]
    Si il vus mort,
    La plaie vus dura mun fort.
    Milfoyl, sau[f.234v]ge destemprét
    E la plaie de ce lavét.
    Amprés ce pernét la plantaine
    E egremoyne plein la main,
    Ensemble ben la triblét
    Aubun de l'hef e mel hi metez
    Ou veil wnt od la plantaine:
    Cet oynement vus fra tut seyne.

55. Pur let a noruse: [66]
    Quant let a la noruse faut,
    Un beivre facét ke munt vaut.
    Prenge fenoil, prenge la ruwe [MS rumle],
    Prenge eruke, prenge letu[e];
    La flur de aube aspine
    Metre devét a la medisine.
    Si ele se(it) beivre use [e fet],

El avera grant plenté de let
...

56. *Contra venas:* [67]
    A veine rump[u]e restreindre
    Ne se deit nu[l] home feindre.
    Pur aver sa garisun
    Plantayne beyve e jus de kersun.

57. Pur fevre terceyne: [68]
    Beive treis plauntes de plantain(e)
    Devant sun assez, si ert sein,
    Treis al matin e treis al seir
    .ix. jurs, si il vout sancté aver.

58. Pur fevre .iiii. [69]
    Perné[t] un of ke seit mol quit,
    Del blanc versét hors hun petit;
    Une femme venge [avant]
    Ke norise un male enfant,
    Tres gutes de let i degute,
    Le feverus lé deit humer tut,
    Mes hitant coyntement le face,
    Ke le malade ne le sace.

59. *Contra plagas:* [70]
    A plaie ke vout saner
    E tout la mortte char ocster:
    A ce pernét hastivement
    Munt bon encens he arnement,
    Trestus en poudre les batét
    E sur la playe les poudrez.

60. *Contra sanguinem:* [71]
    A stancher seynante playe
    Dunt meint home naufré s'emmaye:
    A ce ne vus ubbliét mie
    Les ciuns de la roche ortie,
    Od un cutel tut demincez,
    En fort aysil lé moyllét.
    Ki a la plaie tout mettra,
    Ja un soul point ne seynera.

61. *Contra plagas,* [72] ad celu ke batu est e naveré:
    A ce pernét herbes plusurs
    Pur asuager si grant dolurs:
    Pernét bucle e confir(i)e,
    Sanicle n'i seit mie a dire, [MS S. n'ert mi a dire]
    Consaude pernét he avence
    E vetoine ke munt l'avance,
    Lavendre he la tanesie,

    Homunde ne obbliez mie,
    En bone serveise quisez
    Ces herbes he le beivre usez.

62. *Contra ossa fracta*,[73] item:
    Si os remeine en la plaie, [MS en la pl. remeine]
    N'i ad home ki ben traye,
    U fer u fut ke dedens [f.235r] seit,
    Ke l'en [ne] set ne l'en veit,
    De ditayne deit beivre le jus
    E le pastel lier desus
    Ov la viole en ewe quite,
    Ce est une herbe bene elite.
    Sur les pez metét le pastel,
    Si en istera hors hos u quarel.

63. Item:[74]
    Autre a plaie ke vus serve:
    Pernét plantaine e quinquenerve,
    Goute de mel e flur de forment,
    Tut creu le metét simplement.

64. *Pur fere entrete*:[75]
    Si volét aver autre entrete,
    Si gardét ben ke dunt seit feit:
    De segle pernét la ferine,
    Jus de hache e mel a la medicine
    E le haubun de l'ef hi metét,
    Si avét bone entrete asét.

65. *Contra plagas*:[76]
    Un beyvvre pur plaie vus voil dire:
    Ce cevent mires [MS miuz] plusur
    Ke entre mil ne n'at meilur:
    Pernét plein poin de la parele,
    Un erbe ke est munt net e bele,
    La plaie espurge e nie,
    Ke ordure ne rement mie.
    De sauge me pernét [et] le tim
    Ke garit [MS karit] de palesim,
    La violete od la flur
    Ke essuage la dolur
    E la vetoine ke tout fevere
    Ke en plaie sout estre enrevre,
    Lancelé ke creste al f(r)anc
    Pur ce ke ele restrei[n]t le sanc,
    Plantaine ke crest en chimin
    Ke sout dechasser le venim,
    He metét hi piloseite
    Ke en neie [MS vere] plaie e fet nette,

E egrimoine; ces herbes touz les pernét,
Triblét ben, pus lé quisét
En bone serveise ou en vin,
Si beive al seir e al matin.
Mel hi metét pur enducir [MS enducer],
Si pur plus longe [poét] tenir.

66. *Contra plagas:*[77]
E geres si vus prent talent,
Fere poét bone oynement
De meimes hiceus jus
Des herbes dunt ay dit desus,
For sul hitant ke remuerét [MS rement],
La pilosete he[n] osterét,
Kar si cete herbe mise hi seit,
La playe vus aneyt.
Metét y mel, oyle e cire,
Seu de motun, ce voil dire,
Issi fetes vostre oiniement,
La plaie garra finement.

67. *Pur fer entrete,*[78] un entrete:
La manere de une atrete
Vus dirrai ben dunt ce est fete.
De segle ferine pernét
E aloyne munt ben trinblét
Od oyle de olive e bon veil unt
E mel atut i ceeit ajoynt.
Deuz fethe le remuét le jur
Pur asuager la grant dolur.

68. *Pur fer beivre a plaié:*[79]
Un beivre a plaié vus dirai:
Pernét viole e egrimoine
E tanesie e la vetoyne,
Ere teretre, bug[l]e e plantain(e),
S'il cet beit, si sera sein.

69. La diete al malade; [80]
Le livre apertement le comaunt
Ke il se garde [f.235v] de viaunt,
Herbes, furmage e let e frut.
Si il femme hauntte, si est destrut.
Kar de castriz ke ceit poudré,
Ou ke il seit salé e fumee,
Grase geline, fesaunt, perteris,
Si ce mangut, si est gari.
Munt se garde ben de coureser,
Sa plaie purra le meuz saner,
Hu seit par grant ou par petit

Le sang del cors li boyt he frit
En chalur, en ire e en fu,
Lors est li sanc tut commu.
La plaie rugit, si li dout,
Sovent enfler e rancle[r] sout.
Sages [MS sagas] est ki garder se pout
Quant issi est k[e] fere l'estout.

70. Contra . . . fract . . .:[81] La medicine Hubert Gernun de Ewardestouer [82] pur
gambe depessé ou bras: Primes pernét un canevas e fort. Si trinble l'of creu e le
aubun e le mouuel, si outét lé escales, si moilés cel canevas dedens, si envolupez entur la gambe, si lesét demorer al meyns treis jurs taunt tost u quatre. Esplentés sant plus. E pus l'entrete fete[s] de sire e de gumme e de su e de mel, si
garra. Quant oster voderez le canevas, od euue chaude le otterét.

71. De homine vulnerato,[83] essprove:
Pilosette donét a beivre
Pur quey vus volét aperceyvre
Si le navré devera garir
Ou de playe deit morir;
Si la retent, garir en pot,
Si il vomit, morir l'estot.

72. A yceus ke sunt aroué,[84] essprove:

Ore vus [dirai] ke jo ay loé	Ore vus dirai que ai loé
A yceus ke sunt aroué.	A ces que sunt aroué.
E[n] vin facent boiller savine	En vin facent boiler savine
E mel medlét a la medicine,	E mel metét a la medicine,
Od feves, ce dit nostre escrit,	Od feves, ce dit nostre acrit,
Od ayl mangét en breses quit.	Ail mangét en brese quit.

73. Autre: [85]

Un autre uncore, ce mey semble,	Un autre uncore, ce me semble,
L'enterus pernez del tremble	L'entrus pernét del tremble,
. . .	E de eble la racine.
	En vin quisét cete medecine.
	Useir deit matin e seir,
	Que vodra santé aver.

74. [f.237r] Pur touce de cheval e destresse del pis: [86] Pernét pé de leun e espurge
e quisét en vin vermail e si la destemprét. Si vus n'avét vin, si pernét ewe, si li
donét a beivre.

75. De homine vulnerato: [87]
Si vus volét saver [si murra]
Li [MS si] home playé (murra) ou garra,
Ces herbes li donét a beivre,
Il ne vus pura pas deseivre:
Le jus li donét de la pimpernele
Ou de cerfoyle ke munt est bele.
Quant il od beu, si ist [MS iuit] hors

Par la plaie k'il ad al cors,
Sachez ben par nule [re]sort
Pur la plaie avera la mort
. . .

76. **[f.238v]** *Medecine esprové encuntre teine:* [88]
Teyne est un mal de male manere,
Pur cee medecine dirom chere.
Pur male garde sovent avent
[. . .]
Pernét un herbe ke ad a nun
[. . .] pé de liun,
Triblé seit e ben quite(s)
En lessive bone [elite]
Dunt raét le chef tot nettement.
Pur sancke en [MS ne] isse ne lerrét pas,
Mes la teyne tot otteras.
E dunt l'erbe ke jo dis
Come enplatre desur seyt meis,
Ne seit trop freit ne trop chaud,
Mes teve emplastre a ce mult vaut.

77. *Autre:* [89]
Key en la teste teigne avera,
Si de see garrir vodera,
Si seit sa teste ben lavé
E pus rese e a pomiz naee.
Dunt prenge piz e virgine cire
E facez tout ensemble frire
E [metez] [MS ke] sur la teste chaud
E ben sachét ke cee mult vaut.
.ix. jurs tut enterement
Girra sur sanz remuement.

78. *Pur roine otter:* Pernét la racine de ruge docke, si la quisét trés ben e les neirs li-maceu[n]s quisez ovece bure de may. Pus si tortét parmi un drap, si metez en boites, si en oignét encontre le fu suvent tant deches il seit garri.

79. *Si vus volét aver linge teile teint rouge:* Pernét tan de chene e fetes ben boyler od clere ewe de fontaine. E pus se[é]t le licour en un pot par sey e dunt moylez votre drap en le jus. Pus pernét alun, si fetes quire e quant serra ben boylé mol-lét leinz vostre drap. E pus pernét brasile, si le(n) fetes ben quire cum char de motoun e pus moillét votre drap en cele licur quant vus l'averét colee par sei tant ke cee seit asét roche.

80. *A fere colur de ynde:* Metét primes en alum e pus pernét brasille, si le fetes quire en forte lessive, si l'entemprét od savun e verdegris.

81. *A fere jaune colur:* **[f.239r]** Pernet wildewolde, si le fetes quire en forte lessive e metét en ce votre drap, si le pernét sus tantot.

82. A *fere vert colur*: Plungét le primes en le flur de wade, pus le metét en le jus de jaune.

83. A *fere neir colur*: Pernét tan de chene e fetes ben quire e pus moillét vostre drap cum vus fetes le roge. E pus pernét l'escorce de aune e le molur des cotels e de autres armes. Si fetes ensemble quire e pus moillét [en] le juz vostre drap, e sachét ke vus ne le devét leisser gisir en nule saus fors en le tan . . .

84. [f.240v] E ki les euz lermanz avera, le jus de betoine prendra, ens as euz metera; les lermes tout e les euz cler fra.[90]

Chapter Eight

THE COLLECTION OF MEDICAL RECEIPTS IN MS OXFORD, BODLEIAN LIBRARY DIGBY 69

MS Digby 69 in the Bodleian Library, Oxford, is an interesting, if disordered, manuscript which was once owned by William Marshall, Fellow of Merton College, Oxford (d.1583) and later in the possession of Thomas Allen (d.1632) whence it passed to Kenelm Digby. Measuring approx. 200 x 138 mm and numbering 222 folios, it represents a sprawling compendium of medical extracts copied by many different hands c.1300. It seems, from the paucity of printed references, never to have been studied, so that a preliminary description of its contents is indispensable.

1. ff.1r–11v a miscellany of medical prescriptions and notes with red rubrics throughout, together with marginal titles, headwords etc. It begins with receipts, then continues with sections on birds (f.2r/v *De passere, De gallina* etc.), a short treatise *De aquis medicinalibus* (ff.2v–3r), another *De virtutibus quaru[n]dem herbarum* (ff.3v–6v; marginal indications *contra tumores, ad ossa fracta* etc.) and *Contra infectionem pannorum*, followed by a charm:

> [f. 6v] Incaustum vino lexiva dilue vinum [Walther, *Initia* 9164]
> Stillas ymbre laves oleumque liquore fabarum [Walther, *Initia* 18625]
>
> Jhesu Crist wes in erþe istunge In nomine Patris +
> So ne wes þet wrd te hevene ysprunge In nomine Patris +
> His wunden oken and þine ne mocen In nomine Patris +
> His wunden sual and þine ne sal In nomine Patris +
> His wunden icten and þine ne micten. In nomine Patris +
>
> Carmen istud dicatur ter super plagatum et vulnus non dolebit postea.

Then follow more receipts on ff.7r–11v.[1]

2. f.12r [red rubr.] *Incipit de virtutibus quarumdem herbarum*, an index in three columns beginning with *Arthemesia*.

3. f.12v an Anglo-Norman receipt:

Encuntre chalde maladie fesuns nus cele ewe durthike que depart la chalde maladie sicum en chal tens et en chaud eage. Chaud eage apele tuz cels ki sunt dedenz .xxxv. anz. Nus pernuns semences de curcuns et de meluns et de cur(ur)des et de cucumbres, si lé bat l'en bien en un morter ensemble. Pus les fesum buillir en ewe. Pus la culuns et la dununs a beivre al malade quant ele est refreidie.

En freit tens et en freit esté encuntre freide matire dunum nus la decoctiun de semence de ache et de persil et de fenuil et de bruc. Dunums nus a beivre od la decoction de lur rcines si ço est en esté et de freide matire o en iver et de chalde. Altrement des chaldes choses cum des freides nus l'aturnums solunc ço k'il est fort. Si li donuns a beivre des chaldes et des freides semences.

Par ces signes cunuissums quant la matire de la chalde maladie est departie par l'acession. Si l'acession prent au tens que ele ne sout, et mains dure et tant est li malades
meins grevez. Et notez que la chalurs de quor est cumparé a la chalur del feu: sicume li
feus de muilliés busches ars rent greignur chalur que de secche busche, altresi la chalur
de la crue matire est chalde et plus lungement dure que de la matire qui est legere a
defire. E pus ke la matire est embrasee, et ço porez vus veer aprés le cinckime jor que li
malades serra mult malades, gard li mires qu'il ne doinst nule purgaciun, kar issi
desturbereit il nature et cetera.

This is followed by Latin verses *Contra omnem guttam* (Walther, *Initia* 1278) with two receipts
and another receipt *De paralisi lingue* (red rubr. f.12v).

4. ff.13r–14v [red rubr.] *Hec sunt capitula de curis sequentibus*, an index written in two columns
per page.

5. ff.15r–22r passages on the medicinal application of various plants (beginning *De zipulis*)
followed by red rubrics *De sale et eius speciebus* (f.17v), *Hic agit de animalibus silvestribus* (f.17v),
De animalibus domesticis (f.18r), *De extremitatibus membrorum* (f.18v) together with miscellaneous passages on milk, butter, cheese, birds, and Latin medical verses (ff.20v–21r), ending
with *De pane et eius diversitatibus* (f.21r) and short sections on fruit and herbs (f.21v). On f.15r
zipule is glossed 'crespeus' and *orobum* 'musepese'.

6. ff.22r–23v medical receipts and charms incl. *Ad farcim equi*.[2]

7. ff.23v–25v [red rubr.] *Incipit liber de naturis animalium* by Johannes Mesue, inc. 'Auctor est
filius Messye. [E]x eis itaque quod filius Messye dixit in libro de animalibus . . .'[3] presenting a
series of receipts introduced by 'Dixit Galenus', 'Dixit Tabariensis', 'Dixit Belbelis' etc. Indications 'De . . .' and 'Contra . . .' are found in the margins.

8. ff.26r–27r short Latin cauteries with red rubrics, blue and red initials, each indication
being followed by 'Incenditur sic . . .'

9. ff.27r–28v [red rubr.] *Epistola Ypocratis Mecenati suo salutem* inc. 'Yppocrates mecenati suo
salutem libellum quem roganti tibi promisi omni cura adhibita descriptum . . .'[4] with expl. in
red *Explicit epistola Ypochratis ad Mecenatem.*

10. ff.28v–30r [red rubr.] *Incipit Epistola Anthonii Muse ad Agripp(ip)am de virtutibus herbe
betonice* inc. 'Antonius Musa Agrippe magno Cesari Augusto salutem . . .'[5] with expl. in red
(f.29r) *Epistola Anthonii Muse explicit de herba betonica* and (f.30r) *Explicit de betonica.*

11. ff.30r–61v [red rubr.] *[I]ncipit Epistola Platonis ad cives suos de herba plantagine* [i.e. Ps.–
Apuleius] inc. 'A Grecis dicitur arnoglossa, Galli vocant tarbidolopius . . .',[6] ending incomplete on f.61v with 'Nomen herbe scholismos'.[7] Blank spaces have been left for the
illustrations, never executed.

12. ff.62r–65v medical receipts with red rubrics incl. (f.65v) *Hec sunt capitula de curis precedentibus* (the list occupying ff.62–65), followed by two receipts. The receipt *Ad fistulam*
(f.63v) includes 'succum herbe que dicitur banewrt'.

13. ff.66r–84vb a text of Macer's *De viribus herbarum* inc. 'Herbarum quasdam dicturus
carmine vires . . .' with much interlinear glossing (often of a grammatical nature) and an
extensive marginal commentary.[8] The text, which is sometimes written in two columns, is
provided with red rubrics.

14. ff.84vb–92r a chaotic set of medical extracts incl. *Laus phisicorum*[9] and passages on the
humours, fevers and the convalescent.

15. ff.92r–94v [red rubr.] *Incipiunt synonime* inc. 'Alphita farina ordei idem', short entries
written in three columns, no vernacular items, ending 'zipule: crispelle' and (in red) *Expliciunt
synonime.* There follow passages on mandragora, squinantia etc. A folio is missing at the end.

16. ff.95r–115v medical receipts with red rubrics, marginal headwords, and red and blue initials.

17. ff.116r–124r [red rubr.] *Incipit tabula de herbis constrictivis* followed by long extracts on numerous herbs, their medicinal properties and application. On f.121r there is a red rubric *Tabula .xii. de herbis contra toxicum.*

18. ff.124r–125v [red rubr.] *Epistola Ypocratis ad Filominum de conversacione medici(s)* [10] with another red rubric *Eiusdem de visitatione infirmi* followed by miscellaneous prescriptions and (f.125r) *Potio Aristolabii regis.*

19. ff.126r–127v acephalous index of medical extracts which follow on ff.128r–183v. The receipt on f.128r 'Incisionem venarum' is not part of the works indexed, the first entry of the index 'Paralisi cura in secundo folio postea' corresponding with *De paralisi* on f.130r. Similarly, in the index the heading *Incipiunt anathomie* (f.126ra) corresponds with the section on f.138v (same rubric) and on f.126rb *Epistola regis Egyptionum de virtute taxonis* [11] corresponds with the rubric and text on f.151r. This large and heterogeneous collection includes the two frequently copied treatises *Incipiunt summa de conferentibus et nocentibus* [12] (ff.168v–172r, 'Conferunt cerebro fetida . . .') and *Incipit summa quid pro quo* [13] (ff.172v–173v, 'Pro aristologia . . .'). The vernacular receipts are included in the index, but without vernacular headings. For the text of these see below.

20. ff.184ra–191ra a compendium of medical preparations incl. antidotes, electuaries, purgatories, plasters, trochisks, embrocations, ointments etc. The collection is written in a distinctly new hand, in two columns, and there are green initials, and it begins 'Super carbunculum aut mala nascentia inpositum' and includes (f.187ra) 'Epistola Ypocratis de catarticis'.[14]

21. f.191rb/va measures and weights.

22. ff.192ra–195r a Latin verse treatise on the virtues of herbs and stones, inc. 'De plantagine: Antidotumque salubre di arnaglossa fit inde' and ending with 'De sarcofago', followed by prose sections on the protective properties of stones when inscribed with certain signs and symbols.

23. ff.195v–196r miscellaneous receipts.

24. ff.196r–201r [red rubr.] *De la terre de Inde* inc. 'La terre de Inde est issi apelee de Indun, un flum ki devers occident la aceint . . .'. A prose work in Anglo-Norman which covers the marvels of India incl. stones, animals and fruit.

25. f.201r/v miscellaneous receipts and 'experiments'.

26. ff.202r–208v 'De derivatione nominum partium humani corporis'.[15] No rubrics, but marginal headwords in another hand.

27. ff.208v–211v miscellaneous receipts.

28. ff.212r–213r [red rubr.] *De apostematibus et eorum generibus* inc. 'Infigit, pungat, extendit et aggravat . . .' [16] On f. 213r there is a red rubric *Stupha optima pruritum pacientibus.*

29. ff.213r–214r [red rubr.] *Secreta Ypocratis,* [17] and in brown *Experimenta Ypocratis vite et mortis et in ultimo folio libri de eodem*, ending (f.214r) 'Expliciunt secreta pronosticorum Ypocratis'.

30. ff.214r–220v miscellaneous medical extracts, with red rubrics including *Litargia* and *Cura* (f.214v), *Columpna secunda de vomitis fortibus* (f.215r), *De vomitis forinsecis* (f.215r), *De arboribus constrictivis* (f.215v) etc.

Aside from the vernacular receipts drawn from the collection on ff.128r–183v, which are edited below, there are a few vernacular words [18] and three other vernacular charms [19] which are found in the miscellany on ff.208v–211v.[20]

A number of vernacular plant names are found as glosses, beginning with the text of Ps.–Apuleius: They are of the thirteenth century (fourteenth-century glosses are marked with an asterisk):

[f.31v] sanguinaria .i. stanche / bursa pastoris, anglice stancheblode* / [f.32r] simphoniaca .i. hennebane / [f.33v] arthemesie .i. mugwert / [f.34v] lapatium .i. clote / drachontea .i. dragance / [f.35r] gentiana .i. veldwort / ciclaminos .i. panis por[cinus, anglice hirthnot*] / [f.36r] aristologia .i. wuderove / nasturcium .i. kersun / [f.37r] camedris .i. quercula minor vel cerula minor, anglice mederatel / [f.37v] camedafne .i. ermentilla, grant morele vel burnette / ostriago, anglice stikwurt / [f.39r] oxylapatium .i. docke / [f.40r] ibercus .i. bissopeswert / nomen herbe frage .i. fraser / [f.41r] nomen bulbis cillicidi, bulbus .i. batracion, hoc est gledene / cotulidion: umbilicus veneris, hoc est voystel / marrubii .i. horhune / [f.41v] gallitricum .i. feterwert / [f.47r] felicem: filix, farn / nomen herbe gramen, herba communis que habet angulum in medio, anglice quychen / [f.48r] pastinaca silvatica, achorus, mader silvestris/ mercurialis, zenozostis idem, kerlekes / [f.49r] millefolium: millefole / [f.50r] ebulum .i. walewort / [f.50v] pulejum: puliol / [f.51v] saxifraga .i. stonwrt / [f.52r] cardi silvatici: wilde þistel / [f.54v] eptafilos .i. brunwrt / apium .i. ache / crisocantis .i. atriplex, hoc est methe / [f.55r] anetum: anis / [f.56r] petrosilium .i. persil / basilica .i. feldwert / [f.57r] afrise .i. freses / [f.58v] samsucon: elren / [f.60v] linozostis .i. mercurialis, kerlekes.

The following glosses occur in the text of Macer on ff.66r–84vb:

[f.66r] arthemesia: monoclos, mugwert: tagantes, helde; leptaphilos, hemelech / [f.68v] althea, eviscum .i. mersmalue / [f.69v] mercurialis herba, bete idem / [f.71ra] acidula: surdocke / [f.71rb] De nasturciis: kersuns / [f. 71va] eruca: skirewrt / [f.73vb] De origano: puliol real / [f.74va] bischopwert .i. andre / [f.76ra] De vulgagine .i. foxesglove / [f.78ra] De paratella .i. docke, parele / De lolio .i. nigella, kockel / [f.78vb] De cicuta .i. herba benedicta, hemelec / [f.80vb] De maurella, strignum .i. morele.

Amongst the miscellaneous medical receipts in Latin vernacular items are found as follows:

[f.96r] accipe succum morsus galline .i. chikemete / [f.96v] [red rubric] Contra sinantiam valet scabiosa et anglice dicitur goldwert / allea quam romano vocant wimalve / [f.97r] accipe warance / interl. gl. mader / et chanve / interl. gl. henep / et tanecetam / interl. gl. tanesi / [f.100r] Ad paralisim: Accipe avenciam, lavendulam, salviam, orticam griache et duas herbas paraliticas .i. primerellam salvage, fraser salvage . . . / [f.100v] Ad omnimodam infirmitatem membri virilis: Gileis anglice dicitur wodewise / Ad vulneratum sanandum per potum: Accipe buglam, pigle, senicle, avenciam, spargiam, coperun de runces / [f.110v] Ad sanguinem stringendum . . . pulverem crulle lupini .i. wlvesfist / [f.145v] radices de glagel / [f.181r] urtica griache.

There is a fragment of English in the following charm:

[f.100v] Ad verrucas tollendas: Missa de Sancto Spiritu debet celebrari. Quotiens ad illam missam Oremus dicitur, totiens et in illa hora adiutor nominet nomen pacientis .N. et dicat '.N. verruces tue cadant in honore Patris et Filii et Spiritus Sancti'. Ista verba dicantur lingua latina vel romanice vel anglice. Pater Noster .iii. Ave Maria .iii. Ad idem: Accipe ramum aliquem de ligno juniperi et habeas aliquem qui tibi respondeat et dicas primo 'Sindo'. Dicat alius 'Quid scindis tu?' Respondeas – .N. nominetur ubicumque sit – '.N. yive werten awei in nomine Patris et Filii et Spiritus Sancti, amen'. Sic dicatur ter et totiens respondeatur. Et dicatur Pater Noster ter, Ave Maria ter.

1. [f.175r]²¹ Carmen ad matricem: In nomine Patris etc. usque Amen. 'Joe te cun-

jur estomac e mere e mariz el nun del Pere e del Fiz e del Seint Esperit, e el nun
de Nostre Dame seinte Marie la preciuse virgne, e des quatre ewangelistes Dam-
nedeu, ce est asaver de seint Johan e de seint Luc e de seint Marc e de seint
Matheu, e de seint Michel le bon aungle e de tuz aungles e de tuz archangles, e
de seint Johan le Batiste e de seint Pere e de seint Pol e de tuz apostles, e de tuz
martirs, confessurs, virgnes e de tuz feals Dampnedeu; joe te cunjur par tuz clers
ordinez, par eveskes, abbez e par tuz prestres ordinez come de messes chanter e
par moynes encloistré e par meimes Dampnedeu, mal de l'estomac e de mere e
de mariz, ke tu n'ees poesté de mal fere a cele femme .N. Deu la garisse de cele
enfermeté, amen.[22] Uncore te cunjur, estomac e mere e mariz, par la halte deité
de tutes creatures del ciel e de terre, de rusee, de herbe e par le aver aie
paterne [23] ke tu ne gisez en son penil ne en son umbil ne al quor, mes en drait
liu esteez si ke en nul liu n'eez poesté de mal fere a lui ne de lui encumbrer, mes
lui doint verrai sauntét nostre Pere ki est al ciel e la gloriuse mere Marie e tuz
les seinz Dampnedeu, amen'. In nomine Patris et Filii et Spiritu Sancti, amen.

2. *Contra vermes*: 'Adiuro vos vermes per Dominum Patrem omnipotentem et per
omnes sanctos eius, per sanctam crucem de quocumque genere sitis, ne amplius
huic equo noceatis, increatus Pater, increatus Filius, increatus Spiritus Sanctus
et inmensus Pater, inmensus Filius, inmensus Spiritus Sanctus, eternus Pater,
eternus Filius, eternus Spiritus Sanctus +' In nomine Patris et cetera. Pater noster ter dicat . . .

3. [f.175v] *Ad ficum sanguinolentem*, por le fi senglant: Pernez herbe en engleis apelee hilgars dunt li berbiz morent. Une bevee batez en un morter, si destemprez
od un poi de ewe e colez. E metez od tot lait de chievre e autant de lait de
vache, e bure de may autant, e farine de orge semé en marz. E fetes (pa)pelotes
de totes ces choses, si donez al malade par noef jors, le premer jor .i.,[24] le secund
jor .ii., le tierz .iii., le quart .iiii. eissi cressant .i. deske a noef jors. . . .

4. *Experimentum bonum:* [25] [f.176r] La Sarazine de Meschine garist une dame
veont plusurs que tote fu calve e out perdu les sorcilz. Ele prist persil salvage e le
tribla forment e builli en blanc vin e i mist un poi de seim de porc. Quant fu
bien builli, ele cuilli la gresse que fu sore en un altre pot e prist cumin e mastic e
tribla od les muels des oes quit en ewe. Pus les builli tot ensemble e devint cum
oignement. Si en oint la teste e sorcilz e li peil revint.

Dirichef[26] ele prent toz les chefs de petiz oisels ke ele poet aver e plein poin de
forment e altretant des oes e lea art tot ensemble e fist pudre. E oint la teste e
sorcilz de l'escume de blaunc miel e mist la pudre desore.

Si vus les volez fere luns e espés, pernez brionie, si le quisez en vin ou en aisil e
lavez la teste cum funt les dames de Salerne.[27] . . .

5. *Contra ictum de quarel*, por cop de quarel: Pernez semence de ache, semence de
ortie de ultre mer e flur de segle, de toz oele mesure. E destemprez o(l) le blanc
de l'oef, ke il seit espés cum miel. Pus fetes tente de canve ou de lin e moillez
cele tente en la destemperure. Se la tente seit aforcee de alcun estike pur tenir
red deskes l'un vienge as funz de la plaie, mielz valt. Quant bien est purgé, metez
i oignement sanatif.

6. [f.176v] *Ad dislotionem pedis vel gambe vel alicuius*, si pié ou jambe ou altre menbre seit aloché: Pernez un wastel .i. une manere de pain, si le gratez en une

grate, pus le batez en un morter lungement. Pus le destemprez od blanc vin fort, si l'eschaufez al feu ke il seit teve, sil metez sor le mal. Si trera hors la dolor e le sanera. . . .

7. *Si capud vel aliud membrum inflatum fuerit pro ictu aliquo*, si teste ou altre membre seit emflé par angoisse de cop: Pernez deliees estupes e moillez en ewe, si metez entor la teste ou altre membre u la maladie est. Pus metez la tente dé estupes moillees el jus de ache.[28]

8. *Ad auditum recuperan[dum]*, a celui ki ad perdu la oie: Pernez la gresse de angoille rostie e vin blanc e jus de hundestunge oele mesure e metez en la oreille malade. Si metez la oreille vers val, k'il pusse bien entrer, e sanera.

9. *Contra febrem acutam*, regula, ki est en ague: Pernez safran e les flurs de solsequie, si destempre od cerveise o ewe e beive. Pus suera e turnera.[29]

10. *Contra paralisim acutam et apoplexiam*: Ki use safran petite porciun, le jor ke il le use ja ne sera feru de parlesie ne de ague ne de apoplexie.

11. *Carmen contra fluxum sanguinis*, ad fluxum sanguinis de naribus vel aliud carmen: 'Nostre Sire fu nez en Bethleem, baptizez el flum Jordan e la ewe a ses piez restut. Issi vereiement estanche cest hom de sa seignee'. Ter dicatur carmen. Si presens sit qui patitur, dicatur modo predicto, si absens, eodem modo exeat. . . .

12. *Por alochure de pié ou de main ou de altre menbre e por rancle e a plusurs choses est precius*: Pernez canve delié e metez en une paele. Pus estramez siel sore le canve. Pus pernez brianie [sic] sec e taillez menu e metez sor le siel. Pus i versez vin vermail a mesure ke tot seit covert. Sil quisez k'il seit bien espés. E metez entor le menbre e le sanera e trera hors la anguisse. Primes fetes trere le menbre ke il venge en son dreit liu.[30] Avaunt de meimes çoe. Chose est prové.[31]

13. *Por bleceure de cutel ou d'arme*, si cors de home ou menbre seit trenché de cutel ou de altre arme: Beive le jus de filipendula, si sanera les plaies.

14. *De l'oisel ki est apelé nutehech*: Un oisel est ki l'en apele en engleis nuteheht, ki fet trous el cheene a fere son ni. S'il avient ke les trous seent forment estupez de kivil, si va icel oisel quere un herbe ke l'om apele quartfoille – icele ne crest aillurs ke el liu ou li pulein est novelement pulené. Iceste herbe porte li oisel e met sor la closture de ses trouse e les overe. Icest herbe est preciuse e cil ki en sa main la porte ne serra de nul veu.

15. *Por festre saner*, por saner festre: Pernez avence, wilde tasel, consolide mendre. Donez a beivre. Si metez le past sor le mal. Si saver volez si cancre seit vif dedenz, pernez crudden de leit, si metez sor le mal; s'il seent percé, si est par cancre. Pus pernez clofyunke [f.177r] .i. c[el]idonie, si quisez en breses. Pus triblez od miel e od crudden ou cerveise seit mise. Metez sor le mal, si istra le verm veablement.

16. *A gute chaude*, a gute chaude: Pernez les burjuns de popuiller muntant de un galun, demi quart de miel, un potel de vin egre, si metez ensemble en un pot e lessez ester .ix. jors. Pus pernez sus le pot, si triblez bien les burjuns. Pus pernez

bure de may e gresse de porc e gresse de owe e quisez ensemble. Pus colez parmi .i. drap. . . .

17. *Stupha ad guttam* eiciendam:[32] Accipe moleine, pié de pulein, chanelee .i. hundestunge, manipulum **[33] vel jusquiami mani . . ., marruil manipulum **, celidoine manipulum **, hedere terrestre manipulum **, reste bovis manipulum **, kersuns de ewe manipulum **, foilles de sauz ruges manipulum **, foilles de blanc pruner manipulum **, primerole de pré manipulum **, dent de leon manipulum **, feniculi manipulum **, ortie griache manipulum **, de pié de pulein altant cum de tuz les altres. Partut manipulum .i. Totes ces choses seent quiz en ewe. Pus seit estuvé. Celui ki avera gute as jambes ou braz ou altre membre del cors seit estuvé et mette la sustance des herbes sor le membre malade, si suera hors tote la gute.

18. *Ad dolorem dentium*, por la dolor des denz: Pernez herbe ki est apelé bacuncele,[34] si la triblez e la metez en la palme de la main del malade e la (la) liez tote jor e la nuit si mester seit. Se la maladie seit de la destre part, liez la de cele part, si de la senestre seit, en la senestre main la liez e sein serra si la dent ne seit purrie.

19. *Ad cancrum*, a cancre: Pernez la racine de l'erbe avant dite .i. bacuncele e la reez ke ele seit nette. Si la metez dedenz le cancre deskes[35] as funz. Ja ne crestra tant cum la racine i serra.

20. *Por gute enossee*, por gute enossee: Pernez miel e pain egre, si trenchez aleskes, si fetes bien toster. Pus triblez od le miel e od ail en un morter od vin egre. Si l'eschaufez bien e metez sor la gute. Pus li donez a beivre conseude mendre, herbive, avence quit en cerveise, calketrappe chald.

21. *Por gute eiuere*, por gute eiuere .s. noli me tangere, oignement: Recipe coperuns de runces, cerfoil, le vert chardun, chardun salvage, wderove, horselle .i. henula campana, vif sufre, peivre mulu, gresse de porc. Quisez ensemble, pus culez parmi un drap. Pus oignez le mal, si garra.

22. *Por mal de mamele*, por mal de la memele ki est emflee e neire e dure e ne prent mie a teste crever: Fetes beivre petite conseude, [f.177v] avence, solsequie. Pus metez le past là [ou] vus volez sor la mamele, si depescera. Pus li donez a beivre kersuns de ewe.

23. *Por esquinancie*, por esquinancie: Pernez pié de pulein, betonie, fenoil e poi de jusquiamo, si quisez ben, si le[36] fetes estuver utre le pot quant il seit quiz. Iço valt a cancre e a depescer apostume en la gorge.

24. *Por parlesie*, por parlesie: Pernez ambrosie .i. sauge salvage, primerole de pré, primerole de herber, planteine, gupillere .i. foxesglove, pelusee, maroil, nepte, rue, fenoil, herbe seint Johan, centoire, saxifragie. Quisez en un jalun de vin vermail deskes al tierz. Si li donez a beivre trei fie le jor: matin, aprés manger e al seir chald. Pus li fetes bain de ces herbes: menu ache, luvesche, fenoil, tanesie, moleine, foilles de sauz e de pruner, pié de pulein, malves de curtil, seneçun, chikemete, morun. Si le fetes baigner chescun altre jor par .v. jors. Pus fetes oignement: recipe luvesche, petite ache, wimalve, ortie griache, maroil, waronce, aloine. Triblez bien ensemble bone poignee. Pus pernez gresse

de porc, recopee, fiel de porc. Si en fetes oignement e oignez le malade dous fie le jor.

25. *Por mal de fundement,* por mal del fundement .s. amorroides e manjue [de] le fundement: Pernez chanlee .i. jusquiamum e porette de curtil, bilre, waterbil, kersuns de funtaine, faverole. Quisez les bien en veu vin ou en vin egre. Pus fetes le malade ser sur un eschamel percé. Si s'estuvet bien. Pus fetes oigne-ment: pernez chanlee, brionie, waterbilre, veil gresse de porc. Quisez en-semble, si preignez parmi un drap. Si oignez le fundement dous fie le jor.

26. *Por berbelez des jambes,* por berbelez ki cressent as jambes e devenent lez: Fetes emplastre de jubarbe manipulos duos, aloine manipulos quinque, rue manipu-los quinque. Triblez od le jus, metez sor le mal. Si ensechera, si garra, mes ke il seit enfestré.

Por cel meimes: Quisez bien arkangelicam herbe. En cele ewe baignez la jambe u altre menbre. Pus metez l'emplastre sure tant cum mester est. E pus emplastrez le liu des moeus des oes.

27. *Por dolur des [denz],* por la dolur des denz: . . .[37]

28. **[f.178r]** . . .[38] *Contra fevre ague:* Pernez la flur de cremel .i. edocke, si en fetes ewe sicum l'en fet ewe rose. Pus par cel ewe si moillez la funtaine de la teste celui ki est en ague e les temples, piz, mains, piez desus e desuz e l'eschine e totes les jointes du cors, si tornera le tierz jor.

29. *Pur gutes rungesuns,* pur gutes rungesuns: Pernez brianie [sic], chersuns de ewe, faverole, farine de aveine, siu de mutun. Batez tot ensemble. Pus le quisez bien, si metez sor le mal si chald cum il purra sufrir, si garra.

30. *Pur plaie garir,* pur plaie garir e por oster morte char: Pernez une manere de pere cum coperose, seez la e la pudre metez en la plaie une feiz le jor.

31. *Contre morte subite:* Pernez herbe orible .s. papwrt, si la destemprez od ewe u od vin, si li versez en la buche. Primes li overez les denz.

32. *Contre le mal de flanc:* Pernez cumin un quarter, si triblez en un morter. Pus per-nez une livre de miel e metez le pudre od le miel, sil quisez par resun. Pus le versez sor un canevaz e fetes emplastre, si metez sor le mal si chald cum il le poet sufrir. Pus pernez la racine de orible e la semence de luvesche, si triblez ensemble e metez en ses viandes.

33. *Pur estancher fresche plaie:*[39] Pernez les menues plumes desuz les eles de geline, si metez en l'entree de la plaie e pus si beive eufrasie, sicum avant est dit.

34. *Encontre gute crampe:* Pernez celidonie, matefelun, avence, autant de celidonie cum des altres herbes. Pus les triblez bien ensemble e pernez oille de olive, siu de mutun, seim de pork, mastic, encens, sil quisez un poi, si le metez sor un canevaz, pus sor le mal si chald cum il le purra sufrir.

35. *A home eschaudé de ewe:* Pernez fiens de owe e oille, cerfoil. Quisez ensemble un poi. Pus metez sor le mal alkes tieve, si sanera.

36. *Pur fere collirie as oilz:* Pernez freses muntant d'un galun e les metez en un pot

de areim, si le metez en terre.[40] Pus coverez le pot [f.178v] e metez desus bone quantité de terre. Lesez estre en terre quarante jors. Pus pernez sus le pot, si metez hors les freses, les colez parmi un drap. Si pernez vin blanc, la tierce part del vin seit od le jus. Pus pernez lard, sil trenchez menuement e metez en altre vin blanc. Lesez estre une nuit. Pus pernez bure de mai autant cum del lard, fundez ensemble. Aprés ce pernez calamine, si l'ardez en feu .ix. feiz, pus si l'esteignez en vin blanc ausi sovent. Pus brusez tot en pudre, pesez la quarte part de coperose blanc encuntre les treis parties de calamine.[41] Si pernez encens, mastic, aloen epatik e autant de perre sanguin cum de encens e de mastic e aloen epatik. Suz ciel n'at meillure.

37. *Por emfleure de face ki sudeement avient:* Pernez maroil, herbe beneite, leveine de past, foilles de sui .i. elren, avence. Pernez le past od les herbes triblez ensemble. Fetes emplastre sor la face, si garra. Metez od l'emplastre si mester seit, vin ou cerveise, si il seit dur.

38. *Por le mort mal:* Pernez foilles de sui .i. elren, si les brusez bien e a tote la sustance liez sor le mal e issi seit .iii. jors. Le quart jor ostez le e le renovelez e issi seit .iii. jors, si sanera.

39. *A nerf trenché u veine:* Pernez filipendulam, donez la racine a beivre. Cest tret ensemble nerf e veine (e) sane.

40. *A nerf copé:* [42] Pernez pudre de sauge e le verm ki l'en apele madoc. Triblez ensemble, metez sore. Si filipendula i seit, mielz valt. Ele sule le fet.[43]

41. *A nerf engurdi:* Pernez malvas, solsequie, gresse de chapun ou de geline, cire virgine. Triblez ensemble, sil quisez, colez parmi un drap, oignez le liu.

42. *Por brusure de coste ou pur quel os ki seit depescé:* Pernez spalet, en iver la semence, en esté l'herbe. Brusez la, si la destemprez od le jus de ache. Metez i gleire, ferine de furment, sil fetes espés cum mel. Metez sor un drap linge tenue, pus sor le mal al matin e al seir si chald cum sufrir le purra.

43. *Por manere de rumpure ki vient hors as esues cum pelote:* Pernez comfirie, senicle, petite conseude. Pus pernez la cue de lievre, si mincez le peil de cele cue menuement. Triblez bien ensemble. Pus quisez en miel. Sil metez en boiste. Pus li donez a manger muntant a .iiii. feves al matin e al seir. Pus metez "l'entrete as chivalers' sor le mal, si garra.

44. *Pur rumpure:* Pernez ysacle, la batez e la destemprez od let de vache, colez parmi un drap, donez al malade a beivre. Si li liez sus les pendant, k'il entrent en lor liu.

45. *Item:* Moleine, la teste de ail sechez bien. Pus le ardez en pudre. Triblez en un morter, metez la pudre sor le mal.

46. *A nerf copé e a veine e as altres copeures:* [44] Pernez le verm ki est apelé madoc, mastic, encens fronc, sauge. Destemprez tot el jus de crops de runces, si metez sore.

47. *A mors de chien:* Pernez planteine, veil oint, batez ensemble, metez sor le mal.

48. *Pur rumpure e boel entamé*: Si buel seit entamé, pernez senicle, si la batez, le jus li donez a beivre dous [45] fie le jor par noef jors, e sanera.

49. *Pur les oilz ki sunt ruges*: Pernez une cuiz ruge, si frotez quivre desore. Pus pernez calamine e frotez aprés sor la perre. Pus pernez blanc vin en un veissel, si plungez el vin a chescune feiz le quivre e ausi le calamine deskes le vin seit bien espés. Pus pernez .iii. [f.179r] ou .iiii. gutes, metez as oilz, si garra.

50. *Pur fere la face blanche e vermeille*: Pernez nef salvage, ostez l'escorce dehors, si pernez le blanc dedenz, frotez entre vos mains. Pus frotez la face, pus lavez la face de ewe tieve.

51. *A la maladie le rei*: Pernez le fund de pork,[46] la racine de avence. Batez bien ensemble en un morter, metez l'enplastre al matin e al seir noef jors, si garra.

52. *A nerfs retrez*: Pernez mawe, espurge, cire virgine, gresse de geline. Quisez bien ens[e]mble, metez en boiste, si en oignez les ners retrez.

53. *Pur gute aragee ke va par tot le cors*: Pernez blanc chaudun [sic] .i. metteleve. Triblez en un morter, sil destemprez od vin ou cerveise. Colez parmi un drap, si li donez a beivre. Avant ke il le beive entre en une mesun sul od . . .[47] u oisel u beste, kar il en serra quite, l'altre avera la maladie.

54. *Pur gute*: Pernez avence, kalketrap, matefelon, herbive. Brusez lé ke vus en eez le jus. Bevez le al matin freit, al seir chald.

55. *Pur gute chaive*: Pernez wi de cheine .i. ok-nistle. Pendez al col celui ki ad gute cheive e ke il le porte tute sa vie, si serra garri. Le premer jor die Pater Noster noef feiz, Ave Maria noef feiz e dous jors suant.

56. *Pur gute festre chaude*: Pernez filipendulam, herbe Robert, sauge salvage, agrimoniam, avence, herbe cruisee, cinquefole, [MS vq; fol.] de ces oele porciun. Pus pernez de warance autant cum de totes les altres herbes, si li fetes beivre. Aprés ce pernez la foille de runce u la foille de cholet, triblez, si metez sor la plaie dous fie le jor.

57. *Pur gute festre*: Pernez un herbe k'est apelee angelica,[48] tunde herbam, bibe succum eius e la drasche metez sor le festre, si l'ocira.

58. *Pur gute artatik ki vient as juintes*: Pernez avence, seneçun, heihove, ortie griache. Triblez ensemble ke vus en eez le jus. Metez le jus sor un drap, liez entor le mal. Le tierz jor garra.

59. *Pur estancher sanc de buche u de nés*: Pernez creie e d'oustant de flur, mastic, encens, le blanc de l'oef. Pus metez cele emplastre sor un drap e pus al frunt deskes [49] as temples. Si estanchera le sanc.

60. *Pur tuer le cancre*: Pernez miel e chauz, en fetes un tortel. Pus le metez el feu ke il seit si chald cum feu ardant. Pus metez siel sor un drap, si metez el feu bone pose. Aprés pernez le siel e le turtel. Triblez ensemble. Pus metez le pudre sor le cancre.

61. *Pur tuer cancre*: [50] Pernez les membres de la grue .s. la teste od le col, les piez, entrailles. Metez en pot de terre, sil coverez bien, sil metez en un furn deskes il seit en pudre. Pus metez le pudre sor le cancre, si l'ocira.

62. *Pur oster dertes e roine*: Pernez la racine de ruge parele, la racine de roge ortie, racine de regal .i. kukuspitte, racine de elena campane. Triblez les bien en-semble. Pus pernez veil oint, sil quisez bien ensemble, colez parmi un drap, metez en boiste, oignez dertes e roine.

63. *Pur malveis aleine*: Pernez le fust aloen, galingal, gilofre, vin blanc, piç. Quisez ensemble. De cest pernez le peis de un dener, metez as narilles u en la buche .iii. feiz le jor. Pus en fetes gargarisme.

64. *Por la piere gareisun*: Pernez fiens de colums blans u neirs. Quisez le en vin, ke il seit bien espés. Li donez a beivre al matin freit, le seir chald, si garra en noef jors.

65. **[f.179v]** *Pur brusure*, pur brusure de piez u de mains: Pernez verveine, siel bone partie, triblez ensemble. Metez sor le mal, pus moillez un cince el blanc de l'oef e la cince metez ultre .ii. fie le jor.

66. *Por brusure e por dolur*: Pernez sparge, seneçun, avence, coperun de runce, de ces oele mesure. Triblez ke vus en eez le jus. Pus pernez cire virgine, oille de oes[51] oele mesure. Quisez tot ensemble. Colez parmi un drap, metez en boiste, oignez le mal e s'empartira.

67. *Esperement a dissinterie*: Pernez comfirie, brisez la bien. Pus pernez leit de vache ki seit de une colur, destemprez tot ensemble, colez parmi un drap. Aprés per-nez flur de furment e la terce part de mole creie, si en fetes pulment sicum l'en fet as enfanz. Si le seignez in nomine Patris et cetera. Sil quisez aukes e priez Deu ke si il devera vivre ke la viande pusse bien turner. Si li donez a manger, se altrement se turne, ne li donez mie.

68. *A femme ke ne poet enfanter e l'enfant malement turne*: Pernez un eschamel per(e)cé en milliu, si metez vis charbuns desoz e sor les charbuns metez la rasure de l'ungle del pié de chival. Pus sece la femme sor l'eschamel a nues nages e receive cele fumee deske ele se sente estre amendee.

69. *A home ki est eschaudé* [52] *de femme u de sa nature demeine*: Pernez planteine, chi-kemete, semence de linois, veil oint, flur de furment. Quisez ensemble, fetes emplastre, metez sor le mal si chald cum il le poet sufrir.

70. *A cel meimes*: Pernez leit de vache, ferine d'orge, siu de mutun, pudre de tan, vin vermeil, linois. Quisez ensemble a l'espesor de miel. Metez sor un drap espés si chald cum il le puet sufrir. Si i volupez le menbre e les pendanz, si garra.

71. *Por rancle de mamele de home u de femme*: Pernez morun,[53] gresse de pork, gresse de mutun oele mesure. Triblez ensemble, metez sor le mal.

72. *Pur apostumes*: Pernez linois. Quisez en ewe ferine de aveine, vin, leit de vache, de ces chos[es] oele mesure. Pus pernez siu de mutun, sil trenchez me-nuement, metez od tot. Sil quisez bien, metez sor un drap cum emplastre, pus sor le mal dous feiz le jor si chald cum il le puet sufrir.

73. *A crestre bone char u ele crut avant*: Pernez porrettes, si les triblez. Pus pernez siu de mutun e d'oustant de gresse de pork. Triblez tot ensemble, metez sor un drap, pus sor le mal, si crestra bone char.

74. *Por morsure de chien aragé*: Pernez mente, siel, triblez ensemble.

75. *Por le verm ki est apelé fich*: Pernez herbe seinte Fiacre .s. kukuspitte [54] muntant une feve, si metez entre dous oblees. Pus metez en vostre buche, sil tranglutez si tost cum vus poez. Fetes cest .iii. jors e le verm murra.

76. *Item*: Pernez le neir limaçun, si le liez vif sor le umblil. Liez le ferm un jor e une nuit deske il seit percé, e garra.

77. *Por le fich senglant*: Pernez siu de buk, semence de canve, triblez ensemble. Pus fetes noef pelotes si grosses cum une nugage. Pus pernez .iii. tueus, si les metez el feu ke il seent bien chald. Pus fetes une fose en terre, si metez la tuele leinz. [f.180r] Pus metez une pelote desure. Si pernez le muel de la charette, le gros chef ver val, e sece le malade sore si tost cum une pelote est refreidie. Renovelez les treis pelotes e les .iii. tueles par .iii. jors. Issi fetes ke les noef pelotes seent degastees en .iii. jors, si garra.

78. *Al leu vel lupum*: Pernez les cheels u le cheel de levrer ki seit dedenz noef jors veil. Purfendez le ventre e le piz, ostez les entrailles e si chald metez sor la plaie. Liez le ferm. Si il est gentil home, pernez lise de levrer, si vilain, pernez lise mastive. [55]

79. *A teste depescé u kakenele bon beivre*: Bugle, pigle, senicle, avence, de ces herbes seit ewe fete cum ewe rose, chescune herbe par sei. E dunc seent mis ensemble totes oele mesure.

80. *A teste depescee e kakenele descendue resordre*: Pernez violette, si la triblez bien. Pus la metez desuz la plante del pié un jor e une nuit, si resurdra le test.

81. *Emplastre a teste depescee*: Solsequie, encens, mastic, poi reisin, cire virgine, de poi reisin autant cum de toz les altres. De ces fetes sicum l'en fet [corr. l'entret?] cirante. Metez sor un drap, pus sor la teste, si resurdra le test ki fu avant descendu par le cop. Pus li donez a beivre bugle, pigle, senicle, warance autant cum de totes les altres herbes.

82. *A ruine*: Pernez le moel de l'oef e le blanc ot tot, sil movez bien. Pus pernez ache, si en fetes jus, flur de furment, miel. Triblez ensemble. Metez tenve sor une foille, pus sor le mal. E si est bon a plaie e a felun.

83. *A fere chevoz crestre*: Pernez le ruge limaçun, sil quisez, coille la gresse. Pus pernez le neir ars ki est desoz le plum u chaudere as funz, si mellez od la gresse. Pus oignez le liu u volez k'il cressent.

84. *Item*: Pernez la joefne racine de ache, si la triblez bien. Pus pernez pur miel, mellez od tot, si oignez le liu. Si fetes garser le liu u volez ke il cressent.

85. *A home ki est gros de ventre*: Pernez egrimoine, fumiterie. Li donez a beivre, si garra. S'il seit costive, il se delivera.

86. *Ki emfle e asuage entur le cors*: Pernez wisminte, [56] febrifugie, aloine. Triblez ensemble oele quantité. Pus pernez ferine de segle e fetes le espés cum past. Eschaufez le en une paele. Metez sor un drap e pus sor le ventre si chald cum il purra sufrir. Treis feiz le jor le renovelez.

87. *Por maladie ke est apelé elfkechel ki greve entur le piz*: Pernez orge, si le metez en ewe .iii. jors. Pernez cele ewe, si i quisez hennebane a l'espesisor de miel. Pus

bien chald en oignez le mal. Icest est bon a la maladie k'est apelé elfkechel, une maladie entor le quor.

88. *Pur jointe aloché*: Pernez feves mulues, si les quisez ben. Pus pernez cumin demi poignee e autant de vin egre cum entreit en dous oes. Triblez cest ensemble, si metez od les feves, metez sor un drap e pus sor la juinte. Si trera hors l'angoisse e garra. Metez l'emplastre dous fie le jor.

89. *Por plaie saner hastivement*: Pernez jus de ache, planteine, jus de por, de ces oelement. Pus pernez blanc de l'oef, flur de furment, pudre de tan, sauge, miel, fetes alkes espés. [f.180v] Metét sur un clutet tenve, pus sor la plaie, si sanera.

90. *A brisure de jambe* u braz: Pernez osmunde, confirie, conseude mendre. Donét a beivre al malade od vin u cerveise dous fie le jor.
  Emplastre a mettre sur le mal: [57] Pernez ache, kersun, en esté le herbe, en yver la semence, stanche, henne[bane], kersun. Triblez ensemble. Pus pernez flur de furment e le blanc de l'oef. Sil fetes espés cum miel. Metez sor un drap. Pus pernez feltre, metez environ la jambe u braz, aprés ce les esplentés.

91. Si pié ou main seit percé parmi de clo ou cutel: Pernez herbe verte cumune, si est ele greele. Metez le jus en la plaie e la sustance pardesure deske seit gari. [all written in left-hand margin]

92. *Si verm (ki) est en oreille*, si verm .s. erwigge seit en orille a l'home: Pernez oille de granz noiz, si metez en l'altre oreille e issi gice une pose sor l'altre coste, si istra le verm u murra.

93. *Ad malum mortuum*:[58] Entrete cirante est bone a mort mal e fiel de tor ausi a cel meimes.

94. *A la maele de l'oil*: In nomine Patris et Filii et Spiritus Sancti, Amen. Ter dicatur. Et face le signe sor les oilz. 'Joe vus cunjur, gute maele, el nun del Pere, del Fiz, e del seint Esperit, e de ma dame seinte Marie e dé .xii. apostres e dé .iiii. ewangelistes ki sustenent le throne, Johan, Luc, Marc, Mathieu e par la merite seint Leger, de Eve, de Adam, de flum Jordan e de kanke Deu fist en ciel e terre, se vus estes neire, Dex vus deseivre; se vus estes ruge, Dex vus derumpe; se vus estes blanche, Dex vus deface. El nun del Pere, del Fiz e del Seint Esperit'. Li malade die .iii. Pater Noster e celui ki dit le charme die .iii. Pater Noster. Pus pernez un . . .[59] ke l'en apele . . . Pernez ent .v. Triblez les en ewe beneite, si li metez . . . Pus altres .v. destemprez cum les altres. Li donez a beivre. Quant vus nomez les .iiii. ewangelistes, a chescun nun donez la beneiçun sor les oilz al malade. Noef jors le face l'en issi e garra.[60]

95. *Ki ne poet a femme aver afere*: Pernez valeriene a bast[?], la racine en iver, en esté la foille. Li donez a beivre en vin, si fra son plaisir.

96. *A la gute artatike*: Heyhove, broke-lemeke, chikemete, herbe beneite, moleine, herbive. Triblez les, si les friez en siu de mutun e metez entor le menbre malade.

97. *A teine*: Pernez veil oint, vif argent, mellez bien ensemble, si oignez.

98. *A fere cancre*: Pernez savun e chauz, si metez là u vus volez, si resemblera cancre e nel serra mie. Se volez ke le mal dure lungement, oignez le un poi de seim freis. Si tost volez estre gari, pernez oille des oefs, si oignez e garra.

99. A *fere felon*: Pernez herbe corruble dorré e metez en une eschale de petite noiz, si metez là [u] vus volez e resemblera felun, si nel sera mie. Oignez le de seim, si durra lungement. Si tost volez estre sein, oignez le de oille des oes.

100. Entrete as chivalers:[61] Pernez encens .i. quarter, cire .i. livre, dragagant .i. quarter, gume arabic .i. quarter, aloen epatic .i. quarter, mastic .i. quarter, feingré dimi libra, cumin .i. quarter, de bol .ii. unces, sarcocol .ii. unces, neire peiz demi livre, poresin[62] .ii. livres, de musge le pois de dous deners. La confectiun: primes fundez la cire en une paele, pus pernez le poresin e movez ensemble. Primes veez ke les gumes e les semences seent bien triblez a pudre en un morter. Pus pernez les pudres od la cire e od le poresin e la neire peiz, si movez toteveis od .i. esclice. Pus colez parmi .i. drap, si lessez estre em pes une nuit. Pus pernez e metez en quir u . . .[63]

101. [f.181r] . . . Ad plagam, por saner estraite plaie: . . .[64]

102. A chescune manere de ru[ine]:[65] Pernez feniil, persil, maroil, chikemete ki crest desuz terre, jusquiamum .i. hennebane, herbe beneite, lemeke, de totes oele mesure de chescune dous bones puignees. Pus fetes le patient ser tot nu en une grant cuve sanz ewe sor un eschamel percé en mulliu. Pus metez des herbes d'une part de lui en la cuve e de l'altre part e devant li. Pus fetes eschaufer .iii. tueles si chald cum feu ardant, si metez sor les .iii. munceaus des herbes. Issi seit estuvé. Quant les tuel[es] sunt refreidies, pernez altres, si metez sor meimes les herbes. Pus suera a merveilles e le purgera de tote la maladie, mes ke il feust lepre. Il serra mut travaillé. Pur çoe le fetes alkes manger avant ke il i entre. Issi le face .iii. jors.

103. *Por arsure de feu*, por arsure de feu u de ewe: Pernez oille comun, cerfoil, fiens de owe u de columb. Quisez ensemble, metez sor le mal si chald cum sufrir le purra.

104. A *felun en liu perilleus*, ki ad le felon en liu perilleus e remuer le vodra: Prenge .i. oistre vel .ii. crues e lie desoz la plante de pié .i. jor u .i. nuit e le felon saldra iloec, u en quel liu mener[66] le volez, metez ce e le liez. Pus le lavez.

105. [f.181v] Ad sannarium:[67] Herbe dent de leon frotez en vos mains. Pus metez as narilles ke vus en eez la sentine. Pus si esgardez le herbe une pose, si estanchera le sanc del niés. Mescine vereie esprovee est.

106. *Por fevre ague*, por fevre ague mescine vereie: Le jus de herbe celidonie li donez une fie a beivre. E si il git de une part, fetes le torner de l'altre. Pus comencera a dormir. Quant s'en veillera, si demandera a manger. Si la maladie seit si forte ke il ne puse ne ne voille estre tenu u ausi cum il se arage, pernez la racine del seu .i. elren, si ostez l'escorce dehors e pernez cel dedenz ki[68] est tendre tant cum poet entrer en demi eschale d'un oef. Si destemprez od la racine avant dite de celidonie, si li donez a beivre, si serra par la Dex grace tot sein. . . .

107. Ad memoriam animi:[69] Pernez le busard .i. eicute, si le lesez .iii. jors gisir mort. Pus pernez sa lange, si la metez .iii. jors en miel. Pus la metez desoz la lange celui ki ad perdu memorie, si la recuvera.

Chapter Nine

MEDICAL RECEIPTS AND THE *ANTIDOTARIUM*

The celebrated medical MS, Cambridge, Trinity College 0.1.20, contains two small miscellanies of medical receipts which the scribe may have thought to be part of other works which he was copying.[1] Despite uncertainty about their origin, they are included in the present study in illustration of the *antidotarium* as contrasted to the *receptarium*: the receipts are more complex (with not a few *exotica*) and the drug compounds are headed by names rather than by medical indications, serving as remedies for a whole constellation of ailments. Their debt to the *Antidotarium Nicolai* is obvious. The first collection (A) begins with a series of ointments (*unguenta*) (ff.30rb–32vb) set out in double columns with alternating red and blue initials and red rubrics. At f.33r the scribe changes to long lines and single columns for what is a set of conventional receipts roughly grouped according to their indications (ff.33r–36v). The occurrence of the word *ramese* 'ramsons' suggests an English origin. The possibility that the texts of MS 0.1.20 were transcribed from continental copies containing some words of insular origin cannot be dismissed. There now follows (ff.37r–44v), without any distinguishing mark, the 'Lettre d'Hippocrate' shorn of its prefatory matter on humours and urines which is found later on ff.53r–55r. Between these two parts of the *Lettre* comes a short treatise (B) composed of receipts with the character of an *antidotarium*, written in single columns, with red rubrics and alternating red and blue initials (ff.45r–52v). These two miscellanies give us some idea of the vernacular treatment of *materia medica* as found, for example, in the *Compendium medicinae* of Gilbertus Anglicus which was composed in the first half of the thirteenth century and incorporated much of the *Antidotarium Nicolai* and other medical works.[2]

A.

1. **[f.30rb]** APOSTOLICOM CIRURGICOM [3]
Apostolicum cirurgicom est faite en tele manere: Pernez pois dont om englue nefs demie livre, pois gregoise une livre, galbanon, amoniacon, serapiron, apopanac, de chescun demie once et de chire .iii. onces, aizil une livre. L'aizil [corr. l'oignement] est fait issi: l'aizil seit mis en un vassel d'esteim ovec les goumes, lesqueles ne devent mie estre tribleez. Quant eles serront deffaites, .i. poi seit mis en freide ewe et quant eles se tendront et auront mués lor color, pois gregois, mastic, encens, de chescun demie once triblé en poudre seit mis avec ce ke jo ai dit devant en le vas **[f.30va]**sel d'estaim. Et movez tousjors de le spatele et quant il ert mué de blanc en

jaune, signe est de parfaite decoction. L'esteim ostez et metez une once de terbentine. Totes icés choses seient mellés ensemble. Colez totes icés choses sor froide ewe parmi un drap. Oigniez vos mains en oile d'olive ou en autre licor et estraiez hors l'oignement de l'ewe et espressez hors l'ewe et faites torteus. Cest oignement vaut a l'esplen et a os lier. Aprés le reliement de l'os il onie l'os et polist, il oste le dolor del piz de froisseure.

2. APOSTOLICOM BASTART

Apostolicom bastart vaut a dolor oster et rancle ocire et a plaie saner. Pernez cire virge .vi. onces, une poignee d'ache, une poigne d'aloi [f.30vb]ne,.i. poine d'ortie, .i. poigne de vetoine, .i. poigne de sanicle, .i. poigne de eble, une poigne de bugle, .i. poigne de doke. Si triblez totes ces herbes ensemble mult bien et quisez en .i. noef pot ovec la cire et puis le colez parmi .i. drap. Et metez autretant de neir pois com de la cire. Et pernez l'entresuc de le neire espine une livre (et de l'entresuc) et saim de geline et blaunc saim de porc et quisez tot ensemble mult bien et laissez refreidir. Et coillez tote la gresse que flotera desus et le batez en un vassel et coillez bien et bel. Et puis pernez franc encens, mugue, gilofre et metez ovec vostre gresse et mellez tot ensemble d'une verge mult tresbien sauf, kar ce flaire mult bien et si fait le vis mult net et mult . . .[4]

3. [f.31ra] DE L'OIGNEMENT POR TOTES DOLORS

Oignement por totes dolors et por totes angoisses et por totes plaies: Pernez bugle, sanicle, consoude le petite, egremoine, pigle, plantain, ache, quintefoille et treifoil, lancelee, pervenke, avance, fraziere, simarin vert, osmonde, foiles de poret. Icés herbes seient pris novelement et triblés et frites en bure de mai. Et seient bien quites et colees parmi .i. drap et le jus seit remis en la paele. Et pernez blanc encens et virge cire et seient mis en cel jus et boillis ensemble et refroidies et en sauf mis. Totes plaies, totes dolors et touz rancles enoignez et serront garriz sauns doute. Esprové chose est. Et seient icés herbes quillés en mai.

4. A FAIRE DIAUTÉ[5]

A faire diauté: Pernez oint de [f.31rb] capon et oint de geline et saim de mene de porc, la sisime part de virge cire. Pernez les noiaus de l'argentine qui sont en la racine et de l'herbe autresi et de l'ormiel. Et pernez del seu de cerf tant com vous volez, mes ke il n'en i ait trop. Fondez tot ce ensemble fors les herbes. Triblez les herbes et premez hors le jus et mellés ovec le saim qui fondu est. Et puis laissez refroydir. Si il vous semble ke ele seit trop mole, metez autretant de cire come devant et autretant de siu de cerf. Et si il vous semble ke ele ne flaire assez suef, metez autretant de pois blanche come il(l) i a d'encens. Et si vous n'avez blanche pois, si metez encens.

5. (A)POPELION[6]

A faire popelion: Plantain [f.31va], jubarbe, oinzerole, ronce, lettue, olie de[7] violet, morele, canellie, frazier et del poplier le plus et oint de porc masle freis. Et quant vous le quisez, si metez de l'aisi[l].

6. [. . .][8] Herbe que ad a non ramese et cresson d'ewe, ache, et pernez autretant de l'un com de l'autre et faites jus. Si ce est en esté, donez a beivre au malade. Si vous le volez garder en yver, quisez le en zucre, si le garderez le saison.

7. OIGNEMENT SANATIF

A oignement sanatif faire: Pernez avance qui douce medecine avance, esparge qui tous les maus esparde, et tormentine qui tous les maus define. Or pernez pigle, bugle et senicle. Et pernez herbe(r) Robert, herbe [f.31vb] Wautier et consoude et confire et launcelee et plantain, mirfoil et herbe yve et folle, chierfoil et leusavon.[9] Triblez les herbes ensemble et si pernez saim de porc et siu de moton autretant de l'un com de l'autre et quisez ensemble et colez parmi .i. drap. Et cele coleure metez en une paiele et metez vostre cire et vostre encens et faites tot boillir ensemble et quire et si est fait.

8. COMENT VOUS DEVEZ TENIR VOS HERBES

Si vous volez vos herbes tenir et garder tot l'an entier, si les coillez en mai et puis si les lavez bien en ewe et puis en bon vin et les essuez un poi au solein. Et puis si les batez bien en un mortier et puis les metez au solein secchier. Et puis les remetez en le mortier et bon [f.32ra] vin ovec et rebatez tot ensemble et metez au solein. Et ce fetes .ii. fiez ou .iii. Et quant vous averez ce fait, si pernez bel mie tot cru, si metez vos herbes ens et movez bien ensemble. Et puis si faites pelotes reondes ausi grant come om fait torteus de gaide et puis si les (t)essués mult tresbien au solein. Et puis les metez en un bel sachel de teile en sauf, ke [10] l'air i poet avenir. Et quant vous volez doner a beivre, si en metez en un sachet de teile temprer en bon vin une nuit ou un jor. Et puis torgiés en un bel hanap et donez vostre malade a beivre.

9. OIGNEMENT

A feire oinement: Pernez la racine de lovache, de wimauve, de fenoil et parez totes ces racines bien et trenchés me[f.32rb]nu. Et metez sor le fu boillir et laissez quire tot a leisir a poi de fu. Et quant ce sera assez quite, pernez hors le grasse ewe et per-nez blanc siu de moton et saim de chevre [11] et siu de cerf et saim de capon, del pome dé bos un livre et une livre de ere et .i. livre de warance et une livre de cen-toire. Totes ces choses quisez bien en aisil, en un noef pot, et metez i plaine es-quiele de corne de chievre menue taillé et quisez tot ce tant ke les .ii. pars seient quit ens. Puis si le colez parmi un drap et puis metez al jus .iii. onces de ewe rose et une once de miel bien espurgé. Puis le boillez tant ke bien seit [. . .] Et puis si metez la cire et l[e] pois. Si le faites boillir ensemble un poi a bon [f.32va] fu de carbon et metez avec .iii. onces d'aloine et .iii. onces de mastic et .iii. onces de blanche re-isine et .iii. onces de franc encens mult delié molu. Et movez tot ce mult bien en-semble et puis metez une once d'oile laurine et puis metez tot ce en un drap linge et secchez sor le fu .viii. jors. Et sachez que ce vaut son peis de fin or.

10. ESPERMENT CONTRE FESTRE ET CANCRE

Ci a esperment esprové contre festre et encontre cancre: Pernez orpiment et flor d'araim ou de verdegrece, arrement, saugeme, corne de cerf arse, (dens de livre ars) les cheveus des aus ars, sanc de dragon, gallitricom, tartaron, escreviches de douce ewe arses, fiente arse, chaus vive, herbe linaire [12] secke, si en fetes poudre. Et blanc [f.32vb] et neir (et) encens et mastic et nitre poudree et vieuz semeles de vieuz sou-lers et les os de morte gent arses et alum, de totes icés choses pernez owellement et les poudrez ensemble. Et après lavez le festre de vin egre ou de urine d'enfant ke seit oncore virges. Après pernez la poudre et poudrez sor le cancre, et si ele est mangé si parfont que la poudre n'i puisse entrer, si le confisez od miel quit et la qui-sez a petit feu. Et si lavez le cancre ou le festre dedens et dehors. Et après botés cele licor dedens. En tele maniere garira.

11. POR ESTRAIRE ESPINE SANZ FER

A traire espine del pié sans fer mettre: Pernez polipode et racine de rosel, si le batez [13] ensemble, et reez de miel et vieuz oint. Et estendez sor .i. drap et metez sor la plaie, si l'entraira sans dolor.

12. [f.33r] [14] POUDRE POUR LA PIERE

Poudre por piere receit semence de persil, de fenoil, de ache, de lovache, les semences de chascon une once, camedreos, dauques, asara, esparge, fregon, de glaios la racine, ireos, ameos, sirmontein, semence de genoivre, ciperon, cassialigne, quintefoille, grumil, sausefrage, melons, citru[lis], [15] concungres, cucubbites [. . .] de l'une et de l'autre, alaustelogie la reonde et la longe, baie de luvercost, [16] coe de porcel, meu, walerien, orobes, anetes, squinant, calament, espic, polipode, anis, caparis, tamarin, eruc blanc, oignion de mer ars, titoloses, de fruit de basme et le fust garengal et gingebre. La libre de cest pudre [vaut] treis souz.

13. POUDRE PUR LA PERE DEPESCIER

Autre poudre por la piere depescier receit mire, ceperon, piç, valeriene, racine de glaiol, de chascone drame et demie, piere de sponge, semence de pavaut blanc, semences de laitues, les quatre semences froides mondees, scolopandre, cassialigne, canele, semence de pannaie, de chascon dous drames et demie. Et de ce face la poudre et en use en son mangier tant come il en porra prendre a treis dois. Le [livre] vaut dous souz.

14. SIROP CONTRE LA PERE

[f.33v] Syrop contre le piere receit grumil et fenoil, coriandre, carvi, peresil macedoine, anis, genoivre, semence de ortie griesse, quintefoille, saxifrage, burnete, lange de oisel, noiels de cerises, espic, poivre blanc, de chascon dous onces, lapi[s] lincis, ciperon, foille de loriers, vetogne, pimpernele, valeriene, esquinant, semence de basilicon, (c)origane, de chascon une once. Et puis meller ensemble et boivre en vin.

15. POUDRE PUR LA PIERE DEPECER

Poudre contre la piere depeccier: Pregnés noiaus de cerises une libre, semence de ortie griesce, sené, caparis, anes une once, brusc, spararge, aura dous drames, peresin, ache, la quarte part de chascon, garingal, nois muscades, pincenart, gariofilat, de chascon la quarte partie de une drame, reubarbe quatre crupes et demie, saffran une drame, grumil, agaric, ana de chescon une drame, saxifrage cinc drames, fenoil [. . .] de chascon une drame, zucre une livre, de l'eue assees. Et de cest faces cirop en tele manere: le zucre boillés par soi en ewe, les choses devant dites pudrees soient mises od la decoction. Estués le en un vassel de voire et donés li pleine escalli de oef en l'eue de la decoction, de l'eue [f.34r] et de ache quite par soi au matin et au soyr.

16. POR TENIR URINE

Si aucune ne poet tenir sa urine, pregne ces choses: mirre, encens, glans de cheine. Et quisés en vin et donez au malade a boivre. Derechief pregnez sanemonde et se le quisez en vin blanc, si le liez sor le penil.

17. ENCONTRE RUMPURE PREMEREMENT

Encontre rumpure premerement: Purgiez tot le cors solonc les humors de l'home et de la femme .iii. jors. Aprés le quart jor baigneez le et aprés le fetes seigner del bras de cele part ou la rumpure est ou de l'autre. Aprés fetes une emplastre. Prenés un pel de levre ot tot le peil et quisez le en ewe tant que ele soit decorue. Et aprés pregnez les poudres que il dira. Se mellez ensemble avec la decoction moumie, bol, sanc de dragon, colofonie, cire, pois, silmoniac, mastic, encens, dragagant, consoude menue et grant, vers de terre, sanc de gent, de chascon .i. once, galbanon, almoniac, de chascun demi once. Et plusors pels de levre soient quit o totes ces choses devant dites et o la decoction. [f.34v] Et puis fetes emplastre et puis baigniez le malade et couchiés. Et puis botés ariere les bouels dedens et metez l'emplastre sus et la pel de levre sus et un platin de plum a la mesure de la rumpure par desus l'emplastre. Et gise li malades en cele partie ou la rumpure est et tiegne en haut ses quisses, que li bouels puissent le plus legerement aler en lor leu. Et ensi gise par .xviii. jors ou par .xx. Si la rumpure est veille, gise en leu repos et soit en pes et se garde de coroz et qu'il [17] ne rie. Et se gard de mauveises viandes que les lieures ne departent par un mois ou par .ii. tresc'a tant qu'il [18] soit gariz. Et il soi gard de luxurie et de viandes enflans tot l'an aprés.

18. CLISTERE EN CHAUDE CAUSE
Ensi fait om clistere en chaude cause et en froide cause. En chaude cause en tele manere: pregnez violete, mauves, aluine, mercuriale. Batez ensemble et puis quissés en ewe o bren de forment et puis les colés et metez ovec sel et oile. Et de cele coleure pregnez .i. livre, si en fetes clistere.

19. CLISTERE EN FROIDE CAUSE
[f.35r] Encontre froide cause si faites clistere en tele manere: Pregnez aluine et averone, calament, origane, mercuriale, mauves, rue. Totes ces choses soient quites en ewe o bran de forment. Se les colés et en cele coleure soient mises .iii. drames de oile commune et une de saugemme. Et de totes celes choses pregnez une livre, si en fete[s] clistere.

20. CLISTERE COMMUNE
Autre clistere commune faites en tele manere: Pregnez mauves et mercuriale et sel et oile et miel et ewe et quisiez ensemble et les colez. Et de cele coleure pregnez une livre, si en faites clistere.

21. CONTRE CANCRE
Encontre cancre: Pregnez suie et alum blanc et arnement [et] vert de grece. De ces faites poudre. Et metez sor le cancre, si le ocirra en poi de hure. Derechief pregnez orpiment et alum et suffre et savon de outre mer. Mellez ensemble icés choses et metez sor le cancre, si garra.

22. CONTRE ARTETIKE
Contre artetique et autre goute: Pregnez le fiel de boef et traiez fors la liquor. Et prenez oignons rouges et boilliez ensemble une poi de hure. Et aprés le colez parmi .i. drap et enoignez le malade contre le feu.

23. [f.35v] ENCONTRE ARTETIKE
Encontre artetike: Pernez corne de cerf et si la raez par dehors. Et puis le decoupez menu et quisez en .i. pot ovec bon vin vermail. Et emplez les .ii. pars de vin et la tierce de oile violat et le quisez bien .iii. jors tot adés. Et si com le vin quirra ens, le reemplez tousjors ariere.

24. CESTE POUDRE EST PRINCIPALE ACONTRE PIERE ET GRAVELE

Ceste poudre receit mugue, ambre, de chescune .ii. drames, oile musceline, oile nardus, oile sanguine, cost, de chescune .ii. drames et demie, reubarbe, reupont, le fust
de basme et le fruit de basme, cubebes, de chescune .iiii. drames, gingembre, spic,
racine de glaiol, canele, mente, peivre lonc, peivre neir, saxifrage, de chescune .x.
drames, gilofre, licoriz, ciperon, dragagant blanc, peresile macedoine, germendree,
ameos, semence de ache, semence de sparge, semence de basilicon, semence de
ortie de outre mer, escorce de citre, de chescune .x. drames, sinocassia, croc, squinant, dellion, mastic, ireos, amome, semence de lovasche, gromil, semence de
peresil, sirmontain, [f.36r] cardamome, semence de anet, euforbe, de chescune .x.
drames, feie de butor, char de lion, sanc de bouc, balsami, de chescune .x. drames,
brioine, fenoile, mauves, semence de aresces, arostrologie reonde, centoire,
dauques, foilles de lorier, de chescune .x. drames, puliol, petre, pioine, savine, de
chescune .x. drames, peivre blanc .iiii. drames, carvi, fisalidos, esternue, erostro-
logie longe, titolose, de chescune .i. once, lapis lincis, piere d'ermenie, agapis, lapis
lazuli,[19] limaille d'or pure et de argent, ausi de chescune demie once, gravele de vin
blanc, limaille de fer bien lavee et nettié en vin egre par .ix. fois et puis bien assués
au solein, et zucre de alisandre blanc .ii. livres, et face poudre et melle tot ensemble. Et en use sor sa viaunde au matin et al seir. La livre de ceste poudre vaut
.xx. souz.

25. A GINGEMBRE CONFIRE

Gingembre conduit receit eringes bien reses a un coutel et aprés quites en ewe. Et
quant eles seront quites, l'en (les) deit priendre hors le jus entre les mains [f.36v] et
puis oster a un coutel l'escorche par dehors. Et puis trencher les par menues pieces et
puis batre en un morter de quevre. Et puis prendre .iii. livres pesant de les peces de
eringes apareilleez si come nous avoms devant dit et .x. livres de mel blanc bien
escumé et quite tant ke ele deviegne tot rouge. Aprés pernez demi livre de gingembre sec et decoupez a un coutel par pieces et puis le metez boillir od le mel et od les
eringes a petit fu. Et quant ele sera espesse, le metez a tere et puis metez ces herbes
d'espices: gingembre .iii. onces, galingal demie once, gilofre demi once, canele demi
once, nois muscades demi once, cardamome demi once, pignons mondés .iiii. onces.
Ceste lectuaire conforte le pis et le stomac et les reins et le chief. La livre vaut .iii.
souz.

26. ENCONTRE SORDESON DES OREILLES

Pernez oile de forment et oile de moeus des oes et saim de anguille. Icés .iii. choses
mellez ensemble et puis les degotez en l'oreille.

27. A CE MEIME

Vaut l'oile del freine par sei degotee en l'oreille.

B.

[f.45r]
I . . . medicines s . . . s a doner medicine . . .
Quant vodrés doner medicine a malades, se regardé[s] la quele humor li abunde el
cors et quele maladie il ad. Se ce est fleume, vus le devés atraire par oximel donier

et quant la matere ert apparillé, que vus le conustrés par l'especeté ou par la color de l'urine, se li dietés, ainz que vus li donés medicine, par troi jors de bones viandes et solubles, et si mangut porees que soit fait de mauves et de mercuriale, et se i metés char de porc. Si vus n'avés poree, si pregnez oignions et metés ovec la char de porc. Et se ce est en tens que on ne doit mie manger char, se mangut teles viandes, c'est asavoir menuise, perches, luz, roches, poissons a grosse escardes de mer et de duce ewe. Aprés ceste diete [se li donés] paulin en piles [20] au pesant de sis drames al soir. Et se vus veez que il alasce dou fois ou trois ou quatre ou plus par iceste medicine, aprés cest jor prenés beneoite [21] et gerapigre [22] et se l'agusés de une crupe de esule et d'escamomie, le pesant d'une maille, poudree desus, et si lé mellés ensemble o trois dois et si en faces piles, et si les faites le jor que vus vodreés doner. Et si vus veés qu'il [f.45v] alasce par le paulin, se prenés quatre drames de la medicine devant, si l'agusiés de une crupe d'esula et de une d'escamonie. Aprés ce, fai piles ensi come vus ai dit et si les donés au malades en (es)niules et en vin aprés covrefeu. Aprés ce le fetes aler par la maison esbatant, si que la medicine descende et aprés ce voit dormir. Et maintenant qu'il s'esveillera, si se veste et chauce et il sentera les pressons del ventre. Si(l) allie par la maison et se il crient a vomir, mete une poume a son nes ou une croste de pain brouslé et arousee de vin egre et se li fetes lier les quisses de une fort coreie et soit auques apareillé sodainement qu'il [23] li gete ewe salé enmi le front et se gart quant il irra a chambre qu'il ne se efforce mie. Se il a soif, gart qu'il ne boive, et se il a mult grant soif, si masche l'escorce de la poume et gete fors. Et se il ne va a chambre si come il dot, chauve une tieule et mete a son ventre tote caude ov le drap ploié ou un orillier bien chaut si com il le porra suffrir par trois fois ou par quatre ou par plusors fois, si mestiers est. Et si il n'eust lassiés si com il doit, si destemprés encore de la medicine en vin ou en ewe et li soit donee la polipode triblee et quite en ewe et agusiés d'esule le pesant de un denier. [f.46r] Se vus ne volés ce faire, donés li laituaire douz noef deners pesant, einsi alascera. Et s'il ne alasce assés, mulliés un drap linge en ewe bien chaude et metez sur le ventre par trois fois. Et se tot ce ne vaut, se le metés en un bai[n]g tiede, et si ce est chose qui (e) alasce si que sans i viegne par gemisement qu'il face, prenés la mie d'un pain d'orge, si le boilliés en vin egre et puis le metés tiede sor le ventre.

Aprés ce que vus verrés que la medicine lascera et que il ne sentira ne pressons ne griefteez, c'est signe qu'il n'irra plu a chambre. Aprés ce li donés del bruet de la geline ou autre ewe tieve, si que li ventres et li boiés soient bien espurgé. Aprés ce si le faites jeuner dusque aprés noune, si se gard de dormir si il poet. Et ce sache qu'il ne doit pas dormir dusque le ventre soit tous voides de la medicine, si que la medicine par la force de dormir ne perde sa vertu. Aprés ce qu'il aura jeuné, se li donés une membre de geline o le comin ou un poi d'almandele ou un pou de poisson solunc ce que li tens l'aporte a bovre un petit hanap plein de vin ov les dous pars de ewe et gard qu'il ne mangut glutement ne ne boive, que fievres ne li pregne. [f.46v] Au secund jor le faites baignier et si li gard de froit. Et au tiers jor le faites seignier se il ne soit mult febles. Si se gard de travaillier les trois jors et se mangut bones viandes qui engendront bones chafs [24] et bones humors.

2. CONTRE CHAUDE HUMOR

Si il a chaude humor el cause, si come colere, apparilliés vostre matere de sirop acceptous [25] ou de autre qui soit frois, si com sirop violat, se il est serés, ou de sirop rosat, [26] si il a le ventre soluble. Et quant vos verrés vos signes apareilliés, si come l'urine espesse entor le novisme jor ou le disme, appareilliés vostre medicine en tele manere. Mais premerement li donés trois drames de trife zarazine[27] a essaer, si li covient a doner fort medicine ou legiere. Et se il vet a chambre par trois fois ou par quatre par ceste medicine, donés li le moine medicine et se vus ne veés que soit soluble par ceste, donés li greignors et plus fort.

3. MOINE MEDICINE[28]
Moine medicine si est tele: Prenés trois drames de cartatique emperial[29] et l'agusiés de une crupe de escamonie et d'une crupe d'esule. Et si mellés ensemble et un peu ains jors le destemprés de ewe caude se il est feverus, et se ce non, se le destemprés de vin chaut et donés au malades et li faites si en avant. Et si li [f.47r] baigniés quant vus devrés et si le seigniés quant vos devreés et se li faites les autres choses si com vus devrés.

4. MEDICINE A GENT HAITIÉ
Il avient qu'aucon home est sains et veut prendre medicine, kar nuls n'est parfitement sains qu'il n'ait el cors aucune humor plus que li convendroit. Et ce li meine maladie se ele n'en est ostee ou par travail ou par medicine. Et por ce devons nus esgarder quele humor li abonde plus qu'il ne deust al cors et porgier cele humor: si il est frois, de medicine que purge froide humor, si come benoite et de gerapigre et de semblables choses; et si il i a chaud humor, si come cartatique emperial ou trife sarazine ou laitu[ai]re de jus de roses[30] ou de semblables choses.

5. DE DEUS HUMORS A OSTER SI L'EN LES A EN LE CORS
Se il a dous humors el cors, une chaude et l'autre froide, qui peschent ensemble si come sausefleume, que est comprise de colere et de fleume ensemble, nus le devons purgier de medicine doble, l'une que regart la colere, l'autre que regart le fleume, et en santé et en maladie ensi doit estre. Donc prenés une drame et demie de benoite, kar ele purge fleume, et aprés une drame [f.47v] et demie de cartatique emperial, por ce que ele espurge colere, et mellés bien ensemble ces agusemens. Si il est fors hom, une drame d'escamonie et une de esle [mellez] ensemble et faites piles si come jo vos ai dit. Et si le donés si come jo ai devant dit ou en vin ou en ewe.

6. CONTRE FEVRE AGUE
Se aucons a fevre ague, vos [le] devés dieter en tele manere. Se vus veés premerement qu'il soit grossement malades et sa urine soit clere et blanche et il ait le pous petit ignel et se vus veés qu'il ne soit pas bien solubles et pisse a peine et que il se pleine a peines et ait grant soif et que il mangut povrement et ne dort pas, ne le prenés mie en cure, kar ces sont morteles signes. Et se vus veez qu'il soit fors et sa urine coloree et espesse et qu'il mangut et qu'il soit bien solubles et qu'il[31] ait ses conduiz et qu'il ne resue pas, recevés le en cure et puis le dietés si come vus savés.Donés li un sirop violat a boivre, si il est serrés, ou sirop rosat, s'il est solubles. Et si il est povres, qu'il[32] ne poet avoir ces sirops, si poez quire des violettes et des roses et de ceste decoction se li poés doner trois quilliérés. Et aprés ce li donés a manger gruel [f.48r]. Et alemande et nieules et poires et pomes quites et prunes li poés vus doner. Et se li oigniés les temples et le pous de populeon et de lait de femme que norice femele mellé ensemble avec (a) juis de plantaine et de morele et de jubarbe. Et se boive tisane et si ce soit en yver et si il passe le quarte jur ou la disme que il ne sut et vus avés pour de sa feblesse, vus li poés doner caudel, geline et vin feble. Et quant vus verrés que la maladie iert terminee, par dous jors dietés le

ausi come devant. Et aprés se li porrés doner la char de un pucin et groin de porc et piés et oreilles et perches et cominees. Et quant vus aurés ce fait, se li poés doner plus grosse diete. Et se il sent amertume en sa buche aprés la quinte jur et l'urine soit encore teinte, ce est signe de renchair en la maladie. Se il est serrés, se li faites suppositure de mel et de sel et de saugeme. Et se il avient[33] qu'il ne puisse dormir, prenés la semence de kenillie et semence de laitues et de pu[r]celeine et batés et destemprés de vin egre et puis le enoignés le pous et les temples et ces sont suffisantes choses a fevre ague.

7. [f.48v] OXIMEL DIURETIC

Oximel diueretic receit de vin egre un sester et de mel demi-sester, racine de fenoil, de peresil, de ache, de nifle et de bru et de sparage, de chescone racine quatre onces, semence de fenoil, de peresil, de ache et de anis les semences et polipode. Et prenés ces racines et lavés et raez a un coutel et traés la moele fors et metés en un morter et batés. Et quant il seront bien batus, temprés les dous jors et dous nuis en vin egre. Et les semences mesmement metés en un morter et triblés ensemble et puis metés tot ensemble sor le feu. Et quisés tant que les racines soient moles et puis coler et metre a require tant que il devienent espés. Et quant vus vodrés savoir qu'il ert quis, metés le sor le ongle, et s'il se tient, bien il est quit, et metés en un vassel, se le estuez.

8. SIROP CONTRE MESELERIE ET ROINE

Ceste sirop est bons a gent a boivre qui sont ente(n)chié de meselerie et a tote roine et nettie mult le stomac et les reins et le foie et le chief. Ce receit mirabolans citrins et quiebles et indes,[34] de cheson dis drames, et [e]pitimes et tiegne de lin [f.49r] et aloine et sauge savage, semence de borage, racine de ache, racine de fenoil, de chescon vint drames; belcriques, anbliques, ricolice, polipode, de chascon dis drames; thamarindes, cassia-fistule, de chascon quatre onces; roisins de utre mer quatre onces; roses demie once; manne demie once; violettes demie once; gingebre demie once; prunes de outre-mer quarante quatre livres;[35] jus de fimetere et jus de bourace, de chescon une quarte. Et quant vus vodrés savoir si il est quis, metés une goute sus un coutel; s'il se tient, bien i est quit. Et que l'en broit en poudre les mirabolans en un morter, et puis le cassiafistule et les tamarindes colés parmi un drapel. Et quant li sirop sera refroidi, mellés tot ensemble et puis le poudre de mirabolans encorporés[36] tot tens et puis estués et metés en sauf.

9. ESTUVE CONTRE TOTE MANERE DE ROINE ET A MORT MAL,[37] A DERTRES

Fetes estuve en tele manere encontre tote manere de roigne et a mort mal et a dertres: Prenés les racines de hieveles et les couperons de seus et les racines de auné et de l'irre des arbres et fenoil et ache et peresil. Ices chose[s] batés ensemble en un morter et quisés en ewe avec un poi [f.49v] de vin et se i metés plein poigné de sel et de ces choses fetes estuve en tele manere.

10. ONGNEMENT A CEL MEIME CHOSE

Ognement a ce meime: Prenés les racine[s] de l'auné et si les descoupés par piecetes et metés temprer en vin egre une nuit. L'endemain les quisés en cel vin meisme[38] desc'a tant qu'il sera degasté et le remanant geter poés. Et aprés le mellés et quisés ovec vieus oint de porc au doble. Si i metés vif argent esteint.

11. ESTUVE CONTRE [YDRO]PISIE

Encontre ydropisie fetes estuve en tele manere. Prenés fenoil, peresil et ache, cala-

ment, origane, averoyne, rue, les .ii. cressons, ciperon, sauge, foilles de lorier, savine, genoivre. Depeciez les et batez et puis fetes estuve.

12. ISSI COMENCENT LES OIGNE[ME]NS P . . . ENT POP . . .[39]
Popelion vaut a celui ke ne poet dormir por la pesantume de la chalor de la fevre
ague. Et mellez a oile violat ou a oile rosat et l'oignez contre le foie et sor le ventre,
si hastera a suer.

13. AGRIPPE[40]
Vaut a totes ydropisies et a totes enfleures ou ke eles seient. Et ce vaut a ners ke
sunt retrait et si fait pisser, et oigne son ventre et alaschera.

14. MARCIATON[41]
[f.50r] Vaut al freideure del pis et a l'estomac et a l'esplen et al foie et a la dolor
des loines, si il seit oins au fu ou al solein. Et vaut a paralisie et a totes goutes ke
vienent de freit. Et si asiet totes emfleures et totes dolors. Si vaut a totes choses que
vienent de freit.

15. ARRAGUN[42]
Vaut a totes froidures d'ome et de femme. Et metez l'oignement en une escaille
d'oef deske il seit fondus. Et oignez la maladie et la dolor. Si vaut a celui qui ne
poet torner de sa ni de la et a la dolor des loignes et a artetike et as flauns et as os
qui sunt secchié[s] de goute et a la quartaine. Et l'oignez encontre l'eschine avant
ke la fevre li pregne.

16. DIAUTÉ[43]
Vaut a la dolor del pis qui vient de freit et a la dolor des costes. Metez en l'escaille
d'oes desi que il seit fondus. Et oigniez et metez l'emplastre sor la dolor des costes et
liez desus. Et ce vaut a tous les ners desecchié[s].

17. DIACALAMENT[44]
Diacalament est bons a la freidure del chief et a la freidure del pis et la touz. Aprés
diner et aprés souper en use en vin. Cest lectuaire receit calament, peivre long, sirmontain, semen[f.50v]ce de peresil, de chescun .i. drame et .ii. deners pesant;
semence [. . .] une drame et .i. denier pesant, semence d'ache .i. denier pesant,
ameos .ii. drames, tim .ii. drames avec .ii. drames de canele, .ii. onces gingembre
(.ii. onces) poivre neir .ii. onces. Tot ice confisez en miel. La livre de ceste lectuaire vaut . . . deniers.

18. DIADRAGANT[45]
Diadragant freit vaut a totes les enfermetez del pis et a la chalor del pis et a tousse
ke vient par chalor et meimement a celui ki [a] la langue secche. Cest lectuaire receit dragant blanc .ii. onces, gome arabic blanc .i. once et .ii. drames, amidon demi-
once, penides .iiii. onces, concongre, coordes, melones et citrins,[46] de chescun .ii.
drames. Et puis le confise l'en od cirop de zucre. De ceste lectuaire le livre vaut .ii.
souz. Et ki le met en sa bouche al seir et au matin ausi gros com une chastaigne
tant seit fundus en sa bouche.

19. DIAPENIDION[47]
Diapenidion vaut a totes les enfermetez del pomon, a la tousse secche et a l'esreiement de la vois. Cest lectuaire receit penides .xvi. [f.51r] drames et demie.

20. DRAGIE DE PARIS

Dragie de Paris receit gingembre bien trenché a .i. coutel par menues piecettes .iiii. onces, anis bien poudree demie-livre, fenoil .iiii. onces, ricolice .i. livre, gilofre .i. once, macis une once.

21. DIAUTÉ[48]

Diauté receit racine de wimauve .ii. livres, semence de lin, finegrec, de chescun .i. livre, oignion de mer demie-livre. Ces racines seient bie[n] lavés et triblees tot ensemble. Si metez tot en .ii. livres de ewe par .iii. jors. Au quart jor le metez sor le fu et le laissez boillir tant ke il deviengne espés. Et aprés le metez en .i. sac petit (et petit) et quant vous le vodrez priendre, metez de l'ewe bien chaude en le sac a traire hors le jus. De cel jus pernez .ii. livres et metez en .iiii. livres d'oile et laisiez boillir tant ke il seit degastee deske a la quantité del jus. Aprés si metez une livre de cire ou une livre de bure. Quant ele serra fondue, si i metez terbentine .ii. onces et galbanum .ii. onces et gome de ere .ii. onces et metez i au meins demie-livre de **[f.51v]** poudre de colofoine et de la poiz resine demie-livre. Et quant il sera bien quit et refreidie, si le metez en .i. barel. Proprement vaut a la dolor del piz ke vient de freidure. La livre de cest oignement vaut .xii. deniers.

22. CLARÉ[49]

Claré receit gingembre, canel, galingal, peivre lonc et peivre neir, espic, ciperon, folion, piretron, esquinant, maimuine, cardamome, gilofre, de chescun .iiii. onces, [de] miel .i. sester. Et puis batre et mettre en une chauche quant le miel sera quit et escumé et melle la poudre et le miel et le vin ensemble et puis coler et si il(l) i a poi de miel, metez i plus oncore et si il(l) i a trop, metez i de la poudre plus.

23. DIAMORON[50]

Diamoron vaut a totes les enfermetez del palais et por la luvette relever. Il receit jus de moures douces .ii. livres et de miel escumé .ii. livre et vin douz demie-livre. Et confisez le jus et le miel ensemble et le vin douz en .i. vassel de areim ou en .i. paiele et le quisez a lent fu tant ke il deviengne espés. Si vous volez saveir quant il sera assez quit, metez ent une goute sor le marbre et si la **[f.52r]** goute lieve del marbre sanz tenir, bien est quit. Puis l'estuez en un vassel et quant mestiers sera, s'en oignez le palais.

24. ENCONTRE SAUSEFLEUME, SCABIE, ROIGNE, DERTRE, MANJUE ET TESCH ET AUTRE[S] CHOSES

Pernez arguel, si le triblez mult menu et puis le metez en .i. linge drap et le liez. Puis le metez en un esquiele, si versez desus vin egre fort taunt com il veut beivre, si le laissez ester issi une nuit. L'autre jor si le metez en fu de carbons, si l'ardez mult bien deske il seit tot jaune com le feu et puis le laissez refreidir et le triblez autre fiez et le metez en .i. esquiele de freine. Puis metez le esquiel en .i. basin od une poi d'ewe, si ke rien ne entre en l'esquiele. Si le metez en mult moiste liu, ou vent ni air ni puisse avenir, deske il comence a relentir. Puis le metez en une puscette et metez un basin desuz et veez ke nul vent ni aproche. Puis corra tost. Et le licur metez en .i. viole de veir ou de esteim, kar il est mult persaunt.

25. OIGNEMENT A CE MEIME

Pernez la racine de auné et de rouge parele et de wimauve et **[f.52v]** de rouge ortie et de parelle d'ewe. Si les quisez en vin egre et puis les triblez mult bien. Puis pernez amedeus les aches et la petite consoude et seneschon et launcelé owellement de chescun, si les triblez od vieuz oint de porc. Puis metez les racines o tot en le vin egre, si laissez ester en .i. basin .iii. jors et .iii. nuiz. Puis le quisez en un poscenet de areime. Aprés le colez parmi un drap, si le laissez refreidir. Puis pernez soufre et vif argent, taunt com vous veez ke mestiers est, et metez od vostre oignement en une boiste bien enciré. Cest oinement vaut encontre vermine autresi bien come encontre les choses avant dites. Lavez le liu de l'oile et lassez secchier et puis le oinez de cest oinement.

26. AUTRE
Pernez tendrons de runce et lovasche et quisez en gresse de capon. Puis metez en .i. boiste enciré.

27. OINEMENT A GOUTE ROSE
Pernez demie-marc peisant de blanc de Puille et demi-marc pesant de blanc plum et demi-marc pesant de blanc alum et demi-marc pesant de franc encens et .i. marc pesant d'oile d'olive et .i. marc pesant de vif argent et .i. livre de vieuz oint.

Notes

Notes to Preface

1   *Anglo-Saxon Leechcraft: an historical sketch of early English medicine/Lecture memoranda, British Medical Association, Liverpool 1912* (London etc., 1912).
2   See below pp.24f.
3   For the useful works of Talbot and Rubin see below p.348 n.160–61.
4   *Medieval Medicus: A Social History of Anglo-Norman Medicine* (Baltimore/London, 1981).
5   R. M. Clay, *The Medieval Hospitals of England* 2nd ed. (London, 1966).
6   See the severe reviews of M. Carlin, *Medical History* 31 (1987), 360–62; F. M. Getz, *Bulletin of the History of Medicine* 61 (1987), 455–61; C. Rawcliffe, *Social History of Medicine* 1 (1988), 93–95 (cf. the reviewer's own article 'The Profits of Practice: The Wealth and Status of Medical Men in Later Medieval England', *ibid.*, 61–78).
7   R. H. Robbins, 'Medical Manuscripts in Middle English', *Speculum* 45 (1970), 393–45.
8   For a selection of publications see R. P. Steiner (ed.), *Folk Medicine: The Art and the Science* (Washington, D.C., 1986); E. Grabner (ed.), *Volksmedizin: Probleme und Forschungsgeschichte* (Darmstadt, 1967); M. Bouteiller, *Médecine populaire d'hier et d'aujourd'hui* (Paris, 1966); P. Ribon, *Guérisseurs et remèdes populaires dans la France ancienne* (Le Coteau, 1983).
9   J. M. Riddle, 'Theory and Practice in Medieval Medicine', *Viator* 5 (1974), 157–84 has stressed the continuity of medical practice from Roman times to the Middle Ages and shown how the rise of more theoretical or speculative medicine had the effect of driving a wedge between theory and practice. Medieval pharmacognosy was derived from ancient medicine but made advances of its own, notably through the importation of drugs from the East.
10   T. Hunt, 'The "Novele Cirurgerie" in MS London, British Library, Harley 2558', *Z.f.rom.Phil.* 103 (1987), 271–99.
11   See, for example, J. Scarborough, 'Theophrastus on Herbals and Herbal Remedies', *Journal of the History of Biology* 11 (1978), 353–85 and J. M. Riddle, *Dioscorides on Pharmacy and Medicine* (Austin, 1986).
12   See J. M. Riddle, 'Folk Tradition and Folk Medicine: Recognition of Drugs in Classical Antiquity' in J. Scarborough (ed.), *Folklore and Folk Medicines* (Madison, 1987), pp.33–61 and J. Stannard, 'Medieval Herbalism and Post-Medieval Folk Medicine', *ibid.*, pp.10–20.
13   See, for example, J. Scarborough, *art. cit.* and *id.*, 'Adaptation of Folk Medicines in the Formal Materia Medica of Classical Antiquity' in *Folklore and Folk Medicines*, pp.21–32.
14   J. M. Riddle, 'Ancient and Medieval Chemotherapy for Cancer', *Isis* 76 (1985), [319–30] 320.
15   A good overview of aspects of medicinal plants in therapy is given by papers read at the Second International Congress on the History of Medicinal and Aromatic Plants held at Alexandria (Egypt) 15 Dec. –19 Dec. 1980 and published in *Hamdard Medicus* 25 (1982), 11–216. See especially Ahmed Ali Aboolenein, 'Back to Medicinal Plants Therapy', pp.40–44.
16   A. Nelson, *Medical Botany* (Edinburgh, 1951), p.376.

[17] See J. L. Hartwell, *Plants used against Cancer: A Survey* (Lawrence, Mass., 1982).

[18] Of the innumerable publications on 'green medicine' see especially M. B. Kreig, *Green Medicine. The Search for Plants that Heal* . . . (London etc., 1965); F. Bianchini & F. Corbetta, '*The Kindly Fruits*', Engl. adapt. by M. A. Dejey (London, 1977); P. Delaveau, *Histoire et renouveau des plantes médicinales* (Paris, 1982); B. Griggs, *Green Pharmacy: A History of Herbal Medicine* (London, 1981); M. Howard, *Traditional Folk Remedies: A Comprehensive Herbal* (London, 1987); G. Usher, *A Dictionary of Plants used by Man* (London, 1974). A fundamental reference work is W. Schneider, *Pflanzliche Drogen: Sachwörterbuch zur Geschichte der pharmazeutischen Botanik*, 3 vols (Frankfurt a. M., 1974) = Bd V, 1–3 of the same author's *Lexikon zur Arzneimittelgeschichte*. On the pharmaceutical use of minerals see D. Goltz, *Studien zur Geschichte der Mineralnamen in Pharmazie, Chemie und Medizin von den Anfängen bis Paracelsus* (Wiesbaden, 1972).

[19] The present study includes some plant names not recorded in that monograph which was based exclusively on unpublished lists of *synonyma herbarum*.

[20] See J. M. Riddle, 'Theory and Practice in Medieval Medicine', *Viator* 5 (1974), 157–84, who comments that drug therapy 'is how most medicine was practised'.

[21] See J. B. Simmons et al., *Conservation of Threatened Plants* (N.Y./London, 1976), p.vii.

[22] Much more comparative work needs to be done on popular medical practices throughout the world. O. von Hovorka & A. Kronfeld, *Vergleichende Volksmedizin*, 2 vols (Stuttgart, 1908–9) is now, of course, out of date. See Y. Otsuka, 'Comparative Study of Materia Medica' in T. Ogawa (ed.), *History of Traditional Medicine. Proceedings of the First and Second International Symposia on the Comparative History of Medicine – East and West [1976 & 1977]* (Tokyo, 1980), pp.65ff.

[23] Some idea of the scale of unpublished materials may be gained from, for example, S. Miyahita, 'A Historical Analysis of Chinese Formularies and Prescriptions: Three Examples', in *History of Traditional Medicine* . . ., pp.101–15 who points out that the largest Chinese formulary, from the period 1403–24, contains 61739 prescriptions to cure 1960 diseases. Knowledge of Armenian medicine is still undervalued. Of some 20739 catalogued Armenian MSS 1074 are pharmaceutical or medical MSS and influenced both the Islamic world and the West in the Middle Ages, see G. M. Enezian, *Les connaissances médico-pharmaceutiques de l'Antiquité au Moyen Age à travers les manuscrits arméniens* (Rheinfelden, 1982). For the case of medieval India see P. V. Sharma, 'Contributions of Sarngadhara in the field of materia medica', *Indian Journal of the History of Science* 16 (1981), 3–10 and D. K. S. Chauhan & R. N. Singh, 'Contribution of Medieval India to Āyurvedic materia medica', ibid., 17–21. Our knowledge of ancient Egyptian medicine has been immeasurably enriched by the nine volumes (Berlin, 1954–73) of H. Grapow's *Grundriss der Medizin der alten Egypter*.

[24] Cf. the mixture of Gaulish, Greek and Latin in a fifth-century prescription from Poitiers recommending the use of centaury, R. Le Moniès de Sagazan, 'Une ordonnance médicale du Ve siècle en Gaule', *Revue d'Histoire de la Pharmacie* 32 (1985), 49–52.

Notes to Chapter One

[1] The standard authority is now J. Büchi, *Die Entwicklung der Rezept- und Arzneibuchliteratur*, 3 pts., Veröffentlichungen der Schweizerischen Gesellschaft für Geschichte der Pharmazie Bde 1, 4 & 6 (Zürich, 1982–86). Part 1 deals with Antiquity and the Middle Ages. See also H. E. Sigerist, *A History of Medicine* 2 vols (New York, 1951/61) and the

under-appreciated study of D. De Moulin, *De Heelkunde in de vroege Middeleeuwen* (Leiden, 1964).

2   W. R. Dawson, *Magician and Leech: a study in the beginnings of medicine with special reference to Ancient Egypt* (London, 1929), p.137. Cf. the rich materials in R. C. Thompson, *The Assyrian Herbal* (London, 1924) who discusses the 250 vegetable drugs known to the Assyrian botanists, and *id., A Dictionary of Assyrian Botany* (London, 1949).

3   See D. Goltz, *Studien zur altorientalischen und griechischen Heilkunde: Therapie – Arzneibereitung – Rezeptstruktur,* Beihefte zu Sudhoffs Archiv 16 (Wiesbaden, 1974).

4   For a comparison of some formulae used in Latin, Middle English and Anglo-Norman receipts see below pp.18ff.

5   See I. M. Lonie, 'A Structural Pattern in Greek Dietetics and the Early History of Greek Medicine', *Medical History* 21 (1977), 235–60. Cf. J. H. Kühn, *Die Diätlehre im frühmittelalterlichen Kommentar zu den hippokratischen Aphorismen* (I, 1–11) (Neustadt/Weinstr., 1981).

6   For a recent survey see *La Collection hippocratique et son rôle dans l'histoire de la médecine: colloque de Strasbourg (23–27 octobre, 1972)* (Leiden, 1975) and W. D. Smith, *The Hippocratic Tradition* (Ithaca/London, 1979).

7   That this dichotomy of schools constitutes a false perspective on the *Corpus* is argued by A. Thivel, *Cnide et Cos? Essai sur les doctrines médicales dans la collection hippocratique* (Paris, 1981).

8   General studies on Greek medicine include F. B. Lund, *Greek Medicine* (New York, 1936; repr. 1978); O. & C. L. Temkin (eds.), *Ancient Medicine: selected papers of Ludwig Edelstein* (Baltimore, 1967); E. D. Phillips, *Greek Medicine* (London, 1973). For Byzantine medicine see the papers in J. Scarborough (ed.), *Symposium on Byzantine Medicine,* Dumbarton Oaks Papers 38 (1984) & also R. Volk, *Gesundheitswesen und Wohltätigkeit im Spiegel der byzantinischen Klostertypika* (München, 1983).

9   See J. Ducatillon, *Polémiques dans la collection hippocratique* (Lille/Paris, 1977). Cf. J. Scarborough, 'Theoretical Assumptions in Hippocratic Pharmacology' in F. Lasserre & P. Mudry (eds.), *Formes de pensée dans la collection hippocratique: actes du IVe colloque international hippocratique . . .* (Genève, 1983), pp.307–25.

10   See J. Desautels & M. -C. Girard, 'Les végétaux dans le Corpus Hippocraticum' in *Formes de pensée . . .* pp.187–201, (material recognised as incomplete). Still of value is J. H. Dierbach, *Die Arzneimittel des Hippokrates* (Heidelberg, 1824; repr. 1969) who lists 283 medicinal plants, animal drugs and minerals. See also J. Stannard, 'Hippocratic Pharmacology', *Bull. Hist. Med.* 35 (1961), 497–518.

11   For a list of the works see G. Fichtner, *Corpus Hippocraticum: Verzeichnis der hippokratischen und pseudo-hippokratischen Schriften,* Institut für Geschichte der Medizin (Tübingen, 1985) which numbers 169 items. Also useful is J. -H. Kühn & U. Fleischer, *Index Hippocraticus* fasc.1– (Göttingen, 1986–).

12   See I. Mazzini, 'Le traduzioni latine di Ippocrate eseguite nei secoli v e vi . . .' in *Formes de pensée . . .* pp.483–92.

13   See P. Kibre, 'Hippocrates Latinus: Repertorium of Hippocratic Writings in the Latin Middle Ages' in *Traditio* 31–38 (1975–82).

14   See I. Temkin, 'Geschichte des Hippokratismus im ausgehenden Altertum', *Kyklos* 4 (1932), 1–80. See also D. Jacquart, 'Quelques réflexions sur ce que le moyen âge occidental a retenu de la Collection Hippocratique' in *Formes de pensée . . .* pp.493–97.

15   On Galen generally see O. Temkin, *Galenism* (London, 1973). 323 items are listed by G. Fichtner, *Corpus Galenicum: Verzeichnis der galenischen und pseudogalenischen Schriften,* Institut für Geschichte der Medizin (Tübingen, 1985). See also J. Scarborough, 'The Galenic Question', *Sudhoffs Archiv* 65 (1981), 1–31.

16   See C. Fabricius, *Galens Exzerpte aus älteren Pharmakologen* (Berlin/New York, 1972). See also Büchi, *op. cit.* 1, pp. 32–64. For Galen's transmission of material from Asclepiades see J. Scarborough, 'The Drug Lore of Asclepiades of Bithynia', *Pharmacy in History* 17 (1975), 43–57.

17 *op. cit.*, p.110.

18 *supra*, p.121.

19 See L. Winkler, *Galens Schrift 'De Antidotis'*: *Ein Beitrag zur Geschichte von Antidot und Theriak* diss. Marburg an der Lahn, 1980.

20 See L. Israelson, *Die 'Materia medica' des Klaudios Galenos* diss. Jurjew (Dorpat), 1894. See also J. Scarborough, 'Early Byzantine Pharmacology' in *id., Symposium on Byzantine Medicine*, [pp.213-32] 215-21.

21 See G. Baader, 'Galen im mittelalterlichen Abendland' in V. Nutton (ed.), *Galen: Problems and Prospects* (London, 1981), pp.213-28.

22 For general studies see G. Penso, *La Médecine romaine: l'art d'Esculape dans la Rome antique* (Paris, 1984). Penso lists the *medicamenta* known to the Romans on pp.433-44. See also J. Scarborough, *Roman Medicine* (London, 1969) and F. Kudlien, *Die Stellung des Arztes in der römischen Gesellschaft (Stuttgart, 1986)*. See too J. André, *Etre médecin à Rome* (Paris, 1987). For the archaeological evidence of medical treatment available to the Roman legions see R. W. Davies, 'Some Roman Medicine', *Medical History* 14 (1970), 101-6. For texts and translations see H. Leitner, *Bibliography to the Ancient Medical Authors* (Bern etc., 1972).

23 The standard text of F. Marx (1915) is reproduced, with few exceptions, by W. G. Spencer in the Loeb Classical Library, 3 vols (London, 1935-38). For recent bibliography see Ph. Mudry, *La Préface du 'Medicina' de Celse: texte, traduction et commentaire* (Rome, 1982). Also useful is W. F. Richardson, *A Word Index to Celsus, De medicina* (Auckland, 1982). On Celsus's sources see A. Pazzini *et al., Fonti Celsiane* (Roma, 1958).

24 See S. Sconocchia (ed.), *Scribonii Largi Compositiones* (Leipzig, 1983) and *id, Per una nuova edizione di Scribonio Largo* (Brescia, 1981). Still of value are W. Schonack, *Die Rezeptsammlung des Scribonius Largus: eine kritische Studie* (Jena, 1912) and *id., Die Rezepte des Scribonius Largus zum ersten Male vollständig ins Deutsche übersetzt und mit ausführlichen Arzneimittelregister versehen* (Jena, 1913). See also J. S. Hamilton, 'Scribonius Largus on the Medical Profession', *Bull. Hist. Med.* 60 (1986), 209-16.

25 See J. Scarborough, 'Nicander's Toxology', *Pharmacy in History* 19 (1977), 3-23 and *ibid.* 21 (1979), 3-34, 73-92.

26 See S. Sconocchia, 'Le fonti e la fortuna di Scribonio Largo' in I. Mazzini & F. Fusco (eds.), *I testi di medicina latini antichi: problemi filologici e storici . . .* (Roma, 1985), pp.151-213.

27 See R. Pépin (ed. & transl.), *Quintus Serenus (Serenus Sammonicus), Liber medicinalis* (Paris, 1950) and F. Lombardi (transl.), *Il 'Liber medicinalis' di Quinto Sereno Sammonico* (Pisa, 1963).

28 See J. H. Phillips, 'The Incunable Editions of the *Liber Medicinalis Quinti Sereni*' in Mazzini & Fusco, *I testi di medicina . . .* pp. 215-35.

29 See I. Mazzini (ed. & transl.), *Q. Gargilii Martialis, De hortis* (Bologna, 1978) who summarises what can be gleaned from the sources about Gargilius's life.

30 See R. M. Tapper, *The Materia Medica of Gargilius Martialis* diss. Wisconsin-Madison, 1980, who also translates the receipts of the *Medicinae*.

31 See M. Niedermann (ed.), *Marcelli, De medicamentis liber*, 2nd rev. ed. by E. Liechtenhan, 2 vols (Berlin, 1968). On the background cf. A. Pelletier (ed.), *La Médecine en Gaule* (Paris, 1985) and W. H. S. Jones, 'Ancient Roman Folk Medicine', *Jnl. Hist. Med. & Allied Sciences* 12 (1957), 459-72.

32 See J. Stannard, 'Marcellus of Bordeaux and the Beginnings of Medieval Materia Medica', *Pharmacy in History* 15 (1973), 47-53 with rich bibliography.

33 See Stannard, *art. cit.*, esp. 50f.

34 Cf. A. Delatte, *Herbarius. Recherches sur le cérémonial usité chez les anciens pour la cueillette des simples et des plantes magiques* (Bruxelles, 1961³).

35 See A. Önnerfors (ed.), *Plinii Secundi Iunioris, De medicina libri tres* (Berlin, 1964) and *id.*, *In medicinam Plinii studia philologica* (Lund, 1963). For a late-medieval expansion see J.

Winkler, *Physicae quae fertur Plinii Florentino-Pragensis, Liber Primus* (Frankfurt a. M. etc., 1984) and W. Wachtmeister, . . . *Liber Secundus* (Frankfurt a. M., 1985).

36　See U. Capitani, 'La tradizione indiretta: limiti della sua utilizzazione nella costituzione dei testi di medicina latina' in Mazzini & Fusco, *I testi di medicina* . . . pp.23–61.

37　On the numerous problems associated with this figure see G. Sabbah, 'Observations préliminaires à une nouvelle édition de Cassius Felix' in Mazzini & Fusco, *I testi di medicina* . . . pp. 279–312 who also discusses the 'African School' of medical translators in the 5th C. AD. See also G. Bendz, *Studien zu Caelius Aurelianus und Cassius Felix* (Lund, 1964).

38　See I. E. Drabkin (ed. & transl.), *Caelius Aurelianus On Acute Diseases and On Chronic Diseases* (Chicago, 1950) and also M. F. & I. E. Drabkin, *Caelius Aurelianus, Gynaecia. Fragments of a Latin Version of Soranus, Gynaecia from a Thirteenth-Century Manuscript*, Suppl. to Bull. Hist. Med. no.13 (1951). See also J. Pigeaud, 'Pro Caelio Aureliano', *Mémoires du Centre Jean Palerne* 3 (1982), 105–17.

39　See C. G. Nauert Jr., 'Caius Plinius Secundus' in F. E. Cranz & P. O. Kristeller (eds.), *Catalogus translationum et commentariorum: Mediaeval and Renaissance Latin Translations and Commentaries* IV (1980), pp.297–422.

40　See J. Stannard, 'Medicinal Plants and Folk Remedies in Pliny, *Historia Naturalis*', *History and Philosophy of the Life Sciences* 4 (1982), 3–23 and id., 'Pliny and Roman Botany', *Isis* 56 (1965), 420–25. On the 'doctrine of signatures' cf. S. Mahdihassan, 'A Pahlavi Antecedent of the Doctrine of Signatures', *Hamdard Medicus* 24 iii–iv (1981), 31–35 (see also 36–38).

41　See J. M. Riddle, 'Dioscorides' in F. E. Cranz & P. O. Kristeller (eds.), *Catalogus translationum et commentariorum: Mediaeval and Renaissance Latin Translations and Commentaries* IV (1980). pp.1–143.

42　See id., *Dioscorides on Pharmacy and Medicine* (Austin, Texas, 1985).

43　But not necessarily 'Far Eastern', as scholars have tended to think, see J. Scarborough, 'Roman Pharmacy and the Eastern Drug Trade', *Pharmacy in History* 24 (1982), 135–43.

44　Cf. J. Berendes, *Des Pedanios Dioskurides aus Anazarbos Arzneimittellehre in fünf Büchern* (Stuttgart, 1902) which has useful notes.

45　See E. Dubler, *La 'Matéria Medica' de Dioscórides: transmisión medieval y renacentista* 1–6 (Barcelona, 1953–59).

46　See H. Mørland, *Die lateinischen Oribasiusübersetzungen* (Oslo, 1932) and id., *Oribasius Latinus*, pt.1 (Oslo, 1940) (=*Synopsis* Bks 1–2). See also B. Baldwin, 'The Career of Oribasius', *Acta Classica* 18 (1975), 85–97 and J. Scarborough, 'Early Byzantine Pharmacology', pp.221–24.

47　See L. Voigts, 'The Significance of the Name Apuleius to the *Herbarium Apulei*', *Bull. Hist. Med.* 52 (1978), 214–27. On the tradition of illustrations see H. Grape-Albers, *Spätantike Bilder aus der Welt des Arztes* (Wiesbaden, 1977).

48　See H. J. De Vriend, *The Old English Herbarium and Medicina de Quadrupedibus* EETS O.S. 286 (London, 1984).

49　See J. M. Riddle, 'Pseudo-Dioscorides' *Ex herbis femininis* and Early Medieval Medical Botany', *Journal of the History of Biology* 14 (1981), 43–81.

50　See F. Adams, *The Seven Books of Paulus Aegineta* vol.3 (London, 1844–47) and J. Scarborough, 'Early Byzantine Pharmacology', pp.228–29. See also J. Stannard, 'Aspects of Byzantine Materia Medica' in *Symposium on Byzantine Medicine*, pp.205–11.

51　See H. Schipperges, *Die Benediktiner in der Medizin des frühen Mittelalters* (Leipzig, 1984); E. Patzelt, 'Moines-médecins' in *Etudes de civilisation médiévale (IXe–XIIe siècles): Mélanges offerts à Edmond-René Labande* (Poitiers, 1974), pp.577–88; J. Semmler, 'Die Sorge um den kranken Mitbruder im Benediktinerkloster des frühen und hohen Mittelalters' in P. Wunderli (ed.), *Der kranke Mensch in Mittelalter und Renaissance* (Düsseldorf, 1986), pp.45–59.; R. Schnabel, *Pharmazie in Wissenschaft und Praxis, dargestellt an der Geschichte der Klosterapotheker Altbayerns vom Jahre 800 bis 1800* (München, 1965).

52　See A. Beccaria, *I codici di medicina del periodo presalernitano (secoli IX, X e XI)* (Roma,

1956). See also F. -D. Groenke, *Die frühmittelalterlichen lateinischen Monatskalendarien* diss. Berlin 1986, pp.7ff.

53 See *id.*, 'Sulla tracce di un antico canone latino di Ippocrate e di Galeno', *Italo Medioevale e Umanistica* 2 (1959), 1–56 and *ibid.* 4 (1961), 1–75. See also G. Baader, 'Zur Überlieferung der lateinischen medizinischen Literatur des frühen Mittelalters', *Forschung, Praxis, Fortschritte* 17 (1966), 139–41.

54 See J. Oroz Reta & M. A. Marcos Casquero (eds.), *San Isidoro de Sevilla, Etimologías: edicion bilingüe* 1 (Madrid, 1982), pp.482–507 and W. D. Sharpe (transl.), *Isidore of Seville: The Medical Writings*, Trans. Amer. Philos. Soc. 54, ii (1964). See also *Isidorus Hispalensis, Ethimologiarum liber IIII De medicina* (Masnou, 1945).

55 See J. Duft, *Notker der Arzt. Klostermedizin und Mönchsarzt im frühmittelalterlichen St Gallen* (St Gallen, 1972; 1975²). See pp.30–32 for MSS of 9th–11th C. See also P. Köpp, *Vademecum eines frühmittelalterlichen Arztes* (Aarau, 1980).

56 See R. Payne & W. Blunt, *Hortulus: Walahfrid Strabo* (Pittsburgh, 1966) and H. -D. Stoffler, *Der Hortulus des Walahfrid Strabo* (Sigmaringen, 1978).

57 See H. E. Sigerist, 'The Latin Medical Literature of the Early Middle Ages', *Jnl. Hist. Med.* 13 (1958), 127–46; W. Puhlmann, 'Die lateinische medizinische Literatur des frühen Mittelalters. Ein bibliographischer Versuch', *Kyklos* 3 (1930), 395–416; L. C. MacKinney, *Early Medieval Medicine with special reference to France and Chartres* (Baltimore, 1937). See also F. Kerff, 'Frühmittelalterliche pharmazeutische Rezepte aus dem Kloster Tegernsee', *Sudhoffs Archiv* 67 (1983), 111–16 and R. Reiche, 'Einige lateinische Monatsdiätetiken aus Wiener und St Galler Handschriften', *ibid.* 57 (1973), 113–141.

58 See E. Landgraf, 'Ein frühmittelalterlicher Botanicus', *Kyklos* 1 (1928), 114–46.

59 See M. Wlaschky, 'Sapientia artis medicinae. Ein frühmittelalterliches Kompendium der Medizin', *Kyklos* 1 (1928), 103–13 and R. Laux, 'Ars Medicinae. Ein frühmittelalterliches Kompendium der Medizin', *ibid.* 3 (1930), 417–34. For early medical treatises from MSS in the Vendôme and Montpellier see H. E. Sigerist in *Bull. Hist. Med.* 14 (1943), 68–113 and *ibid.* 10 (1941), 27–47.

60 See L. C. MacKinney, ' "Dynamidia" in medieval medical Literature', *Isis* 24 (1935–36), 400–14.

61 A selection of ancient and medieval treatises by named authors including Strabo, Crispus and Macer are printed in Italian translation in *Corpus scriptorum medicorum infimae latinitatis et prioris medii aevi* 1 (Roma, 1958).

62 See for English translation and notes J. Stannard, 'Benedictus Crispus, an Eighth-Century Medical Poet', *Jnl. Hist. Med.* 21 (1966), 24–46. Some of the information in this article needs to be revised in the light of the work of Bernabeo and Galvani (see next note).

63 See R. A. Bernabeo & S. Galvani, 'Il "Medicinae Libellus" del diacono Crispo e le sue fonti' in Mazzini & Fusco, *I testi di medicina* ... pp.365–74. As 'secondary' sources the authors identify Cassius Felix and Ps.-Apuleius.

64 See J. Jörimann, *Frühmittelalterliche Rezeptarien.* (Zürich/Leipzig, 1925; repr. 1977) and H. E. Sigerist, *Studien und Texte zur frühmittelalterlichen Rezeptliteratur* (Leipzig, 1923).

65 Cf. G. Baader, 'Die Anfänge der medizinischen Ausbildung im Abendland bis 1100', *Settimane di Studio* 19 (1972), 669–742 and *id.* 'Die Entwicklung der medizinischen Fachsprache im Mittelalter' in G. Keil & P. Assion (eds.), *Fachprosaforschung. Acht Vorträge zur mittelalterlichen Artesliteratur* (Berlin, 1974), pp.88–123.

66 The standard authority is M. Levey, *Early Arabic Pharmacology: an introduction based on ancient and medieval sources* (Leiden, 1973). See also S. Hamarneh, 'A History of Arabic Pharmacy', *Physis* 14 (1972), 5–54 and *id.*, *Origins of Pharmacy and Therapy in the Near East* (Tokyo, 1973). There is a great deal of repetition in Hamarneh's published work. Most of his articles cited in the following notes have been reprinted in M. A. Anees (ed.), *Health Sciences in Early Islam: Collected Papers by Sami K. Hamarneh* 2 vols (San Antonio, 1983). See, more recently, S. Hamarneh, 'Modern Historiography and Medieval Arab-Islamic Pharmaceutical Literature', *Hamdard Medicus* 28, iii (1985), 3–26.

Earlier literature will be located in Hamarneh's *Bibliography of Medicine and Pharmacy in Medieval Islam* (Stuttgart, 1964) & R. Y. Ebied, *Bibliography Of Mediaeval Arabic and Jewish Medicine and Allied Sciences* (London, 1971). See also C. A. Storey, *Persian Literature: A Bio-bibliographical Survey* 2, ii (London, 1971).

67   See H. Kamal, *Encyclopaedia of Islamic Medicine, with a Greco-Roman Background* (Cairo, 1975); M. Ullmann, *Die Medizin Islam (Leiden/Köln, 1970)*, and a shorter work, *Islamic Medicine* (Edinburgh, 1978) (references in the notes below are to the German work); S. Ammar, *Médecins et médecine de l'Islam* (Paris, 1984); S. K. Hamarneh, *Directory of Historians of Arabic-Islamic Science* (Aleppo, 1979). For illustrations see M. J. Sinclair, *A History of Islamic Medicine* (London, 1978). For the medical profession see F. R. Hall, 'Die Bildung des Arztes im islamischen Mittelalter', *Clio Medica* 13 (1978–79), 95–124, 175–200 & *ibid.* 14 (1979), 7–33.

68   See H. Schipperges, *Die Assimilation der arabischen Medizin durch das lateinische Mittelalter* (Wiesbaden, 1964) and *id.*, 'Arabische Medizin im lateinischen Mittelalter', *Sitzb. d. Heidelb. Akad d. Wiss.*, math.-naturwiss. Kl. 1976, Abh.2. (192 pp.).

69   Kamal, *op. cit.*, pp. 755–838 provides a Latin-Arabic and Arabic-Latin dictionary of Islamic *materia medica*.

70   See S. Hamarneh, 'Origins of Arabic Drug and Diet Therapy', *Physis* 11 (1969), 267–86 and *id.*, 'Sources and Development of Arabic Medical Therapy', *Sudhoffs Archiv* 54 (1970), 30–48.

71   See Ullmann, *op. cit.*, pp.115–19 and *Hunayn ibn Ishāq: collection d'articles publiée à l'occasion du onzième centenaire de sa mort* (Leiden, 1975).

72   See M. M. Sadek, *The Arabic Materia Medica of Dioscorides* (Quebec,1983) who lists (pp. 48–50) the works influenced by Dioscorides. See also C. E. Dubler & E. Terés, *La 'Materia Médica' de Dioscórides: transmisión medieval y renacentista* 2 (Barcelona, 1952/7).

73   See S. Hamarneh, 'The Rise of Professional Pharmacy in Islam ', *Medical History* 6 (1962), 59–66. and *id.*, 'The Climax of Medieval Arabic Professional Pharmacy', *Bull. Hist. Med.* 42 (1968), 450–61. On the *practice* of medicine see M. W. Dols, *Medieval Islamic Medicine: Ibn Ridwān's Treatise 'On the prevention of Bodily Ills in Egypt'* (Berkeley, 1984).

74   See M. Meyerhof, 'Esquisse d'histoire de la pharmacologie et botanique chez les Musulmans d'Espagne', *Al-Andalus* 3 (1935), 1–41, repr. in *id.*, *Studies in Medieval Arabic Medicine* ed. P. Johnstone (London, 1984). A number of important articles by Meyerhof appeared in *Ciba Symposia* 6, v & vi (1944).

75   See S. Hamarneh, 'Development of Arabic Medical Therapy in the Tenth Century', *Jnl. Hist. Med. & Allied Sc.* 27 (1972), 65–79 and id. & G. Sonnedecker, *A Pharmaceutical View of Abulcasis al-Zahrāuī in Moorish Spain* (Leiden, 1963), pp.23–33 on the reception in the West.

76   G. Karmi, 'A Mediaeval Compendium of Arabic Medicine: Abū Sahl al-Masīhī's "Book of the Hundred" ', *Jnl. Hist. of Arabic Science* 2 (1978) [270–90], 270–71.

77   See M. Meyerhof, 'Alī at-Tabarī's 'Paradise of Wisdom'; one of the oldest Arabic Compendiums of Medicine', *Isis* 16 (1931), 6–54.

78   See W. Schmucker, *Die pflanzliche und mineralische Materia Medica im Firdaus al-Hikma des Tabarī* (Bonn, 1969).

79   See S. Hamarneh, 'Contributions of Alī al-Tabarī to ninth-century Arabic Culture', *Folia Orientalia* 12 (1970), 91–101.

80   See K. M. Habib & H. N. Zubairy, 'The Materia Medica in the 'Canon' of Ibn Sina: An Evaluation', *Hamdard Medicus* 29, i–ii (1986), 82–92 and M. H. Shah, *The General Principles of Avicenna's Canon of Medicine* (Karachi, 1966) app.2.

81   See H. A. Hameed (ed.), *Avicenna's Tract on Cardiac Drugs and Essays on Arabic Cardiotherapy* (New Delhi/Karachi, 1983). For a general assessment and bibliography see U. Weisser, 'Ibn Sīnā und die Medizin des arabisch-islamischen Mittelalters – Alte und Neue Urteile und Vorurteile', *Medizinhist. Jnl.* 18 (1983), 283–305.

82   F. R. Seligman's account (1859) of the Viennese codex Österr. Natbibl. A.F.340 together
     with a facsimile and an introduction by C. H. Talbot has been reissued (Graz, 1972).
83   See F. Moattar, Ismā'īl Ǧorǧānī und seine Bedeutung für die iranische Heilkunde insbesondere
     Pharmazie (Marburg an der Lahn, 1971) and R. Schmitz & F. Moattar, 'Zur Biobiblio-
     graphie Ismā'il Gorgani (1046–1136)', Sudhoffs Archiv 57 (1973), 337–60.
84   See G. Nebbia, 'La materia medica contenuta nel "Liber el Havi di al-Rāzī" ', Estratto
     dagli Atti e Relazioni dell'Accademia Publiese delle Scienze 23 (1965), 311 ff. See also J.
     Ahmad, A. H. Farooqui & T. O. Siddiqi, 'Zakariya Al-Rāzī's Treatise on Botanical, Ani-
     mal and Mineral Drugs for Cancer', Hamdard Medicus 28, iii (1985), 76–93 who list 131
     drugs mentioned by al-Rāzī.
85   S. K. Hamarneh, 'The Pharmacy and Materia Medica of al-Bīrūnī and al-Ghāfiqī – A
     Comparison', Pharmacy in History 18 (1976) [3–12] 6.
86   See H. M. Said, Al-Bīrūnī's Book on Pharmacy and Materia Medica, 2 pts. (Karachi, 1973);
     id., (ed.), Al-Bīrūnī: Commemorative Volume (Karachi, 1979) esp. the art. by K. M. Habib,
     pp. 458–73, who emphasises the value of al-Bīrūnī's treatment of synonyms; K. M.
     Habib, 'Some of the Problems of al-Bīrūnī's Kitāb al-Saydanah fi al-Tibb with special
     reference to drug synonyms, systematics and substitutes', Hamdard Medicus 23 iii–iv
     (1980), 74–94; H. M. Said & A. Z. Khan, Al-Bīrūnī: His Time, Life and Works (Karachi,
     1981).
87   See Hamarneh, 'The Pharmacy and Materia Medica . . . ', p.8.
88   Other encyclopaedic works are the medical synopsis, Taqwīm, and Minhāj of ibn Jazlah.
     The Minhāj al-Bayān discusses simple and compound drugs and diets, listed in alpha-
     betical order, and includes a treatment of substitutes. For a listing of the materia medica
     see J. S. Graziani, Arabic Medicine in the Eleventh Century as represented in the Works of Ibn
     Jazlah (Karachi, 1980).
89   See Levey, Early Arabic Pharmacology, pp.146 ff.
90   See L. Norpoth, 'Zur Bio- , Bibliographie und Wissenschaftslehre des Pietro d'Abano,
     Mediziners, Philosophen und Astronomen in Padua', Kyklos 3 (1930), 292–353.
91   See S. Hamarneh, 'Sabur's Abridged Formulary, the First of its Kind in Islam', Sudhoffs
     Archiv 45 (1961), 247–60 and id., 'A new light on Sabur's Formulary', Hamdard Medicus
     22 (1979), 16–30.
92   See M. Levey, The Medical Formulary or Aqrābādhīn of Al-Kindī (Madison etc., 1966) and
     id., Early Arabic Pharmacology, pp. 72 ff; K. M. Habib, 'Pharmacology and Materiae Medi-
     cae in the Medical Formulary of al-Kindī', Hamdard Medicus 24, i (1981), 92–101; S. K.
     Hamarneh, 'The Life and Ideas of al-Kindī', ibid. 29, iii (1986), 61–72. In his edition
     Levey discusses in detail 319 items of materia medica.
93   See P. Sbath & C. D. Avierinos, Deux Traités Médicaux (Cairo, 1953), pp.7–75.
94   See M. Levey & N. Al-Khaledy, The Medical Formulary of Al-Samarqandī and the Relation
     of Early Arabic Simples to those found in the Indigenous Medicine of the Near East and India
     (Philadelphia, 1967) with excellent indices.
95   Latinized as grabaddin, see L. J. Vandewiele, De Grabadin van Pseudo-Mesues en zijn In-
     vloed op de Farmacie in de zuidelijke Nederlanden (Gent, 1962).
96   See Levey, Early Arabic Pharmacology, pp.146 ff.
97   See Ullmann, op.cit., pp.280–83.
98   See M. Meyerhof (ed. & transl.), Un glossaire de matière médicale composé par Maïmonide,
     Mém. prés. à l'Inst. d'Egypte 41 (Le Caire, 1940), English version by F. Rosner, Moses
     Maimonides' Glossary of Drug Names (Philadelphia, 1979). See also F. Rosner, 'The Medi-
     cal Writings of Moses Maimonides', Clio Medica 16 (1981), 1–11 and H. Ackermann,
     'Moses Maimonides (1135–1204) ärztliche Tätigkeit und medizinische Schriften', Sud-
     hoffs Archiv 70 (1986), 44–63.
99   See P. Kahle, 'Ibn Samagun und sein Drogenbuch . . . ', Documenta Islamica 1952, pp.
     25–44.
100 See B. Lewin, The Book of Plants of Abū Hanīfa ad-Dīnawarī, Part of the Alphabetical Section

A–Z (Uppsala, 1953) and id., ... *Part of the Monograph Section* (Wiesbaden, 1974). See also M. H. Allah, *Part 2 S–Y, al Qāmus al Nabāfi* (Cairo, 1973).

101 See Levey, *Early Arabic Pharmacology*, pp.131–45.

102 See M. Levey, *Mediaeval Arabic Toxicology: The Book of Poisons of Ibn Wahshīya and its Relation to Early Indian and Greek Texts*, Trans. Am. Philosoph. Soc. N.S. 56, pt.7 (Philadelphia, 1966). On pp.8–10 there is a list of works on toxicology prior to Maimonides. See also Hamarneh, *Origins of Pharmacy* ... , pp.101–15 & Th. Holste, 'Vom Dosis–Problem zum Arzneimittelbegleitschein: Wege der Vulgärisierung bei der Theriak-Diskussion', *Medizinhist. Jnl.* 13 (1978), 171–85.

103 See M. Levey & S. S. Souryal, 'The Introduction to the *Kitāb al-Musta 'inī* of Ibn Biklārish (fl.1106)', *Janus* 55 (1968), 134–66.

104 For an example of the tables see Levey, *Early Arabic Pharmacology* ... , pp.156–59.

105 By about 1000 AD less need was felt to supply the four degrees of cold, warmth, moist or dry humour for simples. Galenic theory was diminishing in influence.

106 See M. Levey, *Substitute Drugs in Early Arabic Medicine with special Reference to the Texts of Māsarjawaih, Al-Rāẓī and Pythagoras* (Stuttgart, 1971). Levey provides English translations of three texts, supplementary information about which will be found in a postscript by the editor of Levey's (posthumous) work. Levey points out that the substitutes contained in 'Operation of the Apothecary' (1260 AD) are still in use together with the book itself.

107 On constrasting tendencies towards caution in the prescription of compound medicines on the one hand, and drug abuse on the other, see S. Hamarneh, 'Ecology and Therapeutics in Medieval Arabic Medicine', *Sudhoffs Archiv* 58 (1974), 165–85 and id., 'Pharmacy in medieval Islam and the History of Drug Addiction', *Medicine in History* 16 (1972), 226–37.

108 There are also, of course, individual receipts copied singly or in small groups, cf. A. Diaz Garcia, 'Three Medical Recipes in Codex Biblioteca Medicea-Laurenziana Or. 215', *Jnl. Hist. Arabic Science* 4 (1980), 265–86.

109 The standard history of the school of Salerno is still S. de Renzi, *Storia documentata della scuola medica di Salerno* (Napoli, 1857²; repr. Milano, 1967). The first of a series of fundamental revisions by Kristeller was 'The School of Salerno: Its Development and its Contribution to the History of Learning', *Bull. Hist. Med.* 17 (1945), 138–94, repr. in Italian in id., *Studi sulla scuola medica salernitana* (Napoli, 1986), pp.11–96; see also 'Sources of Salernitan Medicine in the 12th Century', *Salerno* 1, i–ii (1967), 19–26.

110 See A. Pazzini, 'The History and Records of the Medical School of Salerno', *Salerno* 1, i–ii (1967), 5–17.

111 See V. Nutton. 'Velia and the School of Salerno', *Medical History* 15 (1971), 1–11.

112 See A. Z. Iskandar, 'An Attempted Reconstruction of the Late Alexandrian Medical Curriculum', *Medical History* 20 (1976), 235–58 & J. Longrigg, 'Superlative Achievement and Comparative Neglect: Alexandrian Medical Science and Modern Historical Research', *History of Science* 19 (1981), 155–200.

113 For the medical literature see P. Giacosa, *Magistri Salernitani nondum editi* (Torini, 1900). C. H. Talbot, 'Some Notes on Anglo-Saxon Medicine', *Medical History* 9 (1965), 156–69 has shown that both the *Passionarius* and the *Practica* were already known in ninth-century England and have no special Salernitan connection.

114 See N. Acocella, 'The Archbishop Alfano 1 ... ', *Salerno* 1, iv (1967), 61–65 and A. Pazzini, *I santi nella storia della medicina* (Roma, 1937), pp.323–28.

115 See the art. by M. McVaugh in C. C. Gillispie (ed.), *Dictionary of Scientific Biography* 3 (New York, 1971), pp.393–95 and Schipperges, *Die Assimilation* ... , pp.15–54.

116 See K. Sudhoff, 'Konstantin der Afriker und die Medizinschule von Salerno', *Arch. Gesch. Med.* 23 (1930), 113–98 and 'Constantin, der erste Vermittler muslimischer Wissenschaft ins Abendland ... ', *Archeion* 14 (1932), 359–69.

117 On the Arabic background see M. Steinschneider, 'Constantinus Africanus und seine arabische Quellen', *Virchows Arch. Path. Anat.* 37 (1866), 351–410. See also F. Gabrieli,

'The Arabian Medicine and the School of Salerno', *Salerno* 1, iii (1967), 12–23, which also appeared in Italian, 'La cultura araba e la scuola medica Salernitana' in *Rivista di Studi Salernitani* 1 (1968), 7–22.

118 On linguistic aspects of his influence see G. Baader, 'Zur Terminologie des Constantinus Africanus', *Medizinhist. Jnl.* 2 (1967), 36–53 and id., 'Die Entwicklung der medizinischen Fachsprache im Mittelalter' in J. Koch (ed.), *Artes Liberales* (Leiden/Köln, 1959) esp. 97–110.

119 See P. O. Kristeller, 'Beiträge der Schule von Salerno zur Entwicklung der scholastischen Wissenschaft im 12. Jahrhundert' in Koch, *Artes Liberales*, pp.84–90.

120 See P. O. Kristeller, *La scuola medica di Salerno secondo ricerche e scoperte recenti* (Salerno, 1980) and id., 'Bartholomaeus, Musandinus and Maurus of Salerno and Other Early Commentators of the *Articella*', *Italia Medioevale e Umanistica* 19 (1976), 57–87, repr. in Italian in id., *Studi* . . . , pp.97–151. See also M. H. Saffron, *Maurus of Salerno, Twelfth-Century 'Optimus Physicus' with his Commentary on the Prognostics of Hippocrates*, Trans. Am. Philosoph. Soc. N.S. 62 (1972). On p. 9 Saffron comments 'The texts included in the earliest versions of the *Articella* were carefully chosen to blend with the so-called Galenic tradition of the school, and thus enabled such later conservatives as Matthew Platearius and Musandinus to offer some resistance to Arabic infiltration'.

121 See B. Lawn, *The Salernitan Questions: An Introduction to the History of Medieval and Renaissance Problem Literature* (Oxford, 1963) and the revised Italian edition *I Quesiti Salernitani* ([Cava dei Tirreni], 1969).

122 Edited by de Renzi in vol. 5 of his *Collectio Salernitana*, they comprise 12 tables in 50 columns and list simples according to their quality and their effect. See also G. Caturegli & G. P. Della Capanna, *La Tavola 'Salernitana' della Biblioteca Governativa di Lucca (secolo XV)* (Pisa, 1968) & E. Pifferi (transl.), *Maestro Bernardo Provenzale, Commento alle Tavole di Salerno* (Roma, 1962).

123 See S. Musitelli, 'To the Origin of "Regimen Sanitatis" 1.', *Salerno* 1, iii (1967), 25–47 and ibid., 1, iv (1967), 23–59. The Italian original on the facing pages is preferable. For an English translation of the *Regimen* see P. W. Cummins, 'A Salernitan Regimen of Health', *Allegorica* 1 (1976), 78–101.

124 Cf. G. Ongaro, 'La questione degli antidotari salernitani', *Galeno* 15, i (1967), 1–14, repr. in Ital. & Engl. in *Salerno* 2, i–ii (1968), 34–43.

125 See A. Lutz, 'Der verschollene frühsalernitanische Antidotarius magnus in einer Basler Handschrift aus dem 12. Jahrhundert und das Antidotarium Nicolai', *Veröff. d. Int. Ges. für Gesch. d. Pharmazie* N.F. 16 (1960), 97–133 and id., 'Chronologische Zusammenhänge der alphabetisch angeordneten mittelalterlichen Antidotarien', in *Aktuelle Probleme aus der Geschichte der Medizin. Verhandlungen des XIX. Intern. Kongr. für Gesch. d. Medizin* ed. R. Blaser & H. Buess (Basel/New York, 1966), pp.253–58.

126 It was quoted by Simon of Genoa c.1300. Cf. A. Lutz, 'Aus der Geschichte der mittelalterlichen Antidotarien', *Veröff. d. Int. Ges. für Gesch. d. Pharmazie* N.F. 40 (1973), 115–22.

127 See E. Müller, *Der Traktat Liber Iste (die sogenannten Glossae Platearii) aus dem Breslauer Codex Salernitanus*, Inaug. Diss. Berlin 1942 (Würzburg, 1942). See also K. Goehl, 'Kurzindex zum pseudoplatearischen "Liber iste" ' in *Festschrift zum 70. Geburtstag von Willem Diems* (Pattensen, 1982), pp.655–66.

128 See the thorough study by D. Goltz, *Mittelalterliche Pharmazie und Medizin dargestellt an Geschichte und Inhalt des Antidotarium Nicolai, mit einem Nachdruck der Druckfassung von 1471* (Stuttgart, 1976).

129 Cf. G. Keil, 'Zur Datierung des Antidotarium Nicolai' in K. O. Kern (ed.), *Wissenschaftliche Verbindung Cimbria zu Heidelberg: Festschrift zum 100 jährigen Bestehen* (Heidelberg, 1976), pp.28–36.

130 e.g. *diamoron, diaciminum, diapenidion* etc.

131 In the Venice print of 1471, which contains 147 receipts, 72 receipts have nothing on preparation at all and others provide exiguous information.

132 Goltz suggests that the average number of ingredients per receipt is 20–30, whilst the highest number is over 70! Details concerning application are given in 95 receipts.

133 See P. Dorveaux, L'Antidotaire Nicolas: deux traductions françaises de l'Antidotarium Nicolai (Paris, 1896); W. S. van der Berg, Eene middelnederlandsche Vertaling van het Antidotarium Nicolai (Leiden, 1917); W. Braekman & G. Keil in Sudhoffs Archiv 55 (1971), 257–320.

134 For literature see G. Keil in Die Deutsche Literatur des Mittelalters, Verfasserlexikon ed. K. Ruh et al., vol.1 (Berlin/New York, 1978), cols 1282–85. F. J. Anderson, 'New Light on Circa Instans', Pharmacy in History 20 (1978), 65–8 examines an early MS (c.1190), possibly from Montpellier, with 258 items and a second MS (early 13th C.) with 211 items. The Venice editio princeps has 273 chapters. I have not seen E. D. Robertson, 'Circa Instans' and the Salernitan materia medica diss. Bryn Mawr Coll. 1982.

135 See C. Opsomer, Livre des simples medecines (Codex Bruxellensis IV.204) transl. E. Roberts & W. T. Stearn 1 (Antwerp, 1984), pp.10–13. For other translations see P. Dorveaux, Le Livre des simples medecines: traduction française du Liber de simplici medicina dictus 'Circa Instans' de Platearius . . . (Paris, 1913) and L. J. Vandewiele, Een middelnederlandse versie van de Circa Instans van Platearius (Oudenaarde, 1970).

136 See H. Schipperges, 'Zur Rezeption und Assimilation arabischer Medizin im frühen Toledo', Sudhoffs Archiv 39 (1955), 261–83 repr. in G. Baader & G. Keil (eds.), Medizin im mittelalterlichen Abendland (Darmstadt, 1982), pp.151–76.

137 See R. Lemay in C. C. Gillispie (ed.), Dictionary of Scientific Biography 15, suppl. (1978), pp.173–92.

138 See C. Vieillard, Gilles de Corbeil médecin de Philippe-Auguste et chanoine de Notre Dame 1140–1224? (Paris, 1909) and G. Rath, 'Gilles de Corbeil as Critic of His Age', Bull. Hist. Med. 38 (1964), 133–38.

139 Edited in L. Choulant, Aegidii Corboliensis carmina medica (Lipsiae, 1826), excerpts in Vieillard, op. cit., pp.337–59, modern German translation in J. Schönen, Die Medikamentenverse des Gilles de Corbeil diss. Bonn, 1972. Schönen lists the materia medica on pp.168–90.

140 For other works see Vieillard, op. cit. and P. Kliegel, Die Harnverse des Gilles de Corbeil diss. Bonn, 1972.

141 See J. L. Pagel (ed.), Die Areolae des Johannes de Sancto Amando (Berlin, 1893) and Die Concordanciae des Johannes de Sancto Amando (Berlin, 1894); H. Ehlers, Zur Pharmakologie des Mittelalters unter besonderer Berücksichtigung der Areolae des Johannes von St Amand diss. Berlin, 1895.

142 These and the following biographical details are taken from L. M. de Rijk, 'On the Life of Peter of Spain, the Author of the Tractatus, called afterwards Summule logicales', Vivarium 8 (1970), 123–54.

143 See M. H. Da Rocha Pereira (ed.), Obras médicas de Pedro Hispano (Coimbra, 1973), pp.77–301.

144 For later collections of vernacular receipts including those of Jean Sauvage, Jean Pitard and the abbé Poutrel see C. de Tovar, 'Contamination, interférences et tentatives de systématisation dans la tradition manuscrite des réceptaires médicaux français: le réceptaire de Jean Sauvage', Revue d'Histoire des Textes 3 (1973), 115–91 & ibid. 4 (1974), 239–88. See eadem, 'A propos de la Chirurgie de l'abbé Poutrel', Romania 103 (1982), 345–62.

145 See Jörimann, op. cit., pp.1ff; J. Stannard, 'Rezeptliteratur as Fachliteratur' in W. Eamon (ed.), Studies on Medieval 'Fachliteratur' (Brussel, 1982), pp. 59–73; O. Zekert, Das ärztliche Rezept (Ingelheim am Rhein, 1960), pp. 5ff; D. Goltz, Studien . . . pp.14–24; J. Telle, 'Das Rezept als literarische Form', Med. Monatschrift 28 (1974), 389–95; B. D. Haage, 'Zum hypothetischen Rezepteingang im Arzneibuch des Erhart Hesel' in G. Keil (ed.) Fachprosa-studien (Berlin, 1982), pp.363–70; L. Buchheim, Geschichte der Rezepteinleitung: Horusauge – Jupiterzeichen – Recipe diss. Bonn, 1965.

146 The first three categories are also represented in veterinary receipts. For literature see T. Hunt, 'Horses and Courses', French Studies Bulletin 22 (1987), 1–4. The earliest printed

veterinary treatise in French appears to be Lozenne [= 'le bon maistre mareschal de Lozenne'], *La Medecine des chevaulx et bestes chevalines* (Paris: Vérard, 1506).

147 A verse collection in French is found in MS Cambridge, Trinity College 0.1.20 (s.xiii) ff. 236r–39v (172 octosyllabic couplets), whilst MS Cambridge, St John's College D.4 (s.xiv[1]) ff.85vb–86va includes the same cosmetic receipts within a text of the *Physique rimee* (see below pp.204 ff.). The subject of cosmetics has not received the treatment it deserves, but see B. Grillet, *Les Femmes et les fards dans l'antiquité grecque* (Paris, 1975); J. Pagel, 'Geschichte der Kosmetik' in M. Joseph (ed.), *Handbuch der Kosmetik* (Leipzig, 1912), pp.71 ff; S. K. Hamarneh, 'The First Known Independent Treatise on Cosmetology in Spain', *Bull. Hist. Med.* 39 (1965), 309–25; W. Gramm, *Die Körperpflege der Angelsachsen* (Heidelberg, 1938). Further refs. in G. Simon, *Kosmetische Präparate vom 16. bis 19. Jahrhundert* (Braunschweig, 1983).

148 PR = *Physique rimee* (see below pp.142 ff.). References to receipts in the following pages include the manuscript and the number of the receipt as it occurs in the relevant chapter below.

149 Cf. W. Eamon, 'Books of Secrets in Medieval and Early Modern Science', *Sudhoffs Archiv* 69 (1985), 26–49.

150 See my *Teaching and Learning Latin in 13th C. England*, forthcoming (D.S. Brewer)

151 Cf. L. C. Mackinney, 'Medieval Medical Dictionaries and Glossaries' in J. L. Cate & E. N. Anderson (eds.), *Medieval and Historiographical Essays in Honour of James Westfall Thompson* (Chicago, 1938), pp.240–68.

152 See T. Hunt, *Plant Names of Medieval England* (Cambridge, 1989).

153 References are often exact. See, for example, the charm in MS B. L. Sloane 2584 (s.xv) f.31r 'For þe crampe: + Thebal + Ech + Guth + Et + Guthanay + þes names schul be write in parchemyn wit crosses. Whoso beriþ hem on hym schal not have þe crampe, os maister Jon Cattesdene seiþ in þe floure of medicynes, in þe secunde boke, in þe 22 chapeter, in þe ende of þe crampe'. Cf. the abbreviated redaction of the *Rosa* in MS Add.33996 f.170v 'Carmen contra crampam: + Thebal Et Guth Guttanay. Ista nomina scribantur cum cruce in pergameno et quamdiu has litteras super se portaverit non nocebit ei crampa nec spasmus, quod idem est. Istud est sine r[atione ?], tamen expertum est et nisi sint nomina alicuius sancti vel sanctorum aliquorum non adhibeo fidem. Tunc enim erit carmen domino nostro in cuius virtute omnia sanantur'.

154 See esp. no.141* which provides a detailed illustration of almost all aspects of the therapeutic receipt.

155 The ultimate source is Galen's *Antebalomena*.

156 There is a French text in MS B.L. Sloane 962 (s.xv) f.153v–r and an English one in MS Oxford, Bodl. Lib., Ashmole 1392 (s.xv), pt.2, pp.25–9.

157 See E. Schöner, *Das Viererschema in der antiken Humoralpathologie*, Sudhoffs Archiv Beiheft 4 (Wiesbaden, 1964).

158 See Hunt, *Plant Names*.

159 These are listed in W. Bonser, *The Medical Background of Anglo-Saxon England* (London, 1963), pp.24–7 and described more fully in H. J. de Vriend (ed.), *The Old English Herbarium and Medicina de Quadrupedibus* EETS 286 (London, 1984), pp.xi–xlix.

160 See C. E. Wright, *Bald's Leechbook*, Early English MSS in Facsimile V (Copenhagen, 1955) and Cockayne, vol. 2. There is a discussion in S. Rubin, *Medieval English Medicine* (London, 1974), pp.55–61.

161 'Some Notes on Anglo-Saxon Medicine', *Medical History* 9 (1965), 156–69 and id., *Medicine in Medieval England* (London, 1967), pp.18–20.

162 See M. Löweneck (ed.), *Peri Didaxeon. Eine Sammlung von Rezepten in englischer Sprache aus dem 11./12. Jahrhundert*, Erlanger Beiträge zur englischen Philologie 12 (Erlangen, 1896) (note the gloss on p.15, no.22 *croh, safran gallice*). See also Rubin, pp.65–7.

163 J. H. G. Grattan & C. Singer, *Anglo-Saxon Magic and Medicine: illustrated especially from the semi-pagan text Lacnunga* (London, 1952). See also Rubin, pp.62–5.

164 See de Vriend, *ed. cit.* and Rubin, pp.46–50.
165 See above p.6 and de Vriend, *ed. cit.*, pp.lv *et seq.*
166 de Vriend, *ed. cit.*, pp.lxii *et seq.*
167 See Rubin, pp.50–55.
168 See C. Singer, 'A Medical Compendium of the First Half of the Twelfth Century' repr. from *Bull. of the Soc. of Medic. Hist. of Chicago* (1917) and revised as 'A Review of Medical Literature of the Dark Ages, with a New Text of about 1110', *Proceedings of the Royal Society of Medicine* 10 (1916–17), 107–60. In a list of *nomina herbarum* we read 'papaver id est pouncel'.
169 'Anglo-Saxon Plant Remedies and the Anglo-Saxons', *Isis* 70 (1979), 250–68. A comprehensive treatment of botanical terminology will be found in P. Bierbaumer, *Der botanische Wortschatz des altenglischen*, Grazer Beiträge zur englischen Philologie 1–3 (Graz, 1975–79).
170 A beautifully written codex of the twelfth century with fine historiated initials is MS B.L. Royal 12 E XX which has the following charm on the last folio (f.162v): 'Ad dentium dolorem: in nomine domini nostri Jesu Christi, Patris et Filii et Spiritus Sancti, cheilei, cecce, becce, upservicce, slamone, puer, innaco[?], dicapron, sed noli et coli. Þanne hyt an yerþe hates byrnet suum famulum dei .N. Pater Noster .ix.'
171 See below pp.64 ff.
172 See L. Demaitre, 'Scholasticism in Compendia of Practical Medicine, 1260–1450', *Manuscripta* 20 (1976), 81–95.
173 See H. E. Handerson, *Gilbertus Anglicus: Medicine of the Thirteenth Century* (Cleveland, Ohio, 1918). Further bibliographical details in C. H. Talbot & E. A. Hammond, *The Medical Practitioners of Medieval England: A Biographical Register* (London, 1965), pp. 58–60. For a general discussion see C. H. Talbot, *Medicine in Medieval England*, pp.72–82 and Rubin, pp.200–04.
174 See M. Kurdziałek, 'Gilbertus Anglicus und die psychologischen Erörterungen in seinem *Compendium Medicinae*', *Sudhoffs Archiv* 47 (1963), 106–26.
175 See pp.325 ff. and notes.
176 The largest books are the first, on fevers (75 folios), and the last which covers the sexual organs, menstruation, gynaecology, childbirth, leprosy and snakebites (80 folios). Books 2, 3 and 6 average 50 folios. The two shortest books are Book 4 on cardio-thoracic problems (30 folios) and Book 5 on the digestive system (29 folios).
177 See F. M. Getz, 'Gilbertus Anglicus Anglicized', *Medical History* 26 (1982), 436–42. Dr Getz is to publish an edition based on MS London, Wellcome Historical Medical Library 537 (c.1460).
178 It begins 'Incipit liber morborum tam universalium quam particularium a magistro Gilberto Anglico editus ab omnibus auctoribus et practicis magistrorum extractus et excerptus, qui compendium medicine intitulatur, et est primus liber de febribus'.
179 For details of his life see A. B. Emden, *A Biographical Register of the University of Oxford to 1500* vol. 2 (Oxford, 1958), p.739 and Talbot & Hammond, *The Medical Practitioners .* . ., pp.148–50.
180 Gilbertus: 'vetulae provinciales dant purpuram combustam in potu. Habet enim occultam naturam curandi variolas. Similiter pannus tinctus de granno.'
181 Cambridge, Corpus Christi Coll. 261 (s.xv), ff.1r–232r; Edinburgh Univ. Libr. 168 [Laing 180] (s.xiv) ff.1r–305r; Exeter Cathedral 3506 (s.xiv²) ff.1r–239r; London, B.L. Sloane 134 (s.xv) ff.48r–49v (index), 50r–168v ('Explicit rosa medicine abreviata'); Sloane 280 (s.xv) ff.9ra–261vb ('Explicit practica m. Johannes de Catesden'); Sloane 1067 (s.xv) ff. 4ra–5va (index), 6r–280r ('Explicit rosa medicine magistri Johannis de Gadesden'); Sloane 1612 (s.xiv/xv) ff.125ra–340va ('Explicit rosa medicine magistri Johannis de Gatesden'); B.L. Add. 33996 (s.xv) ff.149r–210v (a heavily interpolated abridgement, acephalous and imperfect; 'Explicit rosula medicine secundum m. J. de Catesden'); Oxford, Bodl. Lib. e Musaeo 146 [S.C. 3619] (s.xv) ff.1r–348r; Bodley 362 [S.C. 2463]

(s.xv) ff.1r–246v; Bodley 608 [S.C. 2059] (s.xv) ff.v^r–407r; Corpus Christi Coll. 69 (s.xiv ex.) ff.1r–191r; Merton Coll. 262 [C.2.13] ff.1r–237r.

182   See G. Dock, 'Printed Editions of the Rosa Anglica of John of Gaddesden', *Janus* 12 (1907), 425–35.

183   See L. Demaitre, *Doctor Bernard de Gordon, Professor and Practitioner* (Toronto, 1980).

184   For a general discussion see H. P. Cholmeley, *John of Gaddesden and the 'Rosa Medicinae'* (Oxford, 1912); Talbot, *Medicine in Medieval England*, pp.111–15; Rubin, pp.204–7.

185   These are often indicated by marginal rubrics along with terms like *diffinitio, dieta, localia remedia* etc.

186   See W. Wulff (ed.), *Rosa Anglica seu Rosa Medicinae Johannis Anglici: An Early Modern Irish Translation of a Section of the Mediaeval Text-Book of John of Gaddesden*, Irish Texts Society 25 [1923] (London, 1929). On pp.1–lvi Wulff gives a useful list of unpublished Irish medical MSS.

187   The same receipt is found (in prose) in MS Sloane 146 no.153 and as part of the *Physique rimee* in MS Cambridge, St John's College D.4 f.89ra. It is preceded by two receipts *contre morsure de chien* which are also found, again in prose, in MS Sloane 146 nos 150 & 151, and in verse in MS Sloane 3550 nos 53 & 54 and in MS St John's College D.4 f.89ra, see below p.212.

188   See the *Physique rimee* ll.1157–90.

189   See *Lettre d'Hippocrate* no.47.

190   See *ibid.* no. 35.

191   On f.168v there is a reference to a cure, 'sic fuit vicarius de Northleye [i.e. Northleigh in Oxfordshire] curatus cui anus egressus fuit.'

192   Matth. 17, 20 'Hoc autem genus non eiicitur nisi per orationem et jejunium'. There is an Anglo-Norman version of this rite, attributed to Constantine the African, in MS Edinburgh, N.L.S., Advocates' Libr. 18.6.9 (s.xiv^1) f.93v.

193   See A. B. Emden, *A Biographical Register of the University of Cambridge to 1500* (Cambridge, 1963), p.270.

194   There is a Latin section on the signs of the Zodiac, including some charms, on ff.183vb–184vb and a Middle English treatise on urines on f.185ra–b and *signa mortis* on f.185va.

195   It is followed by 'ista sunt nomina autorum in phisica scilicet Ipocras, Galienus, Alexander, Johannisius, Theophilus, Philaretus, Aristotiles, Constantinus, Ysak, Hilarius, Plinius, Diascorides, Macer, Oribasius'.

196   See Talbot & Hammond, *The Medical Practitioners*, p. 41.

197   For these see below pp.86 ff.

198   A receipt on f.4rb combines three languages: '*Pur rancle ou festre*; ou verme: Pernez heyhof et suwet de motoun et triblés et metez chaud et ditez cest orisoun: "Omnipotens, sempiterne Deus, sicut potes per sanctam graciam et per sanctam dulcissimam misericordiam tuam et per sanctam Mariam virginem matrem tuam, sana hunc egrotum .N." ' The Middle English receipts are found on ff.179va–180ra, 180vb, 181ra, 181vb. Some English words occur sporadically e.g. [f.187va] medicine contra emigraneam et *ache* in capite causa emigranei [f.179ra] Contra *buyles* . . . contra *ache* pro gutta [f.178va] pro *ache* parve mentis ex frigidate . . . pro *ache* in dorso . . . unguentum *for ache* . . . *for ache* in brachiis.

199   See OED sub *blast sb*.6c [1547!].

200   The word is not in the dictionaries.

201   *alectorius* = 'stone found in gizzard of cock'.

202   Cf. f.187ra 'medicina pro auditu recuperando . . . a quantite of life hony wel clarified'.

203   See OED sub *warden sb.*^{2}.

204   At the bottom of f.150r the English rubric *Medycyn for a mannes lywer þat ys grown to hys rybbus* is followed by a Latin receipt. In the *stupha ydropicorum* on f.152ra all the ingredients are in English, but the directions are in Latin. On f.177va we have 'For rennyng of heres: Tak garlek þat haþ bot on clowe on þe hed and meddele hit wiþ þe poudur of cirmoyntayne et pone in aure et extrahetur.'

205   See OED sub *angletwitch*.

206   meaning unclear.
207   i.e. *troglodytus.*
208   i.e. cammock (plant), though the spelling is more usual for cammock = curved stick.
209   The word is not in the dictionaries.
210   i.e. perce-pierre. Cf. OED sub *pierce-stone* (=samphire).
211   The normal sense is 'an affection of the bones' or 'a disease of the mouth' (see MED sub *bon-shaue*) in which sense the word appears in the same column (*contre le bonchawe*) and on f.182rb (*For ache of bonchawe*).
212   See R. H. Robbins in *Med. Stud.* 32 (1970), 282–98.
213   See Walther, *Initia* 18083.
214   See *ibid.* 19692.
215   See P. H. -S. Hartley & H. R. Aldridge, *Johannes de Mirfield of St Bartholomew's, Smithfield: His Life and Works* (Cambridge, 1936) and F. Getz, 'John Mirfield and the *Breviarium Bartholomei*' in *Society for the Social History of Medicine, Bulletin* 37 (1985), 24–26.
216   MS Harley 3 f.304 represents the first leaf of another copy of the *Breviarium*, whilst f.3 is also a leaf from the second copy, and corresponds to the contents of ff.12vb–13rb of the complete copy.
217   And progressing to Part 9, dist. 7, c.4.
218   He uses a variety of commentaries, including that of Johannes de sancto Amando on the *Antidotarium Nicolai*, see MS B.L. Sloane 2268 (s.xiv), ff.18ra–41ra (inc. 'Medicine composite sunt diverse que deteriantur in antidotario Rasis et Avicenne et Serapionis et in Antidotario Nicolai de quo ad presens est intentio'). On ff.1ra–15vb of the Sloane MS is a work which concludes 'Explicit antidotarius magistri Johannis Albi dicti de sancto Jacobo'.
219   See my 'Popular Medical Practices in John Mirfield's *Breviarium Bartholomei*' to appear in *Folklore.*
220   See R. T. Gunther, *Early Science in Oxford* 3 (Oxford, 1925), p.9 who misinterprets this passage as implying that Tingewick (who died in 1339) had read Mirfield! See Talbot & Hammond, pp.229 ff. On Tingewick see A. B. Emden, *A Biographical Register of the University of Oxford to 1500* 3, p.1877. For another misinterpretation of the passage in Mirfield see Hartley & Aldridge, p.21.
221   i.e. 'tan-dust'.
222   corr. *stubbewort?*
223   See S. de Renzi, *Collectio Salernitana* 2 (Napoli, 1852), p.471 ll. 787–805 (a composite and artificial text!). For an important Salernitan text from the celebrated Breslau codex see E. Benndorf, *Der Liber de confectione medicinarum im Breslauer Codex* diss. Leipzig, 1920. See also the *modus medendi* in Renzi, *Collectio* 4, pp.415–38. For simples there is the *Circa instans* and Johannes de sancto Paulo, *Liber de simplicium medicinarum virtutibus* (ed. by G. H. Kroemer in a Leipzig diss. of 1920) which I have seen in MS Oxford, Bodl. Libr. Bodley 761 (s.xiv) ff.42v–57v where it is called *Liber de virtutibus herbarum* and begins 'Cogitanti michi de simplicium medicinarum virtutibus earum quod idem operantur nomina in unum colligere visum est utile ... ' This work simply follows the Galenic *doctrina de gradibus,* enumerating the qualities and degrees of each plant (four degrees of heat, moisture, coldness and dryness). There is an Old French version of the work in MS Princeton University Library, Garrett 131. I have not seen M. McVaugh, *The Mediaeval Theory of Compound Medicines* diss. Princeton 1965, but see *id.,* (ed.), *Arnaldi de Villanova opera medica omnia* II *Aphorismi de gradibus* (Granada-Barcelona, 1975), pp.13–87; *id.,* ' "Apud antiquos" and Mediaeval Pharmacology', *Medizinhist. Jnl.* 1 (1966), 16–23; L. Thorndike, 'Three Texts on Degrees of Medicines (*De gradibus*)', *Bull. Hist. Med.* 38 (1964), 533–7.
224   Little work has been done on vernacular medical terminology. Cf. G. Caturegli, *Espressioni mediche latine e greche dal 'De medicina' di A.C. Celso* (Pisa, 1966); M. L. Altieri Biagi, *Guglielmo volgare: studio sul lessico della medicina medioevale* (Bologna, 1970); B. Quemada, *Introduction à l'étude du vocabulaire médical (1600–1700)* (Besançon/Paris, 1955); G.

Sigurs, 'La langue médicale française: nouvelles datations', *Le Français Moderne* 33 (1965), 199–218; R. Arveiller, 'Médecine et matière médicale', *Rev. de ling. rom.* 34 (1970), 179–85; Ö. Södergård, 'La langue médicale française: quelques nouvelles datations', *Etudes de langue et de littérature du moyen âge offerts à Félix Lecoy* (Paris, 1973), pp.541–50.

225 See below pp.79 f.

226 Cf. Bonser, *op. cit.*, pp.314–25.

227 See R. T. Gunther, *The Greek Herbal of Dioscorides: Illustrated by a Byzantine AD 512, Englished by John Goodyear AD 1655, Edited and First Printed by Robert T. Gunther* (New York, 1934; repr. 1959, 1968), p.3.

228 *ibid.*, p.4.

229 W. R. Dawson, *A Leechbook or Collection of Medical Recipes of the Fifteenth Century* (London, 1934), p.143.

230 R. Flower, 'Popular Science in Mediaeval Ireland', *Ériu* 9 (1921), [61–67], 65–67.

231 E. Wickersheimer, 'Sur le temps de cueillette des simples: deux textes inédits' in *Homenaje a Millas-Vallicrosa* II (Barcelona, 1956), pp.523–7. The first text is drawn from MS 3174 (s.xv) of the Bibl. de l'Arsenal and consists of short Latin precepts attributed to 'Rasis' and mentioning 24 drugs. The second treatise is an eighteenth-century copy (MS 3060–3062 of Bibl. Roy. de Bruxelles) of an earlier German treatise covering c.100 plants.

232 E. Wickersheimer, 'Nouveaux textes médiévaux sur le temps de cueillette des simples', *Archives internationales d'histoire des sciences* 29 no.11 (1950), 342–55. The treatise is also found in Erfurt, Amplon. Q. 174 (s.xiv¹) f.123v.

233 *ibid.*, 343.

234 E. Wickersheimer, 'Epistola Ypocratis ad Alexandrum de tempore herbarum', *Janus* 41 (1937), 145–52.

235 W. F. Daems & G. Keil, 'Die Solothurner Fassung des "Tractatulus de collectione medicinarum" ' in G. Schramm (ed.), *Neue Beiträge zur Geschichte der Pharmazie. Festschrift für Herrn Dr. Phil. Hans-Rudolf Fehlmann zur Feier des 60. Geburtstags* (Zürich, 1979), pp. 47–57.

236 See Galen (ed. Kühn) Lib.19, c.xii and Isidore, *Etym.* Lib.16, c.25–7.

237 See H. E. Sigerist, 'Masse und Gewichte in den medizinischen Texten des frühen Mittelalters', *Kyklos* 3 (1930), 439–44.

238 Cf. B. Kisch, *Scales and Weights: a Historical Outline* (New Haven/London, 1965); E. A. Moody & M. Clagett, *The Medieval Science of Weights (Scientia de ponderibus)* (Madison, 1952; repr. 1960).

239 Sigerist, *art. cit.* suggests the equivalents libra = 327.45 gr.; uncia = 27.288 gr.; drachma = 3.411 gr.; scripulum = 1.137 gr.; obolus = 0.568 gr.; siliqua = 0.189 gr.

240 Renzi, *Collectio Salernitana* 1 (Napoli, 1852), pp.482 f, ll.1136 ff.

241 MS = *consurgit ter triplicatus*. In MS Oxford, Pembroke College 10 f.35rb following line 7 the lines read 'Dat scrupulum nummus, scrupulos tres dragma, sed octo/uncia dat dragmas, duodena dat uncia libram.'

242 In the preceding treatise (f.58r–v) the dragma is given as 'octava pars uncie'.

243 MS = *quem*.

244 i.e. farthing.

245 See Hartley & Aldridge, p.92.

246 See W. Hinz, *Islamische Masse und Gewichte* (Leiden, 1955); I. Fellmann, 'Arabische Medizinalmasse und -Gewichte in lateinischen Übersetzungen arabischer medizinischer Literatur', *Sudhoffs Archiv* 69 (1985), 228–31.

247 See S. Hamarneh, 'The First Recorded Appeal for Unification of Weight and Measure Standards in Arabic Medicine', *Physis* 5 (1963), 230–48.

248 See W. van Zeist, 'Prehistoric and Early Historic Food Plants in the Netherlands', *Palaeohistoria* 14 (1968 [1970]), 41–173 with rich bibliography.

249 See D. Gay Wilson, 'Goldsmith House site, Goss Street, Chester, 1972. II.Plant Foods

and Poisons from Medieval Chester', *Journal of the Chester Archaeological Society* 58 (1975), 55–67.

250 Cf. p.62 'Confusion could also arise from the variety of plant names in popular use before recent attempts at standardisation. Many plants have different popular names in different regions, and mistakes could easily be made if a person from one region used or gathered plants on the instructions (or written receipts) of one from a different region'.

251 See J. Harvey, *York* (London, 1975), p.112.

252 See G. W. Dimbleby, 'The Seeds' in C. Platt & R. Coleman-Smith, *Excavations in Medieval Southampton 1953–1969* 1 (Leicester, 1975), pp.344–46.

253 See J. E. Mellor & T. Pearce, *The Austin Friars, Leicester*, Leicestershire Field Unit Report, CBA Research Report 35 (1981), pp.170–71.

254 See M. Fraser & J. H. Dickson, 'Plant Remains' in J. C. Murray (ed.), *Excavations in the Medieval Burgh of Aberdeen 1973–81*, Society of Antiquaries of Scotland, Monograph Series 2 (Edinburgh, 1982), pp.239–43.

255 B. O'Riordain, 'Excavations at High Street and Winetavern Street, Dublin', *Medieval Archaeology* 15 (1971) [73–85], 77.

256 See B. Moffat (ed.), *SHARP PRACTICE 1: The First Report on Researches into the Medieval Hospital at Soutra, Lothian Region* (1986); id., 'S.H.A.R.P. Practice The Search for Medieval Medical Treatments', *Archaeology Today* May, 1987, pp.22–28; id., 'An Investigation of Medieval Medical Treatments', *Proc. Roy. Coll. Phys. of Edin.* 18 (1988), 80–86.

257 Here the importance of tormentil (Potentilla erecta) as an astringent was established. See Moffat's as yet unpublished paper 'Insights into a Medieval Medical Practice, using Plant Microremains. An Exploration using material from Jedburgh, Scotland' (1986).

Notes to Chapter Two

1 Cf. C. H. Talbot, 'A Medieval Physician's Vade Mecum', *Jnl. Hist. Med. & All. Sc.* 16 (1961), 213–33 and for illustrations of 'portable' MSS incl. volvellae, calendars, almanacs etc. M. P. Cosman, 'Medieval Medical Malpractice and Chaucer's Physician', *New York State Jnl. of Med.* 72 (1972), [2439–44] 2442 f.

2 A. Beccaria, *I codici di medicina del periodo presalernitano (secoli IX, X e XI)* (Roma, 1956), pp.261–6 describes the MS and dates it s.XI ex./XII in., whilst suggesting a 13th C. date for the French additions. A dating c.1100 is proposed by C. M. Kauffmann, *Romanesque Manuscripts 1066–1190* (London, 1975), pp.58f who discusses the pen outline drawings of cautery figures (nos 19 & 20). Further reproductions of the drawings can be found in K. Sudhoff, *Beiträge zur Geschichte der Chirurgie im Mittelalter*, Studien zur Geschichte der Medizin 10 (Leipzig, 1914), Tafel XVII.

3 See L. Thorndike & P. Kibre, *A Catalogue of Incipits of Mediaeval Scientific Writings in Latin*, rev. & augm. ed. (London, 1963), 264 & P. Kibre 'Hippocrates Latinus ... (V)', *Traditio* 35 (1979), 276–7.

4 The initial letter seems to be followed by eight minims, but the MS is indistinct.

5 Printed in T. Hunt, 'The Medical Recipes in MS Royal 5 E VI', *Notes & Queries* 231 (1986), 6–9.

6 These include 'le fi ki seine', 'la gute chaive', 'la gutefestre', 'la piere', 'le huf', 'le cursun', 'le rancle', 'verms', 'jurneles fiefres', 'le cancre', 'pur aveir solucion' etc.

7 Amongst the more interesting plant names which here receive early attestations are

aluidne, boniface, cefrefuil, centorie, erre terestre, esclaire, febrefuie, galinga, nuiz galges, os-munde, puliol, peletre, sanicle, scamonie, senechun, vetonie, uiterole (for *uinterole* ?). Medical terms include *ampulle, letuarie, eximel* (corr. *oximel*) *real.*

8   The MS clearly has here, and later, *iunt*, though *uint* is what is required by the sense.

9   The rest of the line in the MS is blank.

10   See T. Hunt, 'Early Anglo-Norman Recipes in MS London, B.L. Royal 12 C XIX', ZFSL 97 (1987), 245–54. Here, too, we have early, often the earliest recorded, attestations of interesting botanical names and other words e.g. *amblette, amorosche, aristologe, arraces, buterice, centoine, cherlokes, flambe, glagel, guarance, materace, melden* (ME), *opium, pelu-seite, pigle, poucel* (*poncel*) *, puliel, raffe, sageterole* (& *saiterole*), *sarré, scamonie, slecfritgres,* (& *siecfritgres;* ME), *turmentine, chanette, cochuns, curance, cursun, espuint(r)es, esvertun, ferthing, giste, jute, leituarie agut, leye, mal volant, mortrel, sancmeslure, soluble, undee, vun-ches.*

11   I intend to publish these on another occasion.

12   A. Bell, 'A Thirteenth-Century MS Fragment at Peterborough', M.H.R.A. (*Bulletin of the Modern Humanities Research Association*) III, vii (June, 1929), 132–40.

13   S.C. 2355.

14   For a description see N. Ker, *Medieval Manuscripts in British Libraries* 1 (Oxford, 1969), pp.199–201 (referred to as no.227a, but this is no longer correct).

15   Other vernacular names appear as follows: f.157r cape radicem herbe que gallice vocatur *pauier et trumel* ... erbam que gallice vocatur *cerfoyl;* sume radicem herbe que gallice vocatur *glay;* f.157v cape succum *launceleie;* f.160v cape florem arboris que gallice vocatur *genet;* f.161r cape pomum de quercu, poma de *botoiner,* radicem de *glay;* f.164r cape herbas que vocantur *morele, barbion, laytues et cycoré;* f.168v grana de *bay de lorer;* sume erbam que vocatur *jubarbe;* f.169v bibe *puliol* distemperatum cum vino; f.171v cape novam ollam et fac in fundo quasi unum lectum de herba que gallice vocatur *mouron* et alterum de erba que gallice vocatur *lacon;* f.174r cape erbas que gallice vocantur *[hen]belle et cresson.*

16   See above p.29; ff.76v–148v contain a collection of Middle English receipts edited by F. Heinrich, *Ein mittelenglisches Medizinbuch* (Halle, 1896).

17   See T. Hunt, 'Horses and Courses', *French Studies Bulletin* 22 (1987), 1–4.

18   i.e. *salve.*

19   For *septmere?*

20   For a Latin text of the 'Lettre d'Hippocrate' see below pp.124 ff. For a description of the MS see G. F. Warner & J. P. Gilson, *Catalogue of Western Manuscripts in the Old Royal and King's Collections* 2 (London, 1921), pp.13–15.

21   i.e. 'horseheal'.

22   read *teinne de la teste* or *teinuse teste?*

23   i.e. 'brooklime'. There are a few vernacular names amongst the Latin receipts e.g. f.108r accipe herbam *bogie;* f.110r levisticum: *lovasche;* f.135r succum radicis palladie .i. *prim-erole;* f.144r seminum macedonici .i. *bissopesworth.*

24   See T. Hunt, 'The "Novele Cirurgerie" in MS London, British Library, Harley 2558', *Z.f.rom. Phil.* 103 (1987), 271–99, esp. 271–3.

25   See *Catalogue of the Stowe Manuscripts in the British Museum* 1 (London, 1895), p.632. The poems are incompletely recorded in J. Sonet, *Répertoire d'incipit de prières en ancien français* (Genève, 1956), see nos. 311, 432.

26   See below p.143.

27   See Warner & Gilson, *Catalogue* ... 1, pp.284–6.

28   See T. Hunt, 'Recettes médicales en vers français d'après le manuscrit 0.8.27 de Trinity College, Cambridge', *Romania* 106 (1985), 57–83 and see also below p.144.

29   See N. R. Ker, *Medieval Manuscripts in British Libraries* 2 (Oxford, 1977) pp.828–32.

30   The Latin receipts contain a good number of vernacular words: f.135v herbam que dicitur *crousope;* f.138v cape saponem et *ache* minorem; cape *aloyne, mauve* minorem, *morele* maiorem ... la racine de *gladene* ... une poygne de *grounde[s]welie.* The intermingling of Middle English and Anglo-Norman is illustrated on almost every page: f.140v le jus de

chykenmete; f.141v vyolette menue .i. chykenmete; f.145v la meule de syu .i. ellerne; f.146r le jus de wylde tesle; la racyne de hermodache; f.146v verge a pasturs .i. wald iceole [corr. wild tesle ?]; f.151r une porciun de blakeberye; un herbe ke l'en apele stondefast .i. ragde wrt; f.152r la racyne de savuner .i. crowesope; ardez rathles a pudre; f.152v amer dé boys .i. wodesoure; f.157v pernez stychewert, wodesure, herbyve, plantayne, eble e fane; f.159r suette de bausun; f.162v averoynt, c'est en engleis southernewode; puliole .i. hulwurt; morele c'est(e) atterloþe; f.163r une herbe qe est apelé ungle de chyval .i. lappatum rotundum anglice feldhove; f.166r une herbe qe est apelé gallice [sic] groundeswilie; f.168v mangez letuse .i. slepewrt; un herbe qe ad a noun en engleis popi. Interesting words include oculescunse (f.125v), blyayus (f.134r), estrictorie/strictorie (= strictorium, f.137v), enfloures genitories (f.141r), wasteline (f.142v), escore de bogie (f.155v), coupere (f.148r), la racine de le lepre .i. suffoigne neir [= Helleborous niger] (f.165v), amblete (f.169r), diatine est la racine de une herbe qe [est] apelé mesmes le noun.

31   Italicized rubrics are in red in the MS.
32   This compound (electuary) occurs regularly in the receipts in MS Nat. Libr. Scotland, Advocates' Libr. 18.6.9 (s.xiv) ff.128v, 133r, 134v, 136r, 140r, 143r. See also MS London, B.L. Sloane 134 (s.xv) f.67r (John of Gaddesden). It is recorded in the Antidotarium Nicolai.
33   The MS has piiins. For the same receipt see below p.121 no.135.
34   The text as transmitted is obviously corrupt. It seems to derive from a dieta, but some material has obviously dropped out.
35   Cf. below pp.267 (Sloane 146 no.1) and 324 (Digby 69 no.100).
36   i.e. dragmes. After 'un vert unement' the abbreviation is uncertain, looking rather like an s. Perhaps the sign for unce is intended.
37   There is a superscript insertion merche (ME).
38   Another treatment for horses is found on f.159v: 'Pur chival pursif: Ly donetz a manger segle vert per ebdomadam, pus bure e aile, e meretz ensemble e fetes trangluter chaud treys jurs ou plus. Convalescet'.
39   Cf. f.144r 'Pernez la racyne de pamphet .i. wudeþonge'.
40   Cf. f.147v 'ortye savage .i. griesche'.
41   corr. may butere.
42   See F. Kudlien, 'Early Greek Primitive Medicine', Clio Medica 3 (1968), 305–36; G. Majno, The Healing Hand: Man and Wound in the Ancient World (Cambr. Mass., 1975); O. Weinreich, Antike Heilungswunder: Untersuchungen zum Wunderglauben der Griechen und Römer (Giessen, 1909; repr. 1969); D. W. Amundsen, 'Medicine and Faith in Early Christianity', Bull.Hist. Med. 56 (1982), 326–50; W. J. Sheils, The Church and Healing (Oxford, 1982); H. C. Kee, Medicine, Miracle and Magic in New Testament Times (Cambridge, 1986), esp. pp.95–121; V. Nutton in J. Scarborough (ed.), Byzantine Medicine . . . pp.8f.
43   Cf. S. Noorda, 'Illness and Sin, Forgiving and Healing: The Connection of Medical Treatment and Religious Beliefs in Ben Sira 38, 1–15' in M. J. Vermaseren (ed.), Studies in Hellenistic Religions (Leiden, 1979), pp.215–24.
44   See M. C. Martini, Piante medicamentose e rituali magico-religiosi in Plinio (Roma, 1977) and J. Stannard, 'Medicinal Plants and Folk Remedies in Pliny, Historia Naturalis', History & Philosophy of the Life Sciences 4 (1982), 3–23.
45   See J. Stannard, 'Marcellus of Bordeaux and the Beginnings of Medieval Materia Medica', Pharmacy in History 15 (1973), 47–53 and A. A. Barb in Folklore 61 (1951), 20–23.
46   See H. Biedermann, Medicina magica: metaphysische Heilmethoden in spätantiken und mittelalterlichen Handschriften (Graz, 1972); J. Stannard, 'Magiferous Plants and Magic in Medieval Medical Botany', Maryland Historian 8 (1977), 33–46; G. Keil, 'Zauberpflanzen und Wunderdrogentraktate', Leuvense Bijdragen 57 (1968), 165–75; M. T. Caffaratto, Storia, magica e virtù delle piante medicinali (Torino, 1976).
47   B. Thorpe (ed.), The Homilies of the Anglo-Saxon Church I (1844), p.477.

48 *Canterbury Tales* ed. F. N. Robinson, 2nd ed. (London, 1957), p.247, X (1) 605.
49 W. Bonser, *The Medical Background of Anglo-Saxon England* (London, 1963), p.120. Cf. E. Stürzl, 'Die christlichen Elemente in den altenglischen Zaubersegen', *Die Sprache* 6 (1960), 75–93.
50 See, for example, J. F. Borghouts, *Ancient Egyptian Magical Texts* (Leiden, 1978). The texts often exhibit the same parallelism of present case with mythical/historical precedent. Word-play is important. There are spells against dangers during the epagomenal days, specific demons, common ailments, problems of childbirth, and formulae to accompany the administration of medicine. Cf. the modern Syriac texts in H. Gollancz (ed.), *The Book of Protection, being a Collection of Charms* (London, 1912). See also A. Delatte, *Anecdota Atheniensia* 1 (Paris, 1927), *passim*.
51 All writers acknowledge their dependence on the pioneering work of T. O. Cockayne, *Leechdoms, Wort-cunning and Starcraft of Early England* 3 vols (London, 1864–6; repr. 1961). See J. F. Payne, *English Medicine in the Anglo-Saxon Times: The Fitz-Patrick Lectures for 1903* (Oxford, 1904), pp.94–142; F. Grendon, 'The Anglo-Saxon Charms', *The Journal of American Folklore* 22 (1909), 105–237 (repr. separately 1930); G. Storms, *Anglo-Saxon Magic* (The Hague, 1948), an edition and discussion of 86 charms, 24 of which are in Latin, but lacking 16 items included by Grendon; J. H. G. Grattan & Ch. Singer, *Anglo-Saxon Magic and Medicine, illustrated especially from the semi-pagan Text Lacnunga* (London, 1952); W. Bonser, *The Medical Background of Anglo-Saxon England: A Study in History, Psychology, and Folklore* (London, 1963), pp.213–27; C. H. Talbot, *Medicine in Medieval England* (London, 1967), pp.18–23; S. Rubin, *Medieval English Medicine* (London, 1974), pp.109–118; L. M. C. Weston, 'The Language of Magic in Two Old English Metrical Charms', *Neuph. Mitt.* 86 (1985), 176–86. For the German materials see B. Murdoch, *Old High German Literature* (Boston, 1983), pp.45–54. I have also seen H. L. Stuart, *A Critical Edition of Some Anglo-Saxon Charms and Incantations* PhD. thesis, Flinders, NSW, 1973.
52 'Some Notes on Anglo-Saxon Medicine', *Medical History* 9 (1965), 156–69.
53 Whilst relaxing the chronological limits of my survey in this section I have not sought to record all the ME charms which I have found, since both Professor D. Gray and Dr. S. Sheldon have announced their intention of producing editions of the ME charms: see D. Gray, 'Notes on some Middle English Charms' in B. Rowland (ed.), *Chaucer and Middle English Studies in Honour of Rossell Hope Robbins* (London, 1974), pp.56–71 and S. Sheldon, *Middle English and Latin Charms, Amulets and Talismans from Vernacular Manuscripts* diss. Tulane, 1978 (I have been able to obtain a copy of this work, which prints for the first time 84 charms out of a total of 140 ME and Latin charms from 26 MSS. I have deliberately refrained from using those MSS). See also F. Holthausen, 'Rezepte, Segen und Zaubersprüche aus zwei Stockholmer Handschriften', *Anglia* 19 (1897), 75–88; J. M. McBryde Jr., 'Some Mediaeval Charms', *Sewanee Review* 25 (1917), 292–304; I. B. Jones, 'Popular Medical Knowledge in Fourteenth-Century English Literature 1', *Bull. Hist. Med.* 5 (1937), esp. 430–40; C. F. Bühler, 'Prayers and Charms in Certain Middle English Scrolls', *Speculum* 39 (1964), 270–78; T. R. Forbes, 'Verbal Charms in British Folk Medicine', *Proceedings of the Am. Philos. Soc.* 115, iv (Aug. 1971), 293–316.
54 *Herbarius: recherches sur le cérémonial usité chez les anciens pour la cueillette des simples et des plantes magiques* 3e éd. rev. & augm. (Brussel, 1961). See also Bonser, pp.314–24.
55 Delatte, pp.39–72. Cf. Storms, pp.88–90.
56 See p.123 no.153.
57 Delatte, pp.73–87. Cf. Add.15236 no.27*.
58 Delatte, pp.88–117. Cf. Storms, pp.86f. & 92–6.
59 See Storms, pp.235 & 243; Add.15236 no.104*.
60 See R. Heim, *Incantamenta graeca latina* (Leipzig, 1893) & Storms, pp.243ff.
61 See Payne, p.112 & Grendon, p.143. See in general W. Boudriot, *Die altgermanische Religion in der amtlichen kirchlichen Literatur des Abendlandes vom 5. bis 11. Jahrhundert* (Bonn, 1928; repr. 1964).

62 See for examples of the Credo, Pater Noster, Benedicite, Psalms, Litany etc. Storms, pp.224f & 258f. See also Grendon, pp.150ff.

63 Migne, *PL* 140, 961C.

64 See Ch. Joret, 'Les incantations botaniques', *Romania* 17 (1888), 337–54 and Grattan & Singer, pp.45f. See also E. Norden, 'Über zwei spätlateinische precationes', *Festschrift zur Jahrhundertfeier der Universität Breslau* (Breslau, 1911), pp.517ff.

65 See Delatte, pp.148–63.

66 See Delatte, pp.164–88.

67 See Grattan & Singer, pp. 36f. & p.101 n.3; Bonser, p.229; Storms, pp. 77f.

68 See below LH 135, Add.15236 no.15.

69 See below 47.

70 See Delatte, pp.188–97.

71 See A. L. Meaney, *Anglo-Saxon Amulets and Curing Stones*, B.A.R. Brit. Ser. 96 (1981); L. J. A. Loewenthal, 'Amulets in Medieval Sculpture', *Folklore* 89 (1978), 3–12; L. Hausmann & L. Kriss-Rettenbeck, *Amulett und Talisman: Erscheinungsform und Geschichte*, 2te Aufl. (München, 1977).

72 See F. Dornseiff, *Das Alphabet in Mystik und Magie*, 2te Aufl. (Berlin, 1925; repr. 1975) and Payne, pp.119–25. For examples see 77 above, and below LH 168, Sloane 3550 f. 224r (see below p.139), Sloane 146 no.155. Provençal examples are found in P. Meyer, *Romania* 32 (1903), 273 & 292 and in C. Brunel, *ibid.* 83 (1962), 152ff, 157, 165 & 170.

73 For gibberish see below 37, 49, 73 and above (receipt) 76.

74 See below n.117 and H. Meroney, 'Irish in the Old English Charms', *Speculum* 20 (1945), 172–82 and R. E. McNally, ' "Tres linguae sacrae" in Early Irish Bible Exegesis', *Theological Studies* 19 (1958), 395–403. See also Storms. pp. 274f.

75 See below 10, 12, 42–44, 89, Add. 15236 nos 11*, 27*, 28*, 45*, 51*, Sloane 146 no.160, Digby 69 no.2.

76 On 'foilles de lorer' in LH 158 and on hosts in note 119 below. See also 29 below (lead plate; see also MS Wellcome Hist. Med. Libr. 407 ff.19v–20r).

77 See below 54, 85, 86 and notes 117 & 119. See also Add. 15236 no.44* (tetragrammaton), below 28 (cross) and note 132 (cross). On the use of the cross see W. G. Black, *Folk-Medicine: A Chapter in the History of Culture* (London, 1883), pp.85–87.

78 See Payne, pp.125–8; 36 below and note 117; Digby 69 nos. 1 & 94.

79 See Payne, pp.128–32; Grendon, pp.158f; Bonser, p.242.

80 Bonser, p.241. General references to the Life of Christ are found in 47 below and in Sloane 146 nos. 175–6. For Susanna see 32 below, and for Nicodemus 57 below.

81 See Gray, 64f; Storms, pp.150–54; Bonser, pp.252f; Black, pp.122f; A. A. Barb, 'Animula Vagula Blandula . . . ', *Folklore* 61 (1951), 19f & 28f; C. F. Mayer in *Bull. Hist. Med.* 7 (1939), 385; A. Lindgren (ed.), *Ein Stockholmer mittelniederdeutsches Arzneibuch aus der zweiten Hälfte des 15. Jahrhunderts* (Stockholm, 1967), pp.117f and no.138. Examples below are 3, 4, 5, 7, 13 (diminishing and augmenting), 16, 48, 74 (augmenting and diminishing). Cf. also 9 below (daily recitation of the Pater Noster beginning with 12 and reducing daily) and 45 (recitation of 'Quicumque vult' starting with 9 and diminishing daily). In 64 below the charm normally associated with Job is applied to St John (through palaeographical error ?) and in 74 to Raphael. For the background see G. Von der Osten, 'Job und Christ', *Jnl. of Warburg & Courtauld Inst.* 16 (1953), 153–8.

82 See Gray, 62; Black, pp.79f; Bonser, pp.243f; McBryde, 293–6; Lindgren, p.91 no.4; Holthausen, 80–81; O. Ebermann, *Blut- und Wundsegen* (Berlin, 1903), pp.42–52; R. J. Peebles, *The Legend of Longinus . . .* (Baltimore, 1911), pp.72–80. See below 19, 20, 29, Add. 15236 no.43*; MS Sloane 3160 (s.xv), f.162r (ME).

83 See below 54–56, 67 and note 117.

84 See below 30, 39, 41, 69, Add. 15236 nos. 15–16.

85 See below 6, 29, 52, 84; MS Wellcome Hist. Med. Libr. 406 (s.xv) f. 4v (ME).

86 See Gray, 62f; Bonser, p.243; Black, p.76; McBryde, pp.299f; Holthausen, 81; Robbins, *Speculum* 45 (1970), 405 and note 34 (with ref. to 14 texts). See below 23, 25, 26, 51, 53,

55, 76, Digby 69 No.11. On the background see A. A. Barb, 'St Zacharias the Prophet and Martyr: A study in Charms and Incantations', *Jnl. of Warburg & Courtauld Inst.* 11 (1948), 38 n.2–3 & 53ff. See also Ebermann, pp.24–35; MS Wellcome Hist. Med. Libr. 406 (s.xv) f.4v.

87 See below 11. The same charm is also adapted for fevers, see Holthausen, 79–80; P. Meyer, *Romania* 32 (1903), 293; C. Brunel, *Romania* 83 (1962), 150 & 153; Black, pp.77f; A. A. Barb, *Folklore* 61 (1951), 17; MS B.L. Lansdowne 680 (s.xv) f.41r/v.

88 See Gray, 63f; B. R. Townend, 'The Narrative Charm with Special Reference to the Cure of Toothache', *British Dental Journal* 85 (1948), 29–34. See MS Oxford, Bodl. Libr. Digby 69 f.7r/v.

89 See Gray, 63; Bonser, pp.244f; Holthausen, 84; Lindgren, p.99 no. 51; K. Eriksson, 'Pyhä Apollonia – neitsyt ja marttyyri', *Hippokrates* 2 (1985), 33–43; E. F. Frey, 'Saints in Medical History', *Clio Medica* 14 (1979) [35–70] 46f & 62f; H. Nux, 'Sainte Apolline, patronne de ceux qui souffrent des dents', *Revue d'odontologie, de stomachologie* 3 (1947) 113–53. See below 27, 87, Add. 15236 no.91*, Sloane 146 f. 69r; also MS Harley 2558 (s.xiv) f.166v.

90 See J. Guiraud, *Du culte de saint Blaise, le miraculeux guérisseur des maux de gorges* 2e éd. (Pézenas, 1892) & MSS B.L. Harley 3 f. 82va and Sloane 962 f.10r.

91 See Barb, *Jnl. Warb. & Court. Inst.* 11 (1948), 42f and note 132 below. See also below Add. 15236 no.30*.On saints and healing see C. L. P. Trüb, *Heilige und Krankheit* (Stuttgart, 1978) with tables arranged by disease (pp.249ff). See MS Wellcome Hist. Med. Libr. 407 (s.xv) f.45r ('Ad sanguinem narium')

92 See W. Bonser, 'The Seven Sleepers of Ephesus in Anglo-Saxon and later Recipes', *Folklore* 56 (1945), 254–6 & *id., op. cit.*, p. 226; Storms, pp.163–73; Holthausen, 79; C. Brunel, *Romania* 83 (1962), 153 & 166; L. B. Pinto, *Bull. Hist. Med.* 47 (1973), 518f; P. Meyer, *Romania* 22 (1903), 293; Holthausen, *Archiv* 99 (1897), 424. See below 12, 35. See also MS B.L. Royal 12 E XX (s.xii) f.162v.

93 See P. Meyer, *Bull. SATF* 1906, 32; Holthausen, 85; Grendon, p.159. See below 37, 38, 46, 49, LH note 71, Sloane 146 no. 90, Sloane 3550 no. 36.

94 See McBryde, 296–8; Ebermann, *op. cit.*, pp. 35–42; 50 above (receipt) and 65 below; MS B.L. Royal 12 G IV (s.xiv) f.178ra.

95 See Gray, 68; Holthausen, 82 (seynt Ewstas); P. Meyer, *Romania* 37 (1908), 515 (seynt Willame); Add. 15236 f.29r (see below p.224; Susanna); Sloane 3564 f.41r (see below p.91); Sloane 146 no.214.

96 See Add. 15236 no.46*.

97 For the role of candles see Holthausen, 83f; 27 (receipt) above; Add. 15236 no.162* (cf. no.46*).

98 On transferential charms see Black, pp.34–48, and 21 and 51 below (and notes 115 & 118).

99 See J. M. McBryde Jr., 'Charms for Thieves', *MLN* 22 (1907), 168–70 & *id.*, *Speculum* 34 (1959), 637–8; J. Daniel Vann III, 'Middle English Verses against Thieves: A Postscript', *Speculum* 34 (1959), 636–7; C. F. Bühler, 'Middle English Verses against Thieves', *Speculum* 33 (1958), 371–2 and *id.*, 'Three Middle English Prose Charms from MS Harley 2389', *N & Q* 207 (1962), 48. See 59–60 below.

100 See R. E. Bader, 'Sator arepo: Magie in der Volksmedizin', *Medizinhist. Jnl.* 22 (1987), 115–34 who traces its remote origins and also prints an English charm (p.119). The possible translations are listed on pp.130f, the most commonly preferred being 'Der Sämann Arepo hält mit Mühe die Räder'. See also L. Balletto, *Medici e farmaci, scongiuri ed incantesimi, dieta e gastronomia nel medioevo genovese* (Genova, 1986), pp.156–65. For further examples below see 89, LH note 71, Sloane 3550 no.36. See also Brunel, *op. cit.*, p.92 no.550 and p.93 note, and MS Sloane 2584 f.25v.

101 See Beccaria, *op. cit.*, pp.255–59.

102 Beccaria, p.255 argues 'alcune caratteristiche ortografiche communi all'uno e all'altro [viz. the two parts of the MS] (ad es. velud, faciebad, concipiad) e l'accenno a c.112v

Audivi abbate de superiori Scothia cum magna adfirmatione quod postea, quando creverit infans, possit discernere omnes voces cornicum et significationes earum, ne additano come probabile l'origine in territorio britannico'.

103   I have expanded abbreviations. The two preceding receipts are *Ad vermes qui in homine sunt* and *Potio ad ipsos vermes.*

104   Other texts in the MS are an incomplete copy of Macer (ff.1ra–11rb, 13ra–17va), a fragment of Oribasius (ff.19r–34r), and Hippocrates, 'Dinamedia' (ff.34r–40r; *De cattina*).

105   See A. C. Svinhufvud, *A Late Middle English Treatise on Horses edited from British Library MS Sloane 2584 ff.102–117b* (Stockholm, 1978), pp.99, ll.194f; B. Odenstedt, *The Book of Marchalsi: A 15th C. Treatise on Horse-Breeding and Veterinary Medicine edited from MS Harley 6398* ... (Stockholm, 1973), p.73 (note); Gray, 65.

106   On this MS see E. Stengel, *Codicem manu scriptum Digby 86* (Halis, 1871) and B. D. H. Miller, 'The Early History of Bodleian MS Digby 86', *Annuale Mediaevale* 4 (1963), 23–56.

107   In the left-hand margin is written 'et .iii. Pater Noster et Ave Maries'. The Psalm beginning 'Dixit Dominus' is Psalm 109.

108   Psalm 108, 2.

109   At the bottom of f.28v is written 'Que en fin de may le quart jour ou le quint saunc amenusez de amdeus ses braz, jamés fevers n'averraz'. There follows a series of receipts for fevers, with vernacular headings and Latin texts.

110   The following receipts have French rubrics but Latin texts.

111   They were twin brothers, of Arabic origin, martyred under Diocletian c.300 AD. In the West Cosmas came to be regarded as the patron saint of physicians and Damian of pharmacists. See E. F. Frey, *art. cit.*, 49f, 64–6; D. W. Artelt, *Kosmas und Damian, die Schutzpatrone der Ärzte und Apotheker* (Darmstadt, 1954); A. Wittmann, *Kosmas und Damian: Kultausbreitung und Volksdevotion* (Berlin, 1967); P. Julien & F. Ledermann (eds.), *Saint Côme et saint Damien, culte et iconographie ... colloque Mendrisio 29–30 IX 1985* (Zurich, 1985); M. Modig, 'St Cosmas and St Damian Patron Saints of Medicine and Pharmacy: Their Cult in the Nordic Countries', in G. Schramm (ed.), *Neue Beiträge zur Geschichte der Pharmazie: Festschrift für Herrn Dr. phil. Hans-Rudolph Fehlmann zur Feier des 60. Geburtstags* (Zürich, 1979), *pp.119–27. See also W. Artelt, 'Kosmas und Damian - ein Literaturbericht', MJ* 3 (1968), 151–55.

112   Cf. MS London, B.L. Royal 12 B XII (s.xiii[2]) f. 176r *Contra mures*: Accipe .v. garbas primas que intrant in orreum et dic supra primam 'Conjuro te, murem, ne habeas maiorem partem in hoc blado quam sacerdo(ti)s habet in missa dominicali'. Et dic ita per .iii. vices. Postmodum .iii. Pater Noster, in nomine Patris et Filii et Spiritus Sancti. Et ita super unamquamque garbam. See Storms, pp.181f.

113   After a set of receipts with rubrics (f.33r/v) the collection ends with a group of Latin receipts on f.34r which are without rubrics and which are concerned with the following subjects: 'Ut appareat aliquibus quod flumen set in domibus'; 'Si vis eligere meliorem porcellum'; 'Ad muscas necandas'; 'Si vis facere aliqua mortua cantare'; 'Si vis haboundare apibus'.

114   Preceded (f.137va) by *Contra dolorem dentium*: Domine Jesu Christe, Fili Dei, vini [sic] miserere famulo tuo .N. hodie et cotidie, omni nocte et omni tempore, de ista persecutione doloris dentium. Liberet nos Deus de omnibus persecutionibus Messias, Sother, Emanuel, Sabaoth, Adonay, Panton, Craton, Permocraten, Iskiros, agios, ymas, eleyson, Otheos, Athanatos, Alpha et Omega, leo, vermis, vitulus, agnus, homo, aries, usion, serpens, primus et novissimus, finis, Pater et Filius et Spiritus Sanctus, amen. 'Crux bona, crux digna, lignum super omnia ligna / me tibi consigna redimens a morte maligna' [Walther *Prov.* 3818]. 'Crux fugit omen malum, crux est reparacio rerum / Per crucis hoc signum fugiat procul omen malignum' [Walther *Prov.* 3823 & 21192]. Petrus, Paulus, Andreas, Johannes, Jacobus, Philippus, Bartholomeus, Simon, Tadeus, Matheus, Marcus, Lucas, Mathias. 'Sint medicina tua pia crux et passio Christi, amen'. On the trisagion (Iskiros, Otheos, Athanatos) see Bühler, *Speculum* 34 (1959), 637f. Cf. similar names of

God in a charm in MS Sloane 2458 (s.xv) f.8r attributed to 'Seynt Johan l'apostyl de Rome' in which it is said 'Set sunt les nomys Nostre Seignur Jesu Christ que nul homme ne doyt nomer si il ne seist en perel de ewe ou de few ou de batayle ou en jugement'.

115 Preceded (f.156rb) by Carmen contra febres: Sanctus Architriclinus sedebat super scannum et tenebat in sinistra manu runceam portantem 'hupes' et scindebat per medium et tradidit partes duobus hominibus ut springerent fortiter. Et benedixit cum manu dextra et sacra verba loquebatur et dixit 'Pater et Filius et Spiritus Sanctus, adjuva hominem istum de ista febre calida vel frigida et partes jungent'. Et dummodo jungunt dic Pater Noster et Ave. Et tunc scinde in medio partium conjunctarum quantum potes capere manu sed non attingant terram. Et suspende illam partem in medio scissam ad collum infirmi per septem dies. See Holthausen, 84 and note 118 below. On architriclinus see D. A. Trotter, MAe 56 (1987), 258 & 261ff.

116 See above p.34.

117 Preceded (f.162va) by Contra inmundum spiritum: Medicina a sancto Luca inventa. In nomine domini nostri Jesu Christi. Recipe absinthium cum vino, aceto, butiro, ture et oleo. Coque et unge totum corpus infirmi per tres dies et istas tres literas grece, latine et ebraice scribe: a.v. hely heli heloy - quod intrepretatur 'Jesu in manus tuas commendo spiritum meum'. Hos fac in veteri luna. Item ad eiciendum demonem de corpore hominis scribe in manu dextra ou in manu sinistra tetragramaton, in collo in parte posteriori Emanuel, in pectore suo a parte anteriori Sabaoth, et in fronte Agla'. On agla see Balletto, op. cit., pp.152–5. After the vernacular charm for staunching blood comes (f.162vb) the following widespread example: Longius miles lancea latus domini nostri Jesu Christi perforavit et inde exivit sanguis et aqua, sanguis redempcionis et aqua baptismatis. 'In nomine Patris stes, sanguis, in nomine Filii resistes, sanguis, in nomine Spiritus Sancti ne exeas, sanguis. Pater Noster'.

118 Cf. MS Sloane 962 f.38r Item pur fevers un charme: Archidecline syttes on hye and holdes a vergyne 3erde of hesil in his hande and seys 'Also soth os þo prest makes Godes bodi in his handes, and also soth os God blessed is moder Mari, and also soth I conjure þe, vergin 3erde of hesil, þat + þu close and be bote of þis evel fever to þis man .N.' In nomine Patris et Filii et Spiritus Sancti, amen. See 79 & 85 below and note 115 above.

119 Earlier (f.175ra/rb) there are two Latin charms for fevers: Recipe tria oblata. In primo scribe in circuitu dorsi oblati + on + Jesu Crist + on + leo + on + fili + , in medio + A + g + 1 + A; in secondo + on + ovis + on + aries + on + agnus + , in medio + te + tra + gra + ma + ton; in tertio + on + pater + on + gloria + on + numerus (?) + Scribe in dorso Jesu Crist Nazarenus + crucifixus + rex + Judeorum + 'Sit medicina mei'. Et dicat cotidie .v. Pater Noster et Ave . . . Item alia: Cape tria oblata. In primo oblato in dorso scribe ista duo nomina in modo crucis Pater Pantager; in secundo oblato scribe ista duo verba in modo crucis Filius Melchior; in tertio scribe eodem modo Spiritus Sanctus Saday, et in circuitu tertii oblati scribe in circuitu dorsi versum 'Vulnera quinque Dei sint medicina mei'. Et post comestionem uniuscuiuscumque oblati dicat .v. Pater Noster et Ave +. Cf. Gray, 59.

120 Cf. D. Gray, 'The Five Wounds of Our Lord', N & Q 208 (1963), 50–59, 82–89, 127–34, 163–8. For the compilation of which this receipt is a part see M. Benskin, Neuph. Mitt. 86 (1985), 200.

121 See H. L. D. Ward, Catalogue of Romances in the Department of Manuscripts in the British Museum 1 (London, 1883), pp.587f; A. de Mandach, Naissance et développement de la chanson de geste en Europe 1 (Genève/Paris, 1961), p.389; C. Segre (ed.), Li Bestiaires d'amours di maistre Richart de Fornival et li response du bestiaire (Milano/Napoli, 1957), pp.lvi–lviii; and for a thorough account R. N. Walpole, The Old French Johannes Translation of the Pseudo-Turpin Chronicle: a critical edition. Supplement (Berkeley etc., 1976), pp.29–40.

122 I edit this in French Studies Bulletin 30 (1989), 9–11.

123 See Holthausen, 81. Cf. P. Meyer, Romania 37 (1908), 516f.

124 There follows in a later, 14th C. hand, an isolated receipt beginning with a large red

initial: Pur restreindre sang: Fetez poudre de sangdragoun, bol, mastik, piere sanguyne e goutez dedenz la gouture del sang ou dedenz la playe ou lyez a la playe.

125 On this ubiquitous verse see Gray, *N & Q* 208 (1963), 165 n.14.

126 On f.212v there is a red rubric *Icés deus oresouns deit l'en dire pur le tonere treis feiz*, the succeeding text being in Latin.

127 All but the prayer itself is underlined in red.

128 Again, the text is underlined in red with the exception of the prayer.

129 Cf. Sloane 146 no.155 and Sloane 3550 no.22.

130 corr. Porcarius, Sambatius, Cecilius/Gesilius (for Gelasius) ?

131 Cf. W. Bernfeld, 'Eine Beschwörung der Gebärmutter aus dem frühen Mittelalter', *Kyklos* 2 (1929), 272–74. In MS Harley 273 the charm is followed by two receipts: Pur dolur de denz: Pernez plantayne e suwe [f.213v] de muton, si le batez ensenble, le metez là u le mal est, e la dolur eswachera; Pur mal des ees: Pernez siwe de capun e le jus de eufrosie, si le friez en une payle ensenble, si le metez en une vescel ki seit net, si unez ov tut un petit, kar il est fort. E cel est apelé collirie.

132 Other charms include [f.46r] *Charme*: Escryvés en sa destre [f.46v] palme iceotes letres del sanc mesmes + pal + pal + pal. Super hiis et super has 'Veronica sanguis siue gurna statim restringet'; Item contra fluxum sanguinis secundum Gylbertum ad (?) Theolotum [corr. Theodoricum?]: Scribe hoc nomen Veronica in fronte cum sanguine pacientis et dic orationem istam, *oratio*: 'Deus qui solo tactu fimbre vestimenti tui mulierem in fluxu sanguinis constitutam sanare dignatus es(t), te suppliciter exoramus, domine Jesu, qui solus langores [f.47r] sanas, ut fluxum sanguinis istius pro quo vel qua preces effundimus restringere et sistere facias, dexteram tue potencie et pietatis extendendo. In nomine Patris et Filii et Spiritus Sancti, amen'.

133 e.g. ff.44v/45r 'Pernez verms de terre que sount appellez *angeltuactes .i. maddok*'; f.47v 'pié(1) de levere, *hennebane et wynekerson*'; f.50v 'Pur maladie que vent a costez *.i. stych*'.

134 For this and the following two receipts cf. A. Boucherie, *Rev. lang. rom.* 7 (1875), 67. Cf. MS Wellcome Hist. Med. Libr. 407 (s.xv) f.20v.

135 The Latin [f.55r] is: Scribe in pane vel in caseo [f.55v] 'Ogor Secor Vagor. Exi foras, in nomine Patris etc.'. Item aliud: Escrivez en une poume, si li donez a manger: 'De virga virgine ubi oritur radix Jesse. Anna peperit Mariam, Maria salvatorem. In nomine domini Jesu Cristi, infans, exi foras, sive sis masculus sive femina. Pater Noster et Ave Maria et Credo. In nomine Patris etc. Sicut vere credimus quod beata Maria peperit infantem, unum verum deum et hominem. Item et tu, ancilla Cristi, pare infantem. In nomine Patris etc'.

136 Walther, *Prov.* 13046.

137 See notes 115 and 118 above.

138 *ne* may be a misreading of *.iii*. MS Sloane 2584 f.78v has 'say þis charme þries ʒif þou canst his name'. The version printed by Gray, p. 62 has 'say þis charme thris; thare ye never reke whar þe man bee bot þow conne þe name'. Holthausen, 81 prints 'And þis charme seye thre sythys. And þanne tharst nozt recchyn, where þat þe man be or þe women, so þat þou knowe þe name'. See also 84 below.

139 See also MS Sloane 2584 f.78v.

140 Psalm 26, 1–2.

141 MS = *medium*. See the text of MS Oxford, Bodl. Libr. e musaeo 243 in McBryde, *MLN* 22 (1907), 170.

142 Exodus 15, 16.

143 MS Sloane 2584 f.73v has 'Pro latronibus et inimicis meis'. There is a ME version in MS Sloane 56 f.100r.

144 MS = *medium*. See the text printed by McBryde, *MLN* 22 (1907), 168 from MS Add. (incorrectly given as Arundel) 36674 f.89r and Sloane 2584 f.73v.

145 MS = *espaunde*.

146 Cf. T. Hunt, 'Horses and Courses', *French Studies Bulletin* 22 (1987), 1–4; M. Gaster, *Rumanian Bird and Beast Stories* (London, 1915), pp.348–54 ('Rumanian Incantations

against the Illnesses of Animals'); S. Drury, 'Herbal Remedies for Livestock in Seven-
teenth- and Eighteenth-Century England: Some Examples', *Folklore* 96 (1985), 243–47.
147 Printed (with a number of errors) by Gray, p. 64.
148 The apparent gibberish is uncertain.
149 Charms for staunching blood which refer to the Jordan exhibit endless variations e.g. MS
Harley 2378 (s.xv) f.118r/v Pur sanc estanger dites cest orison: Ce flum Jordan ad
cinckante funtaynes e tu as cinckante veynes. Estanchés [MS estancher], veyne, a la
[f.118v] vertu ke Deux ad soy. Seynt Marie tent enter ces bras Jesu Crist – veray mere,
veray enfant, veray veyne retent ton sanc, amen.
150 There is a blank in the MS.

Notes to Chapter Three

1   See, for example, A. Salmon, 'Remèdes populaires du moyen âge', *Etudes romanes dédiées
à Gaston Paris le 29 Décembre 1890 . . . par ses élèves . . .* (Paris, 1891), pp.253–66 (MS
Cambrai, Bibl. Mun. 351); P. Meyer, 'Recettes médicales en français', *Bull. SATF* 1906,
pp.37–52 (MS Paris, BN nouv. acq. lat. 356 on pp.46–52); P. Meyer & Ch. Joret,
'Recettes médicales en français publiées d'après le manuscrit 23 d'Evreux', *Romania* 18
(1889), 571–582; L. Wiese, 'Recettes médicales en français', *Mélanges de linguistique et de
littérature offerts à M. Alfred Jeanroy par ses élèves et ses amis* (Paris, 1928), pp.663–71; R.
Reinsch, 'Maître André de Coutances, Le Roman de la Résurrection de Jésus-Christ',
Archiv 34 Jhg., 64 Bd. (1880) [161–96] 170–76 (MS London, B. L. Add. 10289); Haust,
op. cit.
2   Mme de Tovar's unpublished thesis was completed at Strasbourg in 1970. I am grateful to
her for information supplied.
3   C. de Tovar, 'Contamination, interférences et tentatives de systématisation dans la
tradition manuscrite des réceptaires médicaux français – le réceptaire de Jean Sauvage',
Revue d'Histoire des Textes 3 (1973), 115–191 and *ibid.* 4 (1974), 239–88. Cf. also her
study 'Les Versions françaises de la *Chirurgia parva* de Lanfranc de Milan. Etude de la
tradition manuscrite', *ibid.* 12/13 (1982–83), 195–262.
4   C. Brunel, *Recettes médicales, alchimiques et astrologiques du XVe siècle en langue vulgaire des
pyrénées*, Bibliothèque Méridionale l série, t.xxx (Toulouse, 1956), pp.81–118.
5   O. Södergård, *Une Lettre d'Hippocrate d'après un manuscrit inédit*, Acta Universitatis
Lundensis, Sectio 1 Theologica Juridica Humaniora 35 (Stockholm, 1981).
6   'Contamination . . .', p.136 (Mme de Tovar is in error in dating the MS to the 13th C.).
7   'Contamination . . .', p.116.
8   See P. Kibre, 'Hippocrates Latinus: Repertorium of Hippocratic Writings in the Latin
Middle Ages (VIII) xlvi.', *Traditio* 38 (1982), 165.
9   See G. F. Warner & J. P. Gilson, *Catalogue of Western Manuscripts in the Old Royal and
King's Collections* vol. 2 (London, 1921), pp.13–15.
10   For the text see below pp.124ff.
11   Not least because it contains the famous Reading Rota 'Sumer is icumen in'. A description of the contents of the MS was published by C. L. Kingsford, *The Song of Lewes*
(Oxford, 1890), pp.xi–xvii and there is also a concise survey in R. Baum, *Recherches sur
les oeuvres attribuées à Marie de France*, Annales Universitatis Saraviensis, Reihe
Philosophische Fakultät 9 (Heidelberg, 1968), pp.45–47.
12   The different hands are identified by Baum, *supra*, p.46.

13 See E. H. Sanders in *The New Grove Dictionary of Music and Musicians* ed. S. Sadie, vol.18 (1980), pp.366–68.

14 See J. B. Hurry, *Reading Abbey* (London, 1901), p.111 for a brief description of the Harley and Cotton MSS and a list of the *obits* in the Harley calendar. At the bottom of Harley 978 f.16r we read: [in red] Post stellam terne domini lux tercia lune / [in brown] En la tierce lune aprés la tiffeine est le jur de paske le tierce dimeine / [in red] Efter þe sterre þe þridde sunedai i þe þridde mone is estre dai.

15 See Walther, *Proverbia* 774 & 810.

16 See H. Suchier, *Denkmäler provenzalischer Literatur und Sprache* Bd. 1 (Halle, 1883), pp. 473–80 & 530–31; P. Möller, *Hiltgart von Hürnheim. Mittelhochdeutsche Prosaüberset-zung des 'Secretum Secretorum'*, Deutsche Texte des Mittelalters 56 (Berlin, 1963); L. Thorndike, 'John of Seville', *Speculum* 34 (1959) [20–38] 24–27; M. A. Mazalaoui, *Secretum Secretorum: Nine English Versions* I, EETS 276 (1977), pp.xiv–xv.

17 See R. H. Robbins, 'Signs of Death in Middle English', *Mediaeval Studies* 32 (1970), 282–98 (Latin and French texts on p.283) and R. Woolf, *The English Religious Lyric* (Oxford, 1968), pp.78–82, 530–32. The Latin verses are drawn from the *Flos medicinae scholae Salerni*. For the French verses see also P. Meyer in *Romania* 4 (1875), 384 and T. Hunt in *Le Moyen Age* 87 (1981), 45 n.1.

18 See Th. Wright & R. P. Wülcker, *Anglo-Saxon and Old English Vocabularies* vol.1 (London, 1884), cols 554–59. The editors print only the vernacular *synonyma*, omitting the description of the herbs' properties. In 556,6 read *saliunca*; 557,11 corr. *Cuscute*; 557,34 read *grumil*; 559,6 read *psillum*; 559,23 read *Dragagantum*; 559,24 read *mirobalauns*. The last two rubrics in col. 559 are really descriptions of the preceding headwords. After the vernacular entries cease there is a red rubric *Electuarium calidum* and a list of Latin names until the rubric *Des especes* on f.27va.

19 See Walther, *Initia* 7108 and *Proverbia* 10190b. See also Warner & Gilson, *Catalogue . . .* pp.52–3.

20 See Walther, *Proverbia* 3428.

21 Including Walther, *Initia* 10472 and *Proverbia* 14095, 605a, 22111a, 22101.

22 See Walther, *Initia* 19692. The first five verses are found in a Peterborough fragment, see A. Bell, 'A Thirteenth-Century MS. Fragment at Peterborough', MHRA 3, vii (1929) [132–40], 138. There are also texts in MSS Sloane 3550 f.76v (with added line 'Purgat pulmonem, servat laterum regionem'), Sloane 3525 f.259r (with added line p.p. purgat l. lesionem), Royal 12 B XII f.151ra and Exeter Cathedral Library 3519 f.199r/v. Variant readings include *nescivit vim sc.* (Sloane 3550), *per se* (Royal, S3550), *comprimit* (Royal), *apostema* (Royal, S3525), *emplastrata* (Royal, S3550, S3525, Exeter), *evacuatus* (Exeter), *langoris* (Sloane 3550), *pedum* (Exeter), *de languore* (Exeter, S3550, S3525). Lines 5–7 are missing in the Royal MS, line 5 alone in S3525. Different verses on the virtues of *scabiosa* are found in MS Oxford, Bodleian Library, Digby 86 f.201v.

23 There follows an erasure.

24 See Walther, *Initia* 13306.

25 See Walther, *Initia* 15306. Cf. MS B. L. Add 12195 f.112r and D. Thomson, *A Descriptive Catalogue of Middle English Grammatical Texts* (New York / London, 1979), p.205.

26 See Walther, *Initia* 12243.

27 See H. L. D. Ward, *Catalogue of Romances in the Department of Manuscripts in the British Museum* 1 (London, 1883), pp. 408–15. At the top of the page is 'Ssci cumence le ysope'.

28 See Th. Wright, *The Latin Poems commonly attributed to Walter Mapes*, Camden Society 16 (1841), pp.95–106.

29 See Walther, *Initia* 91.

30 See Walther, *Initia* 627.

31 Ending on ff. 99va–100va with the *Praedicatio Goliae* (Walther, *Initia* 11395).

32 See Walther, *Initia* 18404, followed on ff.102va–103ra by *Initia* 11427.

33 See A. Sakari, *Doctrinal Sauvage publié d'après tous les manuscrits*, Studia Philologica

Jyväskyläensia 111 (Jyväskylä, 1967), p.52 and T. Hunt, 'Le Doctrinal Sauvage – another manuscript', French Studies Bulletin 17 (1986), 1–4.

34   See Walther, Initia 18302.

35   See Kingsford, op. cit, pp.154–58 and E. Stengel, Codicem manu scriptum Digby 86 (Halis, 1871), pp.35 & 118–25.

36   See Kingsford, op. cit.

37   A legendary account of Becket's eastern descent found interpolated in some copies of Edward Grim's Life and in the chronicle bearing the name of John Bromton, see J. C. Robertson, Materials for the History of Thomas Becket, Archbishop of Canterbury, RS 67,ii (London, 1876), pp.453–58.

38   See G. Tilander, 'Fragment d'un traité de fauconnerie anglo-normand en vers', Studier i modern Språkvetenskap 15 (1943), 26–44. The surviving 176 verses display an obvious relation to Daude de Pradas's Roman dels auzels cassadors.

39   See Baum, op. cit., pp.47ff.

40   See C. de Tovar, 'Contamination . . . ', p.130.

41   The limits of the text were not discerned by P. Meyer in Romania 32 (1903), 82ff.

42   Additional receipts are indicated by an asterisk. Receipts found in MS Sloane 3550 are indicated by Sd$^{1-3}$.

43   On the MS as a whole see Stengel, op. cit. and B. D. H. Miller, 'The Early History of Bodleian MS Digby 86', Annuale Mediaevale 4 (1963), 23–56.

44   See N. R. Ker, Medieval Manuscripts in British Libraries II (Oxford, 1977), pp.828–30.

45   For a description of the MS see T. Hunt, 'The "Novele Cirurgerie" in MS London, British Library, Harley 2558', Z.f.rom.Phil. 103 (1987) [271–99], 275–79.

46   'Contamination . . . ', p.136.

47   For the vernacular receipt at the bottom of f.219r see appendix, p.137.

48   English equivalents in the text include: f.223r mauve anglice hockes; f.224r le jus de morele: anglice chokenemete; la menue consoude: anglice brosewort; f.224v la racine de glajol: anglice glade; parele: anglice redockes.

49   See P. Meyer, 'Notice du MS Sloane 1611 du Musée britannique', Romania 40 (1911), esp. 536–39. There are some interlinear English glosses in a later hand: f.143v eble: malwort [corr. walwort]; f.144v troncons: stok; gars: en engleis gandre; f.145v aloine: wormout en engleis; f.146r semence d'ache: merch en engleys. On the other hand receipt no. 82 on f.146r contains 'maroil que est apellé horehune' and 'senescon, c'est asavoir grondeswilie en englais'.

50   The text of the 'Lettre d'Hippocrate' is preceded (ff.69r–142v) by Ci commence Avicennes selonc fisique inc. 'Ceus qui par sa grant puissance tot le monde establi . . .' The following interlinear glosses, also in a later hand, are found: ff.80v/81r foie: splene; f.83r de sanguissegis [sic] .i. waterleche; f.91v en printans: veer; f.91v poree d'arreches: arage; lus: pik. At the bottom of f.11r a later hand has added two verses (Walther, Initia 17188) with vernacular equivalents: salvia: sauge; castorium: en l'espeiserie serra trové; lavendula: lavendre; primula: cousluppe; nasturs: watercurse; avencia: avence. On the prayers to St Margaret on ff.146v–147r see K. V. Sinclair, Prières en ancien français (Hamden, Connecticut, 1978), p.55, no.469.

51   i.e. the 'Réceptaire de Jean Pitard', see C. de Tovar, 'Contamination . . . ', pp.125f. and in Romania 103 (1982), 357–59. The text of the 'Lettre d'Hippocrate' contains an interesting selection of regional terms from N. E. France: f.32r bautemore; f.34v chanellade; f.37v jombarde; f.39v racine qui a non rigaut; poutricon; f.50r une herbe qui est apelé corage; f.50v une herbe qui est apelee tete soriz; ff.51v/52r pie collum que l'en apele espargoute; f.54v catiatour; f.56r clavelate; f.59v fineterne (i.e. 'fumeterre') c'est une herbe que l'en apelle conchanu [MS conchani]; f.59v racine que l'em apele rigaut; ciconaut; f.60r follion .ii. drames; carteton.

52   MS Sloane 706 (s.xv) ff.95r–96r offers a 'Dieta Ypocras' which has the discussion of the humours and then simply four sections on the seasons. MS Sloane 2584 (s.xv) ff.9r–12v has the treatises on the humours and urines in an amplified version. MS Sloane 3258

(s.xv) ff.73r–74r has a verse introduction (10 lines) and the sections on the humours and urines. These MSS are therefore incorrectly recorded by Kibre, *art. cit.* as versions of the 'Lettre'.

53 See R. H. Robbins, 'Medical Manuscripts in Middle English', *Speculum* 45 (1970), 393–415.

54 References in square brackets to MS Sloane 3550 indicate the corresponding vernacular receipt where there is no equivalent in MS Harley 978. For the sake of comparison I print those Latin versions of 'Lettre' receipts which are found in MS Sloane 146: these, where short, are printed after the Royal MS text with MS references in square brackets and, where longer, in these notes.

55 MS = *emplastrum multum prodest super capud.*

56 There is no rubric in MS Harley 978, but MS Harley 2558 f.176r has *Item a tuz lé mals de chef.*

57 Though not in MS Harley 978, the last three words are in MS Harley 2558 f.176r which also has the rubric.

58 This receipt is found in MS Harley 2558 f.176r.

59 This receipt is found in the vernacular in MS Digby 86 f.11r (see appendix), which also has (like MS Sloane 3550 f.219r) another receipt from the Royal MS at this point: *Aliter ad capillos longos faciendos: Accipe radicem ungule caballine, coque in aqua et inde lava capud et procul dubio capilli elongabuntur.*

60 Cf. MS Sloane 146 f.15r 'Ad faciem decorandam: Conmisce sagimen porcinum et albumen ovi dimidium cocti. Et adde parum pulveris baccarum lauri et faciem inunge'.

61 See also MS Digby 86 f.11r (see appendix) where it is preceded by another receipt also found in the Royal MS: *Aliter ad faciem lentulosam: Sepe inunge faciem sanguine leporino.*

62 Cf. MS Sloane 146 f.15r 'Ad faciem albificandam: Conmisce pinguedinem porcinam et gallinaceam et unge sepius et bibe succum fimiterre'.

63 Cf. MS Sloane 146 f.15r 'Aliter ad idem: Coque simul per optime recens lardum et salviam et sepum arietinum et thus liberum in vino [f.15v] et in olla nova, et cum infrigidatum fuerit, proice vinum et de reliquo faciem perunge'.

64 Cf. MS Sloane 146 f.16v 'Item contra siccam tussim: Tere semen apii et semen feniculi ana et in vino decoctum cum liquiricia bibe'.

65 Cf. MS Sloane 146 f.16v 'Contra dolorem et stricturam pectoris: Tere nigras prunellas de bosco et infunde cervisiam triticeam recenter colatam. Et conmisce et pone sub terra in olla nova bene cooperta per .ix. dies. Postea utere inde cotidie, in mane tepidum et in sero frigidum donec cureris'.

66 Cf. MS Sloane 146 f.21r 'Ad idem et ad omnia mala interiora: Multum valet semen canabi coctum in lacte caprino et tribus diebus in potu sumptum'.

67 Cf. MS Sloane 146 f.19r 'Item contra vomitum et contra sputum sanguinis: Coquatur farina ordeaca in aqua et fiant inde pultes et dum coquitur inmittatur pungnum plenum de crota caprina in pulvere redacta. Et comedat inde patiens donec curetur'.

68 Cf. MS Sloane 146 f.21r 'Contra duriciem et dolorem ventris: Bibat patiens de succo pentaphilon duo coclearia plena'.

69 Cf. MS Sloane 146 f.21r 'Vel bibat sepius rutam in vino vel cervisia distemperatum'.

70 The rest of the receipts as far as *Ad scabiem* are found in Södergård's edition, pp.18–19.

71 See p.358 n.100.

72 MS London, B. L. Harley 273 (s.xiv) f.214r–v has LH 27–30, 33, 34; MS B. L. Royal 12 B III (s.xiii²), of continental origin, transmits on ff.6r–9r LH 8, 16, 21, 31, 41, 62, 83, 86, 105, 120, 128, 130, 146, 147, 152, 153, 160.

Notes to Chapter Four

1   See K. Sudhoff, *Beiträge zur Geschichte der Chirurgie im Mittelalter. Graphische und textliche Untersuchungen in mittelalterlichen Handschriften*, Studien zur Geschichte der Medizin Heft 10 (Leipzig, 1914), pp.33–42 and Tafel v–vii; W. Dressendörfer, 'Französische Apothekendarstellungen aus dem 13. Jahrhundert', *Beiträge zur Geschichte der Pharmazie* 31, viii (1980), 57–61.

2   It is striking, for example, that the word *bibuef* (see below *Physique rimee* ll.718 & 1605), which points to the Picard-Walloon area, is missing in the first instance in two insular witnesses (see notes) and in the second instance is replaced by *artimese/artemese*.

3   See M. R. James, *The Western Manuscripts in the Library of Trinity College, Cambridge: a descriptive catalogue* III (Cambridge, 1902), pp.23–8 and P. Meyer, 'Les Manuscrits français de Cambridge', *Romania* 32 (1903) [18–120] 75–95. Supplementary indications will be found in C. de Tovar, 'Contamination, interférences et tentatives de systématisation dans la tradition manuscrite des réceptaires médicaux français: le réceptaire de Jean Sauvage', *Revue d'histoire des textes* 3 (1973) [115–191] 132.

4   The prologue is printed by Meyer, *art cit.*, 75–7 and Tovar, *art cit.*, 171–3.

5   The first two and last two receipts are printed by Meyer, *art cit.*, 77–8.

6   For a recent review of the literature on Roger Frugardi see K. Goehl, *Guido d'Arezzo der Jüngere und sein 'Liber Mitis'*, Teil 1 (Pattensen/Hann., 1984), pp.9–14. The Latin text and commentaries / glosses are in K. Sudhoff, *Beiträge zur Geschichte der Chirurgie im Mittelalter*, Teil 2 (Leipzig, 1918), pp.148ff. There is a modern Italian translation of most of the text (a few chapters are omitted) in M. Tabanelli, *La Chirurgia italiana nell'alto medioevo* 1 (Firenze, 1965), pp.23–99. There is a good critical study by A. Pazzini, *Ruggero di Giovanni Frugardo, maestro di chirurgia a Parma, e l'opera sua* (Roma, 1966). The Anglo-Norman translation is edited by D. J A. Ross, *Some Thirteenth-century French Versions of the 'Chirurgia' of Roger of Salerno*, PhD thesis, London, 1940. Ross considers that this translation may be of continental origin and dates it to c.1250, considering it superior to the second vernacular translation found later in the same MS. Ross edits the first translation on pp.234–64. A few excerpts are printed by Meyer, *art. cit.*, 78–82.

7   A few excerpts are printed by Meyer, *art. cit.*, 83–4.

8   The text was first printed at Ferrara in 1488. I have consulted *Practica Jo. Serapionis dicta breviarium . . . Practica Platearii . . . Impressum Venetus mandato et expensis nobilis viri domini Octaviani Scoti civis Modoetiensis per Bonetum Locatellum Bergomensem .17. kal. Januarias 1497* (pp.169ra–185va). On sources see P. Diebgen, *Gualteri Agilonis Summa medicinalis* (Leipzig, 1911), p.9.

9   Overlooked by Meyer, *art. cit.*, 86–7, who mentions only the *De adventu ad aegrotum*.

10 A few extracts are printed by Meyer, *art. cit.*, 87.

11 See now the important article by J. F. Benton, 'Trotula, Women's Problems and the Professionalisation of Medicine in the Middle Ages', *Bull. Hist. Med.* 59 (1985), 30–53. See also M. H. Green, *The Transmission of Ancient Theories of Female Physiology and Disease through the Early Middle Ages* diss. Princeton, 1985.

12 Some extracts are printed by Meyer, *art. cit.*, 91–5. The whole text is edited by Ross, *op. cit.*, pp.15–187. The text is sometimes careless and inaccurate as a translation. Its English origins seem assured by the appearance of English words in the text e.g. 'pernez de la semence jusquiami que en englés est apelé *hennebaire*' (f.261r); 'la semence de chenillé qui est apelee *hannebanne*' (f.265v); 'les verms que issent hors del ventre de l'homme(e) que li anglés apelent *maddokes*'; 'gipsus qui est en englés apelé *cockel*' (f.267r).

13 M. Faribault, 'La Chirurgie par rimes: problèmes de compilation de recettes médicales en français', *Fifteenth-Century Studies* 5 (1982), 47–59.

14 See Tony Hunt, 'The "Novele Cirurgerie" in MS London, British Library, Harley 2558', *Z. f. rom. Phil.* 103 (1987), 271–99.

15 A. Salmon, 'Remèdes populaires du moyen âge', *Etudes romanes dédiées à Gaston Paris le 29 Décembre 1890 . . . par ses élèves . . .* (Paris, 1891), pp.253–66.

16 See Tony Hunt, 'Recettes médicales en vers français d'après le manuscrit O.8.27 de Trinity College, Cambridge', *Romania* 106 (1985), 57–83.

17 See C. de Tovar, *art. cit.*, (hereafter *art. cit.* 1) and its continuation in the *Revue d'histoire des textes* 4 (1974), 239–88 (hereafter *art. cit.* 2).

18 See M. R. James, *A Descriptive Catalogue of the Manuscripts in the Library of St John's College, Cambridge* (Cambridge, 1913), pp.105–7.

19 See S. de Renzi, *Storia documentata della scuola medica di Salerno* (Milano, 1857; repr. 1967), pp.166–7.

20 The text of Petrocellus is found in Renzi's *Collectio Salernitana* IV, pp.185–286. From the *Physique rimee* one might compare ll.97ff with a receipt on p.193, ll.121ff with a similar, *ibid.*, and ll.307ff with a receipt on p.198.

21 Including nos 7, 8b, 9, 21, 14, 38, 39, 31, 35, 47, 50, 51, 56, 57, 58, 60, 59, 62, 41, 42, 43, 45, 65, 66, 68, 69, 79d, 79b, 79a, 82, 83, 88, 132, 147, 148, 149, 151, 160, 161, 168 followed by a large number of the 'extra' receipts found in the third copy in MS Sloane 3550 printed above in the Appendix and ending with 93, 97, 98, 102, 105, 107.

22 On f.100rb there is a charm which is found in the Latin version of the 'Lettre d'Hippocrate' (see above p.133): 'A femme ki travail de enfant: Liez a sun flanc ceste escrit: Maria peperit Christum + Anna Mariam + Elizabet Johannem. Sator arepo tenet opera rotas'. It is accompanied by a further popular practice for the same condition: 'Escrivez le Pater Noster en le funz de une mazelin e(l) lavez od vin od ewe chaud, si li done[z] a beivre, si gettera l'enfant vif u mort'.

23 The cosmetic receipts (nos 1–7) which are part of the *Physique rimee* in the St John's MS are found as a separate item in MS Trinity College O.1.20 ff.236r–39v the readings of which I print beside the St John's text, which throughout is very corrupt.

24 See Tovar, *art. cit.* 1, p.184. 'Pour avoir longs cheveux' (= MS Paris, B. N. fr. 1319).

25 See MS Sloane 146 no.160 below. There is obviously a line missing in the St John's MS. See also Tovar, *art. cit.* 2, p.247.

26 See Tovar, *art. cit.* 2, p.246.

27 Cf. MS Sloane 146 no.96 below.

28 See MSS Sloane 146 no.150 and Sloane 3550 no.53 below.

29 See MSS Sloane 146 no.151 and Sloane 3550 no.54 below.

30 See MS Sloane 146 no.153 below.

31 See *ibid.* no.14.

32 See *ibid.* no.15.

33 See *ibid.* no.17.

34 See *ibid.* no.16.

35 See *ibid.* no.132.

36 See *ibid.* no.133.

37 See *ibid.* no.152.

Notes to Chapter Five

1   For a full description see Tony Hunt, 'The Botanical Glossaries in MS London, B. L. Add. 15236', *Pluteus* 4.

2   For a discussion of MSS of Irish provenance see A. McIntosh & M. L. Samuels, 'Prolegomena to a Study of Mediaeval Anglo-Irish', *Med. Aev.* 37 (1968), 1–11. See also A. Zettersten, *The Virtues of Herbs in the Loscombe Manuscript. A Contribution to Anglo-Irish Language and Literature*, Acta Universitatis Lundensis, Sectio 1, Theologica, juridica, humaniora 5 (Lund, 1967). See also Hunt, *Plant Names*, p.xxxvi.

3   This is the earliest of the surviving copies: see MSS B. L. Add. 15236 (c.1300) ff.172v–187v; Sloane 5 (s.xiv[1]) ff.4ra–12va; Sloane 405 (s.xv) ff.7r–17v; Cambridge, Gonville and Caius College 200 (106) (s.xv) pp.196–214; Oxford, Bodleian Library, Digby 29 (s.xv) ff.38r–44v.

4   Such an index is obviously essential for gaining access to the different receipts, though it is not always provided in receipt collections. A similar index is found in MS Add. 33996 (s.xv) ff.76v–80r. In the present instance I have supplied the modern folio references, even when I do not reproduce the receipt, in round brackets. Italics are used strictly in accord with underlining in the MS, however arbitrary it may appear.

5   The Irish glosses in the third glossary (ff.172v–187v) are as follows: [f.174v] ciclamen: colueran; [f.178v] lapacium rotundum: pobel; [f.179v] malum terre: colranis; [f.182r] peucedanus: colranis; [f.184v] sigillum sancte Marie: hibernice mas tork; [f.185v] siclamen: colranis; [f.186r] trifolium: samrok.

6   There is a blank space in the MS.

7   At the bottom of the page a contemporary hand has inserted a receipt *Medicina ad omnia vicia oculorum* inc. 'Quere has herbas: apium .i. merche, funiculum . . .'

8   There follow (f.78r) two receipts in the hand of the one added to f.76r (see note 7 above) *Contra morbum caducum* and *Carmen contra morbum caducum probatum, contra guttam caducam.*

9   There is no heading or underlining. A red paragraph mark precedes *Veez* and a green one is placed before *In nomine Patris*. See G. Müller, *Aus mittelenglischen Medizintexten. Die Prosarezepte des Stockholmer Miszellankodex* X. 90, Kölner anglistische Arbeiten 10 (Leipzig, 1929) pp.105–6 where the charm is attributed to 'Seynt Ewstas' (in Henslow's collection it is sent by 'aungyl Gabriel to Sanctus William'). See D. Gray, 'Notes on some Middle English Charms' in B. Rowland (ed.), *Chaucer and Middle English Studies in Honour of Rossell Hope Robbins* (London, 1974) [pp.56–71] p.68. See above pp.90f.

10 All but the first two words of the rubric have been added, along with the phrase 'usque . . . partis', by a contemporary hand which has also added to the rubric of receipt no.10 below. The text is written in two columns, the ingredients appearing as a list (as in receipt no.30 below).

11 In the left-hand margin has been added *pimpemol* which, on the evidence of receipt no.4 below, seems to be a gloss on *fleurt*.

12 At the bottom of the page a later hand has added a receipt *Contra caducos* inc. 'Pulvis vel succus rute vel pigani missus in naribus . . .'

13 All but the first two words of the rubric have been added by a contemporary hand (see note 10 above).

14 MS = *herbas.*

15 At the bottom of the page a later hand has added a receipt *Contra malignum morbum.*

16 MS = *deliveres.*

17 MS = *manga.*

18 MS = *solible.*

19 See for the same receipt Müller, *op. cit.*, p.102.

20 See F. Heinrich, *Ein mittelenglisches Medizinbuch* (Halle a. S., 1896), p.166 and MS Sloane 146, f.56v (no.176 below p.287.)

21 These words are underlined in red in the MS.

22 See Heinrich, *op. cit.*, pp.163ff and O. Ebermann, *Blut- und Wundsegen in ihrer Entwickelung dargestellt*, Palaestra 24 (Berlin, 1903), pp.42ff and 52ff.

23 At the bottom of the page a later hand has added two receipts *Ad potandum pro felone* inc. 'Medefelon, warmot, spinegre . . .' (Cf. *Alphita* p.174a 'Spigurnella . . . angl. spinagre').

24 See Ebermann, *op. cit.*, pp.43ff and 52ff.

25 MS = *garris*.

26 A folio is missing, the medieval foliation moving from 4 to 6.

27 Interlinear gloss in the hand of the text.

28 See the *Lettre d'Hippocrate*, above p.111 no.31.

29 MS = *clescun*.

30 Added in a contemporary hand with red underlining.

31 From *blanc* to *e* has been added in the left-hand margin. See the *Lettre d'Hippocrate*, above p.112 no.39.

32 *.i. mouser* is an interlinear gloss by another hand. The rest, also in another hand, has been inserted in the left-hand margin.

33 MS = *malde*.

34 At the bottom of the page a later hand has added a receipt *Pro calido morbo* inc. 'Quicumque sanitatem de calido morbo desiderat . . .'

35 The ingredients are listed in a single column and bracketed with red lines in accord with the measure of each.

36 These ingredients are listed in a single column.

37 MS = *fuem*.

38 Cf. no. 77 below.

39 MS = *cantra*.

40 The rubric provided, *Ad stranguriam*, has been expuncted and a later hand has inserted the new rubric in the margin.

41 An insertion in the left-hand margin reads 'vel betonicam'.

42 A similar hand to that of the text has needlessly added 'si cerfolium jejunus commederit'.

43 At the bottom of the page a later hand has added a receipt *Ad dolorem aurium* inc. 'Succum edere terene missum in aure . . .'.

44 'Nota' is written in the right-hand margin.

45 At the bottom of the page a later hand has added the receipt *Ad fas[i]diosos (?) vel qui non dormunt nec cibo nec potu dilectant . . .*'.

46 MS = *ungo*.

47 MS = *possum*.

48 See Walther, *Initia* 6423.

49 See the *Lettre d'Hippocrate*, above p.111 no.32.

50 An error for *Walteri*?

51 At the bottom of f.39v has been added in a later hand a prescription . . . *de viro et muliere* inc. 'Si vir et mulier iuncti non possunt habere prolem et vis scire in quo peccat . . .' On f.40r there is a prescription 'Si vis scire aut pregnans genuerit masculum vel feminam . . .' and a receipt *Pro peste porcorum*. Folio 40v, which contains these added receipts, is badly rubbed.

52 A new quire now begins and I have numbered this second part of the collection separately (accompanied by an asterisk in the glossaries at the end of this book).

53 At the bottom of f.41r a charm has been added in a later hand.

54 At the bottom of f.41v the scribe has added 'Ista verba sancta in meo partu juvent me .N. et me a periculo liberent quocumque gloriosissime virginis et matris Dei Marie'. A further text by a later hand is illegible.

55 The receipt is repeated under the rubric *Item pur tote maner de fester*, omitting simply

feltewort, yarou and from *fronkencens* to *couhismarch*. In the right-hand margin is written 'butirum eodem die factum sine gale'.

56   In the right-hand margin there is a pointing finger and the word *mulier*.

57   In the left-hand margin is written in a contemporary hand 'Item ad provocandum menstruum respice infra 21'.

58   Before *lus crey* (*e* added by a corrector) there is an insertion mark relating to *quintefoyle* written by a later hand in the right-hand margin.

59   'albo, si potest habere' is an insertion in the left-hand margin and *rubeo* a superscript insertion for the phrase in brackets which has been expuncted.

60   *Mulier* is written in the left-hand margin and underlined in red.

61   An insertion in the right-hand margin reads *vel albo*.

62   An insertion in the right-hand margin reads *vel feces vini*.

63   See Müller, *op. cit.*, p.58.

64   At the bottom of the page a later hand has added two receipts, *Item experimentum vite et mortis, probatio vite et mortis* inc. 'Super urinam egroti lac mulieris inmitte . . .' and *Item experimentum circumque infirmo*.

65   Interlinear gloss by a contemporary hand.

66   There is a *renvoi* to a note at the bottom of the page 'Et nota quod si non apposueris liquiriciam, apponas post decoctionem herbarum cum liquorem clarificare volueris unum mediocrem discatum de melle et spumetur et .x. vel .xii. ova ad omne magis ad clarificationem eiusdem'.

67   MS = *mūtura*.

68   The words 'tam . . . quam' are a marginal insertion in red. For the charm see Müller, *op. cit.*, p.89 and Ebermann, *op. cit.*, pp.42ff.

69   There follow a number of receipts for electuaries which are simply a list of ingredients and quantities. At the bottom of f.48r a later hand has added a receipt *Pro fatigatione itineris vel belli*. Note the celebrated 'Pulvis imperatoris qui vocatur diapigamon: valet contra omnes humores ex quibus diutine infirmitates proveniunt et pro debilitate stomachi, viscositatem et omnem guttam et parelesim expellit, renum et inferiorum partium dolores mitigat, naturam perditam restaurat et semen coagulat'. The receipt includes 'greyn d[e] Paris' (f.48v), as does the next one (f.49r). Beside the receipt there is a marginal note 'Pocio correspondens respice folio sequenti [= 22, mod. fol. 50v, see no.49 below] and beside that for *diasaturion* 'Potio correspondens respice sequenti folio 22' and the same for the receipt which 'confortat coitum' (f.49v). Also beside *diasaturion* is a marginal note 'Quibus temporibus debeat uti illud electuarium respice infra 22 [= f.50v]'. In the electuary *diasaturion* the word 'satureia' is glossed 'anglice bolyngras'.

70   In the left-hand margin is written *mulier* with red underlining. At the bottom of f.49v is added *Mulier: Item ad restringendum fluxum matricis respice supra 15* [= f.43v, no.13 below].

71   MS = *mentem* here and in no.49 below.

72   There is a *renvoi* to the marginal insertion *maddirrot*.

73   The words 'in . . . poterit' are a marginal insertion.

74   In the left-hand margin there is a pointing finger accompanied by 'Nota'.

75   There follows a receipt for an electuary *ad reddendum hominem potentem in opere venereo experimentum* applied like *diasaturion* and another *Ad reddendum hominem pro suo perpetuo inpotentem quoad opus venereum*. At the bottom of ff.50v and 51r is the following note: 'Nota quod ad unam libram de succura sufficit una uncia cum dimidia ad omne magis de pulveribus zynziberi, galange, piperis nigri, granorum parisiensium .i. greyn de Parys, ita quod de zynzibero / sit una uncia, de pipere nigro una uncia, de grano vero parisiensi et de galanga de quolibet illorum dimidia uncia ad terendum in mortario. Item una uncia cum dimidia de predictis pulveribus sufficit ad unam quartam mellis crudi sive non cocti'.

76   MS = *habentes*.

77   There is an illegible insertion in the left-hand margin.

78   Cf. MS Oxford, Bodleian Library, e Musaeo 219 (s.xiii) f.186r. At the bottom of f.53r is a note 'Hoc experimentum alio modo et in alia forma scribi sol . . .'. The charm is followed

on f.54r by *Ut mulier concipiat* according to which certain letters are written on a lead plate. At the bottom of f.54r there is a note in a later hand with prescriptions for a woman wishing to give birth to a male child.

79   There follows a charm *Contra febres et frigores* in which various formulas are written on three holy wafers or hosts, and the following prognostication: 'Si littere nominum viri et uxoris sue in latino sumpte fuerint equales, senior ex illis semper primo morietur. Si vero littere fuerint inequales, minor ex illis semper primo morietur. *Istud tamen intelligendum est de desponsatis et de morte naturali, non autem accidentali*'.

80   At the bottom of the page is a note on quantities: 'Si receperitis de turbit tamen dimidiam unciam, accipiatis de zucura tamen unciam unam et de gingibero quartam partem tamen unius uncie .i. pondus quinque denarii tamen. Item si receperitis tamen unam dragmam de turbit, accipiatis duas dragmas de zucura et de gingibero, dimidiam dragmam .i. pondus unius denarii cum quadrante'.

81   At the bottom of the page there is a receipt in a later hand beginning 'In nomine Patris et sancte [sic] Raphael . . .' with references to Tobias Bk 3.

82   A later hand has added a receipt at the bottom of the page.

83   MS = *pulvus*.

84   A later hand has added *De isto unguento h. . . infra* 69 . . .' [= f.81r no.141 below].

85   A marginal insertion by a later hand reads '.i. bugyl'. For the Irish see glossary.

86   At the bottom of the page a later hand has added a receipt *Experimentum bonum contra febres*.

87   Written above is the statement 'proved on my selfe 1614'.

88   *et teris* is a superscript insertion in a later hand.

89   An insertion in paler ink.

90   A marginal insertion reads *vel butirum*.

91   A list of properties separated by red and green paragraphs.

92   The explanatory phrase is inserted in the left-hand margin.

93   In the left-hand margin there is a pointing finger in red and on the right the word 'Nota' also in red.

94   A later hand has furnished an insertion mark and further material at the bottom of the page.

95   The phrase is inserted in the right-hand margin.

96   Now follow the signs of death: '*Nota quod in homine infirmo septem sunt signa mortifera* que sunt ista, videlicet, frons rubeus, supercilia declinantur, occulus sinister minuitur, venter defugit, pedes frigescunt, juvenis vigilat, senex dormitat, nasi summitas abligat'. Cf. T. Hunt in *Le Moyen Age* 87 (1981), 45 n.1 and R. H. Robbins, 'Signs of Death in Middle English', *Mediaeval Studies* 32 (1970), 282–98. See also P. Meyer in *Romania* 44 (1915–17), 181.

97   i.e. little hock.

98   In the right-hand margin are the words 'Nota bene pro plagis, pistulis, bilis' accompanied by a pointing finger.

99   There follows an 'experimentum': '*Nota miraculum*. Sume herbam Johannis in festo nativitatis beati Johannis Baptiste et reservetis in mundo loco usque ad natalem domini et pone eam super lapidem in nocte nativitatis et explora bene et videbis eam viridem tota hora qua sancta virgo fuerat pariendo Christum. Et postea redibit ad priorem statum'.

100 Cf. Müller, *op. cit.*, p.130.

101 A later hand has added a receipt at the bottom of the page [*Contra] dolorem dencium*.

102 Cf. Müller, *op. cit.*, p.40 and variations on p.130. See also W. R. Dawson, *A Leechbook or Collection of Medical Recipes of the Fifteenth Century* (London, 1934) nos. 299–301. A similar receipe is found in MS Harley 3407 (s.xv) f.58r 'Here is a makyng of Gracia Dei þat þe ladi Beauchamp used, þe erlys wyf of Warwik' and f.59r 'Here is þe makyng of another Gracia Dei þat þe good erle of Heyford usede þat .J. holde a noble and gracious surgier'.

103 An insertion in the right-hand margin reads '.i. bryswor[t]'.

104 At the bottom of the page a later hand has added a receipt.

105 MS = *testo*.

106 There now follows a charm *Contra fantasmata* (ff.63v–64r) and at the bottom of f.63v, in a later hand, *Ad eum qui non potest dormire*.

107 The opening of the receipt is written out on f.66r and then repeated on f.66v.

108 There follows a prescription for conception, accompanied by the word 'Nota' in red, which is too badly rubbed to permit accurate reproduction.

109 In the left-hand margin is the note 'Nota bene pro uxore 1628'.

110 This last line is very badly rubbed.

111 The missing word is illegible in the MS.

112 As above.

113 As above.

114 An insertion in the left-hand margin has been lost through cropping.

115 There now follow sections in Latin on *fumeterre, absinthium, anisium, apium;* then 'Galienus de fleobotomia' (f.69v) and, on ff.70r–71r, a passage from the ps.-Aristotelian Letter to Alexander corresponding to ll.96–139 in the ed. of H. Suchier, *Denkmäler der provenzalischen Literatur und Sprache* Bd. 1 (Halle, 1883), pp.478f.

116 At the bottom of the page a later hand has added a short receipt *Ad combustionem de foco vel aqua . . .*

117 There is a *renvoi* to the bottom of the page and the following note: '*Idem* facit succus salgee et agrimonie bibitus si in equali proporcione herbe sumantur et post expressionem succi tritura dictarum herbarum ad vulnus posita fuerit'.

118 At the top of the page, which has been cropped, a later hand has inserted a receipt and at the bottom of the page there is *Ad sagitam vel spinam expellendam*.

119 At the bottom of the page a later hand has added a receipt *Ad mamillas*.

120 There is an insertion in the left-hand margin which is too badly rubbed to be legible.

121 From 'Facto igitur isto lexivio' to this point is an insertion at the bottom of ff. 81v and 82r. The margin has been cropped.

122 MS = *illud*.

123 In the right-hand margin, which is cropped, there is an insertion 'Per unum mili . . . prout usque confectio f . . .'.

124 In the right-hand margin, which is cropped, there is an insertion 'vel fiat . . . scribitur s . . . ad hoc ut si non que . . .'

125 An insertion in the right-hand margin reads 'Item inferius in . . . gime'.

126 See f.55v, no.56 above.

127 MS = *exeunten*.

128 Followed by *butirum* expuncted, *butiro* in the left-hand margin.

129 See f.50r, no.48 above.

130 In the right-hand margin is the word *stu* underlined in red.

131 The MS reads *mentem* in both cases.

132 In the right-hand margin is inserted 'folia lorer'.

133 The sentence is inserted at the bottom of f.85v.

134 *recens* is inserted in the left-hand margin.

135 In the right-hand margin is the word 'Nota' underlined in red.

136 The receipts on the rest of f.86r and on ff.86v and 87r are written in a pale grey ink and are so badly rubbed as to make transcription futile.

137 See Müller, *op. cit.*, p.107.

138 At appropriate points in the right-hand margin are the words 'potio', 'locio', 'emplastrum', all underlined.

139 At the bottom of the page a later hand has written 'Experimentum: pones has litteras sub capite mulieris dormientis. . .'.

Notes to Chapter Six

1   Cf. I. Short in *Romania* 94 (1973) esp. 221–31.
2   See above ch.3. In the following notes these receipts are identified by the letters LH and a number.
3   See B. von Lindheim (ed.), *Das Durhamer Pflanzenglossar lateinisch und altenglisch*, Beiträge zur englischen Philologie 35 (1941; repr. 1967) and T. Hunt, 'The Trilingual Glossary in MS London, B. L. Sloane 146 f.69v–72r', *English Studies* 70 (1989), 289–310.
4   MS = *chelepeine*.
5   See L. Thorndike & P. Kibre, *A Catalogue of Incipits of Mediaeval Scientific Writings in Latin*, rev. & augm. ed. (London, 1963) (hereafter ThK) 269.
6   ThK 644 lists Sloane 146 ff.75v–79 as 'De aquis phisicalibus', but this is misleading. Certainly MS Harley 2558 ff.189r–190v, also cited, is a different work, as is MS Add. 28555 ff.36rb–37ra.
7   See E. Wickersheimer, *Dictionnaire biographique des médecins en France au moyen âge* (repr. Genève, 1979) vol. 2, pp.720f and *Suppl.* p.263.
8   ThK 610.
9   ThK 1609.
10 The first begins 'Beata Apollonia . . .'.
11 There is no change of hand or format at f.59v.
12 The page is badly rubbed, rendering some words and phrases illegible. Some of the missing readings can be recovered from the text in MS London, B. L. Royal 9 A XIV f.192ra and Oxford, Bodl. Libr. Digby 69 f.180v, see pp.73 no.64 and 324 no.100.
13 In this receipt, as elsewhere where confidence seems justified, I have expanded the abbreviations used for quantities and weights.
14 The reference is enigmatic, since it is preceded by a list of 37 herbs!
15 There are 5 short receipts in Latin dealing with 'gutta frigida', 'gutta inossata' and 'gutta ubicumque est'.
16 2 short Latin receipts dealing with 'homo gutturnosus' and 'gutta frigida'.
17 MS = *oignēs*.
18 3 Latin receipts dealing with ointments and a plaster for gout.
19 As is the case throughout the MS, the verses are written out as prose with the first letter of each verse splashed in red.
20 See note 19 above.
21 Error for *ovec*.
22 The receipt begins with a red initial decorated with blue.
23 A haplography from *dreskes* to *dekes* has been made good by marginal insertion in the hand of the scribe.
24 MS = *aviez*.
25 MS = *malada*.
26 MS = *olō*.
27 MS = *ol'o*.
28 A number of short receipts in Latin incl. 'Ad purgandum caput et contra dolorem dencium' and 'Contra dolorem capitis'.
29 *seed* has been inserted below the line.
30 The series of Latin receipts includes 4 on scabies and over 30 on diseases of the eye. The latter include Latin versions of LH 26, 28, 29, 30, 32, 33, 34, 28, 31 and are introduced by the heading 'Ad omnes dolores et infirmitates oculorum subiunguntur curationes'. In a receipt on f.11r *camedreos* is followed by '.i. burnete'. Then follow 16 receipts on dental ailments which include Latin versions of LH 51, 56, 57, 59, 60, 62.
31 This receipt is the penultimate of 16 prescriptions for dental conditions.

32   14 Latin receipts on conditions of the ear, including Latin versions of LH 65–69.
33   The preceding heading is 'Si propter vermes fiat dolor in auribus'.
34   4 Latin receipts on 'fetor oris', including Latin versions of LH 47, 49, 50, and 7 (including no. 40 in Anglo-Norman) on facial complexion including Latin versions of LH 78 and 80.
35   8 Latin receipts on hair restoration including Latin versions of LH 70–74.
36   6 more Latin receipts on hair restoration including a Latin version of LH 76, followed by 13 receipts on coughs and constriction of the breast, including Latin versions of LH 83 and 86.
37   A receipt 'Contra malam habitudinem stomachi et epilationem splenis et epatis'.
38   A Latin receipt headed 'Autre' and another 'Contra ardorem cordis'.
39   Throughout the MS the verse receipts are written out as prose, the first letter of each verse being splashed with red.
40   Interlinear gloss in the hand of the text. See also no.190 below.
41   There is no paragraph mark, but the first letter is splashed with red.
42   A haplography from *avant* to *nomez* has been made good by a marginal insertion in the hand of the scribe.
43   Latin receipts 'Contra splenis vicium', 'Contra omnes infirmitates stomachi' and 'Contra indignationem stomachi'.
44   A Latin version of LH 95 'Item contra vomitum et contra sputum sanguinis'.
45   for *entrerus*.
46   8 Latin receipts on catarrh and 'uvula cadens' followed by one 'Contra squinantiam'.
47   4 receipts 'Contra squinantiam' (including 'Bevez *spigurnele* et vus voudra [= vaudra]' on f. 20v), followed by 'Ad tollendum fistulas in gutture nascentes' and 3 receipts 'Contra potiones venenosos [sic]'.
48   A Latin version of LH 90 and of LH 99 + 100 ('Contra duriciem et dolorem ventris'), followed by 3 remedies against constipation in one of which (f. 21r) we have 'accipe radicem yris .i. gladioli ortensis .i. *gledene*'.
49   2 Latin receipts 'Ad idem'.
50   In MSS Cambridge, Trinity College 0.1.20 and 0.8.27 (the 'Physique rimee') this line marks the beginning of a new receipt. As usual the receipt is written out as prose.
51   3 Latin receipts 'Contra tortiones et dolores ventris' and one 'Contra dolorem yliacum et omnem constipationem ex duricia stercorum vel fleumate viscoso', followed by 2 'Ad lumbricos ventris eiciendos'.
52   5 Latin receipts 'Contra dissinteriam'.
53   A Latin receipt: 'Ad idem: saponaria minor anglice *vane* vel herba que dicitur *turmentine* in lacte vaccino cocta valet'.
54   corr. *un noef pot.*
55   A Latin receipt 'Contra fluxum sanguinis ex ventre'.
56   A Latin receipt 'Qui habet ventrem inflatum'.
57   A Latin receipt 'Ad idem'.
58   2 Latin receipts, 'Contra emoroydas' and 'Ad frangendum lapidem in renibus et ad eos qui mingere non possunt'. The first begins 'Recipe tapsum barbastum .i. *moleyne*'.
59   See no.234 below.
60   2 Latin receipts 'Pulvis ad frangendum lapidum et educendum et expellendum', followed by 2 receipts 'Ad eos qui mingere non possunt'.
61   Latin receipts 'Ad idem' and 'Item pur pisser'.
62   A Latin receipt 'Ad virilem virgam si inflata fuerit'.
63   2 Latin receipts 'Contra inflationem testiculorum' and one 'Contra inflacionem virge ex calore coitus'.
64   A Latin receipt 'Ad testiculos inflatos'.
65   2 Latin receipts 'Quando cifac rumpitur ut intestina descendent in oceum .i. testiculos'; 2 'Contra dolorem renum'; 5 'Contra ficum' of which 2 are written out twice (the vernacu-

lar plant name *restebeof* occurs twice on f.28v) including a Latin version of LH 112; one 'Ad exitum ani' and 6 'Ad tumorem mamillarum'.

66 The haplography from *treys* to *treys* has been made good by a marginal insertion in the hand of the text.

67 A Latin receipt 'Si lac mulieris fuerit induratum in mamillis'; another 'Si defecerit lac nutrici'; 2 'Ne mamme nimis crescant'; 4 'Ut mamille puellarum semper sint parve'; 2 'Contra apostema in mamillis'.

68 4 Latin receipts 'Ad menstrua provocanda' including 'fomentum nobile salernitanum'; 2 'Ad menstrua stringenda'; 2 'Ad mortuum fetum vel vivum eiciendum'; 2 'Contra nimium fluxum menstruorum'.

69 A Latin receipt 'Si mulier non se potest purgare post partum' followed by 'Signa conceptus', 'Ad retrahendum matricem lapsam externis', 'Utrum masculum [MS = *marē*] vel feminam hiis signis discernitur', 'Item significatio masculi concepti erit huiusmodi'.

70 8 Latin receipts 'Contra ictericiam .i. jauniz', one of which has 'Da pacienti bibere succum electri .i. saponarie vel nimphee aquatice quod idem est .s. *crousope* gallice [sic]'.

71 2 Latin receipts against jaundice, 2 'Contra antracem'.

72 2 Latin receipts against the 'felun'.

73 MS = *os*.

74 13 Latin receipts 'Contra fistulam'.

75 MS = *chanche*.

76 MS = *tendrur*.

77 Inserted in the right-hand margin.

78 In no.58 above, the meaning hemp seems assured by LH 90 and the Latin version on f. 21r 'multum valet semen canabi'. MS Sloane 962 f.252r has 'acus dyaboly .i. filago, horworth, chanuette' which seems to indicate cudweed (Filago germanica). Cf. *Sin. Barth.* ed. Mowat, p. 21 'Filago .i. chauvet' and n. 4 ('perhaps cudweed'). W. Rothwell in *ZFSL* 86 (1976) 231 identifies *chaunette* with 'pilewort, lesser celandine'.

79 2 Latin receipts 'Ad cancrum sanandum', one 'Contra cancrum virge', 2 'Contra cancrum et fistulam et foramina in virga virili', one 'Ad cancrum'.

80 MS = *os*.

81 A Latin receipt 'Potio probatissima que omnem plagam sine appositione alicuius emplastri curat . . .' and another 'Ad vulnera sananda'.

82 A Latin receipt 'Unguentum mirabiliter vulnera sanans, potenter mundificans et carnem novam regenerans'.

83 7 Latin receipts 'De vulneratis pronosticendis' and one 'Ad vulneratum: succum piloselle .i. *peluette* . . .'

84 4 Latin receipts for extracting splinters etc. from wounds; 3 against bruising followed by 'Secundum magistrum Ricardum contra tumorem pedum et tibiarum . . .'. Then come 'Emplastrum quo domine sepe utantur in transmarinis partibus contra inflationem pedum vel alibi'; 'Pedes inflati: socco [sic] solatri .i. morelle'; 'Narravit Diascorides de quondam qui habuit crura inflata et fecit emplastrum de fimo columbe et farina ordei et aceto et mirabilem habuit effectum', and 2 Latin receipts 'Contra tumorem undecumque accidat'.

85 Latin receipts: 'Ad deponendum ranclum in plaga'; 'Ad articulorum dolorem'; 'Postea ne nimis desiccentur loca nervorum adde emplastrum illud'; 'Ad sedandum dolorem in menbris junccturalibus undecumque accidat'.

86 6 Latin receipts against scabies and one 'Contra malum mortuum et omne genus scabiei in quacumque parte corporis sit'; followed by 'Ad omnia exteriora apostemata', 'Ad omnes tumores et dolores et etiam ad vulnera sananda' and 10 'Ad maturandum apostemata et etiam rumpendum'.

87 2 Latin receipts 'Contra apostema in oculo' and 4 'Ad verrucas'.

88 A Latin receipt 'Ad delendas pustulas in facie et variolas' and another 'Contra pustulas quas habet infans in pedibus et in manibus ultra modum'. A receipt 'Ad pustulas faciei deponendas' has 'herbam alleluia que dicitur ʒekessure' and another 'Ad serpiginem et

inpetiginem .i. *teter* et omnem scabiem' has 'serpigo vero dicitur quia serpit vel idem est quod serpigo quod intensa impetigo et vocatur *dertre* gallice'.

89   3 Latin receipts 'Contra omnimodam arsuram'.

90   The haplography from *bien* [le arsun . . .] to *bien* has been made good by a marginal insertion in the hand of the text.

91   3 Latin receipts 'Contra morsum canis rabidi'.

92   Latin receipts 'Contra morsum scorpionis vel aranee' and 'Ad morsum serpentis', followed by 4 'Pro punctura serpentis'.

93   2 Latin receipts 'Ad conjurandum serpentem ut capiatur et exeat a latebris' and 'Contra puncturam aranee'.

94   2 Latin receipts 'Contra punctiones apum et vesparum'.

95   8 Latin receipts on styptics esp. against nosebleed.

96   A Latin receipt 'Ad necandos siriones' and 3 'Contra pediculos et lentes'.

97   2 Latin receipts 'Ad pediculos auferendos'; 2 'Ad vomitum provocandum' the second of which has 'herbam illam que gallice *tetesuriz*, anglice *stancrop* vocatur'; 2 'Contra vomitum'; one 'Contra ventositatem et indigestionem et acidam eructuationem'; one 'Contra omnes infirmitates stomachi'; one 'Ad regenerationem unguium' and 'Si quis habet ungues incompositos'; 3 'Contra noli me tangere'; one 'Quando aliquis perdit loquelam propter infirmitatem' and 3 'Ad memoriam et sensum recuperandum'.

98   A Latin receipt 'Contra defectionem appetitus'.

99   Latin receipts: 'Ad ebrietatem sedandam'; 'Contra podagram'; 'Unguentum ad hoc'; 'Contra ydropisim calidam'; 'Pillule ad idropisim ex frigido humore'.

100 16 Latin receipts against palsy, one of which (f.54r) has 'peucedani .i. *swinescrasse* . . . ypoquistidos .i. *swom* . . . prassi .i. *maroil*'; 8 against fevers.

101 5 Latin receipts for fevers; 2 against hoarseness; one against buzzing in the ears; one against a fishbone lodged in the throat; one 'Ad unguem male compositum deponendum'; one 'Ad malam habitudinem stomachi et opilationem splenis et epatis'; one 'Ad nimium sudorem restringendum' (incl. on f.58r 'auricule muris .i. *stancrop*').

102 One Latin receipt 'Contra reuma tam frigidum quam calidum'; one 'Contra omnem speciem epilentie'; one 'Contra cardiacam passionem et tremorem cordis'.

103 Latin receipts: 'Contra spasmum .i. *romme*' (incl. on f.58v 'cum pulvere poracis [sic] qui vocatur *bureys* gallice'); 'Nota quod quando aliquis fuerit ductus in profundum sompnum ex usu narcoticorum ut opii, jusquiami et mandragore, taliter potest expergefieri et excitari a sompno: instilletur acetum tepidum vel forte vinum tepidum in naribus dormientis et statim surget'; 'Pillule optime contra caput reumaticum'.

104 In the right-hand margin is written 'Ad sensum perditum'.

105 MS = *matin e seir*.

106 In the right-hand margin is written 'Ad inpinguandum'.

107 In the right-hand margin is written 'Ad macerandum'.

108 In the left-hand margin is written 'Contra scabiem'.

109 In the left-hand margin is written 'Nota'.

110 In the left-hand margin 'Mal del flanc'.

111 In the left-hand margin 'Contra vermes in ventre'.

112 In the left-hand margin 'Ad virgam virilem'.

113 In the right-hand margin 'Silotrum'.

114 In the right-hand margin 'Contre le fei eschaufé'. See no.46 above.

115 A Latin receipt 'Contra vicium matricis'.

116 In the right-hand margin 'Pur mal des costez'.

117 In the right-hand margin 'Pur tecchelure oster'.

118 In the right-hand margin 'Pur tuse'.

119 In the right-hand margin 'A enfans ke plurent', cf. f.102v 'Ne infans multum ploret: medulla cervina [MS corvina] cer[v]ices capitis utrasque et tempora (et) illinies et a tali periculo liberabitur'.

120 In the right-hand margin 'Pur vernes [sic]'.
121 In the left-hand margin 'Pur enroeure'.
122 A Latin receipt 'Ad auferendum paroccismum in febre quartiana' and 'Contra variolas'.
123 Written in the left-hand margin.
124 In the left-hand margin 'Pur enbelir la face'.
125 In the left-hand margin 'Pur la gorge'.
126 The receipt is inserted at the bottom of the page.
127 In the left-hand margin 'Pur crouleure'.
128 In the left-hand margin 'Pur kacie'.
129 A Latin receipt 'Contra malum mortuum fomentatio' (including amongst the ingredients
     'hondestonge, schordocke') and 'Unguentum ad idem' (including among the ingredients
     'summitates tapsi barbasti .i. softe' and 'lapacii acuti .i. scordocke'). In both receipts
     understand 'sourdock'.
130 In the right-hand margin 'Pur cengle'.
131 Latin receipts: 'Contra calefactionem epatis'; 'Contra guttam caducam'; 'Ad dormien-
     dum'; 'Potio qua rex Aristolabius utebatur'.
132 Cf. the English receipt in MS Sloane 2479 f.89v.
133 Latin receipts: 'Collirium contra defectum visus, lacrimas, pannum et ruborem oculorum';
     'Collirium ad vicia oculorum vetustissima et visus obscuritatem'; 'Contra melancoliam et
     tristiciam'.
134 'Item tres dies sunt in anno in quibus si aliquis sanguinem minuerit vel potionem
     acceperit in brevi morietur'; 'Ut scias si mulier possit concipere'; 'Ad sterilitatem proba-
     tam'; 'De ovibus: In nomine sancti Pangracii sume agnum de ovili tuo'; 'De porcis'; 'Est
     avis que dicitur upupa cuius oculi gestanti reddunt hominem gratiosum'; 'Turtur est avis
     cuius cor si feratur in corio lupi ferens numquam habebit appetitum luxurie . . .' [see f.
     87r].
135 In the right-hand margin 'Experimentum'.
136 In the right-hand margin 'Experimentum'.
137 Latin receipts: 'Ut capilli nigri fiant'; 'Ad argentum sophisticum [for whitening hair]'; 'Ad
     eos qui de nocte loquuntur'; 'Ad pilos generandos'; 2 'Ad ferrum ignitum portandum'
     (including 'herba que vocatur walteye vel milteia'); 'Ut lignum ardere non possit'; 'Ut
     pannus videatur ardere et non ardeat'; 'Ardens aqua sic fit'; 'Experimentum [to produce
     silver colour]'.
138 In the left-hand margin 'Pur mosches'.
139 In the left-hand margin 'Pur home afolé'.
140 Latin receipt 'Pro fulmine' ('Si quis jejunaverit in die sancti Johannis et Pauli, non
     morietur ictu fulmineo').
141 In the left-hand margin 'feu gregeys'.
142 MS = mta.
143 'Ut caro cocta appareat sanguino[len]ta'; 'Ut caro cocta apparebit vermosa'; 'Experimen-
     tum' (for making cloth appear to burn without actually burning); 'Ad inhebriandum
     hominem'; 3 'Ad extrahendum vinum de aqua' followed by a miscellany of short prescrip-
     tions dealing with such problems as fish dying in the pond, a candle burning in water,
     invisible writing that can only be seen at night, hardening eggs, ending with 'De diebus
     anni periculosis', 'Realgar sic fit' and 'Ad miscas [cor. muscas] necandas'.
144 In the left-hand margin 'Oignement a gute freide'.
145 There is a change to a larger hand. There is a red rubric Ad hominem ruptum medicina
     probata.
146 = red rubric. For the same charm see MS Add. 15236 f.29r/v.
147 There follows a blue paragraph mark and, in a new, large hand, a Latin receipt 'Contra
     scabiem, porrigines et subitam infirmitatem ovium et rubeum morbum'.
148 Latin receipts for the care of the hair, a collirium etc. There are red rubrics as follows: 'Ad
     oculos purgandos et clarificandos'; 'Collirium probatum ad oculos'; 'Item collirium contra
     albuginem et nebulam oculorum'; 'Ad faciem a vento vel a calore estuatum'; 'Ad surdita-

tem'; 2 'Potio . . .issima ad vocem, ad pectus, ad omnem infirmitatem'; 'Ut omnibus diebus sis sanus'; 'Ad vocis clarificationem'; 'Ad strictionem pectoris'; 'Si cui in gutture spina vel os vel aliudquid inheserit'; 'Contra le felun medicina'; 'Emplastrum ad ranculum auferendum'; 'Si inflatura contigerit in homine'; 'Ad eos qui cibum et potum non possunt retinere'; 'Ad fluxum ventris'; 'Ad clavos pessimos delendum'; 'Ad morbum caducum'; 'Ad dolorem pectoris'; 'Ad guttam'; 'Contra ructus et ventositatem'; 'Ad sompnum phisicum'; 'Ne ebrius sis'; 'Ad muscas effugandum'; 'Ut oves non moriantur'; 'Ut frigus non sencias'.

149 A Latin receipt 'Experta medicina ad gutam omnimodum'.

150 A Latin receipt to determine whether 'gutta calida' or 'frigida' is indicated, followed by 'Unguentum preciosum ad guttam'.

151 Latin receipts: 'Ad eos qui subito obmutescunt'; 2 'Ad fluxum ventris'; and one 'Si vis facere ollas interpungrare [apparently error for interfrangere]'.

152 Latin receipts: 'Ad plagam'; 'Quicumque lumen oculorum clarum habere voluerit'; 'Si vis scire quid jugulator facit' ('sume terram talpe et jacta ultra domum ut nesciat'); 'Ad pulices tollendas'; 'Ad steriles feminas'; 'Ut mulie[r] concipiat'; 'Si mulier voluerit masculum parere'; 'Ut scias si mulier concipere possit'.

153 In this section some of the red rubrics are very badly rubbed. The collection begins with Latin receipts: 'Prius data blacca potione valet diaalibanum [sic]'; 'Optima medicina ad oculos revolutos'; 'Si quis infans habet maculam in oculo'; 'Contra morbum' (including 'herbam que vocatur *primerose*'); 'Si quis habere voluerit distemperatam fluxionem'; 'Ad lippitudinem oculorum'; 'Ad dolorem dentium'; 'Ad paralisim vel caducos'; 'Ad sanguinem restringendum'; 'Si quis serpentes vel quoslibet vermes in ventre habet'; 'Ad cancrum'; the receipts on f.100r all have effaced rubrics. There follow: 'Ad vermes in utero'; 'Ad dolorem cordis'; 'Quibus cibis non delectatur'; 'Ad claritatem oculorum'; 'Si vis scire de aliquo vulnerato si evadet'; 'Ad fistulam'; 'Ad raucitudinem'; 'Ad tussim'; 'Ad dentem cavum'; 'Ad cocturam ignis'; 'Ad cancrum'.

154 For *cheverefoil*.

155 A large number of Latin receipts, many with effaced rubrics, including: 'Ad cancrum'; 'Ad fracturam capitis'; 'Oculus percussus'; 'Dolor aurium'; 'Ad crofas'.

156 The text appears to be corrupt.

157 A Latin receipt 'Qui de nocte loquitur'.

Notes to Chapter Seven

1 See Edward Edwards, *Lives of the Founders of the British Museum* I (London, 1870), pp.274–312; E. St. John Brooks, *Sir Hans Sloane: The Great Collector and His Circle* (London, 1954); G. R. de Beer, *Sir Hans Sloane and the British Museum* (London, 1953).

2 On his life see the *Dictionary of National Biography* 4 (1885), pp.377–78. On his bequest to the Bodleian Library in 1705 of an MS of Tacitus see W. D. Macray, *Annals of the Bodleian Library, Oxford* 2nd ed. (Oxford, 1890), p.174. In attendance at the sale of the considerable Bibliotheca Bernardiana was Jonathan Swift. A catalogue of Bernard's books is found in MSS B. L. Sloane 1694 ff.1r–40r and 1770 ff.212v–245v (dated 1676).

3 William Whitfield was a canon of St Paul's, London.

4 See P. Kibre, 'Hippocrates Latinus: Repertorium of Hippocratic Writings in the Latin Middle Ages (IV) ix. *Capsula Eburnea*', *Traditio* 34 (1978), 194–207. The text is the Arabic-Latin version of Gerard of Cremona. The copy in MS Sloane 282 (s.xv) ff.124r–125r has the red rubric Hic tractat Ypocras de signis mortis inc. 'Pervenit ad nos quod cum

Ypocras moraretur', but contains only the introduction, ending at MS Sloane 3550 f.6r (Kibre, *art. cit.*, 204). MS Sloane 3550 is recorded by Kibre (*art. cit.*, 201).

5 See L. Choulant, *Aegidii Corboliensis carmina medica* (Lipsiae, 1826), pp.14–18 (text) and C. Vieillard, *Gilles de Corbeil, médecin de Philippe-Auguste et chanoine de Notre Dame 1140–1224?* (Paris, 1909), pp. 48ff (the work is his first medical treatise and comprises approx. 352 verses summarizing Salernitan teaching on urines). See also E. Wickersheimer, *Dictionnaire biographique des médecins en France au moyen âge* I (Paris, 1936; repr. Genève, 1979), pp.196f and *Supplément* by D. Jacquart (Genève, 1979), pp.90f.

6 See R. H. Robbins, 'Signs of Death in Middle English', *Mediaeval Studies* 32 (1970), 182ff and T. Hunt in *Le Moyen Age* 87 (1981), 45 n.1.

7 See Wickersheimer, *op. cit.* 1, pp.170–73 and *Suppl.*, p. 80 (this MS misdated to s.xv!). The text in MS Sloane 420 ff.122r–24r breaks off at MS Sloane 3550 f.25v. See L. Thorndike & P. Kibre, *A Catalogue of Incipits of Mediaeval Scientific Writings in Latin* rev. & augm. ed. (London, 1963) (hereafter ThK), 1398.

8 See ThK 1620. Cf. MS Oxford, Bodleian Libr., Digby 79 (s.xiii), ff.142r–144v. There is a considerable number of texts in Latin and the vernacular with the title *De ornatu mulierum* which need to be studied. Cf. P. Ruelle, *L'Ornement des dames (Ornatus Mulierum): Texte anglo-normand du XIIIe siècle* (Bruxelles, 1967).

9 See ThK 89. Cf. MS Sloane 420 (s.xiv) ff.107ra–113va and see Hunt, *Plant Names*, p.xxi.

10 See ThK 1129 (*Pro aristologia ruta*). An early printed text is reproduced in D. Goltz, *Mittelalterliche Pharmazie und Medizin . . .* (Stuttgart, 1976). I have not seen Paul Berges, *Quid pro quo. Geschichte der Arzneimittelsubstitution* (Marburg, 1975). I have noted insular copies in MSS Oxford, Bodleian Libr., Auct. F.5.31 (s.xiv) ff.44v–45vb; Cambridge, Trinity Coll. 0.9.10 (s.xv) ff.119v–120v; London, B. L. Sloane 213 (s.xv) ff.134va–135vb and Sloane 1067 (s.xiv) ff.288ra–289rb.

11 See ThK 589 (*Grana quatuor*, the introduction to Galen's *Antibalomena*) which follows in MS Sloane 3018 f.10rb/c. See above p.60

12 ThK 69.

13 A large number of 'Tabulae Salernitanae' exist in medieval MSS, often with extensive commentary. See S. de Renzi, *Collectio Salernitana* 5 (Napoli, 1859), pp.233–53. See above p.346 no.122.

14 See ThK 274.

15 See ThK 943. Cf. Wickersheimer, *op. cit.*, p.171.

16 See ThK 1583 and above Ch.2 p.82.

17 See above, ch.3.

18 See S. de Renzi, *Collectio Salernitana* 2 (Napoli, 1853), pp. 497–724 and 3 (1854), pp. 205–54. On the development of glosses on Roger Frugardi's *Chirurgia* see Th. Meyer-Steineg & K. Sudhoff, *Geschichte der Medizin* 3rd ed. (Jena, 1928), pp.196ff. In MS Sloane 3018 (s.xiv) we have ff.11ra–32vb 'Cyrurgia Rolandi cum additionibus Rogeri' (ThK 856) and ff.33ra–63vb 'Glosule super Cyrurgiam' (ThK 1383 = MS Sloane 3550 f.100v) ending 'Expliciunt Glosule quatuor magistrorum'.

19 See ThK 1064.

20 See ThK 1482 (= Guido Arenensis on Roger's *Chirurgia*).

21 See ThK 225.

22 Cf. MS London, B. L., Add. 15236 f. 26r and cf. L. E. Voigts & M. R. McVaugh, *A Latin Technical Phlebotomy and its Middle English Translation*, Trans. Am. Philos. Soc. 74, ii (Philadelphia, 1984).

23 See above, ch.3.

24 Cf. MS B. L. Sloane 3018 (s.xiv) f. 36va (bottom of the page). In MS B. L. Arundel 332 (s.xiii) f.230v the verses appear under a red rubric *Hec est ars conficiendi pilas medicinales ad plagas sanandas*. See also P. Meyer in *Romania* 37 (1908), 515.

25 See ThK 246. Cf. the text (s.xiii) in MS Sloane 2584 ff.94r–101r which ends 'Nocent spleni . . . omne nimis ventosum'.

26 See MS Oxford, Bodleian Libr., e Musaeo 219 (s.xiii) ff.124r (pref. on f.123 ult.)–127r. See ThK 1498 and P. Kibre in *Traditio* 35 (1979), 295 who lists our MS mistakenly as 'XII–XIII Century'.

27 ThK 1498.

28 The contents include 'Emplastrum bonum m. J. de Lin' (f.246v) and 'cecretum m. J. de Lin' (f.247r); 'Experimentum secretum Gilberti [= Gilbertus Anglicus?]' (f.248v; cf. 'Gilbertus: pulmo leporis combustus, pul[vis] valet ad idem', f.243v). Vernacular glosses occur as follows: 'urticam silvestrem que gallice dicitur *grezche* et lancelye' (f.245r); 'herba trita que dicitur *plantayne*' (f.245r); 'semen buxi .i. *box* [MS lox] anglice'.

29 = 'sans'.

30 A number of vernacular items are included in the Latin receipts on f.92r: 'utriusque rubi .i. *de l' eglenter e de la petite runce*'; 'ungule caballine .i. *edocke*'; 'flores verbene .i. *vepervoye*'; 'flores de *medewrt*'; 'radicem herbe que dicitur anglice *levres*'.

31 This receipt is part of a section headed *Contra instantiam vigilarum*. The opening is repeated on f. 231v.

32 Rubrics printed in italics are written in red in the MS. This receipt appears in full in MS Sloane 146 (see above p.282 no.130) and in the 'Physique rimee' (see above p.173f., ll. 777ff.). On f.93v there is a vernacular entry 'rubeam parellam: [r]edocke'.

33 The MS has 'Si os en la playe remeine' (see below no.62). The text changes abruptly from *ke l'en* (f.93v) to *bibat levante vomitum provocat* (f.94r).

34 For *trimblét / trinblét* see also nos 8, 67, 70.

35 i.e. *bure de may* (cf. nos 14 & 15), perhaps under the influence of English *may butter*.

36 This form is not attested in FEW 6, i, 377a.

37 Corr. *en yvern* or *iver tens?*

38 In the left-hand margin is the red rubric *Pur suager dolur de play*. Cf. nos. 49 & 70.

39 This is followed simply by a paragraph mark and the next receipt.

40 In the left-hand margin is the red rubric *Pur fer atret encontre felun*.

41 In the left-hand margin is the red rubric *Pur fer ciroine* [= emplastrum ceroneum]. Cf. Meyer, *Bull. SATF 1906*, p. 79 no.1 and FEW 2, i, 597a.

42 i.e. English 'dock' and 'hollyhock'.

43 In the right-hand margin is the red rubric *Contra fluxum sanguinis*. The MS has *Quant sanc remeint en plaie*. See the full text in MS Cambridge, Trinity College, 0.2.5 (s.xiv) (hereafter T) f.117vb where it forms part of the collection of verse receipts known as the *Novele Cirurgerie* see T. Hunt, 'The 'Novele Cirurgerie' in MS London, British Library Harley 2558', *Z.f.rom.Phil.* 103 (1987), 271–99. The next receipt (no. 21) also follows in T with variants *menuement* and *bue en vin*.

44 The words are clear in the MS, but their significance remains obscure. The beginning of the receipts appears to be corrupt.

45 See T f.115vb with variant *i seit mellé* in line 4.

46 See T f.116vb.

47 See T f.115ra with the following introductory lines: 'Pur acumpler ma reison / medecine dirrai pur trencheson / kar mal est mut et anguisous / e al cors mout perilous'. The Latin receipts on f.98r of MS Sloane 3550 contain the following vernacular items: 'malve .i. *mauve*'; 'senescionis: *grundeswelie*'; 'narstucii aquatici .i. *karsuns de euue*'; 'liquerei .i. *licoris*'; 'cinamomi .i. *canele*'; 'seminis apii .i. *h[a]che*'; 'papaveris .i. *popi*'. On f.97v there is 'sanguis hirci .i. *gote bucke*' and on f.97v/98r 'edere arboree, galice [sic] *yvi*'. On f.98v there are three vernacular items: 'neptam .i. *nep[t]e*'; 'febrifuga .i. *vepervoye*'; 'herbam illam que vocatur gallice *recopé* '.

48 In the left-hand margin is the red rubric *De dolore mamillarum*.

49 See T f.113va.

50 Nos 33–35 are found in T f.113va/b.

51 See A. Salmon, 'Remèdes populaires du moyen âge', *Etudes romanes dédiées à Gaston Paris le 29 Décembre 1890 ...* (Paris, 1891) [pp.253–66] no.77; P. Meyer, *Bull. SATF 1906*,

p.52 nos 44 & 45; MS Sloane 146 no.90 (see above p.278) and MS Sloane 2584 f.25v.
See above p.82 and note 100.

52   In the left-hand margin is the red rubric *Contra plagas*. See T f.117ra.

53   Cf. *eschufer* two lines below. In T. f.117ra the receipt ends 'De la plaie seit pure et nette /
ceste entrete i devez mettre'.

54   In the left-hand margin is the red rubric *Contra plagas*. See T f.117rb.

55   In the left-hand margin is the red rubric *Contra tibiam*. The receipt is a 'version dérimée'
of that in MS Harley 2558 f.8vb, as is the following receipt.

56   In the left-hand margin is the red rubric *De sompno*.

57   In the left-hand margin is the red rubric *Contra tussim equi*. Further down the page there
is a Latin receipt with the rubric *Contra jauniz*. On f.233r there is a vernacular gloss
'bibant abrotanum .i. *souþernewode*'.

58   The receipt which follows is in Latin.

59   The rubric, in red, is found in the right-hand margin. Cf. no.12 above & 70 below.

60   *Tut* is written with a nasal bar. Corr. *entrayra*?

61   In the right-hand margin is the red rubric *Contra stomachum*.

62   In the right-hand margin is the red rubric *Pur menesun*. A Latin receipt on f.233v
includes a vernacular gloss: 'enulam .i. *hoshelne*'.

63   In the left-hand margin is the red rubric *Contra singultum*.

64   The red rubric is found in the left-hand margin. See Salmon, *art. cit.*, no.24 and MS
Sloane 146 no.150 (see above p.283) and MS Cambridge, St John's College D.4 no.26
(see above p.212).

65   In the left-hand margin is the red rubric *Autre*. See Salmon, *art. cit.*, no.25 and MS
Sloane 146 no.151 (see above p.284) and MS Cambridge, St John's College D.4 no.27
(see above p.212).

66   In the right-hand margin is the red rubric *Contra defectum lactis*. The receipt is found in
the 'Physique rimee' in MS Cambridge, Trinity Coll. 0.1.20 (see above p.200), hereafter
PR, ll.1635ff. See also MS Sloane 146 no.89 (see above p.278).

67   The red rubric is found in the right-hand margin. In the second line the MS has *nū home*.
The receipt is found in PR ll.555ff.

68   The same receipt is found in PR ll.1331ff. See also MS Sloane 146 no.173 (see above
p.287).

69   In the left-hand margin is the red rubric *Contra febres*. In PR ll.1335ff the receipt begins
'Por cotidiane: La cotidiane fevre / cel est mal et malevre'. See also MS Sloane 146
no.174 (see above p.286).

70   See PR ll.1009ff which has the rubric *A plaie saner*.

71   The red rubric is written in the right-hand margin. The receipt is found in PR ll.753ff,
with the final line reading 'La plaie tost estaunchera'.

72   The red rubric is written in the right-hand margin. The receipt is found in PR ll.761ff,
beginning 'Si home est quassés ne nauvrés / ke ait membres quassés et froissés / prendre
devés herbes plusors'.

73   The red rubric is written in the right-hand margin. The receipt is found in PR ll.777ff,
beginning '*Por os plaié*: Si aucun os est remis em plaie / et vous ne trovés ki l'en traie'.

74   In the left-hand margin is the red rubric *Contra plagas*. In PR ll.787ff the receipt begins
'Emplastre querai que vous serve / . . .'

75   The red rubric is written in the left-hand margin. In PR ll.791ff the receipt begins 'Jo
vous dirai .i. bon entrait / ke en tel guise sera fait'.

76   The red rubric is written in the left-hand margin. In PR ll.811ff the receipt begins '*Beivre
a plaie garir*: Un beivre vous vodrai elire / ke vaut a plaie, ce os bien dire, / kar bons mires
l'ont dit plusurs . . .'. It is clear that on several occasions MS Sloane 3550 condenses by
conflation.

77   In the left-hand margin there is the red rubric *Contra plagas*. The receipt is found in PR
ll.839ff.

78   The red rubric is repeated in the left-hand margin. See PR ll.959ff.

79   See PR ll.965ff.
80   In the left-hand margin there is the red rubric *De dieta*. See PR ll.971ff.
81   The red rubric is in part illegible.
82   Cf. nos. 12 and 59 above.
83   The red rubric is found in the right-hand margin. See PR ll.989ff which has the rubric *Por plaié garir*.
84   The receipt is found in PR ll.1387ff. It is also written out as verse at the bottom of f.235v of MS Sloane 3550 and I print the two Sloane versions in parallel.
85   In the main text the rest of the receipt is in Latin, but the full Anglo-Norman verses are written out at the bottom of f.235v. The same receipt is found in PR ll.1393ff. The following Latin receipt on f.233v begins 'Recipe unam herbam que vocatur peluse, anglice mushere . . .'.
86   In the left-hand margin is the red rubric *Contra tussim equi*.
87   The red rubric is written in the left-hand margin. The receipt is found in T f.116va.
88   See T f.110rb/va '*Pur teigne de la teste*'. The fourth line, missing in the Sloane MS, reads 'La ou se arde fermement se tint' and the sixth line begins 'En romanz . . .' At line 9 T reads 'Dounc sachez tut finement / le chief reez mout nettement'.
89   See T f.110va which reads in line 4 'e byn naee'.
90   This receipt is written in red at the bottom of the page. On the same page there is a receipt headed 'Cura .m. Eruardi de opido contra fluxum lacrimarum cum rubore oculorum'. On f.241r there is 'Experimentum R. de Warwich ad visum accuendum'. There are also three sets of verses: (1) *Ista nocent oculis: faba, lens, piper, allia cepe* (3 verses) (2) *Camphora, sarcolla, licinium, celidonia, ruta* (4 verses) (3) *Feniculus, verbena, rosa, celidonia, ruta* (2 verses; Walther, *Initia* 6423).

Notes to Chapter Eight

1   Individual vernacular items occur as follows: 'accipe herbam que romane dicitur *moleine*' (f.8r); 'pediculus ovis qui anglice dicitur *tike*' (f.9v); 'Contra epilepenciam et palisim et fulgura et tempestates: porta circa collum lignum quod vocatur *wi de cheene*' (f.9v); 'accipe amaruscam herbam .i. *meidene*' (f.9v); 'Contra acutam fe[brem]: carmen istud contra fe[brem] acutam: *Le lit seint Estiefne seit entre mei e le chald mal*. Postea dicat orationem de sancto Stephano et ter Pater Noster et ter Ave Maria' (f.10r); '. . . caprifolii .i. *hunisukeles*, corone regie .i. *medwert*' (f.10v); 'herba *clivre* . . .' (f.10v); 'succus de *fan* et succus de *elfan* magis quam de *clivre*' (f.10v: at the bottom of the page is written 'herba elfan quere in libro de panno nigro et invenies qualis sit').
2   There are five vernacular entries: 'accipe herbam que vocatur *tette soriz* .i. *stonore*' (f.22v); 'accipe muscas magnas que dicuntur *flesfliyen*' (f.22v); 'coquatur herba *ueldfrit*' (f.23r); 'pes caballi .i. *colcrai*' (f.23r); 'accipe vermes terre .i. *madoc*' (f.23r).
3   See L. Thorndike, *A History of Magic and Experimental Science* vol.2 (London, 1923), p.734 n.1 and p.735 n.1. See also L. Thorndike & P. Kibre, *A Catalogue of Incipits of Mediaeval Scientific Writings in Latin*, rev. & augm. ed. (London, 1963) (hereafter ThK) 532.
4   See P. Kibre, 'Hippocrates Latinus: Repertorium of Hippocratic Writings in the Latin Middle Ages (V)', *Traditio* 35 (1979), esp. 280–2 (this MS on p.282).
5   Edited by E. Howald & H. E. Sigerist, *Corpus medicorum latinorum* IV (Lipsiae / Berolini, 1927), pp.1–11.
6   Edited by Howald & Sigerist, *ed. cit.*, pp.13–225.

7   ed. cit., p.177. There are about 35 vernacular glosses inserted beside the red rubrics in the text.

8   As in the case of Ps-Apuleius above there are a number of vernacular glosses.

9   ThK 327.

10 See Kibre, art. cit., 280 (citing this MS).

11 ThK 1360; Howald & Sigerist, ed. cit., pp.227–32.

12 ThK 246.

13 ThK 1129.

14 Kibre, art. cit., 233–34 gives this MS as the sole witness.

15 ThK 901.

16 ThK 743.

17 The 'Capsula eburnea', see Kibre, 'Hippocrates Latinus . . . (IV)', Traditio 34 (1978) esp. 194–207 (this MS on p. 202).

18 Two isolated vernacular glosses are 'suc rute, suc ambrete' (f.209r) and 'herba restolantia .i. clofyunke' (f.209v, left-hand margin).

19 For these and other charms see D. Gray, 'Notes on some Middle English Charms', in B. Rowland (ed.), Chaucer and Middle English Studies in Honour of Rossell Hope Robbins (London, 1974), pp.56–71 and above pp.78ff.

20 There are red rubrics.

21 This marks the beginning of the vernacular receipts proper. On f.173v the receipt Contra paralisim contains the phrase 'duas herbas paraliticum .s. primulam sauvage et fraser sauvage' and on f.175v Ad omnes plagas includes 'medwert' and 'sparge'.

22 In the right-hand margin is written 'tribus diebus dicatur'.

23 In the right-hand margin is written 'si necesse fuerit ter in die'.

24 In the left-hand margin is inserted 'une coilleree'.

25 For the same receipt see P. Ruelle (ed.), L'Ornement des dames (Ornatus mulierum). Texte anglo-normand du XIIIe siècle (Bruxelles, 1967), p.38 no.vii. For the figure of La Saracine see p.34 ll.32ff, p.36 no.iv and p.56 no.xlii. In the right-hand margin of f.176r a gloss to persil salvage reads '.i. stanmar[c]h'.

26 MS = diriches. For the same receipt see Ruelle, ed. cit., p.38 no.ix (Dame Trote).

27 Same receipt in Ruelle, ed. cit., p.40 no.x. Beside this section in the Digby MS is written 'stobile'.

28 In the left-hand margin is written 'experimentum', and also beside nos. 8 & 11.

29 In the left-hand margin is written 'probatum', and also beside nos. 10 & 12.

30 There follows a new paragraph mark in the MS.

31 It looks as if some material has fallen out.

32 'eiciendam' is added in brown ink to the red rubric.

33 All the numerical indications of quantity have been erased in the MS.

34 Above is written as an interlinear gloss 'consol[ida] mi[nor]'.

35 MS = keskes.

36 i.e. the patient.

37 What follows is in Latin.

38 Two receipts with vernacular rubrics (Pur plaie saner ki est perillus and Pur estreite plaie saner) are in fact in Latin, whilst a third, Unguentum ad plagas sanandas mixes Latin and vernacular forms throughout: Accipe avenciam, bugle, pigle, senicle, matefelun, plantaginem, lanceleiam, orpin, senecionem, jubarbe, herbive, coperun de runces, cerfoil, ache, consolidam minor [sic], folia caulis rubei, feniculum, primerole, millefolium, moleine, herbe Water, herbe Robert, mastik, incensum, ceram bonam. Sil movez. Pus metez le mastic, sil movez, pus l'encens, sil movez, pus la cire, sil movez d'un esclice.

39 This receipt is written in the right-hand margin.

40 In the right-hand margin is written 'Eschaufez une tuele al feu bien, si metez sor l'emplastre'.

41 In the left-hand margin is written 'les oilz seent un poi uvert e oint de çoe'.

42 This receipt is written in the left-hand margin.

43   Read 'e l'esule le fet'?
44   This receipt is written in the left-hand margin.
45   MS = *douf.*
46   In the right-hand margin is written 'le fund si est la gresse ki est desuz les costez'.
47   Erasure in the MS.
48   MS = *angelico.* In the right-hand margin is written 'archangelica'.
49   MS = *keskes.*
50   Same receipt, in Middle English, in MS London, B. L. Royal 17 A VIII f.35v.
51   See Ruelle, *ed. cit.* p.62 no.lii, ll.504–6 'Olie de ofs frez issi: triblez ofs quiz mult durs et friez en une paele et muvez durement et puis premez parmi un drap par force'.
52   Corr. *eschaufé?*
53   There is an interlinear gloss 'chikeme' and in the right-hand margin 'chykemete'.
54   MS = *kukusp̄.* The hermit saint Fiacre (d. c. 670) became patron of horticulturalists. His name did not enter the Irish martyrologies until the end of the 12th C. There is little evidence of his being known in England before the late middle ages. See J. Dubois, *Un sanctuaire monastique au moyen âge: Saint-Fiacre-en-Brie* (Genève, 1946) and *XIIIe centenaire de saint Fiacre: actes du congrès Meaux – 1970* (Meaux, n.d.).
55   In the right-hand margin is written the following passage: 'Li leu si est un verm de la lungure de un dei, si ad teste cum chat, le bec lung et agu; .x. et .viii. piez ad, les dous dereins piez sunt crocuz pur tenir sei ferm, ke par aventure ne isse de la plaie. As esues desus le penil est sa mansiun, mes al braun de la jambe ist quant il ist. E iloc li donet l'en a manger quant manger deit, kar si il ne manjiast, il devoreit le home en poi de tens'.
56   At the bottom of the page is written 'A home ki emfle e asuage en toz le cors wsminte'.
57   This is introduced by a new paragraph mark.
58   The second and third words are written in brown. The receipt in the main text has been erased and the present text inserted in the left-hand margin.
59   There are a series of erasures in the MS.
60   The last sentence is written in the left-hand margin.
61   Same receipt in MSS London, B. L. Royal 9 A XIV f.192ra (see below p.73) and Sloane 146 f.1r (see above p.267). Here it is written in the left-hand margin.
62   The scribe writes this as a single word, though it is clearly a form of *pois resin* 'pitch resin'.
63   There is a folio missing. At the bottom of f.180v is written 'Seit colé en une gate u ewe seit mise ke ne se prenge al vessel'.
64   The following receipt is written in Latin.
65   In the right-hand margin is written 'de ruine'.
66   MS = *menez.*
67   The receipt is written in the left-hand margin.
68   MS = *hi.*
69   In the left-hand margin is written 'mirabile'.

Notes to Chapter Nine

1   See P. Meyer, 'Les manuscrits français de Cambridge III', *Romania* 32 (1903) [18–120; 75–95 on O.1.20] 82–4 who recognizes that the receipts on ff. 30r et seq. are not part of Roger Frugardi's *Chirurgia* which precedes them, but fails to realize that those on ff. 37r et seq. are part of the 'Lettre d'Hippocrate'.
2   In the notes I cite from the Lyon edition of 1510, *Compendium medicine Gilberti anglici tam morborum universalium quam particularium nondum medicis sed et cyrurgicis utilissimum.*

The colophon reads *Explicit compendium medicine Gilberti Anglici correctum et bene emen-datum per dominum Michaelem de Capella artium et medicine doctorem: ac Lugduni impressum per Jacobum Saccon: expensis Vincentii de Portonariis. Anno Domini M. D. X die vero vigesima mensis Novembris. Deo Gratias.* The *Compendium* is divided into seven books and extends over 362 numbered folios. For the Latin text of the *Antidotarium Nicolai* I have used the 'Antidotarium Nicolai cum expositionibus et glosis clarissimi physici magistri Platearii' found in *Mesue cum additionibus Francisci de pedemontium . . .* Venice, 1491, pp.223ff. There is a text of the 1471 edition in D. Goltz, *Mittelalterliche Pharmazie und Medizin* (Stuttgart, 1976).

3   The same receipt is found in MS London, B. L. Sloane 962 (s.xv), f.158r. It is found in Gilbertus Anglicus (Lib. 2 f.87va) under the heading *De fractura cranei cum amplo vulnere*: 'Apostolicon: Recipe picis navalis libram semis, picis grece libram semis, galbani, serapini, amoniaci, oppoponaci ana unciam semis, cere uncias tres in estate, in hyeme uncias due, aceti libram semis. Conficiantur sic: galbanum, serapinum, oppoponax, pix navalis in aceto supra ignem in stagnato liquefiant et cum parum de eo in aqua frigida positum se tenuerit et colorem mutaverit in citrinum, pix greca et mastix et olibanum amborum ana uncia semis pulverizentur et cum supradictis incorporentur supra ignem, et cum de subalbo colore in citrinum mutaverit, quod est signum perfecte decoctionis, ab igne removeatur et terbentine uncia una apponatur. Et tunc totum supra aquam frigidam coletur et manibus inunctis oleo laurino vel alia pinguedine malaxetur iuxta ignem quousque aqua effluxerit et consumatur. Et tunc magdaleones formentur et reserventur' [Here and throughout I expand abbreviations, even at some risk]. A different receipt for 'Emplastrum apostolicon' is given on f. 358va/b from the *Antidotarium Nicolai* and corresponds to that in the French translation edited by P. Dorveaux (hereafter AN followed by paragraph no.), p.17, para. 34. See also P. Meyer in *Romania* 44 (1915–17), 170.

4   Here a folio is missing.

5   Many varieties of 'dialthea' (made with marshmallow) are found in receipt collections. This is not the one contained in the *Antidotarium Nicolai*.

6   Like 'dialthea' 'populeon' also exists in many varieties, all using the leaves or buds of the poplar. The present receipt is different from that found in AN 73.

7   MS = *te*.

8   There is a coloured initial but no rubric or indication. Presumably something has dropped out.

9   In '.i. livre de cyrurgie' in MS London, B. L. Sloane 1977 (s.xiii[2]) f.143vb we read 'Pur rapis: rapis est maniere de cranque. Pren herbe Robert et esparge et *leu saulum* et agullie et fai pastel et met sus la maladie. Et si i met miel et vin aigre'. I do not know what the word means. It appears again in our MS in a prose receipt on f.23vb as *lusalveon* and in MS B. L. Arundel 42 (s.xv in) f.95rb 'leusavun: crousope' which clearly suggests Saponaria officinalis.

10   MS = *ki*.

11   MS = *chevine*.

12   MS = *liuaire*.

13   In the MS the phrase *si le batez* is misplaced after *polipode*.

14   From this point the text is written in single columns.

15   MS = *citru*. In this list of the celebrated 'four major cold seeds' *citru[lis]* probably indicated Cucurbita pepo ('pumpkin gourd'). Cf. receipt 13 and B.18.

16   One should probably read 'baie de lorer, cost'.

17   MS = *qui il*.

18   MS = *qui il*.

19   MS = *lapis lazimi*.

20   See Gilbertus Anglicus Lib. 2 ff.119vb–120ra: 'Paulinum: paulinum proprie datur veteri et nove tussi que fit ex discrasia capitis et contra vicia pectoris ex frigiditate; cum vino calido in sero caput et stomachum a flegmate et melancolia et occulorum gravedinem mirabiliter purgat. Datur in modum electuarii vel pillularum . . . Recipe aloes dragmas

undecim et grana quindecim, croci, costi, anacardi, agarici, coralli, mirre, amoni, terebenti, galbani, serapii, oppoponaci. Confice rute, storacis calamite, yrei ana dragmas quattuor
et semis, opii, olibani, masticis, bdellii, corimbri ana dragmas duas et grana quindecim,
balsami, folii ana scrupulum unum et semis, mellisse dragmas duas. Conficiatur sic:
galbanum, serapinum, oppoponax, amonia terantur et in vino odorifero per noctem
ponantur. Mane super ignem liquefiant et colentur et iterum bulliant. Post adde mellis
dispumati uncias tres et coquantur ad spissitudinis inceptionem. Tunc imponatur pau-
latim storax calamita et corimbrum cum pistello calido tunsa et liquefiat. Post addatur
terebenti et cum bene coctum fuerit, et supra marmor gutta posita colligatur et teneat,
addatur mirra, bdellium, olibanum et post reliqua pulverizata ad ultimum cum croco
orientali magdaliones componas, sed non apponatur opium nisi quando datur contra
fluxum reumatizantem. A capite indigestioni et discoloratis ex frigiditate opitulatur'.

21   See AN 9: 'Benoîte est dite, quar ceus qui la receivent la beneissent. El vaut à artetique, à
     poacre; el fait pisser; el purge les rains et la vessie. Pren: esule, once .ii.; turbit, çucre, ana
     dragme .x.; girofle, espic, dragme .i.; safran, saxifrage, lonc poivre, amome, sal gemme,
     garingaut, carvi, fanoil, brusque, groumil, [ana dragme .i.]; miel sofeisant. El soit donee au
     soir ou vin chaud en quantité d'une chastaine'. Cf. Gilbertus Anglicus Lib. 7 f.316rb
     (Benedicta).

22   See Gilbertus Anglicus Lib. 6 f.237ra for 'yera pigra Galieni' and 'yera pigra Constantini'.
     AN 84 has 'Yera pigra vaut à diverses passiuns de chef et à destempramce de euz,
     d'oreilles et de ventrail, et à dolor de faie, et à duresce d'esplain, et à rains et à vesie, et à
     destempramce de mariz. Pren: canele, safran, espic, squinamtum, cassie, ana dragme .ii.;
     violes, alesne, epitin, agaric, roses, turbit, colloquintide, mastic, ana dragme [.ii.]; miel
     sofeisant. Sa dose est dragme .iii. ou eve de coorde. Si tu [le] veuz faire laxatif, [ajuste] i
     dragme .ii. de scamonee'.

23   MS = qui qui li.

24   The MS is unclear.

25   See AN 63: 'Sirop acetus vaut à chalor et fievre ague, et à passion d'esplain et de foie, et à
     constipatium de ventre. Pren: fenoil, ache, scariole l'escorche, ana dragme .x.; espic,
     narde, squinamtum, ana dragme .ii. Icestes atriblees soient mises en .v. livres de vin aigre
     ou .iiii. livres d'eve, et soient dus jorz ensemble, puis boillent à petit feu jusque à la moitié,
     et soit preint et colé, puis soit pendu en un sac linge qu'il degote peti[t] et petit, puis i soit
     mis le çucre, et boille jusque il soit espès . . .'

26   See AN 62: 'Sirop rosat est fait isi: Pren roses fresches et les met en vessel par soi, et met
     eve en une paelle jusque el boille, puis soit mise sus les roses, et soit covert le vessel que la
     fumee ne s'en isse. L'eve fraide, trai les roses, et i meit autres bouillir, et fai isi en muant
     les roses jusque l'eve soit roge, et mest .iiii. livres de ceule eive en .iiii. livres de vin eigre
     et de çucre, et, com ce bouillira, bat aubun d'uef en eve fraide jusque el espument, puis
     pren l'espume et met ou sirop boillant, et, quant il commencera à nercir, oste l'espume
     jusque le sirop soit cler, et, com il fera ausi co[m fil] s'il soit atouchei ou le dai, il est cuit.
     Il vaut à chalor et à soi, et constraint. Ausi est fait sirup violat. Il vaut à feivre, à tisique, et
     amoiste les costivez et lasche ventre . . .'.

27   Gilbertus Anglicus Lib. 6 ff.235vb–36ra 'Trifera sarracenica hic propria est, trifera dicitur
     quia hominem juvenem reddit; sarracenica a sarracenis inventa. Proprie datur yctericis,
     epaticis de calore epatis et de fumositate colere rubee patientibus et patientibus calorem
     capitis et visum tenebratum a calore . . .'. See AN 64: 'Trife sarazine est doné à dolor de
     foie, à jaunice, à sinple tierçaine et à doble, et rent la veu[e] pardue de chalor. Pren: çucre,
     livre .iiii.; mirobolans citrins escorce, de cassia fi[s]tule meolla [et] de tamarindes, ana
     once demie; reubarbe mumdé, mamne, ana dragme [,vi.]; violes, dragme demie; anis,
     fanoil, ana dragme .ii.; mastic, macis, ana dragme .i.; belleriques, enbliques, ana dragme
     demie. Il est confeit isi: en .ii. livres d'eve soient mis once .iiii. de violes, et boillent jusque
     il veingnent à porpre color; puis soient praintes les violes et colees, et en .i. partie de la
     coleure soit lavé cassia fi[s]tulis et tamarindes, et soit colé. En l'autre eve soit mis .i. livre
     de çucre, et soit mis sus le feu, et boille, et, com il commencera à espoisier, soit i mise la

coleure de cassiafi[s]tulis et de tamarindes et puis manna. Il est cuit si il s'aert au[si] comme miel mis sus marbre. A dereinie[r] soit mis la poudre de[s] autres espices en movant totdis. Il est doné au matin en quantité d'une chastaine ou eve chaude'. 'Tryphera Saracenica' is also described in Gilles de Corbeil's *De laudibus et virtutibus compositorum medicaminum* Lib. 4 ll.845ff in L. Choulant (ed.), *Aegidii Corboliensis carmina medica* (Lipsiae, 1826) [hereafter cited as Gilles].

28 I have not traced the source of this receipt.

29 See Gilbertus Anglicus Lib. 1 f.24va 'Katarticum imperiale quod optime purgat caput os bene olens reddit, de stomacho et de toto corpore utramque co. quiete educit. Recipe dyagredii et zuccare amborum dragmas duas, cinamomi, nardi, saxifrage, polipodii, omnium quattuor dragmas quattuor, gariofili, zinziberis, celtice, melanopiperis, macropiperis, cardamomi, amomi omnium septem dragmas tres, mellis quantum sufficit. Datur in modum avellane ante cenam et post cenam. Sed ratio receptionis testificatur eum multum calefacere, quod etiam experientia mihi sepius confirmavit, ideo commutavi pro scamonea reubarbarum, pro cardamomo mirabolani citrini, pro melanopiperis medullam cassiefistule, et addidi seminum frigidorum liquidorum ana dragmas quattuor, confice cum zuccara'. AN 41 has 'Kartacum inpariale vaut à constipatium, à ventosité, et purge sanz moleste. Pren: scamonee, zucre, dragme .iii. et demie; quanele, narde, saxifrage, polipode, ana dragme .ii.; girofle, gingimbre, noir poivre et lon, cardamome, amome, ana dragme .i. et demie; esule, once .i. et demie; mirrobolans citrins, once demie; miel sofeisant. Il soit doné au soir et au matin ou vin ou o eve'. See also Gilles Lib. 3, ll.752ff.

30 See AN 32 'Eletuarium de succo rosarum vaut à goute, et purge cole, et vaut à tierçaine et cotidiane. Pren: zucre, jus de rose, [ana] livre .i.; sandali blanc et roge, gumme arabic, ana dragme .vi.; spodium, dragme .iii.; [s]camonee, dragme .iii.; camfre, dragme .i. Soit doné au matin ou eve chaude en quantité de .i. chastainne'. See also Gilles Lib. 3, ll.542ff and cf. Gilbertus Anglicus Lib. 7 f.314va.

31 MS = *qui il.*

32 MS = *qui il.*

33 MS = *auent* with hairline over second letter.

34 See the *Livre des simples medecines* ed. Dorveaux, 759 '.v. maneires sunt de mirobolanz: citrins et kebles et emblis et indes et belleris. Li citrins, cil qui sunt gros et pesant, sont li mellor, et quant l'en les depiece, qu'il sunt glumous par dedenz. L'en le[s] puet garder .x. anz. Kebles et belleris conoistroiz en tel maniere maiemes: li kebles ne se puet garder que .v. anz; li emblic et li inde [sunt] toz jorz buen, meis qu'il ne seiant (sic) trop vieuz'.

35 MS = *quarante qutre quatre.*

36 MS = *encorporer.*

37 Gilbertus Anglicus Lib. 7 f.335vb has 'Malum mortuum species est scabiei de pura melancolia naturali corrupta et putrefacta; aut de melancolia innaturali cum admixtione fleumatis salsi generata . . .' and recommends a 'stupha' for its treatment.

38 MS = *meisne.*

39 Parts of the rubric are too badly rubbed to be deciphered.

40 See Gilbertus Anglicus Lib. 6 f.265ra/b 'Agrippa valet ydropicis et tumori splenis et omnibus tumoribus in quacumque parte corporis fuerint et ad nervos indignatos, vomitum provocat et, inunctum supra ventrem laxat . . .' and AN 74 'Unguent Agripe vaut à idropiques et à totes emfleumes; il fait uriner. Si il soit oint sus le ventre, il lasche . . .' See Gilles Lib. 4, ll.1306ff.

41 See Gilbertus Anglicus Lib. 7 f.316vb 'Unguentum marciaton facit ad frigiditatem et dolorem capitis et pectoris et stomachi et ad sclirosim epatis et splenis et ad ylii dolorem, ad ignem vel ad solem inunctum statim subvenit. Paraliticis, artheticis, sciaticis, nefreticis et podagricis prodest. Tumores reprimit et contra omnes dolores potenter medetur . . .' and AN 75 'Unguent Marciaton vaut: à fraidor de chef, de piz, de ventrail; à duresce d'esplain, de foie; à paralesie, à artetique, à sciatique, à dolors de rains, à poacre, à enfleumes . . .' See Gilles Lib. 4, ll.1235ff.

42 See Gilbertus Anglicus Lib. 6 f.266rb 'Arogon .i. adiutorium valet ad dolorem ex frigidi-

tate viris et mulieribus ad spasmum et thetanum et dolorem ylii et renum. Valet etiam artheticis et sciaticis, multum prodest quartanariis per spinam dorsi inunctum ante horam accessionis . . .' and AN 76 'Unguent Arogon vaut à fraidor, oint isi: il soit remis en test de uof et soint oint le leu devant, puis i soit mis le test chaut. Il vaut à spasme e[t] à dolor de rains, [à] artetique et à ciatique et à quartainne s'il soit oint sus l'eschine devant l'acession'. See also Gilles Lib. 4, ll.1290ff.

43   See AN 77 'Unguent dialtee . . . il vaut à dolor de piz de fraidor et à pleurisie, eschaufé en un tes[t] de oif et oin[t] sus le piz. Il eschaufe touz les leus freiz et amoleie les seccheiz'.

44   See Gilbertus Anglicus Lib. 5 f.215rb 'Dyacalamentum valet ad omne vicium pectoris ex frigiditate maxime bis qui sunt in senili etate. Et etiam tussientibus et quartanariis et frigiditati stomachi precipue ex matrice. Recipe calamenti, pulegii, melanopiperis, siselei, petrosilinii ana dragmas tres et scrupulos duos, levistici dragma una et scrupulus unus, ameos, thimi, aneti, cinamomi, zinziber ana scrupulos duos, mellis quantum sufficit' and AN 26 'Diacalamentum vaut au dolors dou poumon de fraidor, meesment au veilarz, et à tus de fraidor, et à quartaine, pris après mangier au soir ou vin. Pren: calamente, pulegium, noir poivre, sirmontain, perresil, ana dragme .ii.; levesche, semence d'ache, dragme .i.; ameos, time, anete, quanele, gingembre, ana dragme .i.; miel sofeisant'. See Gilles Lib. 2, ll.442ff.

45   See Gilbertus Anglicus Lib. 4, f.184ra 'Dyadragagantum frigidum valet ad omne vitium pectoris ex calore et siccitate et ad omnem lingue et gutturis asperitatem. Sed cum sumitur in ore teneatur donec solvatur . . .' and AN 23 'Diagragant vaut à vice de piz et de pulmun qui vient de chalor, à etique, à tisique, à tus de chalor et de secheté, à aspresce de langue et de goitrun. Quant il sera usé, soit tenu en la bouche longuement. Pren: dragagant, once .iii.; gumme arabic, once .ii.; amidum, once demie; riquelice, dragme .ii.; penides, semence de melons, de cohordes, de citrules, de cucumer, ana dragme .ii.; camfre dragme demie; sirop julevi sofeisant. Soit doné ou eve de decocciun d'orge et de dragagant'. See Gilles Lib. 2, ll.626ff.

46   See note 15 above.

47   See Gilbertus Anglicus Lib. 4 f.184ra 'Dyapenidion valet ad omnem vitium pulmonis et tussis et ad raucedinem ex siccitate et ptisicum. Recipe penidiarum dragmas sedecim et semis . . .' and AN 21 'Diapenidion vaut contre vice de pulmon et à tus, à esroeure de fraidor et à tisique. Pren penides, dragme .xvii. et demie . . .' See also Gilles Lib. 2, ll.544ff.

48   The receipt is that of AN 77 in all essentials.

49   Cf. Gilbertus Anglicus Lib. 1 f.48rb 'Claretum et pulvis ad quartanam: claretum eis fiat ad vigorationem virtutis cum virtus debilis est . . . Recipe liquiricie, zinziberi, cardamomi, galange, spice, gariofili, cuscute, sene, macis, ciperi, omnium istorum quantum videbitur medico expedire . . .'

50   See Gilbertus Anglicus Lib. 4 f.178rb 'Dyamoron valens ad omnes passiones palati et gutturis et maxime squinantie, uvam cadentem sublevat et humores desiccat. Recipe mori celsi et rubi ana libra una, mellis libram semis, sape libras tres. Omnia coque in stagnato ad prunas lento igne ad perfectionem. Signum coctionis est quod gutta adheret catie . . .' and AN 14 'Diamoron vaut à totes dolors de palais et de goitron: il releve la luete et deseiche icelle moite. Pren: mores de morier, livre demie; mores de buissun, livre demie; miel, livre demie; vin duz, once .iii. Il est confeit isi: met le jus de meures ou le miel et ou le vin douz en un vessel d'araim bien estopé, et fai bouillir à petit feu. Si tu veuz savoir s'il sait cuit, met une gote sus le marbre: s'il aert, il est cuit'. See also Gilles Lib. 2 ll.207ff.

Glossaries

GLOSSARY
to Chapter 2, pp.64–99

Only the receipts are covered in the glossary, which is intended, like the glossaries to the other chapters, to be a guide to the ingredients of the receipts. The Middle English version (no. 90) of no. 89 is not included.

ACHE s. 8, 53, 72, 80, 87 wild celery, smallage (Apium graveolens) [FEW 1, 105a]
AGRIPPE s. 69 an ointment, 'Agrippa' [FEW 24,270b]
AGUILLE s. RUGE A. 8 possibly butcher's broom (Ruscus aculeatus)
AIL s. AYLE 86 garlic (Allium sativum) [FEW 24,333a]
AIS s. 11 ES 66 board
AISIL s. 52, 53 EYSIL 70 vinegar
ALISANDRE s. 80 alexanders, horse-parsley (Smyrnium olusatrum) [FEW 24,313b]
ALOEN s. 6 A. APATICH 64 aloes [FEW 24,345b & 4,403b]
ALOIGNE s. 7, 34, 42 ALOINE 23, 59 wormwood (Artemisia absinthium) [FEW 24,346a]
ALUM s. 78 alum [FEW 24,376b]
AMBRE s. 57 amber
AMBROISE s. 14 wood sage (Teucrium scorodonia) [FEW 24,412b]
ANGUILLE s. 58 ANGUOYLLE 85 eel
ANYSE s. 87 anise, aniseed (Pimpinella anisum) [FEW 24,599a]
APOSTUME s. 19 impostume, abscess
AQUILEIA s. 4 columbine (Aquilegia vulgaris)
ARRACE s. 11 orache (genus Atriplex) [FEW 1,166b]
ARMOISE s. ERMOISE 57 mugwort (Artemisia vulgaris) [FEW 1,149a]
ARREMENT s. 2, 62 oak-gall, gall-nut
AUBUN s. 13, 59 white of an egg
AUNE s. 78 HALNE 8 EAUNE 17 elecampane (Inula helenium) [FEW 4,784b]
AVANCE s. 8, 15, 65 AVENCE 14, 89 AVENCIA 32 AVENZ 77 wood avens (Geum urbanum)
AVEINE s. 25 oats
BERECHEVE (ME) s. 88 barley chaff
BETE s. 1, 38 red beet [FEW 1,344a]
BETOINE s. 15, 67, 73, 80, 87 (wood) betony (Betonica officinalis) [FEW 1,345b]
BIBUEF s. BLANC B. 57 mugwort (Artemisia vulgaris) [FEW 15,i,102a]
BORAGE s. 38, 40 borage (Borago officinalis) [FEW 1,442a]
BRASYL s. 86 brazil-wood, red-wood [FEW 15,258a]
BREN s. 73 bran B. DEL FURMENT 12 wheat-bran
BRU s. 16 BRE 38 broth
BUGLE s. 8, 15, 19, 39, 65, 87, 89 bugle (Ajuga), sometimes confused with bugloss [FEW 1,600a]
BURE s. 10, 26, 68, 89 butter B. DE MAI 8, 15, 36, 39, 65, 68, 70, 77, 89 May butter [FEW 1,663b]

BURNETTE s. 15, 65, 89 BURNET 39 burnet; great burnet (Sanguisorba officinalis), garden burnet (Poterium sanguisorba), common pimpernel (Anagallis arvensis) [FEW 1,563b]

CALAMENTE s. 73 common calamint (Calamintha officinalis) [FEW 2,i,53b]

CAMAMILLE s. 67, 87 common camomile (Anthemis nobilis) [FEW 2,i,148a]

CANCRE s. 86 carcinoma, tumour [FEW 2,i,174b]

CANFER s. 61 hemp (Cannabis sativa) [FEW 2,i,210a]

CASSIAFISTRE s. 9 purging cassia [FEW 2,i,462b]

CAREWY s. 87 caraway (Carum carvi) [FEW 2,i,377b]

CASTOR s. 51 beaver

CASTORIUM s. 32 castoreum, drug extract from glands of beaver [FEW 2,i,474b]

CAUQUETREPE s. 63 caltrops (Centaurea melitensis) or star thistle (Centaurea calcitrapa) [FEW 2,i,65a]

CELIDOINE s. 20, 65 greater celandine (Chelidonium maius) [FEW 2,i,634a]

CENTOINE s. 11 wormwood (Artemisia absinthium) [FEW 11,187a]

CENTOIRE s. CENTORIE 87 CEY[N]TORIE 87 common centaury (Centaureum umbellatum) or yellow centaury (Chlora perfoliata) [FEW 2,i,583b]

CERFLANGE s. 8, 40, 87 hart's tongue fern (Phyllitis scolopendrium) [FEW 2,i,614b]

CERFOIL s. 8, 86 CERFEL 62 chervil (Anthriscus cerefolium) [FEW 2,i,37b]

CERVEISE s. 14, 15, 77 SERVEISE 21, 36 ale SERVEYSE ESTALE 89 clear ale, free of dregs of lees, old and strong

CETERAC s. 87 scale fern (Ceterach officinarum) or bishopweed (Ammi maius) [FEW 19,173a]

CHANVRE s. 89 CHANVERE 15 CAUNVRE 57 CHAUNVRE 70 hemp (Cannabis sativa) [FEW 2,i,210a]

CHARDON s. 15 thistle VERT C. 89

CHIENLANGE s. 8, 87 hound's tongue (Cynoglossum officinale) [FEW 5,362a]

CHERLOKE (ME) s. 11 charlok, 'wild mustard' (Sinapis arvensis)

CHEVREFOYL s. 89 honeysuckle (Lonicera periclymenum / caprifolium) or red clover (Trifolium pratense) [FEW 2,i,308b]

CHOLET s. RUGE C. 15, 57, 89 red cabbage (Rubeus olus) [FEW 2,i,308b]

CIRE s. 5, 27, 43, 52, 64, wax VIRGINE C. 8, 65, 77 VIRGE C. virgin wax

CIUN s. 11 scion, shoot

CLOW s. 68 boil, furuncle, carbuncle [FEW 2,i,771a]

COLLECREIE (ME) s. 21 ? coltsfoot (Tussilago farfara)

COLLERIE s. 6 collyrium, eye-salve [FEW 2,ii,919b]

COLUMBINE s. 14 columbine (Aquilegia vulgaris) [FEW 2,ii,930a]

COMFIRYE s. 15 CUMFERIE 87 comfrey (Symphytum officinale) [FEW 2,ii,1030a]

COMIN s. 64 COMYN 42 cumin (Cuminum cyminum) [FEW 2,ii,1526a]

CONSOLDE s. LA GREINE C. 15 CONSEUDE LE GREINDRE 70 LA GRANT CONSOUDE 89 consound, comfrey (Symphytum officinale) [FEW 2,ii,1076a]

CONSOUDE s. 77 CONSODE 39 CUNSOUDE 8 consound, comfrey (Symphytum officinale) LE MEINDRE CONSOLDE 15, 70 LA PETITE C. 15, 65, 89 consolida minor, daisy (Bellis perennis) LA MENE C. 89 consolida minor, daisy (Bellis perennis) [FEW 2,ii,1076a]

CONSTRICTIF s. 13 having the property of thickening

COPEROSE s. 78 copperas, a metallic sulphate

CORFBIN s. 28 crow

COUDRE s. 52 hazel (Corylus avellana) [FEW 2,ii,1240b]

COUPERE s. 40, 87 COPERE 20 'epatica', 'liverwort' = ? Cf. M. Foerster, Anglia 42 (1918), 160. Cotgrave gives under copiere 'herbe copiere, oeil de cerf' glossing these terms as 'a kind of wild parsnip'. In MS Add. 15236 ff. 3v & 176r coupere glosses epatica, presumably Anemone hepatica. MS Sloane 3126 ff. 51v & 60v has coupiere (also copiere). See Hunt, Plant Names, p.108.

CRAMPE s. 33 cramp [FEW 16,354a]

CRAPOUT s. 86 toad

CRESP MAVE s. 8 curled marrow (Malva crispa)

CROPLESEWORT (ME) s. 15 ? elsewhere it is used to gloss *brigla*, see MSS royal 12 G IV (s.xiv) f.134vb (anglice *cripulwort*) and Sloane 347 (s.xv) f. 81r (*crepleswort*). See Hunt, *Plant Names*, p.55.

CROYSÉ s. 15, 89 crosswort (Galium cruciata) [FEW 2,ii,1379b]

CUMFIRIE s. 8 comfrey (Symphytum officinale) [FEW 2,ii,1030a]

CURSUN s. 11 diarrhoea

CYTRINE a. OYGNEMENT C. 88 a yellow ointment

DAUKE s. 15, 89 wild carrot (Daucus carota / asininus)

DERTRE s. 34 tetter, eczema, herpes [FEW 3,46a]

DIADRAGAUNT s. 72 electuary made with tragacanth

DIAGRAGANT s. 47 electuary made with tragacanth

DIAIRIS s. 47 electuary made with iris

DIAMANT s. 15 ? (ceo est lupyes) hop plant (Humulus lupulus)

DIAPENIDION s. 47, 72 electuary made with barley sugar

DITAUNDRE s. 87 dittany (Origanum dictamnus or Dictamnus albus)

DRACHE s. 14, 66 sediment, lees

DRAGAN(T) s. 64, 73 tragacanth [FEW 13,ii,158a]

DRAGAGANT s. 46 tragacanth [FEW 13,ii,158a]

EBLE s. 10, 38, 87 EYBLE 25 dwarf elder, danewort (Sambucus ebulus) [FEW 3,202a]

EGRIMOINE s. 39, 70, 89 EGRIMONIE 8 EGREMOYNE 15 agrimony (Agrimonia eupatoria) [FEW 24,270a]

ELENA CAMPANA s. 46 elecampane (Inula helenium) [FEW 4,784b]

EMFLURE s. 68 swelling

ENCENS s. 8, 54, 55, 59 incense FRAUNC E. 45, 64, 65 frankincense BLANC E. 69

ENDIV(I)E s. 20, 40 endive, chicory, wild lettuce (Cichorium intybus and endivia) [FEW 4,784b]

ENTRETE s. 64, 69, 77 poultice

EPPARGE s. 15 asparagus (Asparagus officinalis) [FEW 1,156a]

ERE s. 80 ivy (Hedera) E. TERRESTRE 26, 67 ground ivy (Glechoma hederacea) [FEW 13, i, 262a]

ESCLARIE s. 73 CLAREYE 87 clary, clear-eye (Salvia sclarea)

ESTUVER v. refl. 38 to take a steam bath

EUFRAS s. 87 euphrasy, eyebright (Euphrasia officinalis) [FEW 3,249b]

FAVAZ s. 62 bean-straw [FEW 3,339b]

FAVEROLE s. 19, 37 brooklime (Veronica beccabunga) or water parsnip (Sium angustifolium)

FELTRIS (ME) s. 77 probably mullein (Verbascum thapsus), possibly common centaury (Centaurium umbellatum)

FELUN s. 68, 79 abscess, ulcer

FENTE s. F. DE HUMME 86 dung

FENEGREC s. 64 fenugreek (Trigonella foenum-graecum) [FEW 3,461b]

FENOIL s. 11, 38, 53, 57, 73, 87 FONUIL 6, 8 RUGE F. 7 fennel (Foeniculum vulgare) [FEW 3,454a]

FERLINGE (ME) s. 78 farthing

FESAUNZ s. 38 pheasant

FEVREFUIE s. 8, 87 feverfew (Chrysanthemum parthenium)

FI s. 3, 86 ficus, tumour [FEW 3,496b]

FIEL s. 85 gall F. D'UNE LISSE 4 bitch's gall F. DE COC 7 F. DE PESSUN 61

FIENS s. F. DE L'OWE 17 goose droppings

FIGE s. 46, 72, 73 fig

FRASER(E s. 8, 65, 70 strawberry plant [FEW 3,748b]

FUMETERRE s. 8, 36, 38 FEMETERRE 70 fumitory (Fumaria officinalis) [FEW 3,857b]

FUNDEMENT s. 3, 19 anus, fundament

FURMAGE s. 69 cheese
FURMENTs s. 12, 15, 68, 83 wheat
FURMIE s. 74 ant
GALBANUM s. 43 a gum resin extracted from plants of the genus Ferula [FEW 4,23b]
GALINGALE s. 42 galingale, sweet cyperus (Cyperus longus) [FEW 19,61b]
GELINE s. 24, 38 hen
GENEST(E s. 1, 87 GENETTE 89 broom (Sarothamnus scoparius) [FEW 4,100b]
GILOFRE s. 42 cloves (Eugenia caryophyllata) [FEW 2,i,446b]
GLAN s. G. DE CHESNE 16 oak-apple
GLANBRE(S s. 77 glander(s [FEW 4,146b]
GOWME s. 73 gum G. ARABIC(H 46, 64, 73 gum arabic G. DE EDRE 74 gum-ivy
GRATURE s. 36 scratch
GRES(S)E s. 66, 69, 70 animal fat
GROMYLE s. 80 gromwell (Lithospermum officinale) [FEW 2,87a]
GROUNDSWILIE (ME) s. 89 groundsel (Senecio vulgaris)
GUESCHEI s. 84 greek nettle (? Urtica urens / Lamium purpureum) [FEW 4,211a]
GUTE s. 26, 63, 69, 84 gout G. CHAIVE 4 epilepsy, gutta caduca G. ENOS(S)É 25, 69 gout in
    the bone G. FESTRE 1, 12, 14 fistulous sore, gouty swelling
HARPOIS s. 52 pitch [FEW 16,174a]
HENNEMAWE s. 87 ? error for hennebane
HERBE BENOYT s. 81 avens (Geum urbanum) or hemlock (Conium maculatum)
HERBE IVE s. 63, 70 buck's horn plantain (Plantago coronopus)
HERBE JON s. 39, 89 H. JOHAN 15, 29 St John's wort (Hypericum perforatum) [FEW 5,48a]
HERBE ROBERT s. 14, 15, 19, 34, 39, 52, 65, 89 Herb Robert (Geranium robertianum) [FEW
    10,426a]
HERBE SEINT CRISTOFERE s. 29 ? yellow loosestrife (Lysimachia vulgaris)
HERBE WATER s. 39, 65, 89 H. WALTER 15 sweet woodruff (Asperula odorata)
HORSELEN (ME) s. 17 elecampane, horseheal (Inula helenium)
HORHUND (ME) s. 87 HORHUNE 46 horehound (Marrubium vulgare)
JAUNIZ s. 20 jaundice
JAZERE s. 80 ? wild vine (Vitis sylvestris)
JUBARBE s. 2, 41, 52, 58, 87 houseleek (Sempervivum tectorum) [FEW 5,78b]
JUFUS s. 47 ?
JUTE s. 11, 38 vegetable broth
KERSUN s. 87 garden cress (Lepidium sativum) K. EWAGE 37 CARSUN DE FUNTAYNE 38
    CRESSUN D'EAWE 70 water cress (Rorippa nasturcium-aquaticum) [FEW 16,384b]
LANCELÉ(E s. 8, 15, 39, 52, 70, 75, 87, 88, 89 ribwort plantain (Plantago lanceolata) [FEW
    5,158a]
LAVENDRE s. 13 lavender (Lavandula officinalis)
LAVENDULA s. 32 lavender (Lavandula officinalis)
LETUE s. 86 LETUSE 40 lettuce
LICORIZ s. 72, 73 licorice
LILIE s. 8 lily
LIMEKE (ME) s. 19 (?) LYMERCHE 80 brooklime (Veronica beccabunga)
LINGUA AVIS s. 19 stitchwort or great starwort (Stellaria holostea)
LINOIS s. 70, 87 linseed [FEW 5,368b]
LIQUERIS s. 40, 46 licorice
LISSE s. 4 bitch
LORER s. 43, 58 sweet bay tree, laurel (Laurus nobilis) [FEW 5,208b]
LOVESCHE s. 38 LUVESCHE 8 lovage (Ligusticum scoticum) [FEW 5,334b]
LUPYE s. 15 ? hops (Humulus lupulus)
LUSALVEON s. 52 apparently soapwort (Saponaria officinalis), see below p.385 n.9
MALVE s. MAVE 38 mallow
MANJUE s. 36, 37 itch, irritation

MARIUL s. 3 horehound (Marrubium vulgare) [FEW 6,i,377b]

MARRIS s. 55 womb [FEW 6,i,501b]

MASTIK s. 43, 54, 78 MASTICH 64 mastic

MAT(E)FELON s. 14, 63, 70 knapweed, matfellon (Centaurea nigra / scabiosa / iacea) [FEW 6,i,519b]

MATER HERBARUM s. 1 mugwort (Artemisia vulgaris)

MAYDENHER (ME) s. 87 maidenhair fern (Adiantum capillis-veneris or Asplenium trichomanes)

MEGUE s. 54 whey [FEW 6,ii,43b]

MELICE s. 15, 89 (sweet) balm (Melissa officinalis) [FEW 6,i,678a]

MELILOTE s. 15 melilot (Melilotus) [FEW 6,i,661b]

MENEISUN s. 13 MENESOUN 48, 49 MENESON 66 diarrhoea [FEW 6,ii,103a]

MENTASTRE s. 38 horsemint (Mentha sylvestris) [FEW 6,i,731b]

MENTE s. 42,55,56 spearmint (Mentha viridis) NEYRE M. 87 ? Mentha arvensis, Mentha piperita

MERCURIE s. 38 allgood (Chenopodium bonus Henricus) or annual / dog's mercury (Mercurialis annua / perennis) [FEW 6,i,18b]

MIEL s. 7, 53 honey

MILFOIL s. 19,39,65,70, 87 MILFUIL 8 MIRFOIL 52 milfoil, yarrow (Achillea millefolium) [FEW 6,ii,92b]

MIRABOLAN CITRIN s. 9 fruit of Terminalia citrina [FEW 6,iii,315b]

MIRRE s. 55,78 myrrh (Commiphora myrrha) [FEW 6,iii,316a]

MIRTUS s. 87 myrtle (Myrtus communis) [FEW 6,iii,316b]

MODERWORT (ME) s. 89 'motherwort', applied to a variety of plants esp. mugwort (Artemisia vulgaris), motherwort (Leonuris cardiaca) and meadow-sweet (Filipendula ulmaria)

MOLEINE s. 19 mullein (Verbascum thapsus) [FEW 6,iii,52a]

MORELE s. 8, 11, 52, 56, 71, 79, 87 petty morel, belladonna (Solanum nigrum) [FEW 6,i,544a]

MORMAL s. 68 mormal, dry-scabbed ulcer [FEW 6,iii,135a]

MORTREL s. 12 dish of thick consistency incorporating pounded and boiled chicken, fish or pork [FEW 6,iii,148b]

MUEL s. 13 yolk (of egg)

MUGE DÉ BOYS s. 15 sweet woodruff (Asperula odorata)

NASTER s. 32 ?

NINIFAR s. 40 water-lily (Nimphaea / Nuphar)

NOER s. 8 nut-tree

NOIS MUSCADE s. 58 nutmeg (Myristica fragrans) [FEW 19,133b]

OBLEE s. 21 wafer

OCULESCUNCE s. ? see below p.400

OINT s. 53,59, 78 animal fat, grease UINT DE VER 5, 8 O. DE PORC 5, 8, 17, 36, 37, 62, 75 O. DE SENGLIER 34, 61 O. DE TESSUN 69 O. DE TRUIE 75

OINUN s. 30 onion

OLIBANUM s. 78 frankincense

OLIVE s. 8, 31, 32, 56, 57 olive

OPOPONAK s. 43 opoponax [FEW 7,374b]

ORGE s. 19, 42, 73 barley

ORPIMENT ROWGE s. 74 orpiment, yellow arsenic [FEW 1,182a]

ORTIE s. 8, 11, 33, 37 nettle ORTILLE VERMAYLE 87 red nettle (Lamium purpureum) O. SALVAGE 84 O. GRIESCHE 52 ? Urtica urens / Lamium purpureum ROWGE O. 65 red nettle (Lamium purpureum)

OSELE s. 87 wood sorrel (Oxalis acetosella) [FEW 7,451b]

OSEMUNDE s. 80 OSEMOUND 79 OUMUNDE 65 royal osmund (Osmunda regalis)

PAIN ALIS s. 38 unleavened bread

PANIS CUCULI s. 19 cuckoopint (Arum maculatum)

PANWHET s. 84 ? hellebore

PAPILOT s. 83 porridge

PARELE s. 78 sorrel, dock (Rumex acetosa / acetosella) RUGE P. 8, 36, 78 red-veined dock (Rumex sanguineus) [FEW 7,639a]

PARITARE s. 38 pellitory-of-the-wall (Parietaria diffusa) [FEW 7,654a]

PARLESIE s. 30 paralysis

PEIVRE s. 1, 13, 30, 62 pepper

PEIZ s. 5 pitch P. RAISINE 5 P. REYSINE 64 P. REISIN 77 pitch resin NOIR POIZ 64 black pitch

PELETRE s. 8, 87 pellitory-of-the-wall (Parietaria diffusa) [FEW 7,654a]

PELUETTE 89 PULUSETTE 15 mouse-ear hawkweed (Hieracium pilosella) [FEW 8,504a]

PENITES s. 47 barley sugar [FEW 8,188b]

PERDRIZ s. 38 partridge

PERSIL s. 38, 53, 70, 73, 80, 87 parsley (Petroselinum crispum / sativum) [FEW 8,325b]

PES LEPORINA s. 19 wood avens (Geum urbanum)

PIÉ DE LEVRE s. 70 wood avens (Geum urbanum)

PIGLE s. 15, 39, 70, 89 PIGRE 39 stitchwort or great starwort (Stellaria holostea)

PIJUN s. 28 young (of crow)

PIMPRE s. 8 pimpernel, variously applied to Sanguisorbia officinalis, Paxterium sanguisorba and Anagallis arvensis [FEW 8,517a]

PIMPERNELE s. 87 PIMPERNELEE 39 as above

PLANTAINE s. 8, 11, 15, 24, 39, 41, 66, 70, 77, 87, 89 PLAUNTAIGNE (LA GREINDRE ET LA MEINDRE) 49 PLAUNTEIN 52 PLANTEIN 63 PLAWINTEYNE 65 PLAWNTEYNE 66 PLAUNTEINE 75 plantain, waybread (Plantago major) [FEW 9,19b]

PLUM s. BLANC P. 62 white lead

POMME s. P. GARNÉS 40 pomegranate (Punica granatum) P. D'AMBRE 45 'amber ball' (see J. M. Riddle in *Sudhoffs Archiv* 48 (1964), 111–22)

POPIE s. 87 poppy (Papaver)

PORTULAC s. 87 purslane (Portulaca sativa / oleracea) [FEW 9,226b]

PRIMEROLE s. 70, 87 PRIMORELE 8 varieties of the genus Primula [FEW 9,379a]

PRIMULA VERIS s. 19, 32 primrose, cowslip (Primula) [FEW 9,379a]

PRUNE DAMASCENE s. 73 damson (Prunus domestica) P. DAMACIEN 40

PRUNER s. BLANC P. 38 plum-tree

PRUNETTE SAUVAGE s. 82 wild plum, sloe (Prunus spinosa)

PULEGII s. 35 see below

PULIOL s. 67, 73 wild thyme (Thymum serpyllum) [FEW 9,521a]

QUINTEFOIL s. 65 QUINQUEFOILLE 8 cinquefoil (Potentilla reptans) [FEW 2,ii,1481a]

RAIZ s. 17 RAYS 87 radish [FEW 10,27a]

RAVELE s. 53 radish [FEW 10,27a]

REINE s. 8 meadowsweet (Filipendula ulmaria) [FEW 10,211b]

REOUME s. 45,46 ROEME 45 rheum, catarrh [FEW 10,376a]

ROIGNE s. 36, 62 ROINE 68, 81 scabies

ROSE s. 41, 54, 55, 56 rose EUWE ROSE 49 rose-water

RUE s. 3, 6, 7, 26 rue (Ruta graveolens) [FEW 10,597a]

RUNCE s. 8, 11, 39, 65, 89 bramble

SAFRAN s. 22, 24 saffron (Crocus sativus) [FEW 19,202a]

SAIM s. SAUN 5, 10 animal fat, grease

SALGEA s. 32 sage (Salvia officinalis) [FEW 11,132a]

SANGUINARIE s. 87 applied to various plants with styptic properties esp. shepherd's purse (Capsella bursa-pastoris) knot-grass (Polygonum aviculare) [FEW 11,164a]

SANICLE s. 4, 8, 15, 19, 39, 87, 89 SENICLE 65 wood sanicle (Sanicula europaea) [FEW 11,183b]

SAPONERE s. 89 soapwort (Saponaria officinalis) [FEW 17,5b]

SARCACOL s. 64 sarcocol, gum sarcocolla

SAUGE s. 38, 70, 71, 73, 87 sage (Salvia officinalis) [FEW 11,132a]

SAUNDRES s. S. BLAUNCHES ET ROUGES 40, 41 sandalwood (Santalum album / Pterocarpus santalinus)

SAUNK DE DRAGOUN s. 48 dragon's blood, juice or resin of the dragon tree (Dracaena draco) [FEW 11,171a]

SAUSEFLEME s. 61 saucefleme, 'salt phlegm' [FEW 11,108b]

SAVYNE s. 26 savin, creeping juniper (Juniperus sabina) [FEW 11,5b]

SAXIFRAGE s. 70 any member of the genus Saxifraga [FEW 11,258a]

SCABIOUSE s. 40 scabious, various plants incl. Knautia arvensis and Succisa pratensis [FEW 11,263a]

SCLARIOL s. 87 endive (Cichorium intybus and endivia) [FEW 3,245b]

SEL s. 30 SEOOL 48 salt

SENESCIUN s. 89 SENEZUN 8 CENEÇHOUN 15 groundsel (Senecio vulgaris) [FEW 11,446a]

SENEVEY s. 31, 81 mustard (Sinapis arvensis / alba) [FEW 11,638b]

S[E]PTMERE(?) s. 15 ? gum resin from Ferula persica

SILIUM s. 61 fleabane (Plantago psyllium)

SIU s. animal fat S. DE BUC 86 S. DE CERF 8 S. DE BESTE 70 S. DE MUTUN 5, 19, 26, 77

SOLSECLE s. 87 solsecle, marigold (Calendula officinalis) [FEW 12,74a]

SOLUBLE s. 11 free from costiveness

SPARGE s. 89 asparagus (Sparagus officinalis) [FEW 1,156a]

SUCRE s. 46 SUGRE 40 sugar S. ROSET 48

SUFRE s. 61, 78 sulphur

SUMAK s. 49 sumac

SURELE s. 65 sorrel (Rumex) S. DÉ BOIS 8, 39 wood sorrel (Rumex acetosa / acetosella) S. DES CHANS 8

SURSANURE s. 88 scar, cicatrice

TANESIE s. 1, 35, 52, 57, 87 tansy (Tanacetum vulgare) [FEW 13,i,79b]

TAPSUS BARBASTUS s. 19 mullein (Verbascum thapsus)

TAUPE s. 75 mole

TEINE s. 16, 17, 78 ringworm, tinea, disease of the scalp [FEW 13,i,340b]

TERBENTINE s. 43 resin extracted from the terebinth (Pistacia terebinthus), 'turpentine' [FEW 13,i,236a]

TEYE s. 85 cataract [FEW 13,i,302b]

TORMENTILLE s. 15, 89 TORMENTINE 39 TURMENTINE 1, 87 tormentil (Potentilla tormentilla) [FEW 13,ii,44b]

TRIASANDALY s. 24 an electuary composed of varieties of sandlewood

TRIBULER s. 14 mash

TRIFOIL s. 65, 70, 87 clover, plant of the genus Trifolium [FEW 13,ii,295b]

TRUMEL s. 52 ? see below p.398 (crumel)

UNEMENT s. VERT UN. 69, 70 green ointment

UNGEUNT AURIN s. 69 yellow ointment, see Gilles de Corbeil, Carmina medica ed. L. Choulant p.184

UVE PASSE s. 73 raisin

UUDEÞONGE (ME) s. 84 ? black hellebore (Helleborus niger)

VALERIANE s. 4 valerian (Valeriana officinalis) [FEW 14,135a]

VANE (ME) s. 87 ? a variety of iris or 'Saponaria minor' (Saponaria)

VARIOLE s. 34 smallpox

VERGE DE PASTOUR s. 15 wild teasel (Dipsacus sylvestris) [FEW 14,492a]

VERM s. 76 worm

VERT DE GRECE s. 62 verdigris

VESCES s. 15 vetch VESSES 89

VEÞERFOYE (ME) s. 87 feverfew (Chrysanthemum parthenium)

VETONIE s. 8 betony, bishopwort (Betonica officinalis) [FEW 14,360a]

VIF ARGENT s. 37, 59, 61, 78 quicksilver

VIGNEE s. 56 vine
VINEGRE s. 41 vinegar
VIOLE s. 8 violet
VIOLET(TE s. 15, 40, 65, 70, 89 violet
VIRGA PASTORIS s. 89 wild teasel (Dipsacus sylvestris)
WAIDE s. 86 woad (Isatis tinctoria) [FEW 17, 471b]
WARANCE s. 15, 57, 89 madder (Rubia tinctorum) [FEW 17,622b]
WEN s. 18 wen, sore
WORMELE (ME) s. 88 worm-meal
WYLDE TESEL (ME) s. 89 teasel (Dipsacus sylvestris)
WYMAUVE s. 87 marshmallow (Althaea officinalis) [FEW 4,422b]
YRINGES s. 49 yringo, sea holly (Eryngium maritinum) [FEW 3,243b]
YSOPE s. 46, 72, 73, 87 hyssop (Hyssopus officinalis) [FEW 4,629b]
YVURE s. 22, 24 YVERE 40 ivory

GLOSSARY

to Chapter 3, pp.100–124

An asterisk indicates that the word in question is given a considerably later dating in Wartburg, FEW. Further references are to W. Rothwell in ZFSL 86 (1976), 221–60.

ACHE s. 2, 81, 83, 164 wild celery, smallage (Apium graveolens) [FEW 1, 105a]
ADIANTOS* s. 1 maidenhair fern (Adiantum capillus-veneris) [FEW 24, 141a]
AGRIMOINE s. 63 agrimony (Agrimonia eupatoria) [FEW 1,55a]
AGUE* s. 134 ague [FEW 24,128b 'ca. 1380'], Rothwell, 223
AIL s. 79, 122 garlic (Allium sativum) [FEW 24,333a]
ALASCHER v.a. 3 to relax [FEW 5,231a]
ALISANDRE s. 1 alexanders, horse-parsley (Smyrnium olusatrum) [FEW 1,64b]
ALMUCE, AUMUZ s. 10 cap, hood, almuce [FEW 1,75a]
ALOEN s. 38, 97, 110 aloes [FEW 24,345b]
ALOIGNE s. 23, 25, 45, 73, 125 ALOINE 20 (ALIVERNE 16) wormwood (Artemisia absinthium) [FEW 24,346a]
AMENDER v.a. 35, 41, 67 to improve, make better, cure
AMEROCHE* s. 109 stinking camomile, mayweed (Anthemis cotula) [FEW 24,383a], Rothwell, 225
AMIABLEMENT adv. 3 carefully
AMOISTER v.a. 3 to moisten
AMPOLLE s. 25 phial, flask
AMPULLE s. 6 bubble [FEW 24,488b 'ampoulles en l'orine, "signe de maladie des reins" ']
ANDIVE* s. 1 wild lettuce, chicory, endive, scariola (Cichorium intybus / endivia) [FEW 4,784b]
ANDRE s. 89 ? betony (Betonica officinalis), see DMLBS sub andra
ANISE s. 89 anise, aniseed (Pimpinella anisum) [FEW 24,599a]
ANTOS* s. 156 rosemary (Rosmarinus officinalis), see R. Arveiller, Romania 94 (1973), 164 [FEW 24,648b]
ARREIM s. 31 AREIM 38 brass
ARREMENT s. 28 oak-gall, gall-nut

ARTEMISIE* s. 138 ARTEMESIE 154 mugwort (Artemisia vulgaris) [FEW 1,149a]
ASSIDUELEMENT adv. 73 assiduously
ATEMPREMENT adv. 37 sparingly, moderately [FEW 13,i,174a]
ATURNER v.a. 4 to prepare
AUBUN s. 1, 28, 29, 78 white of an egg
AUNE s. 36, 163 elecampane (Inula helenium) [FEW 4,784b], Rothwell, 226
AVENCE s. 111, 123, 132, 133 wood avens (Geum urbanum)
BETE s. NEIRE B. 13 red beet [FEW 1,344a]
BETOIGNE s. 24 BETOINE 35, 58 (wood) betony (Betonica officinalis) [FEW 1,345b]
BOGIE [1], SUCRE B. 1 'bogie' seems to be a place name
BRAIS s. 143, 146, 148 malt
BRUERE s. 134 heather [FEW 1,557b]
BUGLE s. 118, 123 bugle (Ajuga), sometimes confused with bugloss [FEW 1,600a]
BUILLISSEMENT s. 26 ? inflammation
BURAGE s. 3 borage (Borago officinalis) [FEW 1,442a]
BURE s. 4, 25, 150 butter [FEW 1,663b]
CANCRE s. 114, 115, 116 carcinoma, tumour [FEW 2,i,174b], Rothwell, 229
CAPILLUS VENERIS s. 1, 156 maidenhair fern (Adiantum capillus-veneris)
CARBUN s. 62 charcoal
CARCIVE a. fem. 6 ? corrosive (cf. MED corsif)
CARDUN s. 139 thistle [FEW 2,i,368a]
CAREUY s. 2 CAREWY 81 caraway (Carum carvi) [FEW 2,i,377b]
CELIDOINE s. 16 greater celandine (Chelidonium majus) [FEW 2,i,634a]
CENTOIRE s. 1, 33, 92, 160 common centaury (Centaurium erythraea) or yellow centaury
    (Blackstonia perfoliata) [FEW 2,i,583b]
CERFOIL s. 29, 47, 88, 119, 144 chervil (Anthriscus cerefolium) [FEW 2,i,37b]
CERLANGE s. 1, 156 hart's tongue fern (Phyllitis scolopendrium) [FEW 2,i,614b]
CERVEISE s. C. ESTALE 1, 92, 100 clear ale, free of dregs or lees, old and strong (see OED
    sub stale a. [1].) C. FURMENTALE 1 wheat beer [FEW 3,828a with different sense]
CETTRAKE* s. 1 scale fern (Ceterach officinarum), bishopweed (Ammi maius)
CHACIE s. 26, 28 rheum, matter (in eyes) [FEW 2,i,21b]
CHANILEE s. 57 henbane (Hyoscyamus niger, 'jusquiamus') [FEW 2,i,86a], Rothwell, 231
CHANUZ a. 76 white (of hair)
CHANVE s. 90, 126, 127, 143 hemp (Cannabis) [FEW 2,i,210a]
CHAPON s. 31 capon
CHENLANGE s. 146, 148 hound's tongue (Cynoglossum officinale) [FEW 5,362a]
CHOLET s. 30, 76, 127 cabbage (Brassica oleracea) RUGE C. 121, 136 [FEW 2,i,535a]
CICOREIE s. 1 CYCORÉ 156 chicory (Cichorium intybus) [FEW 1,i,665a]
CIRE s. VIRGINE C. 130 virgin wax
COCTIUN* s. 2 preparation by cooking, coction [not in FEW 2,i,832b]
COILLEREE s. 25, 82 CUILLEREE 25, 95 CUILLERÉ 92, 99 QUILLEREE 4 spoonful
COLLIRIE s. 31 collyrium, eye-salve [FEW 2,ii,919b]

---

[1]   Cf. Brunel, *Recettes médicales, alchimiques et astrologiques du XVe siècle en langue vulgaire des pyrénées*
(Toulouse, 1956) 487 'cupre scorsa de Bogia', 671 (= *Lettre d'Hippocrate*) 'de escorssa de Bogia .i. cart de
onza' (glossary, 'La ville de Bougie, peut-être'). In MS B. L. Royal 12 B XII (s.xiii) f.108r a receipt has
'accipe herbam bogie'. MS B. L. Sloane 1754 (c.1300) f.2r has 'cortices bugie'. MS B. L. Sloane 3550
(c.1300) f.249rb has 'zuccara buggte'. In the *Pandectae* of Matthaeus Silvaticus, printed in 1498, we read
in chap. CIX 'Bugee .i. herba de bugea quod est locus barbarie in littore africano .i. abes et guzema et
pulvis bugie' and in chap. CCCCCLXXXI 'Pulvis bugie .i. pulvis de radice arboris berberi'. In Henri de
Mondeville's *Antidotarius* (ed. by J. L. Pagel in his edition of the *Chirurgia*, 1892) we read 'Cortex bugiae
est cortex sicut cinnamomum et dicunt quidam quod est cortex arboris berberis' (p.571, para.173). In MS
Exeter Cath. 3519 (s.xv) f.155v a receipt for redness of the eyes contains 'le escorce de bogie', and a
receipt in MS B. L. Arundel 295 (s.xiv in.) f.110r includes 'stuellum de cortice ligni de Bugea'. Possibly
the bark of the root of barberry (Berberis vulgaris) is indicated by some of the references.

COLOFONIE s. 3 colophony [FEW 2,ii,921b], Rothwell, 232

COMINEE* s. 104 stew flavoured with cumin [FEW 2,ii,152a]

CONFECTIUN s. 4 mixture, compound

CONFERMER v.a. 71 to strengthen

CONSTIPACIUN s. 99 constipation

COPERUN s. 134 top, tip [FEW 2,ii,1555b]

CORF s. 135 crow, raven [FEW 2,ii,1238b], Rothwell, 233

CORNE DE CERF s. 51 C. DEL C. 101 hartshorn

COSTIVURE s. 102 constipation [FEW 2,ii,1083b], Rothwell, 233

COSTUVISUN* s. 104 constipation, Rothwell, 233

COUPERE s. 1 156 in lists of *synonyma herbarum* glosses *epatica* and is in turn glossed by *liver-wort* (? Anemone hepatica). Cotgrave under *copiere* gives 'herbe copiere, oeil de cerf' and glosses those terms with 'a kind of wild parsenip'

COVER v.n. 115 to be brooding (of a hen)

CRASSE s. 6 fat

CROTE s. CROTES DE CHEVRE 95 goat dung

CRUMEL s. 77 read *trumel*? Cf. Sc f. 39v 'Prenez la racine du crumel qui crest en ces eues autrement apelee ongle de cheval [= Nymphaea alba L. or Nuphar luteum Sm.]. See also Meyer, *Romania* 37 (1908), 377 and MS Cambridge, Trinity Coll. 0.1.20 f. 23vb 'flor de trumel', and MS London, Royal College of Physicians 227 (s.xiv) f.157r 'cape radicem herbe que gallice vocatur pauier et trumel'

CRUSTE s. 122m 128 crust (of bread) [FEW 2,ii,1371a]

CURACIUN s. 37, 70 cure, healing

CURS s. 165 flux, running (of the nose)

DECOCTIUN s. 1 decoction, liquid [FEW 3,26a inadequate]

DECURIR v.n. 2 to run down (from), drip

DEFIRE v.a. 3, 4 to melt, dissolve, digest v.n. 112 to dissolve

DESECHER v.a. 25 to relieve dryness of 111 v.a. to dry out

DIOTÉ s. 3 a salve, dialtea Cf. R. Arveiller, *Romania* 94 (1973), 169

DITAUNDRE s. 2 dittany (Origanum dictamnus or Dictamnus albus) [this form not in FEW 3,70b]

DOILLER v.n. 33 to hurt, be painful

DOSSE s. DOSSES D'AIL 79 clove of garlic [FEW 3,120a]

DRAGANCE s. 44 dragonwort, green dragon (Dracunculus vulgaris) and various other plants. Not in FEW

DRAGME s. 81 drachm, dram

EBLE s. 2, 69, 128 YEBLE 16 dwarf elder, danewort (Sambucus ebulus) [FEW 3,202a]

EISIL s. 1, 2, 7, 12, 14, 15, 17, 18, 20, 23, 38, 47, 48, 58, 101, 113, 136 vinegar

EMFLURE s. 59 ENFLURE 26, 59, 100 swelling

EMPLASTRE s. 23, 28, 59, 109, 131, 157 ENPLASTRE 9, 10, 133, 137, 139 plaster (medic.)

ENCENS s. 52 incense

ENTRE-ESCORCE s. 64 middle bark, cambial layer, 'cortex mediana' [FEW 4,763a]

EPETIME s. 1 thyme dodder (Cuscuta epithymum) Not in FEW

ERE s. 10, 14, 18, 42 ivy (Hedera) E. TERESTRE 8, 17, 37, 151 ground ivy (Glechoma hederacea) RUGE E. 142 [FEW 13,i,262a]

ESCALE s. 45, 113 shell (of an egg)

ESCALER* v.a. 81a to scale [FEW 17,77a (16 Jh.)]

ESCLAREIE* s. 1 clary, clear-eye (Salvia sclarea) Cf. MS B. L. Sloane 475 (s.xii^2) f.101r 'sclareie flores'

ESCLARIR v.n. 32 to clear, brighten ESCLARZIR v.a. 36 to clear

ESCLICE s. 2 spatula

ESCOPIR v.n. 3 to spit

ESCORCE s. 16, 136 bark MEINE E. 2 middle bark

ESCUMER v.a. 2, 4, 92 to skim

ESCURER v.a. 1 to scour

ESPESSIR v.a. 3 to thicken

ESPLEN s. 5, 94 spleen

ESPURGE s. 81 spurge (Euphorbia) [FEW 3,314b]

ESPURGEMENT s. 85 purging, cleansing

ESQUELEE s. 79 bowlful [FEW 11,352a]

ESTAMPER v.a. 5, 31, 57, 83, 104, 105, 107, 109 to grind, crush [FEW 17,215a]

ESTANCHER v.n. 163, 165 to dry up, cease flowing [FEW 12,231a]

ESTEMPRER v.a. 13 ? error for *estamper*

ESTOUPES s. 115 ESTUPES 144 fibres of tow [FEW 12,314b] Cf. Rothwell, 238

EUFRASIE* s. 31 euphrasy, eyebright (Euphrasia officinalis) [FEW 3,249b], Rothwell, 238

FARINE s. flour F. DE FEVES 25 F. DE ORGE 95 F. DE FURMENT 105, 131 F. DE SEGLE 113, 120, 131

FARSER/-IR v.a. 5, 104 to stuff

FEL s. gall F. DE LIEVRE 39 F. DE CHEVRE 116 [FEW 3,445a]

FELUN s. 10, 137 abscess, ulcer

FENUGREC, FENEGREC s. 3 fenugreek (Trigonella foenum-graecum) [FEW 3,461b]

FENUIL s. 11, 68, 81, 83, 94, 111 FENOIL 19, 20 FANUIL 1, 2 fennel (Foeniculum vulgare) [FEW 3,454a]

FEVERE s. F. QUARTEINE 6, 155 quartan fever F. TERTEINE 153 tertian fever

FI s. 108, 109, 110, 111, 112, 113 ficus, tumour

FIENTE s. 122 droppings, excrement [FEW 3,496b]

FLUVIE s. 32 river [FEW 3,644b]

FOU s. 48 beech (tree) [FEW 3,371a]

FRASER s. 107 strawberry plant [FEW 3,748b]

FUGEROLE* s. 103 F. DE CHENNE 104 polypody of the oak (Polypodium vulgare) [FEW 3,515a (14.Jh.)], Rothwell, 242

FUMETERRE* s. 80 fumitory (Fumaria officinalis) [FEW 3,857b]

FUNDEMENT s. 109, 111, 142, 144 anus, fundament [FEW 3,863a]

FUR s. 114 oven [FEW 3,902b]

FURBER v.a. 62 to clean, polish (teeth) [FEW 3,882b]

GALBANUM s. 3 a gum resin extracted from plants of the genus Ferula [FEW 4,23b]

GALUN s. 1 gallon jar

GARS s. 130 gander

GELINE s. 45, 79, 104, 115 hen

GINGIBER s. 81 ginger (Zingiber officinalis) [FEW 14,663b]

GLEIRE s. 124 GLERE 30 white of an egg [FEW 2,i,738a]

GLETTE s. 92, 94 mucus, phlegm [FEW 4,157a]

GLETTUNER* s. 129 GLETUNER 147 burdock (Arctium lappa) [FEW 16,330b (14, Jh.)]

GRELEMENT adv. 1 thinly (hapax) [FEW 4,201b]

GRESSE s. 10, 27, 32, 79 animal fat

GRUE s. 14 stork [FEW 4,296b]

GUTE s. 4, 128, 130, 131 gout G. CHAIVE* 135 epilepsy, guta caduca [FEW 4,350a *goutte caduque* 1721] G. FESTRE 132, 133, 163 fistulous sore, gouty swelling

GUTETTE s. 6 droplet [FEW 4,344b]

GUTUS a. 4 gouty

HAGER v.a. 4 to chop up

HANAPÉ s. 1, 86 HANAPEE 25 gobletful [FEW 16,214b]

HERBE YVE s. 4 buck's horn plantain (Plantago coronopus)

HUMER v.a. 4, 51, 99, 104, 152 to swallow

HUVETE* s. 25 uvula [FEW 14,90a *uvette* ca. 1500]

JUNIPRE s. 145 juniper (Juniperus communis) [FEW 5,74b]

KERSUN s. 130 cress K. QUE CREST EN CORTIL 106 garden cress (Lepidium sativum) K. DE EWE 136 common water cress (Rorippa nasturtium-aquaticum) [FEW 16,384b]

LANCELÉ s. 129 ribwort plantain (Plantago lanceolata) [FEW 5,158a]

LAXATIF a. 1 laxative [FEW 5,226b]

LEPRE s. 81 ? black hellebore (Helleborus niger), see MS Exeter Cath. MS 3519 (s.xv) 'le lepre .i. suffoigne neir'

LESSIVE s. 73 lye

LETUE s. 159 lettuce L. SALVAGE 1 wild endive

LETTUEIRE s. 92 LETEWIRE 4 electuary

LICORIZ s. 156 licorice [FEW 4,173b]

LIMAÇUN s. 27, 79, 112 snail [FEW 5,340b]

LIN s. SEMENCE DE L. 72, 102 linseed (Linum usitatissimum)

LINOIS s. 3, 102 linseed [FEW 5,368b]

LORER s. 8, 158 sweet bay tree, laurel (Laurus nobilis) BAIE(S) DE L. 52, 78 laurel berry [FEW 5,208b]

LOVACHE s. 19 LOVESCHE 81 LUVACHE 8 LUVASCHE 1, 3 LUVESCHE 89 lovage (Levisticum officinale, Ligusticum scoticum) [FEW 5,334b]

MAELE s. 37, 38 leucoma [FEW 6,i,13a]

MALVE s. M. ORTEILANE 1 tame mallow (growing in a garden)

MANJUE s. 26 itch, irritation

MARIZ s. 6 womb [FEW 6,i,501b]

MAROIL s. 91 MARUIL 25, 82, 93 horehound (Marrubium vulgare) [FEW 6,i,377a]

MASCHER v.a. 24, 63 to chew

MELANCOLIE s. 37 black bile [FEW 6,i,655a]

MENEISUN s. 105, 106, 107 MENISON 6 diarrhoea [FEW 6,ii,103a]

MENTASTRE s. 66 horsemint (Mentha sylvestris) [FEW 6,i,731b]

MENTE s. 34, 41, 65 spearmint (Mentha viridis) NEIRE MENTES 4 mentha arvensis (?), mentha piperita (?)

MERE DES HERBES s. 143 mugwort (Artemisia vulgaris) [Not in FEW 6,473b]

MIRFOIL s. 56, 105, 107 milfoil, yarrow (Achillea millefolium) [FEW 6,ii,92b]

MOLEINE* s. 108 mullein (Verbascum thapsus) [FEW 6,iii,52a]

MORELE s. 10, 148, 156, 157 petty morel, belladonna (Solanum nigrum) [FEW 6,i,544a]

MORTER s. 79 a mortar

NARILLE s. 60 NARILLES 17, 41, 43, 45, 65, 164 NASRILLES 41, 42 NARIZ 7 nostrils [FEW 7,15a]

NEELE s. 77 darnel (Lolium temulentum) or corn-cockle (Nigella arvensis) [FEW 7,127a]

NOUER v.n. 6 to float

NUMBLIL s. 112 navel [FEW 14,18a]

OCULUSSCUNSE s. 138 ? in MS B. L. Sloane 420 (s.xiv) f.119r glosses 'oculus sconsus' and appears in other MSS as culcunse, ouquelescensce, okelescunse, oskelescunce

OILLE s. O. ROSADE 15 attar of roses [FEW 10,482a]

OINT s. 77,130 OIGNT 31, 70, 74 animal fat, grease, lard

OLIVE s. 37 olive

ORTIE s. 113, 163 nettle

OWE s. 31 goose

OXIMEL s. 2 medicinal preparation of vinegar and honey with herbs [FEW 7,452a]

PELESTRE s. 81 common pellitory (Parietaria officinalis) and commonly applied to a variety of plants [FEW 9,648b]

PELOTE s. 64 ball

PERFUSION* s. P. DE SANG 26 bleeding [FEW 8,239a ca.1390]

PERSIL s. 1, 2, 81, 156 common parsley (Petroselinum crispum / sativum) [FEW 8,325b]

PICHER s. 1, 4 pitcher, jug

PIGUNS s. pl.135 young (of the crow) [FEW 8,556a]

PINPERNELE s. 37, 118 applied to a variety of plants, especially the burnets (Sanguisorba officinalis and Paxterium sanguisorba) and pimpernel (Anagallis arvensis) [FEW 8,517a]

PIONIE s. 98 peony (Paeonia officinalis) [FEW 7,464b]

PLANTAINE s. 16, 107, 137, 156 PLANTEINE 129, 153 plantain, waybread (Plantago major) [FEW 9,19b]

PLEURESI* s. 3 pleurisy [FEW 9,64a], Rothwell, 251

PLUM s. 6, 38 lead

POAGRA s. 135 gout in the foot, podagra [FEW 9,109a]

POLIPODE* s. 1, 2 common polipody (Polypodium vulgare) or oak fern (Thelypteris dryopteris) [FEW 9,139b 'seit 15 Jh.']

PORALES s. 129 sorrel (Rothwell, 252) Cf. *pareles* (varieties of Rumex) [FEW 7,639a]

POTEL* s. 1 small pot, bottle [FEW 9,265a = 1308]

PREMBRE / PREMER v.a. to press (out) [FEW 9,356b]

PREMEROLE s. 60 varieties of Primula [FEW 9,379a]

PUCIN s. 45 chick

PULIOL s. 7, 21, 47, 48, 93 wild thyme (Thymus serpyllum) P. REAL 1 pennyroyal (Mentha pulegium) [FEW 9,521a], Rothwell, 253

PURNELE s. P. DÉ BOIS 38, 86 sloe (Prunus spinosa) [FEW 9,494b]

QUARTEINE see under FEVRE

QUILLEREE s. 4 spoonful

QUINTFOIL s. 99 cinquefoil (Potentilla reptans) [FEW 2,ii,1481a]

QUITURE* s. 29 suppuration, quitter 149 cautery [FEW 2,ii,1166a], Rothwell, 253

RAER v.a. 5, 10, 57, 104 to shave, peel

RANCLE s. 124, 125, 127, 145 impostume, abscess, malignant tumour [FEW 3,151b]

RASURE s. 51 shavings, powder

REELEE p.p. 6 mottled [FEW 10,218b]

REISINE s. 3 resin

REIZ s. 2, 4 radish [FEW 10,27a]

RESCUNS s. R. DEL SOLAIL 153 sunset

REUMATIC* a. 4 rheumatic [FEW 10,379b]

ROCHE s. 132 roach (Leuciscus rutilus) [FEW 16,732a]

ROSE s. 1, 43 rose

RUE s. 8, 9, 11, 12, 16, 19, 36, 41, 53, 100, 162 R. VERTE 162 rue (Ruta graveolens) [FEW 10,597a]

SACEL s. 3 pouch, sachet [FEW 11,23a]

SAIM s. 31, 120, 130 SEIM 31, 32, 75, 80, 102 animal fat, grease [FEW 11,55a]

SANICLE s. 118, 123, 143 sanicle (Sanicula europaea), also applied to plants of various genera

SAUGE s. 15, 16, 22 sage (Salvia officinalis) [FEW 11,132a]

SAUNSUE s. 75 leech

SAUZ s. 129 willow [FEW 11,100b]

SAVINE s. 98 savin, creeping juniper (Juniperus sabina) [FEW 11,5b]

SAXIFRAGE s. 1 any member of genus Saxifraga [FEW 11,258a]

SCAMONÉ s. 81 scammony (Convolvulus scammonia) [FEW 11,276a]

SEIGNEE s. 127 lat. *sanies*, 'Matière purulente liquide, pus séreux qui sort des ulcères ou des plaies non soignées' [FEW 11,184a]

SEL s. 64 salt

SEU s. 2, 16 SU 64, 67 elder (Sambucus) [FEW 11,6a]

SIMPHONIE* s. 88 hellebore or henbane [FEW 12,489a '15 Jh.' and cf. 491b]

SINCFOIL s. 164 see under QUINTFOIL

SIUE s. 122 suet, tallow [FEW 11,358b]

SOLSEQUIE s. 129 solsecle, marigold (Calendula officinalis) [FEW 12,74a]

SPES s. 25 thickness

SQUILLES s. pl. 3 SQUILLIS 3 squills or sea onions (genus Scilla) or the roots or bulbs thereof [not in FEW 12,218a with this meaning], Rothwell, 258

SUREDOCKE s. 129 common sorrel (Oxalis acetosella) or sorrel dock (Rumex acetosa) [FEW 17,289a]

TANSEIE s. 125 TANESEIE 155 THANSEIE 143 tansy (Chrysanthemum vulgare) [FEW 13,i,79b]

TEIE s. 38 TEYE 39 cataract, 'web' [FEW 13,i,302b]

TEIGNE s. 77 ringworm, tinea, disease of the scalp [FEW 13,i,340b], Rothwell, 258

TERBENTIN s. 3 resin extracted from the terebinth (Pistacia terebinthus), 'turpentine' [FEW 13,i,236a]

TERTEINE see under FEVRE

TIUME s. 1 thyme [FEW 13,i,317b]

TIWELE s. 113 tile

TORTEL s. 113 TURTEL 105, 128 a round cake [FEW 13,ii,110a]

TRANSGLUTER v.a. 47 to swallow [FEW 4,172a]

TRESCE s. TRESCES DE AIL 122 bunch of cloves of garlic [FEW 13,ii,262a]

TRIACLE s. 90 theriac, treacle, antidote (to venomous bites) [FEW 13,i,308a]

TRUNS s. 121 stump (of cabbage) [FEW 13,ii,337a]

TRUS s. 136 stump (of cabbage) [FEW 13,ii,333b]

URINAL s. 6 chamberpot [FEW 14,62a]

VEINE s. V. CAPITALE 37 cephalic vein

VERM s. 66, 68, 101 worm

VERVEINE s. 16, 63, 73 vervain (Verbena officinalis) [FEW 14,277a]

VETOINE s. 16 betony, bishopwort (Betonica officinalis) [FEW 14,360a]

VIOLE s. 1, 143 violet

VOMITE s. 94 vomit [FEW 14,631a]

WANTELEINE* s. 59 foxglove (Digitalis purpurea) [FEW 18,507a ganteline 1820]

WYMALVE s. 3 marshmallow (Althaea officinalis) [FEW 4,422b]

YPOCRAS s. 5 wine flavoured with spices, hippocras [FEW 4,629b]

YSOPE s. 1 hyssop (Hyssopus officinalis) [FEW 4,528a]

SELECT GLOSSARY TO APPENDIX

to Chapter 3, pp.136–141

Only unusual words or forms or ingredients are recorded.

MS Sloane 3550 1st Copy:
[a]postolicon s. 136a 'unguentum apostolicon'
genet s. 136b broom (Sarothamnus scoparius)
mastin s. 136b mastiff
tessun s. 136b badger

MS Sloane 3550 2nd Copy:
colcreie (ME) f.219r coltsfoot (Tussilago farfara)
nugage s. 79c walnut, fruit of Juglans regia
plectrom s. 79b ? Centaury (Centaurium erythraea)
ungle de cheval s. f.219r coltsfoot (Tussilago farfara)

MS Sloane 3550 3rd Copy:
amerok s. f.224v stinking camomile, mayweed (Anthemis cotula)
brosewort (ME) s. f.224r daisy (Bellis perennis) or comfrey (Symphytum officinale)
cerflanc s. f. 225r hart's tongue fern (Phyllitis scolopendrium)
chokenemete (ME) s. f.224r chickweed (Stellaria media)
code s. f.224v code, cobbler's wax
cristal s. f.224r cristal

gladen (ME) s. f. 224v gladiolus
glere s. 133a & f. 225r yolk of egg
hockes (ME) s. f.223v plant of genus Malva or Althaea
nugage s. f.225r walnut, fruit of Juglans regia
perche de cerf s. 99a stag's antlers
quiture s. f.224r cautery
radich (ME) s. f.225r radish (Raphanus sativus)
ravene s. f.225r radish (Raphanus sativus)
redockes (ME) s. f.224v sorrel (Rumex acetosa)
sentorie s. 160 common centaury (Centaurium erythraea) or yellow centaury (Blackstonia
     perfoliata)

MS Digby 86:
brockarse (ME) s. f.18v ?
crusie s. f.13v crosswort (Galium cruciata)
hennebone (ME) s. f.20r henbane (Hyoscyamus niger)
hundestunge (ME) s. f.11r hound's tongue (Cynoglossum officinale)
plectrin (en ewe) s. f.11r ? centaury (Centaurium erythraea)
popi (ME) s. f.14v poppy (Papaver)
restebos s. f.13r restharrow, cammok (Ononis repens)
revenesfot (ME) s. f.18v ? orchid (Orchis)
softe (ME) s. f.18v mullein (Verbascum thapsus)
swinekarse (ME) s. f.14v knotgrass (Polygonum aviculare) or hog's fennel (Peucedanum of-
     ficinale)
vic (ME) s. f.12v 'ficus', tumour
wilde tesle (ME) s. f.18r teasel (Dipsacus sylvestris)

GLOSSARY[1]

to Chapter 4, pp.142–216

ACCÉS s. 1332 ACCESSE 1357 attack (of illness)
ACHE s. 1407, 1588, 1601, 1624 wild celery, smallage (Apium graveolens) [FEW 1,105a]
ACHON s. 1583 [cf. f.194r] wild celery, smallage
ACOSTIVEURE s. 492 constipation
AFESTRI a. 1053 festering, ulcerous
AFODILLUS s. 463 ramsons (Allium ursinum) or sometimes sweet woodruff (Asperula
     odorata) [FEW 1,157b]
AIL s. 1687 garlic (Allium sativum) [FEW 24,333a]
AISIL s. 122, 137, 177, 222, 329, 349, 397, 603, 758, 1551, 1559, 1592, 1660, 1666, 1681
     vinegar [FEW 24,101b]
AISTRE s. 871 hearth
AIUUERE a. GOUTE A. 737 dropsy
ALISAUNDRE s. 1303 alexanders, horse parsley (Smyrnium olusatrum) [FEW 24,313b]
ALUIGNE s. 261, 407 ALOIGNE 412 ALOINE 493, 918, 947, 962 wormwood (Artemisia
     absinthium) [FEW 24,346a]
AMAIER v. refl. 754 EMAIER 600 to be dismayed
AMORTIR v.a. 1195, 1199 to destroy

---

[1]   The Appendix is not included.

ANBLETE s. 629 spurge, euphorbia ? FEW 19,7a gives *amblete* as a 13th C. hapax 'centaurée, jaune musquée'; J. L Pagel, *Die Chirurgie des Heinrich von Mondeville* (Berlin, 1892), anti-dotarius cirurgie c.9, para. 185 has 'anabulla herba est communis nota de lactiniis corro-sivis, gallice amblete, crescit copiose in locis sabulosis'. See MSS London, B. L. Add. 10289 (s.xiii) f.127r 'L'amblete triblee oste les vermes' and Royal 12 C XIX f.105r 'Per-nez la racine del time, ço est l'amblette del pré u des marais' (above p.66). See also MS Oxford, Bodleian Library, Digby 69 f.209r 'ambrete'.

ANGUIL(L)E s. 239, 313, 937, 1173 eel

ANIS s. 465 aniseed (Pimpinella anisum) [FEW 24,599a]

APROISER v.a. 75 to praise

ARAIM(E) s. 876, 1110 brass

ARESTBOEF s. 573 restharrow, cammok (Ononis repens) [FEW 1,146b]

ARGENT s. VIF A. 390 quicksilver

ARGILLE s. 1103 clay

ARREMENT s. 166, 221, 284, 512, 1012, 1023, 1077, 1081, 1120, 1148 oak gall, sometimes vitriol [FEW 1,166a inadequate]

ASSAUDRER v.a. 976 to flavour, season

ASSOIGNE s. SAUNS A. 832 without delay

ASTRE s. 138 hearth

AUBE ESPINE s. 1639 hawthorn (Crataegus monogyna)

AUBON s. 101, 1146 AUBUN 179, 795, 869, 905, 1100, 1117 white of an egg

AUNE s. 1412? alder (Alnus glutinosa) [FEW 15,i,14b]; more likely, elecampane (Inula hele-nium) [FEW 4,784b; Rothwell p.226]

AVANCE s. 1067 AVAUNCE 767 wood avens (Geum urbanum)

AVEINE s. GRUEL D'A. 1577 oatmeal

AVEROINE s. 1375 southernwood (Artemisia abrotanum) [FEW 24,48a]

BETE s. 369 here probably error for *amblete* q.v.

BETOINE s. 1544 (wood) betony (Betonica officinalis) [FEW 1,345b]

BIBUEF s. 718 BIBUES 1605 mugwort (Artemisia vulgaris) [FEW 15,i,102a]

BOLACER s. 1032 bullace tree (Prunus insititia) [FEW 1,624a]

BOT s. DE B 180 immediately, completely

BOUTON s. 594 rosehip

BRAON s. 1205 brawn, muscle

BRASIER s. 567 live coals, fire

BREN s. 1720 scurf

BRESE s. 321, 505, 720, 1086, 1104, 1392 embers

BRESIL s. 1709 brazil wood, redwood (Sequoia sempervirens) [FEW 15,i,258a]

BROÇONE s. 702 knot, knob

BROÇONÉ a. 698 knotty, knobbly

BROILLER v.n. 658 to rumble (of stomach)

BRUIL s. 1696 ?

BRUET s. 541 broth, stock

BUGLE s. 765, 969, 1068 bugle (Ajuga reptans), sometimes confused with bugloss [FEW 1,600a]

BULLETER v.a. 564, 1451 to bolt, sift

BURE s. 495, 745, 1072 butter

BUTOR s. 730 bittern

CACHEUS a. 173 rheumy

CACHIE s. 165, 186, 227, 259 rheum [FEW 2,i,21b]

CA(U)NCRE s. 1027, 1047, 1066, 1075, 1099, 1114, 1122, 1125, 1156, 1160, 1183, 1193, 1195, 1197 cancer, abscess, malignant tumour

CANEL(L)IE s. 295, 1323, 1645 henbane (Hyoscyamus niger, 'jusquiamus') [FEW 2,i,86a]

ÇANESON s. 303 groundsel (Senecio vulgaris) [FEW 11,446a]

CAPITAL a. VEINE C. 144 cephalic vein

CHAUNVRE s. 644, 1175 CAMVRE 1150 hemp (Cannabis) [FEW 2,i,210a]
CAUS s. C. VIVE 1051 quicklime
CELIDOINE s. 171, 198, 1480, 1503, 1683 greater celandine (Chelidonium majus) [FEW 2,i,634a]
CENTOIRE s. 488, 580, 1067 CENTOYRE 1361 common centaury (Centaurium erythraea) or yellow centaury (Blackstonia perfoliata) [FEW 2,i,583b]
CERFOIL s. 748, 1695 chervil (Anthriscus cerefolium) [FEW 2,i,37b]
CERISE s. 1233 cherry
CERVEISE s. 681, 711, 735, 771, 891, 1243, 1400, 1505, 1527, 1593 CERVOISE 278, 409, 835 ale
CERVEL s. 152 CERVELE 356 brain
CHASTRIS s. 975 wether
CHAUDEL s. 527, 549 CHAUDELET 544 caudle
CHAUDET a. 1509 warm
CHEINE s. 1030, 1735 oak
CHEÜE s. 857 hemlock (Conium maculatum) [FEW 2,i,668a]
CHIE s. 201, 214 eyelash, eyelid, eyebrow
CHIEVREFOIL s. 167, 1142 honeysuckle (Lonicera periclymenum / caprifolium) or red clover (Trifolium pratense) [FEW 2,i,308b]
CHIN s. 819? china, china root (Smilax china) [FEW 2,i,637a]; more likely error for *thim*, thyme
CHION s. 756 shoot
CHOLET s. 566, 1604 cabbage
CICOREE s. 1443 chicory (Cichorium intybus) [FEW 2,i,665a]
CILECTRE s. 1663, 1668 depilatory
CIRE s. 322, 739, 798, 805, 847, 875, 881, 1655 wax
CIRICER 1316 cherry tree
CIRURGIAN s. 1210 surgeon
CIZRE s. 1436 cider
CLISTERE s. 550 enema, clyster [FEW 2,i,801b]
COIGNE s. 269 block of wood
COLEICE a. GELINE C. 546 chicken broth, cullis
COMIN s. 1229 cumin (Cuminum cyminum) [FEW 2,ii,1526a]
CONDUIT s. 1285 urethra
CONFIRE s. 765, 909, comfrey (Symphytum officinale) [FEW 2,ii,1030a]
CONFIRE v.a. 996 to prepare, concoct
CONFISION s. 252, 622 confection (pharm.), electuary, preparation [not in FEW 2,ii,1032a]
CONSOUDE s. 767, 909, 1366 consound, variously applied, incl. comfrey (Symphytum officinale) and daisy (Bellis perennis) [FEW 2,ii,1076a]
CONTROVE s. 1171 invention, fiction, untruth
CORCHON s. 1463 diarrhoea
CORIAUNDRE s. 1614 coriander (Coriandrum sativum) [FEW 2,ii,1184b]
CORN s. 1055, 1072 horn C. DE CERF 1449 hartshorn
COROSIF a. 268, 1121 caustic
COUDRE s. 380, 677 hazel tree
COUPERON s. 920 top, tip (of herb or plant)
CRESP a. 1671 curly
CRESSON s. 558 cress, watercress
CROES a. 1203 hollow
CROIS s. 1209 hollow
CROSER v.a. 1188 to make a hole in
CROTE s. droppings, dung CROTES DE CERF 607 CROTES DE LIEVRE 1126
CSINCE s. 269, 1615 strip of material, bandage
DAUNGER s. A D. 1500 reluctantly, under duress

DECACHER v.a. 1362 to drive out
DEFUMER v. refl. 1492 to cleanse oneself
DELIÉ a. 206, 245, 248, 1107, 1453, 1514 fine, of fine texture
DESEIVRE s. 1197 difference, distinction
DESEIVRER v.a. 1362 DESEVRER 1461 DESÇOIVRE 274 to separate, remove
DESTEMPRER v.a. 133, 352, 486, 710, 1227, 1287, 1298, 1356, 1439, 1527, 1550, 1606,
    1612 to distemper, dissolve in or combine with another liquid
DIETER v.n. 1380 to diet
DITAIN s. 781 DITAN 1611 dittany (Dictamnus albus) [FEW 3,70b]
DRAP s. 169, 248, 1289, 1290, 1435, 1452, 1485, 1581 cloth D. LINGE 102, 205, 1326
    LANGE D. 393 LINGE D. 1124 linen cloth
DRAPEL s. 324 cloth
EBLE s. 917, 1395 (496) EVELE 429, 717 dwarf elder, danewort (Sambucus ebulus) [FEW
    3,202a]
ECHAUFEMENT s. 1427 inflammation
EGREMOIGNE s. 831 EGREMOINE 967, 1352 agrimony (Agrimonia eupatoria) [FEW
    24,270a]
EFFONDRER v.a. 1213 EFFUNDRER 1219 to pierce, break open
EGRUN s. 973 acrid food
EMAIER v. refl. 600 AMAIER 754 to be dismayed
EMPLASTRE s. 137, 223, 484, 507, 787, 872, 900, 906, 1046, 1063, 1079, 1193, 1319, 1595,
    1644, 1657 ENPLASTRE 893 plaster (med.)
EMPLASTRER v.a. 103, 184, 364, 898, 927, 1075, 1173, 1581, 1649 to cover with a plaster
EMPLASTRIR v.a. 1006 to cover with a plaster
ENCENS s. 957, 1012 incense
ENDAUBER v.a. 1164 to smear
ENDITER v.n. 357, 1580 to indicate, explain
ENGRÉS a. 1048 inflamed, angry
ENGROTÉ p.p. 26 afflicted, made ill
ENNEIRE adv. 1049 forthwith
ENPESTRIR v.n. 999 to knead
ENTAMER v.a. 694, 696, 1167 to pierce, destroy
ENTRAIT s. 791, 796, 932, 959, 995 poultice
ENTRERUS s. 447, 889 middle bark, 'cortex mediana' [FEW 4,763a]
ERE s. 1029 ivy (Hedera helix) GOUME D'E. 1286, 1665 gum ivy
ERE TERRESTRE s. 98, 831, 855, 949, 969 ground ivy (Glechoma hederacea) [FEW 13,i,262a]
ESCALE s. 378, 430, 499, 1496, 1553 (egg) shell
ESCLENDRE a. 457, 474 slim, thin
ESCLICE s. 545 spatula, slice
ESCORCE s. 1024, 1028, 1029, 1039, 1059 bark
ESCORCHEURE s. 287, 337 excoriation, sore
ESCOT s. 1654 share
ESCUMER v.a. 230, 436, 442, 501 to skim
ESMIER v.a. 775 to crumble, render into small pieces
ESPINE s. 641 thorn, prickle NOIR E. 888, 1030 blackthorn (Prunus spinosa)
ESPIS s. 1736 SPIS 1119 ear (of rye)
ESPOUDRER s. v. refl. 1106 to become powder (hapax, cf. FEW 9,562b]
ESROÉ a. 1388, 1421 hoarse
ESROURE s. rubric after 1386 hoarseness
ESSOIGNE s. SAUNS NUL E. 858 without delay
ESTAL s. 1291 urine
ESTALER v.n. 1224 to urinate v.a. 1240 to discharge with the urine
ESTANCE s. 580 shepherd's purse (Capsella bursa-pastoris)
ESTAUNCHER v.a. 760, 1556 to staunch, stop the flow of

ESTEIM s. 254 tin
ESTEINT s. 1732 stain, dye
ESTOPER v.a. 341 to stop, block up 1103 to stiffen, thicken (of mixture)
ESTOUNER v.a. 1568 to deafen
ESTOUPES s. pl. 1133 fibres of tow
ESTREIM s. 1737, 1739 (barley) straw
ESTUER v.a. 120, 253 to store, reserve
ESTUVER v. refl. 647, 674, 1491 to take a steam bath
EUFRASE s. 275 eufrasy (Euphrasia officinalis) [FEW 3,249b]
EWE s. BENOITE E. 1236, 1612 holy water E. ROSE 1307 rose water
FAISIL s. 618, 619 scoria, slag, scale
FAVEE s. F. DE L'EWE 1225 an aquatic plant, perhaps water plantain (Alisma plantago-aqua-
    tica); often used to gloss M.E. *lemke* (brooklime) and Lat. *favida / fabaria*, thus possibly in-
    dicating Veronica beccabunga or Sium angustifolium / latifolium (= water parsnip). FEW
    3,340b suggests Berula angustifolia and Sium angustifolium
FEISAUN s. 977 pheasant
FENOIL s. 166, 188, 417, 479, 1259, 1429, 1624, 1637 fennel (Foeniculum vulgare) [FEW
    3,454a]
FESTRE s. 1052, 1066, 1099, 1122, 1159, 1185, 1189, 1197, 1198 fistula, ulcer
FESTRIER a. 1170 fistular
FEUKEROLE s. 535 royal fern, osmunda (Osmunda regalis) [FEW 3,515a]
FEUTRE s. 1558 felt
FEVE s. 1391 broad bean
FEVRE s. F. AGUE 1301, 1359 ague COTIDIANE F. 1335 quotidian fever (F.) QUARTAINE
    1345 quartan fever F. TERSAINE 1329 tertian fever
FI s. 605, 631, 643, 657, 675, 685, 692, 1463, 1468, 1521, 1532 ficus, tumour FI ARDANT
    633
FIEL s. gall F. DE CHIEVRE 161 F. DE ANGUILE 239 F. DE UN MOTUN 292 F. DE LA PER-
    TRIS 189 240 F. DE TOR 1681
FIENTE s. dung F. DE GELINE 923 F. DE COLUMBE 1655
FINEGREC s. 363 FENUGREC 459 fenugreek (Trigonella foenum-graecum) [FEW 3,461b]
FISIKE s. 877, 1094, 1296 the science of medicine; the first and last examples may indicate
    the title of the source
FLAME s. 495 fat, grease [FEW 3,598b]
FLAOUR s. 157 scent, odour, fragrance
FOIRE s. 518 diarrhoea
FORMAGE s. 601, 1163, 1167, 1402 cheese
FOSSELETTE s. 1482 small ditch, hollow
FOU s. 1059, 1673 beech (Fagus sylvatica)
FRAINE s. 1029 ash tree (Fraxinus excelsior)
FRAINELE s. 629 probably ashweed (Aegopodium podagraria) [FEW 3,772a]
FREINE s. 309 ash tree (Fraxinus excelsior)
FRESCENG s. 946 pig
FRESE s. 229 strawberry
FUMITERE s. 479, 1432 fumitory (Fumaria officinalis) [FEW 3,857b]
FUNDEMENT s. 514, 642, 654 anus
GARGARIME s. 368, 1410, 1426 gargle
GELINE s. 533, 537, 923, 941, 977, 1090, 1116 hen
GEUN a. 134 GUNS 112 JUN 1524, 1629 fasting, on an empty stomach
GINGEMBRE s. 433 GINGIMBRE 238 ginger [FEW 14,663b]
GLEIRE s. 1074, 1129 yolk of an egg
GLETTE s. 405 phlegm, mucus
GOMME s. G. ARABIKE 1445 gum arabic [FEW 4,324a]
GOUTE s. 1114 gout

GOUTE FESTRE s. 1131, 1155, 1180 fistula, ulcer
G[R]ATEISON s. 1722 itching
GRAVELE s. 1285, 1290 gravel (med.)
GRESSE s. 477, 553 GRASSE 599, 941 fat, grease
GRUMIL s. 1230, 1257 common gromwell (Lithospermum officinale) [FEW 2,87a]
HASCHEE s. 1346 affliction, distress, suffering
HELEMEN s. 9 element
HOUS s. 1031 holly (Ilex aquifolium) [FEW 16,261b]
HUMOR s. 373, 406 moisture, fluid
IERRE s. 121 ivy (Hedera helix) [FEW 4,396b]
IVE s. 329 mare
JOUTE s. 551 vegetable broth
JOVENET a. 1056 young
JUBARBE s. 311, 417, 1322 houseleek (Sempervivum tectorum) [FEW 5,78b]
JUNER v.n. 151 to fast
KAUKETRAPPE s. 708, 1070 caltrops (Centaurea melitensis) or star thistle (Centaurea calci-
    trapa) [FEW 2,i,65a]
KERSON s. 1727 cress K. DE EWE 749 water cress (Rorippa nasturtium-aquaticum)
LAINE s. 301 wool
LAIT s. 588, 973, 1401, 1635, 1642 milk L. DE CHIEVRE 595, 1523
LAITEROLE s. 1058 spurge (Euphorbia) [cf. FEW 5,113a]
LARD s. 509, 1025 fat
LARD(R)ON s. 510, 1206 strip of (bacon) fat
LAUNCELEE s. 825, 1351, 1533 LANCELEE 949 ribwort (Plantago lanceolata) [FEW 5,158a]
LAVANDRE s. 769 LAVENDRE 1132 lavender (Lavandula officinalis) [FEW 5,219b]
LAVEURE s. 1731 lotion
LECTUAIRE s. 624 electuary
LEISSIVE s. 1702, 1743 LAISSIVE 1708 lye
LENTILLE s. 1135 lentil
LETUE s. 1637, 1651 LETTUIS 1431 lettuce
LICORIZ s. 1445 liquorice
LIEVRE s. 356, 1263 hare
LIMAISON s. 688, 1061 snail
LIME s. 685 slime
LIM(E)URE s. 879 filings L. D'ARAIM 876, 1110 L. DE CORN 1071
LIN s. 182, 1175, 1591 flax
LINGE a. 102, 205, 269, 1124, 1326, 1616 linen
LION s. 730 lion
LOVASCHE s. 408 lovage (Levisticum officinale) [FEW 5,334b]
LUMOR s. 389 ? error for limon, slime
LUS s. 611 pike (ict.)
MAILE s. 236, 274, M. ENCLOSE 267 cataract, leucoma
MANJUE s. 174, 197, 228, 1719 scabies, mange
MARCIATON s. 1570 a green ointment
MAROBRE s. 1414 black horehound (Marrubium nigrum) or common horehound (Marru-
    bium vulgare) [FEW 6,i,377b]
MAROIL s. 1623 black horehound (Marrubium nigrum) or common horehound (Marrubium
    vulgare) [FEW 6,i,377b]
MASTIC s. 381, 466 mastic, resin
MAUVE s. 551 mallow (Malva sylvestris) or marshmallow (Althaea officinalis) [FEW
    6,i,129a]
MAZELIN s. 712, 1506 drinking cup, goblet of veined maple wood
MEGUE s. 517 whey [FEW 6,ii,43b]
MELLE s. 1037 medlar (Mespilus germanica) [FEW 6,ii,44b]

MENEISON s. 560, 605, 1464 diarrhoea

MENTASTRE s. 1533 horsemint (Mentha sylvestris) [FEW 6,i,731b]

MENTE s. 1226, 1399, 1607, 1645 mint

MIE s. 529 piece of bread (soft part)

MIEL s. 101, 162, 167, 190, 230, 284, 291, 396, 419, 422, 495, 504, 511, 621, 671, 745, 789, 837, 963, 1000, 1016, 1043, 1081, 1164, 1273, 1390, 1402, 1436, 1537, 1597, 1626, 1655, 1661, 1698 MEL 847, 1148, 1299, 1407 honey

MIER v.a. 531 to crumb

MILFOIL s. 485 MIRFOIL 1533, 1677 milfoil, yarrow (Achillea millefolium) [FEW 6,ii,92b]

MIRE s. 813 physician

MIRRE s. 1286 myrrh

MIRSAU s. 554 sea salt, brine, cf. *saumure* [FEW 11,89b]. cf. MED *mere-sauce*

MOEL s. 738, 1145, 1497 yolk of an egg

MOISSE s. 889 sloe (?)

MOLEINE s. 1525 mullein (Verbascum thapsus) [FEW 6,iii, 52a]

MOLESTE s. 1721 discomfort, pain

MORELE s. 858, 1324 petty morel, belladonna, black nightshade (Solanum nigrum) [FEW 6,i,544a]

MORON s. 1537 pile (med.)

MOSCHE s. 1693 fly

MUELE s. 562 millstone, grindstone

MUSART s. 1171 fool, idle chatterer

NAGES s. pl. 666 buttocks

NAVET s. 1073 turnip, neep

NELE s. 1149 corn cockle (Agrostemma githago) or darnel (Lolium temulentum) or Nigella arvensis

NOIEL s. 650 hub

NOIS s. 378 nut

NOMBLIL s. 685, 689 NUMBLIL 484, 507 navel

OIGNON s. 319, 503 onion

OILE s. 122, 271, 738, 847, 870, 875, 881, 1404, 1677, 1689, 1698 oil

OINT s. 477, 1078 fat O. DE CENGLER 946 O. DE CHAR 740 O. DE GELINE 250 O. DE TESSON OU DE BUTOR OU DE LION 729–30 O. DE VER 745

ORGE s. 1137, 1736, 1737 barley FERINE DE O. 395 barley flour FLOUR D'O. 1321, 1591 barley flour

ORPIMENT s. 878, 879, 1119, 1665 orpiment, yellow arsenic [FEW 1,182a]

ORTIE s. 920, 1057, 1557, 1723 nettle ROUGE O. 747, 756, 1258 red nettle

OSMONDE s. 770 OMONDE 910 royal fern, osmunda (Osmunda regalis)

OUQUELESCONSCE s. 1069 ? see above p.400

PAELLETTE s. 1510 small pan, skillet

PALASIN s. 820 paralysis

PANIFEST s. 1508 ?

PARELE s. 815, 1369 sorrel, dock (Rumex acetosa) [FEW 7,639a]

PAS s. P. DE CHEVAL 1413 coltsfoot (Tussilago farfara)

PASTEL s. 782, 785, 1144 poultice

PASTISIER v.a. 467 to knead pastry, to make pastry [FEW 7,751a]

PAUPIERE s. 214, 262 eyelid

PAVOT s. 1653 poppy (Papaver) [FEW 7,573b]

PEIVRE s. 432, 1348, 1404 POIVRE 238, 1152 P. BLANC 1603 BLAUNC P. 1259 pepper

PELOSETTE s. 829, 844, 856, 989, 1069 mouse-ear hawkweed (Hieracium pilosella) [FEW 8,504a with change of suffix]

PELUSELE s. 584 mouse-ear hawkweed (Hieracium pilosella) [FEW 8,504a]

PENIL s. 1251 penis

PENNE s. 163, 191, 742 quill, feather

PERESIL s. 1245, 1258, 1430, 1624 common parsley (Petroselinum crispum / sativum) [FEW 8,325b]

PERTRIS s. FIEL DE LA P. 189 PARTRIS 241, 977 partridge

PERTUIS s. 1052, 1064, 1733 opening, mouth (of wound)

PERVENKE s. 1541 periwinkle (Vinca maior / minor) [FEW 14,461b]

PESCHER s. 363, 1315 peach tree

PESSON s. PORC EN P. 472 pig being fattened

PIERE s. 1247, 1285, 1290 stone (med.)

PIMPERNELE s. 1020 applied to a variety of plants, especially the burnets (Sanguisorba officinalis and Paxterium sanguisorba) and pimpernel (Anagallis arvensis) [FEW 8,517a]

PLACHEUS a. 1691 bald

PLANTAINE s. 558, 1322 PLANTAIN 347, 788 PLANTEIN 827 PLAUNTAIN 969, 1331 PLAUNTAINE 351 PLAUNTEIN 679 plantain, waybread (Plantago major) [FEW 9,19b]

POINDRE v.a. 641 to prick, sting

POIS s. 708, 804 POIZ 739 pitch

POLIPODE s. 521, 734 polipody (Polipodium vulgare) or oak fern (Thelypteris dryopteris) [FEW 9,139b]

POMER s. 1031 apple tree

POPLER s. 155 poplar (Populus) [FEW 9,181b]

PORCHET s. 553 piglet

PORIAU s. 1423 leek (Allium porrum)

PORPÉ s. 275 purslane (Portulaca oleracea) [FEW 9,529a]

POULENS a. 637 stinking

POUME s. P. DE CHAINE 1061 oak apple [FEW 9,155b 'seit 1718'] P. DÉ BOIS 1085 crab apple

PRUNER s. 1032, 1316 plum tree

PULIOL s. 365 POLIOL 414 wild thyme (Thymus serpyllum) [FEW 9,521a]

QUARTER s. 208 quarter segment

QUARTILIER v.a. 204 to cut into (four) pieces [FEW 2,ii,1426b]

QUILLER s. 426, 532, 625 spoon(ful)

QUILLIER v.a. 113, 954 to gather

QUINKENERVE s. 788 ribwort (Plantago lanceolata)

QUINTEFOILE s. 1522, 1549 cinquefoil (Potentilla reptans) [FEW 2,ii,1481a]

RAIRE v.a. 896, 1680 to shave

RAIS s. 669, 1411 radish [FEW 10,27a]

RA(U)NCLE s. 914, 1585, 1598 impostume, abscess, malignant tumour

RANCLIER v.n. 986 to suppurate, ulcerate, rankle

RASTELLER v.a. 1478 to rake over (coals)

RAVENE s. 669 radish [FEW 10,63b]

RAVLE s. 1268 radish [FEW 10,27a]

RETOR s. 1302, 1365 return (to health), recovery

RIERE v.a. 128 to shave

RIEVRE a. 1253 obstinate, recalcitrant (aphetic form of enrievre, FEW 4, 815b)

ROCHE s. 1174 roach

ROELE s. 673, 1270 round slice ROELETTE 667

ROIGNON s. 944 kidney

ROMAUN s. EN ROMAUNS 83, 89 in the romance vernacular

RONCE s. NEIRE R. 919 bramble

ROSEL s. 895 reed

ROUJOR s. 227 redness

RUE s. 97, 121, 129, 159, 188, 198, 276, 407, 947, 1298, 1349, 1601, 1638 rue (Ruta graveolens) [FEW 10,597a]

RUIRE v.n. 658 to gurgle

SABLON s. 1051 sand

SAFRAN s. 1709 saffron (Crocus sativus) [FEW 19,202a]

SAIM s. 477, 500, 524, 800, 801, 803, 1584 S. DE ANGUILLE 313 S. DE PORC 431 S. DE LART 1015 fat

SAISON s. ESTRE S. 92 to be right, fitting, proper

SALLE s. 819 sage (Salvia officinalis) [FEW 11,132a]

SANGUINE s. 1349 applicable to a variety of plants incl. 'bloodwort' or shepherd's purse (Capsella bursa-pastoris). FEW 11,164a cites Middle French examples and glosses 'nom donné à plusieurs plantes astringentes, telles que le polygonum aviculaire ['knotgrass'], le géranium sanguine ['bloody cranesbill'] et le plantain coronope ['buckshorn plantain']'. The name might also be applied to dogwood (Cornus sanguinea).

SANICLE s. 766, 1067 wood sanicle (Sanicula europaea) [FEW 11,183b]

SARREE s. 747, 1322, 1611 savory (Satureia hortensis) [FEW 11,252a]

SAUGE s. 547, 947, 1376 sage (Salvia officinalis) [FEW 11,132a]

SAUGEMME s. 221, 1101 rock salt [FEW 11,77a]

SAU(S) s. 156, 1316 willow (Salix) [FEW 11,100b]

SAVINE s. 1389 savin, creeping juniper (Juniperus sabina) [FEW 11,5b]

SAVON s. 1726 soap

SEGLE s. 715, 793, 901, 961, 1016, 1050, 1119, 1149, 1514, 1715 rye

SEIE s. 699 silk

SEIE s. 700 (horse) hair

SEI(G)NER v. refl. 144, 146 to have oneself bled

SEITE s. 886 arrow

SEL s. 395, 739, 746, 1024, 1101, 1126, 1148, 1299, 1353, 1461, 1513 SEEL 1544 BLAUNC S. 871 salt

SELE s. 661 stool (for evacuation of bowels)

SELETTE s. 649, 1481 stool, small seat (for evacuation of bowels)

SENESÇON s. 1363 groundsel (Senecio vulgaris) [FEW 11,446a]

SENTE s. 56 path

SEONER v.a. 702 to detach, isolate, separate

SEU s. 1472, 1493 SEUZ 447 elder (Sambucus) [FEW 11,6a]

S(O)IRON s. 201, 211, 335, 1712 ciron, itch mite [FEW 17,67b]

SIU s. 740, 805, 944, 1024 SIEUE 1127 S. DE BOUC 645, 746, 799 S. DE CERF 945 S. DE MOTON 352, 848, 1589 S. DE TOR 1685 S. DE VEL 740 suet, tallow

SIUR a. S. PAIN 529 sour

SOFFOIGNE s. NOIR S. 349, 1660 hellebore (Helleborus niger) or henbane (Hyoscyamus niger) [FEW 12,73b]

SOLSECLE s. 1375 marigold (Calendula officinalis) [FEW 12,73b]

SOLUCION s. 451, 456, 519 freedom from constipation

SORDEISSONS s. pl. 332 buzzing (in ears)

SOUFFRE s. 1297 sulphur

SOUPE s. 571 sop

SUOR s. 1367 sweat

SURSANER v.a. 851 SORSANER 873 to cicatrize, scar

TACON s. 1151 sole of a shoe

TAN s. 1098, 1494 tan EWE DE T. 1096 solution of tan

TANESIE s. 769, 968, 1070 tansy (Chrysanthemum vulgare) [FEW 13,i,79b]

TEIGNE s. 1680 tinea, ringworm, scalp disease

TEIGNUS a. 1679 suffering from tinea

TENDRON s. 919, 1394 shoot (of plant)

TENTE s. 1192, 1204, 1211 tent (med.) or pledget

TENUET a. 668 slender, thin

TERMINE s. 275 ? clover [FEW 13,ii,245b]

TESI a. 636 swollen

TESSON s. 729 badger

TIULE s. 648, 664, 1475, 1479 tile
TORMENTINE s. 276, 580 tormentil (Potentilla tormentilla) [FEW 13,ii,44b]
TORTEL(E) s. 646, 651, 719, 723, 726 cake, poultice
TRANSLATER v.a. 80, 89 to translate
TORTELET s. 999 small cake
TOUNER v.n. 308, 1567 to buzz, roar, boom (of ears)
TRAVAIL s. EN T. 18, 19, 21 in a state of agitation
TREMBLE s. 1024, 1031, 1394 aspen (Populus tremula) [FEW 13,ii,245a]
TROCHE s. T. DE AIL 1687, bulb of garlic
TU(I)AL s. 589, 591 pipe, tube
UNGLE s. UNGLES DE PORC 1293 pig's trotters
URINE s. 283, 289 OURINE 659 urine
VEIRE s. 1120 glass
VENEISON s. 597 venison
VENIM s. 914 poison
VENTRAIL s. 403, 405, 658 stomach, belly
VER s. 297, 305, 335, 354, 360, 482, 489, 775 worm
VERDEGRECE s. 244, 1152 verdigris
VERMINE s. 213, 327 vermin (insects)
VERTIN s. 97, 125, 141 vertigo [FEW 14,326a]
VERVAINE s. 194, 1638 vervain (Verbena officinalis) [FEW 14,277a]
VESSIE s. 1223, 1247 bladder
VETOI(G)NE s. 108, 129, 132, 276, 299, 735, 768, 823, 857, 859, 918, 1068 betony, bishop-wort (Betonica officinalis) [FEW 14,360a]
VIAIRE s. AL MIEN V. in my opinion
VIGNE s. 1701 VINGNE 1707 vine
VIN s. 167, 278, 312, 365, 711, 735, 835, 892, 904, 1016, 1081, 1230, 1243, 1261, 1265, 1356, 1385, 1396, 1415, 1606, 1625, 1724 wine BLAUNC V. 133, 629, 710, 1227, 1287 ROUGE V. 585 V. ROUGE 587 V. EGRE 130
VIOLE s. 783, 967 violet
VIOLETTE s. 821 violet
VOMIR v.n. 400 to vomit
VOMITE s. 427, 450, 451, 453 vomitory
VONQUES s. 399 vomiting
WARANCE s. W. ROUGE 1241 madder (Rubia tinctorum) [FEW 17,622b]
WIMAUVE s. 1579 marshmallow (Althaea officinalis) [FEW 4,422b]

GLOSSARY I (Vernacular) [1]
to Chapter 5, pp.217–63

ACHE s. 13, 37, 48* wild celery, smallage (Apium graveolens) [FEW 1,105A]
ACTOUN s. 13* acton, padded jacket or decorative garment worn over armour [FEW 19,102a]; ME 1335

[1] The glossary is selective, its principal aim being to record the ingredients of the receipts. For greater clarity compound words which may appear as single words in the main text are here hyphenated. Abbreviations used are C = the opening charm, O = the first receipt, written in two cols on f.29v Numbers accompanied by an asterisk refer to the second part of the collection (ff.41r et seq.). Datings preceded by ME are supplied from The Middle English Dictionary.

ADIANTOS s. 0, 30, 31 maidenhair fern (Adiantum capillus-veneris) [FEW 24,141a 13th/14th C. *adiantum* 1546]

ALISAUNDRE s. 4 ALIZAUNDIR 6* ALISAUNDIR-ROTE 78 alexanders, horse parsley (Smyrnium olusatrum) [FEW 24,313b] ME 1300

ALLELUIA s. 31, 32, 33 wood sorrel (Oxalis acetosella)

ALOYN s. 73 wormwood (Artemisia absinthium) [FEW 24,346a]

ALYM s. 56*, 141* common or potash alum [FEW 24,376b] ME 1398

ANCLE(ME) s. 153* ankle

ANGUILTWYCH (ME) s. 95* earthworm, lumbricus ME 1200

ANYS s. 48*, 151* aniseed (Anethum graveolens)

ASKEBAN s. 151*. 163* comfrey? henbane?[2]

ATTIRLOUE s. 12* plant used as antidote esp. betony and black nightshade (Solanum nigrum)

ATTIRLOBERY s. 12* ATTIRLOUEBERY 12*, 29*, 99* berry of above. Cf. Zettersten, *op. cit.* p.30

AUST s. 93* August

AVENCE s. 1 AVANCE 52* wood avens (Geum urbanum) ME c.1200

AYSEL s. 127* vinegar

BALL s. 141* ball, pelote

BARCHYS-GREYS s. 79* boar's grease

BAUME s. 92* aromatic oleoresin of the genus Commiphora ME c.1230

BE (ME) s. 47* bee

BEN s. BEN LEVIS 79* bean leaves BEN HELME 141* bean stalk, bean haulm

BET s. BETYN ROTIS 10* roots of the beat

BETOYN(E) s. 52*, 167* BETOYNG 92* wood-betony (Betonica officinalis) [FEW 14,360a]

BIL (ME) s. 82*, 142* (index sub *antrax* & *pistule*) blister, pimple ME 1440

BISSOPWRT (ME) s. 37 betony (Betonica officinalis) [or 'agnus castus' (Hypericum androsaemum)?] ME 1300

BLERYNE[S] s. 79* bleariness, rheumy condition of the eye, eye disease ME 1398

BLODE-BENDE s. 148* ligature or bandage to stop bleeding ME c.1230

BLU-CLOTH s. 26* a kind of blue, woollen cloth

BORAGE s. 39* borage (Borago officinalis) [FEW 1,442a] ME 1300

BOTHUM s. 95* rosemary (Rosmarinus officinalis) ; sometimes corn marigold (Chrysanthemum segetum), ox-eye daisy (Chrysanthemum leucanthemum) etc. ME c.1225

BOTTOUN s. 164*, 166* haemorrhoid, pile (see index sub *anus* & *bottouns*)

BREMMYL (ME) s. 52* briar BREMIL-CROP 4 BREMMYL-CROPPIS 57* BREMMYL-KROP 122* bramble, briar, blackberry (Rubus fruticosus)

BRIDIS-TUNGE (ME) s. 1 stitchwort, 'lingua avis' (Stellaria holostea/graminea) ME c.1300

BRISWORT (ME) s. 18, 163* daisy (Bellis perennis) or comfrey (Symphytum officinale), appears 92* as marginal gloss to *conseude la petite* ME 1300

BROME (ME) s. FLUR OF B. 52* broom (Cytisus scoparius) ME ? c.1125

BROOK (ME) s. 138* BROK 169* (index sub *brook*) boil, swelling ME c.1440

BROUÉ s. 10* broth [FEW 1,550a]

BROUNEWORT (ME) s. BROUNWORT 156* BROUNEWORT MAIOR 7* used of a variety of plants incl. spleenwort (genus Asplenium or Ceterach) and whortleberry (Vaccinium myrtillus) and species of Scrophularia[3]

BUGLE s. 0, 1, 29, 30, 31, 33, 77, 92* BUGIL 39*, 98* BUGYL 52*, 123*, 167* BUGYL SAVAGE 92* bugle (Ajuga reptans) sometimes confused with bugloss [FEW 1,600a] ME 1300

---

[2]   Cf. f.3v where to the entry 'consolida maior .g. confery, .a. muchebrisewort' a later hand has added, in the left-hand margin, '.i. askebane'. Zettersten, *op. cit.*, p.29 comments on the form *eskbam* 'This plant may seem difficult to identify, but it is certainly identical with *henbane*, Hyoscyamus niger, which is found in *Treat. Garden*. 171. It is probably a blend of *iusquiamus* and *henbane*'.

[3]   Sometimes also applied to soapwort (Saponaria officinalis).

BURNET s. 52* BURNETE 77*, 82* BURNETTE 29 burnet; great burnet (Sanguisorba officinalis), salad burnet (Poterium sanguisorba), common pimpernel (Anagallis arvensis), burnet saxifrage (Pimpinella saxifraga)

CALAMYNT s. 151*, 152* common calamint (Calamintha officinalis) ME 1300

CAMAMYL s. 1, 49*, 152* common camomile (Anthemis nobilis) [FEW 2,i,148a camomille 1322, camamile 16th C.] ME 1300, camamille 1425

CARSIN (ME) s. 4 a kind of cress ME 1500, see Zettersten, op. cit., p. 29

CARWEY s. 49*, 111* caraway (Carum carvi) ME c.1390

CAUMBRE s. 52*, 94* hemp (Cannabis sativa)

CA(U)NKRE s. C, 16 KAUNKYR (index sub carmina) tumour, abscess, cancer

CELIDONE s. 92* CELIDOYN 98* greater celandine (Chelidonium majus) [FEW 2,i,634a] ME c.1125

CENTIRGALLE s. 19 wild clary (Salvia verbenaca) ME 1400

CENTOIRE s. 24, 98* CENTORIE 31 CENTORY 34* common centaury (Centaurium umbellatum) or yellow centaury (Chlora perfoliata) [FEW 2,i,583b] ME c.1390

CERFOYLE s. 100 chervil (Anthriscus cerefolium) [FEW 2,i,37b]

CERVEISE s. 13 ale

CETRAC s. 0, 30, 31 scale fern (Ceterach officinarum) [FEW 19,173a 1542] ME 1425

CHAPPOUNYS-GRES (ME) s. 79* capon's grease

CHIK(K)YNMET(TE) (ME) s. 144*, 148*, 153*, 163* chickweed (Stellaria media) ME ?c.1125

CHOLETTE s. cabbage RUGE CHOLET(TE) 15, 52* red cabbage [FEW 2,i,535a]

CHOU s. 20 cabbage (Brassica oleracea)

CIRE s. 92* wax C. VIRGE 3 VIRGINE 92* virgin wax

CLAVYR (ME) s. 52* clover ME ? c.1125

CNAPP (ME) s. 141* bud, rosebud, rosehip ME 1398

COLUMBINE s. COLUMBYN 52* COLUMBINE-ROTE 78 columbine (Aquilegia vulgaris) ME 1325

COLYS s. 10* cullis, strained clear broth [FEW 2,ii,878b] ME 1381

CONFERRY s. 52* CONFORY 163* comfrey (Symphytum officinale) ME 1300

CONSEUDE s. C. LA PETITE 27, 92* consolida minor, daisy (Bellis perennis) [FEW 2,ii,1076b]

COODE s. 142*, 152* code, cobbler's wax, mastic ME c.1150

COPROS s. 79*, 84* (= vitreolum viride) copperas, a metallic sulphate ME 1325

COUHIS-MARCH s. 7* (moel de beuf) ox marrow

COWIL (ME) s. RED COWIL-CROP 4 REED COUL-CROP 122* red cabbage

CRESSUN s. 3 cress C. DE JARDYN 13 garden cress (Lepidium sativum)

CRISTIS-LADDIR (ME) s. 37 common centaury (Centaurium erythraea) or yellow centaury (Blackstonia perfoliata) ME c.1325

CROP (ME) s. 78*, 155* any part of the plant except the root

CROPLESWORT (ME) s. 52*, 120* (vel brounwort) [4]

CROYSRY (ME) [5] s. 52* crosswort (Galium cruciata) ME ? c.1450

DAUKE s. 52* wild carrot (Daucus carota/asininus) ME 1400

DAYSE (ME) s. 0, 31, 98* DAYCE 52* daisy or marguerite (Bellis perennis) ME 1300

DEAUTÉ s. 148*, 153* a salve, dialthea

DENTE DE LYOUN s. 52* dandelion (Taraxacum officinale) ME 1425

DITTOUNDIR s. 52* DYTTAUNDRY 128* dittander (Lepidium latifolium) or dittany (Origanum dictamnus or Dictamnus albus) [FEW 3,70b] ME 1300

DOK (ME) s. DOK-ROTE 36 root of the dock (plant of genus Rumex) [FEW 15,ii,63b] ME 1300

---

[4]   Croplesewort is found in MS Add.33996 in a receipt on f.211r. See also Hunt, Plant Names sub brigla.
[5]   Cf. Hunt, Plant Names sub Cruciata maior/minor.

DRACHE s. 87* lees, dregs, sediment

DRAPLETTE s. 10 cloth [FEW 3,155a–b no fem. form]

EDDYR-GOMME (ME) s. 141* laudanum (resin)

EGREMOY(G)N(E) s. 4, 6, 26, 52* EGYRMOYN 128* agrimony (Agrimonia eupatoria) [FEW 24,270a]

ELSAUNDIR s. 111* GREYN DE ELISAUNDRE 93* alexanders (Smyrnium olusatrum)

EMOROYD s. 7* haemorrhoid

EMOT (ME) s. 126* ant ME 1300

ENDIVE s. 39*, 114* ENDIVIE 48* wild lettuce [FEW 4,784b] ME 1400

ENPLASTRE s. 86* plaster

ENTRET s. 92* salve, plaster

EPATIK s. 48* liverwort (?Marchantia polymorpha) [FEW 4,403b 15th C.] ME epatica ? 1425

ESKEBAN (ME) s. 52*, 149*, 160* ASKEBAN 151*, 163* comfrey? herbane? (see note 2 above)

ESTAL a 13 settled, clear

ESTAUNCHER v.a. 95* to staunch, halt flow of v.n. 13 to dry up

ESTUER v.a. 10 to store, reserve

EUFRAS(E) s. 10, 78, 36*, 79* eufrasy (Euphrasia officinalis) [FEW 3,249b] ME 1425

EYSIL s. 20 vinegar

FEL s. F. DU LEVRE 20 hare's gall

FEL(O)UN s. 27, 21*, 167* (index sub anthrax) abscess, ulcer, suppurating sore RUGE F. 27 [FEW 3,523a]

FELT(E)WORT (ME) s. 7*, 165* the great mullein (Verbascum thapsus) or felwort (Gentiana amarella)

FEN(O)IL s. 10, 9*, 98*, 148* F. -ROTE 0, 31, 78, 39* F. -CROP 122* fennel (Foeniculum vulgare) [FEW 3,454a]

FERINE s. F. de FEVES 13 bean flour

FESTRE s. C, 16 fistula, ulcer FESTYR (ME) 156* (and index sub carmina and festir) ME 1398

FEVRE s. F. AGUE 29 ague

FETHIRVOY s. 155* feverfew (Chrysanthemum parthenium) ME 1300

FILLIS (ME) s. 52* VILLIS 100* chervil (Anthriscus cerefolium) ME c.1125

FLEWRT (ME) s. 2, 4 'fleawort', variously applied (in 4 to pimpernel) ME 1400

FLUX s. 95* flux, discharge

FLUXE s. 13 dysentery [FEW 3,645b]

FORMIE s. 126*, 127* ant

FOXSISBLODE s. 171* blood of the fox

FRANKENCENS s. 92* FRONKENCENS 7* frankincense, olibanum ME 1398

FUM(E)TERE s. 0, 61, 98* (index sub fumeterre) FYMTER 52* FYMETER 83* fumitory (Fumaria officinalis) [FEW 3,857b 1372]

FUNDURE s. 0 FOUNDOUR (index sub foundour) 'fundacio'

GALYRSOUR (ME) s. 79* a disease

GANDIR-SMERE (ME) s. 3 grease of a gander

GARCER v.a. 86* to scarify (to allow bleeding)

GASIR (ME) s. 37 ? opoponax; [6] var. applied incl. to wild vine (Vitis sylvestris)

GLADYN(E) (ME) s. 140*, 153* RACINE DE G. 9* orris-root, rootstock of the iris

GLAVELYE s. 82* 'heyrive', cleavers (Gallium aparine)

GLASSYN KYLLE (Irish) [7] s. 57* bugle, wood betony

GLETENER s. 23* common burdock (Arctium lappa) [FEW 16,330b]

GLETTE s. 25 phlegm, mucus

---

[6] See Alphita ed. Mowat, p.84, 9 (and note).

[7] The glossary on f.15r has 'buglosa, anglice wodeburne .s. bugle, hibernice glaskil'. See the Royal Irish Academy, (Contributions to a) Dictionary of the Irish Language (hereafter DRIA) sub glasar which gives a variety of plants including wood betony. Dinneen's Irish-English Dictionary (1927) p.633 sub lasair gives glasair coille 'the plant common bugle'.

GOMME s. 141* gum, resin ME 1336

G(O)UTE s. C, 3, 4 GOUT 86 gout G. CORABLE C (index sub *carmina*) for *goute coral* = angina[?] or *goute curaunt* = gout that passes from joint to joint (ME 'þe goute mevande')

GOUTFAN s. 144* a type of fane?

GOUTOUS(E) a. 55* inducing the gout (of food) ME c.1425

GRAVEL(E) s. 93* (index sub *arena* & *urina*) gravel (med.) ME 1398

GRES s. G. DE CHEVER 86* goat's grease WYT G. 153* lard ME 1381

GRITTIS (ME) s. 18* 'simila avenatica', oat grains, oat flour

GROMILLE s. 71 GROMYL 106*, 111* common gromwell (Lithospermum officinale) [FEW 2,87a] ME 1300

GROUNDYSWYLY (ME) s. 52*, 145* groundsel (Senecio vulgaris) ME c.1150

HALF(E)WODDE (ME) [8] s. 83*, 167* wood ash

HELRYN-RINDIS (ME) s. 10* bark of the elder (Sambucus ebulus) ME c.1150

HENEBAN (ME) s. 1*, 164* henbane (Hyoscyamus niger) ME 1300

HENNPE (ME) s. 52* hemp HEMP-CROP 122* hemp (Cannabis sativa) ME 1303

HERBE COPPI s. 52* for *herbe copiere* (Cotgrave 'oeil de cerf', kind of wild parsnip)?

HERBE-IVE s. 52* buck's horn plantain (Plantago coronopus)

HERBE JOHAN s. 1, 52*, 87* H. JON 4, 30, 33, 77, 98*, 115*, 151* St John's wort (Hypericum perforatum) [FEW 5,48a 14th C.] ME c.1300

HERBE ROBERT s. 2, 52* Herb Robert (Geranium robertianum) [FEW 10,426a hap. 13th C.] ME c.1300

HERBE WATER s. 52* sweet woodruff (Asperula odorata) ME ? c.1425

HERTIS-TUNGE (ME) s. 0, 30, 31, 33, 77 HERTIS-TONG 34*, 48*, 98* hart's tongue fern (Phyllitis scolopendrium) ME 1325

HEVYR-FERNE (ME) s. 52* oak fern, common polypody (Polypodium vulgare)

HEY(H)OVE (ME) s. 2, 4, 62, 6*, 144*, 148*, 153*, 163* ground ivy (Glechoma hederacea) ME c.1325

HEYREVE (ME) s. 77*, 78* HEYRIVE 82* cleavers (Galium aparine) ME 1400

HOCK(YS) (ME) s. 6*, 10*, 98*, 144*, 153*, 163* various plants of the genera *malva* and *althaea* SMAL H. 138*, 148*, 153* ('malva agrestis') LITYL HOOK [sic] 82* 'malva minor'

HOLYHOKK(YS) (ME) s. 148* marsh mallow (Althaea officinalis) ME 1300

HORHOUND (ME) s. 48*, 69* HORSHUNDE 52* HORHUNNE 52 horehound (Marrubium vulgare) ME c.1150

HORPYN s. 52* orpine (Sedum telephium), sometimes applied to ground ivy (Glechoma hederacea) ME 1325

HORSEL (ME) s. 48* elecampane, horseheal (Inula helenium) ME 1300

HORSMYNT s. 48*, 115*, 150* horsemint (Mentha sylvestris) and other kinds of wild mint

HORWEY (ME) s. 117* (= *mousegras*) an error for *weyhore* (*filago*)

HOUNDEFENYL (ME) s. 20*, 85*, 110*, 113* stinking camomile (Anthemis cotula) ME 1400

HYMMEROLYS (ME) s. 117* a kind of potage

HYND(E)HAL(E) (ME) s. 48*, 52*, 57*, 89* wood sage, hindheal (Teucrium scorodonia) ME 1300

HYPPEBON (ME) s. 148*, 153* hipbone, ilium ME c.1150

HYVE (ME) s. 47* beehive

JARS s. 3 gander

JAUNDIZ s. 159* (index sub *ilyaca passio*) jaundice ME 1387

JUBARBE s. 86*, 99* houseleek (Sempervivum tectorum) [FEW 5,78b]

LACTUCE s. 48* garden lettuce (Lactuca sativa) ME ? 1450

LANG s. 14* sole [FEW 5,361b Cotgrave 1611 cf. TL 5,147b]

---

[8]   See Wright & Wülcker, *Anglo-Saxon and Old English Vocabularies* 1 (London, 1884), p.557, 45 and Zettersten, *op. cit.*, p.30 who cites Wright's *English Dialect Dictionary* 'Woody nightshade, *Solanum dulcamara*, or the clematis or honesty, *Clematis vitalba*'.

LATHYVE s. 46* 'pilosella, mouser', mouse-ear hawkweed (Hieracium pilosella)

LAUNCELÉ s. 27 ribwort plantain (Plantago lanceolata) [FEW 5,158a]

LAVANDIR s. 52* lavender (Lavandula officinalis) ME 1300

LINARY s. 31 LINORY 9*, 39* linary, toadflax (Linaria vulgaris) [FEW 5,369a 'linaria vulgaris' 15th C.] OED 1548

LITHYR FALLINGYS (ME) s. 4* (index sub morsus) = 'male casure' L. PRICHYNGGYS (index sub morsus) painful smarting

LIVERW(O)RT (ME) s. 31, 9*, 39*, 48*, 98* liverwort (?Marchantia polymorpha) ME c.1300

LONGYN (ME) s. (index sub pulmo) lungs

LORER s. 37 LOREL 66* bay (Laurus nobilis) [FEW 5,208b] ME 1381

LOVAGE s. 153* lovage (Levisticum officinale) [FEW 5,334b] ME c.1390

LUS CREY (Irish) [9] s. 13* burnet, speedwell

LUVACHE s. 98* lovage (Levisticum officinale) [FEW 5,334b]

LYMYK (ME) s. 64* 163* plant of genus Veronica, brooklime (Veronica beccabunga) ME ? c.1125

LYN s. 14 flax (Linum usitatissimum) [FEW 5,367b]

MAD(D)IR s. 1, 17, 48*, 52*, 151*, 167* M. -CROP 122* madder (Rubia tinctorum) ME c.1150

MAROL s. 48* black horehound (Marrubium nigrum) or common horehound (Marrubium vulgare) [FEW 6,i,377b] ME 1400

MASTIK s. 92* mastic, resin

MAT(E)FEL(O)UN (ME) s. 81 MADEFELOUN 52* MEDEFELOUN 87* M. - ROTE 30, 77, 20*, 21*, 96* knapweed: greater knapweed (Centaurea scabiosa), lesser knapweed (Centaurea iacea/nigra) ME 1400

MAY (ME) s. RED M. 83*, 85* ('huundefenyl) error for maythe, stinking camomile (Anthemis cotula) cf. Zettersten, op. cit., p.30

MAYDYNHER(E) (ME) s. 25, 30, 31, 34*, 39*, 114* maidenhair fern (Adiantum capillis veneris or Asplenium trichomanes)

MEDWORT (ME) s. 10* a herb, common balm (Melissa officinalis) ? ME 1300

MEL s. 20 honey

MENTE s. 12 mint

MERCHE (ME) s. 13, 29*, 57*, 92*, 108*, 163* wild celery, smallage (Apium graveolens) ME 1150

MERCURIALI (ME) s. 98* mercurial, mercury; the pot herb allgood (Chenopodium bonus Henricus) or annual mercury (Mercurialis annua) [FEW 6,ii,18a] ME ? 1425

MIIS s. pl. 61* breadcrumbs

MILEFOYL s. 52* milfoil, yarrow (Achillea millefolium) [FEW 6,ii,92b]

MISKYN (ME) s. 170* dungheap

MODERWORT (ME) s. 82* applied to a variety of herbs esp. mugwort (Artemisia vulgaris), motherwort (Leonuris cardiaca) and meadowsweet (Filipendula ulmaria) ME 1400

MOLD (ME) s. 110 top or crown of the head ME 1300

MOOL (ME) s. 62* (index sub morfea) sore, chilblain ME 1400

MORELE s. 27 MOREL 7*, 29* petty morel, belladonna, deadly nightshade (Solanum nigrum) [FEW 6,i,544a]

MOSSE (ME) s. ÞE REDE M. OF ÞE MOR 19* a kind of lichen

M(O)USER(E) (ME) s. 0, 4, 25, 30, 31, 33, 61, 8*, 20*, 21*, 46*, 52*, 92*, 96*, 128* mouse-ear hawkweed (Hieracium pilosella) ME 1300

MOUSGRAS (ME) s. 117* a plant (Cotgrave calls it joubarbe sauvage and wild prickmadame) variously identified as several kinds of vetch, as stonecrop (Sedum acre) and tête de souris (Vermicularis maior)

MUCHE CLIT (ME) s. 23* bardana, common burdock (Arctium lappa)

---

[9] See DRIA sub 1 lus (c) lus creidhe 'burnet, speedwell'. See also MS Add. 15403 f.15r 'burneta .i. lus cree'.

MUEL s. M. DE BEUF 7* ox marrow

MUGWRT (ME) s. 17 MOGWORT 48*, 151* M. -ROTE 30, 33, 77, 34*, 98* mugwort (Artemisia vulgaris) ME 1150

MUSSOUROUN s. 170* mushroom [FEW 6,iii,267b] ME 1400

MYNT s. REED M. 83* water mint (Mentha aquatica)

NAVYL (ME) s. 148*, 153* navel, umbilicus ME c.1150

NEDYNGGYS (ME) s. 117* bodily needs

NEPTE s. 48*, 52* catnip, catmint (Nepeta cataria) [FEW 7,93b] ME 1300

NETYL (ME) s. 52* nettle (genus Urtica) WYLD N. 52* RED N. 78* REED N. 83* REED-NETIL-CROP 122* BLYNDE N. 128*

OINT s. 10 animal fat O. DE JARS 3 O. DE CHAT 3 O. DE PORC 3, 7* O. DE COK 10 O. DE GELYNE 10 O. DE BERBIS 7*

OLIVE s. OYL DE O. 86*, 92* olive oil

ORPIMENT s. 141* orpiment, yellow arsenic [FEW 1,182a]

OYNGNOUN s. 3 onion

OYNGNOUR s. 126* ointment

PAPPE (ME) s. 161* gruel or porridge ME 1421

PARALISI s. 2 paralysis

PÉ DE COLUM s. 52* dovesfoot, wild geranium (Geranium columbinum) [FEW 8,299b]

PEDELYUN s. 83 lady's mantle (Alchemilla vulgaris), sometimes also christmas rose (Helleborus niger) [FEW 5,256a 'alchimille' 15th C.]

PELETRE s. 37 comon pellitory (Parietaria officinalis) [FEW 9.648b] ME c.1390

PELUSEL s. 25 mouse-ear (Hieracium pilosella) [FEW 8,504a]

PENIW(O)RT (ME) s. 32, 3* ?pennygrass (Cymbalaria muralis) ME c.1325

PEPELER s. BOURJUNS DE P. 3* poplar buds [FEW 9,181b]

PERCEPERE s. 52* the plant Alchemilla arvensis OED percepier 1610

PERSIL s. PERSOYL 9* P. -ROTE 0, 31, 78, 39* common parsley (Petroselinum crispum) ME c.1300

PERVENK s. 16*, 95* periwinkle (Vinca maior & minor) ME 1325

PESTIRNEP (ME) s. 136* parsnip (Pastinaca sativa) ME c.1390

PIGYL (ME) s. 52* stitchwort or great starwort (Stellaria holostęa) ME 1400

PIMPIRNEL s. 4 PIMPIRNOL 52*, 123* PIMPIRNOLE 92* 'pimpernel' variously applied ME 1400 [FEW 8,517a]

PLANTEYNE s. 13, 52* plantain, waybread (Plantago major) [FEW 9,19b]

PLATEYN s. 142* a paten [FEW 9,48b] ME 1450

POLIPODI s. 9*, 39*, 52* common polypody (Polypodium vulgare) or oak fern (Thelypteris dryopteris) [FEW 9,139b 15th C.] ME 1398

POLLITRICUM s. 0 Maidenhair spleenwort (Asplenium trichomanes)

PORSWORT (ME) s. 14* shepherd's purse (Capsella bursa-pastoris) ME 1400

POUCHE s. 13* pouch, bag

POUKISTHES (ME) s. 170* puffball (Lycoperdon bovista) OED puckfist 1601

POUKSPERE (ME) s. 111* plant with needle-like fruit, storksbill (genus Erodium) or shepherd's needle (Scandix pecten-veneris)

POYSOUN s. (index sub plaga) potion, drink

PRIM(E)ROL(E) s. 52*, 89* primrose, cowslip (genus Primula) [FEW 9,379a] ME c.1325

PULIOL MUNTAYNE s. 37 P. MONTAN 49* PULLEOL MONTAYNE 52* wild thyme (Thymus serpillum) or pennyroyal (Mentha pulegium) ME 1400

PULIOL REAL(E) s. 37, 49*, 52*, 92*, 150* pennyroyal (Mentha pulegium) or wild thyme (Thymus serpyllum) ME 1300

PUREE s. 54* soup or broth (often of leeks and peas) [FEW 9,610b] ME 1325

PURNELE DÉ BOYS s. 93* sloe (Prunus spinosa)

QUARTER s. 92* a unit of dry measure, approx. 8 bushels

QUINTEFOIL s. 1, 52* cinquefoil (Potentilla reptans) [FEW 2,ii,1481a]

RADICH (ME) s. 37, 113* radish (Raphanus sativus) R. -ROTE 0

RAGWORT (ME) s. 52*, 156* ragwort (Senecio jacobaea) sometimes applied to gladdon (Iris foetidissima) ME ? 1425

RAGYDWORT (ME) s. 57* ragwort ?

RAKYNGGYS (ME) s. 120*, 158* ('assensum matricis') displacement (index sub *matrix*)

RA(U)NCLE s. C (index sub *carmina*) RANKYL (index sub *inflacio*) impostume, abscess, malignant tumour

RATHELE (ME) [10] s. 77, 92* one of the germanders; or Rhinanthus crista-galli or Pedicularis palustris

RAY s. 14* fish of the genus Raia, ray or skate [FEW 10,34b] ME 1323

REQUILER v.a. 3 to collect, gather

REUBARBE s. 114* rhubarb (genus Rheum)

RIBBEWRT (ME) s. 17 RIBWORT 12*, 52*, 57*, 79* RYBWORT 158* narrow-leaved plantain (Plantago lanceolata) ME 1440

ROD(DIS) (ME) s. 34*, 39*, 57*, 138*, 167* marigold (Calendula officinalis) ME 1400

ROUNCE s. 52* bramble

RO(Y)SIN(E) s. 92* resin

RUE s. 10, 11, 36, 78 RU 138*, 147* rue (Ruta graveolens) [FEW 10,597a]

RY-MELE (ME) s. 53* rye meal, rye flour ME 1413

SAFRAN s. 79* saffron (Crocus sativus) [FEW 19,202a]

SAGE s. 83* SAUGE 52* WYLDE S. 169* sage (Salvia officinalis)

SAIM s. SEIM 3 S. DE PORC 10 WYT S. 142*, 153*, 165*, 166* seam, fat, hog's lard

SALPETYR s. 141* saltpetre (Potassium nitrate)

SAMROK (ME) s. 52* shamrock OED 1571

SANICLE s. 1, 30, 31, wood sanicle (Sanicula europaea), often applied to plants of various genera [FEW 11,183b]

SAUSFLEEME s. 81* saucefleme, swelling of the face accompanied by inflammation ME 1408

SCABIOS(E) s. 0, 4, 52*, 98* scabious, any of the plants of the genus Scabiosa [FEW 11,263a]

SECRÉ s. S. DE LA MESSE C prayer or prayers said by the celebrant at Mass in a low voice, after the Offertory and before the Preface [FEW 11,376b]

SEGG(YS) (ME) s. 157* sedge, esp. cyperaceous genera Carex and Cladium, often applied to the sweet flag (Acorus) and wild iris (Iris pseudacorus)

SELVEGREN (ME) s. 159* sengreen, most often the houseleek (Sempervivum tectorum), sometimes the sedums ME c.1000

SENÉ s. 80* senna, 'cassia officinalis' [FEW 19,153b]

SENEKYL s. 14*, 52*, 64*, 123* SENICLE 98* wood sanicle (Sanicula europaea) [FEW 11,183b *senicle* 14th C.] OED 15th C.

SEYNTE MARY WORT (ME) [11] s. 158* probably alecost, costmary (Chrysanthemum balsamita)

SKYRWYTT(YS) (ME) s. 132* skirret (Sium sisarum) OED 1338

SLOU (ME) s. 93* sloe, blackthorn (Prunus spinosa) OED c. 725

SNAYL (ME) s. 37* snail

SOLSIECLE s. 27 SOLSEKYL 52* marigold (Calendula officinalis) [FEW 12,73b] OED 1310

SOLUBLE s. 14 free from constipation ME 1400

SOURDOK (ME) s. SOURDOK(K)YS 14*, 138* common sorrel (Rumex acetosa) OED 1325

SOUR MILK s. 14* 'acetosum lac'

SOUTHRINW(O)DE (ME) s. 35, 88* SOUTHIRNEWODE 7* SUTHIRNWODDE 52* southernwood (Artemisia abrotanum) OED c.1000

---

[10] Cf. *Alphita* p.28,6 'mederatele' and MED sub *mede* n.(2) (a). In the glossary on f.3r *rathille* glosses 'Camepitheos, quercula maior'. *Chamaepitys* usually denotes a germander (Teucrium) or ground pine (Ajuga chamaepitys).

[11] Cf. 'erbe Sainte-Marie' in P. Dorveaux (ed.), *L'Antidotaire Nicolas . . .* (Paris, 1896) para. 75.

SPERGE (ME) s. 52* 'pé de colum', dove's foot cranesbill (Geranium molle)
SPINACLE [12] s. 4, 61, 52* SPINAKYL 52* spignel, baldmoney (Meum athamanticum) ?
SPIR (ME) s. 112* stem
STICHEWORT (ME) s. 1, 16* stitchwort (Stellaria holostea) OED c.1265
STIRYNG (ME) s. ANY STIRYNG AS A CREPINDE WORM 156* 'aliquem motum ad modum vermiculi repentis'
STOR (ME) s. 164* incense OED c.1000
STORAX CALAMIT(E) [13] s. 92* storax, resin of Styrax officinale [FEW 12,283a]
STROWBERYWISE (ME) s. 0, 30, 31 STREBERIWYSE 13*, 52* strawberry plant (genus Fragaria) OED c.1000
STRICHIL (ME) s. 109* (index sub uva) uvula
STU (ME) s. 152*, 153* stew, steam bath
SWOLLING (ME) s. 18* swelling
SWOWNYNG (ME) s. 21* swooning
SYNDYR (ME) s. 144* cinder
TANS(E)Y s. 52*, 122* TANESYE 1 tansy (Tanacetum vulgare) [FEW 13,i,79b] ME 1420
TETRYS (ME) s. 63* (index sub scabies & tetris) tetter, eczema [FEW 3,46a]
TEY(E) s. 20 (index sub occulus) web or cataract in the eye [FEW 13,302b] OED 1547
TRANSGLUTER v.a. 95* to swallow
TRET s. (index sub tret) poultice
TUNCARS (ME) s. 13 garden cress (Lepidium sativum) OED 700
TURBENTINE s. 92* TURBENTYN 142* turpentine, resin of the terebinth (Pistacia terebinthus) [FEW 13,i,236a]
TURMENTILLE s. 52*, 147* tormentil (Potentilla tormentilla) [FEW 13,ii,44b]
TYME s. 49* thyme (Thymus serpyllum) [FEW 13,i,317b]
VALERIAN s. 52* valerian (Valeriana officinalis) [FEW 14,135a] OED 1385
VELLE (ME) s. 62* skin, hide
VERLICHE (ME) a. 120* (index sub matrix) dreadful, terrible
VERME s. 16, 25 worm
VERTGRYS s. 64* VRTIDEGRES 7* verdigris [FEW 14,514a] OED 1300
VERVEYN(E) s. 52*, 92*, 151* vervain (Verbena vulgaris) [FEW 14,277a] OED 1390
VILLIS (ME) s. 100* chervil (Anthriscus cerefolium) ME c.1125
VINE s. 92* vine
VIOLET s. 9*, 34*, 39*, 48*, 52*, 66*, 69*, 92*, 156* VIOLET(T)E 0, 30, 31 violet
WAL(LE)W(O)RT (ME) s. 37, 42, 6*, 32*, 112*, 121*, 144*, 153* W. -ROTE 0 danewort, dwarf elder (Sambucus ebulus) OED c. 725
WALM(YS) (ME) s. 141* spell of boiling, wallop OED 1558
WARENCE s. 52* madder (Rubia tinctorum) [FEW 17,622b]
WARMOT (ME) s. 4, 17, 31, 73, 80, 29*, 83*, 98*, 113*, 138*, 139* wormwood (Artemisia absinthium) OED c. 725
WATERCARS (ME) s. 32, 150* WATIRCARS 89* water cress (Rorippa nasturtium-aquaticum)
WERT(IS) (ME) s. 171* wart
WETHWYND (ME) [14] s. 52* WYTHEWYNDE 89* bindweed (Convolvulus arvensis) OED c.1000
WEY (ME) s. 54* whey, serum OED c. 725
WEYBRED(E) (ME) s. 4, 31, 12*, 13*, 99*, 138*, 150*, 165*, 169* WAYBREED 57* waybread, plantain esp. Greater plantain (Plantago major) OED c.700

---

[12] DuCange has spinacellum 'peucedanum' (Peucedanum officinale, 'hog's fennel, sulphur wort'). See Alphita p.174 'Spigurnella g. et ang. spigurnelle vel freydele ... angl. spinagre'. Cf. MS Sloane 146 no.184, p.288 above, MS Sloane 962 f.4r 'spygurnole' and Müller, op. cit., p.70.
[13] See R. Arveiller in Romania 94 (1973), 176.
[14] Cf. glossary on f.6v 'Perichimenon, matris silva, caprifolium g. cheverefoile, a. wythewynde'.

WLAKKE (ME) a. 147* lukewarm, tepid OED 897
WOD-ACSYN (ME) [15] s. 141* ashes of burnt wood to make a lye
WODBYND (ME) s. 52* woodbine, convolvulus, or honeysuckle OED c.875
WODES(O)UR (ME) s. 17, 77, 52*, 92* woodsour, alleluia, wood sorrel (Oxalis acetosella)
    OED 1378
WODETHUNGE (ME) [16] s. 4 WODEÞONG 1*, 64* hellebore ?
WODROVE (ME) s. 52* woodruff (Asperula odorata) OED c.1000
W(O)RT (ME) s. 78, 9*, 39* wort, infusion of malt, unfermented beer OED 1000
WRECHING (ME) s. 18* (and index) retching OED c.1000
WYCHE-HASIL (ME) s. 141* witch hazel, applied to a variety of trees, esp. the wych elm
    (Ulmus montana) OED 1541–2
WYMAWE s. 60* WYMAW 153*, 165* marshmallow (Althaea officinalis) [FEW 4,422b]
WRMELE (ME) [17] 53* 'farina de vermibus'
WYTE (ME) s. 79* white of the eye
YAROW (ME) s. 7*, 13*, 20*, 165* yarrow (Achillea millefolium) OED c. 725
YEKESTERS (ME) s. 1*, 64* cuckoo pint (Arum maculatum) OED 1387
YHORNID (ME) p.p. 16* horned
YHORYDDE (ME) p.p. 57* made white, hoary
YSIFTYTE (ME) p.p. 50* sifted
YSOP(E) s. 78, 1*, 48*, 160*, 163* hyssop (Hyssopus officinalis) [FEW 4,528a]
YSTONEYD (ME) p.p. 163* stunned

GLOSSARY II (Latin) [18]

to Chapter 5, pp.217–63

ABSINTHIUM s. 96, 29*, 41*, 42*, 48*
ACCESSIO s. 104*, 155*
ACCORUS s. 153*
ACETUM s. 38, 47, 69, 89, 13*, 29*, 48*, 58*, 61*, 71*, 75*, 159*, 170*
ACULEUS s. 47*
AGRYMONIA s. 128*
ALBEDO (oculorum) s. 10, 55*
ALBUGO (oculorum) s. 19, 79*
ALBUM (ovi) s. 69
ALBUMEN (ovi) s. 5, 18, 31, 16*, 84*, 108*, 113*, 143*, 144*
ALLIUM s. 58, 55*, 109*
ALOES s. 40*
ALTEA s. 60*, 153*
AMBROSIA s. 37
AMIGDALA s. 129*, 136*
ANETUM s. 38*, 96*, 106*
ANGUILLA s. 65, 80, 87, 53*, 55*
ANISUM s. 80*, 137*
ANTRAX s. 15, 20, 21*, 22*, 77*, 82*, 142*, 167*, 169*

---

[15] See OED sub *woad-ashes*.
[16] Cf. Wright & Wülcker, *op. cit.* 19,9 & 391,40.
[17] See Bosworth & Toller, *Anglo-Saxon Dictionary* sub *wyrm-melu*.
[18] The glossary is largely intended as a checklist of ingredients. This time the Index is not included.

ANUS s. 150*
APIS ALVEARIA s. 47*
APIUM s. 44, 50, 29*, 38*, 106*, 108*
APOSTEMA s. 35, 61, 85*, 170*
ARCHA ANGELICA s. 128*
ARGENTUM VIVUM s. 89
ARSURA s. 58*, 71*, 124*
ARTEMESIA s. 72, 34*, 41*
ATTRAMENTUM s. 79*, 102*
AURIPIMENTUM s. 68*
AUXUGIA s. 60*, 142*
AVELLANUS s. 116* (nuces avellanas)
AVENA s. 69
AVENATICUS a. simila avenatica 18*; stramina avenatica 56*, 112*, 167*
AVENCIA s. 37, 89*
AZORUS a. 26*
BALNEACIO s. 12*
BARBA JOVIS s. 3*, 33*, 41*, 96*
BAUCIA s. 131*, 136*, 137*
BAUCON s. 5*
BETONIA s. 78
BETONICA s. 93, 31*, 75*, 76*
BOMBAX s. 22
BORAGO s. 56, 80*
BRODIUM s. 10*, 121*
BU[L]BUS s. 134*
BULLIUM (?) s. 137*
BURNETTA MAIOR s. 35, 88*
BURSA s. 33, 77, 99*, 112*
BURSA PASTORIS s. 14*
BUTIRUM s. 32, 64, 101, 3*, 8*, 36*, 56*, 57*, 82*, 141*, 142*, 153*, 163*
BUTIRUM DE MAYO s. 1 B. DE MAII 52*, 89*
BUTTUS (?) s. 46
CALAMINA s. 21
CALCULUS (med.) s. 93*, 168*
CALEFACTIO epatis s. 31, 3*, 10*, 99*
CALX VIVUS s. 141*
CAMAMILLA s. 78
CAMPHORA s. 50*
CANABUS s. 1, 37
CANCER s. 2, 9, 35, 88*, 156*, 157*
CANDELA s. 162*
CAPILLUS VENERIS s. 34*
CARDUUS BENEDICTUS s. 145*
CASEUM s. 67, 55*, 111*
CATAPLASMA s. 8*
CATAPLASMARE v.a. 13*, 112*
CAUDA stinccorum s. 137*
CAUDA PULLI s. 84*
CAULA / CAULIS s. 1, 94, 53*
CEDULA s. 2* SEDULA 45* SCEDULA 91*
CELIDONIA s. 79, 35*, 36*, 79*
CENTAUREA s. 37, 34*, 88*, 109*
CENTRUM GALLI s. 74*

CEPA s. 99 SEPA 42*, 55*, 134*
CEPULA s. 134*
CERA s. 64*, 145*
CERA VIRGINEA s. 28, 142*, 164*
CER(VI)FOLIUM s. 53, 41*
CIMINUM s. 22, 55, 29*, 33*, 38*, 96*, 153*, 164*
CINAMOMUM s. 49*, 137*
CLAUSTRUM PUDORIS s. 152*, 153*
COAGULACIO s. 56*, 57*
COAGULUM s. 104
COLLIRIUM s. 10, 52*
COLUMBINA s. 6, 7
CONCUSSUS p.p. 163*
CONFORTATIVUS a. 140*
CONGRUUS s. 14*
CONSOLIDA MINOR s. 1, 18
CONTAGIOSUS a. 15
COPROS s. 79*, 84*
CORNU CERVI s. 73*
CORROSIVUS a. 56*, 57*, 141*
CORVUS s. 35*
COTIDIANUS a. febris cotidiana 61*
CREPATURA s. 103*
CROCUS s. 68*, 80*
CURNELLUS s. 116*
DACTILIS s. 129*
DAUCON s. 163*
DAUCUS s. 49*
DECOCTIO s. 32, 33, 77, 14*, 36*, 88*, 90*, 112*, 114*, 129*, 141*, 167*
DEFECATUS a. 1, 17, 20*, 52*, 83*, 106*, 112*, 117*, 120*, 128*, 140*, 147*, 163*, 167*, 169*
DIADRAGANTUM [19] s. 135*
DIAFORON s. 129*
DIAPIGAMON s. 49*
DIASATURION [20] s. 49*, 129*, 136*
DISTEMPERO s. 55, 73, 76, 27*, 96*, 108*, 136*
DISTILLARE v.a. 109*
DITONIA s. 128*
DRAGAGANTUM s. 40*
DULCIDRIUS s. 78, 39*, 48*, 69*, 106*
DYAGREDIUM [21] s. 40*
EBRIOSUS a. 53
EBRIUS a. 93
EBULA s. 32*
EBULUS s. 30, 37, 42, 97*
EDERA s. 86, 41*, 111*, 141*, 168*
EDERA TERRESTRIS s. 34, 62, 82*
ELECTUARIUM s. 67, 40*, 49*, 50*, 101*, 129*
EMOROIDA s. 164*

[19] See Gille de Corbeil's *De laudibus et virtutibus compositorum medicaminum* ed. L. Choulant in *Aegidii Corboliensis, Carmina medica* (Lipsiae, 1826) p.96, 2, 626ff and Dorveaux, *ed. cit.* para. 23. See also P. Dorveaux (ed.), *Le livre des simples medecines* (Paris, 1913) para. 1120.
[20] See Choulant, *ed. cit.* pp.83ff (2,218ff), Dorveaux, *Antid. Nic.* 16.
[21] See Dorveaux, *Livre* . . . paras. 396–403.

EMPLASTRUM s. 2, 6, 35, 42, 90, 8*, 10*, 12*, 15*, 18*, 20*, 33*, 56*, 58*, 77*, 82*, 96*, 99*, 105*, 112*, 138*, 139*, 153*, 156*, 163*, 170*
EMUNDATUS a. 137*
ENDIVIA s. 48*
ENTRACTUM s. 92*
ENULA CAMPANA s. 48*
EPILENCIA s. 162*
EPITIMUM s. 80*
ERUCA s. 132*, 137*
ESULA s. 40*
EUFORBIUM s. 37
EUFRASIA s. 19
FABA s. 16*, 52*, 58*, 79*, 81*, 114*, 141*
FEBRIFUGA s. 155*
FEL s. arietis 65 galli 65 anguillarum 65 leporis 68, 103 caprinum 98 bovinum 102
FENICULUM s. 30, 34, 37, 50, 66, 78, 36*, 48*, 80*, 106*, 111*, 129*, 143*, 153*
FICUS s. 129*
FISTULA s. 15, 35, 142*, 156*
FLAGRIS s. 157*
FLEOBOTOMIA s. 41
FLEUMA s. 40*
FLORES s. pl. 121*, 151*
FLUXUS s. 23
FORMELLUM s. 83
FORMICA s. 80, 50*
FRAXINUS s. 95, 135*
FRAXINUS a. 56*, 141*
FRENESIS s. 54
FUNDACIO s. 30
GALANGA s. 49*, 149*
GARIOFILUM s. 37
GINGIBER s. 54* ZYNGIBER 128*
GLAREA s. 62*
GLEBA s. 12*
GRANUM SOLIS s. 111*
GRUELLUM s. 1*, 161*
GUMMA s. 37, 5*, 50*
GUTTOSUS a. 55*
HERBA JOHANNIS s. 151*
HERBA ROBERTI s. 1, 9, 88*
HERBA WALDECA (?) s. 88
HERBA WALTERI s. 1
HERMODACTULUS s. 40*
(H)IRCUS s. 132*
IMPEDIGO s. 36
INCENSUM s. 37
INEBRIARE v.a. 92
INFLATIO s. 144*
INFLATIVUS a. 139*
INOSSATUS a. gutta inossata 86
JUNCTURA humeri s. 139*
JUSQUIAMUS s. 3*, 164*, 165*
LAC s. L. CAPRINUM 41, 90* L. DULCE 53*, 55* ACETOSUM L. 14*
LACTUCA s. 54, 57, 48*

LAMINA plumbi s. 15
LAURUS s. 37 OLEUM LAURINUM 5*, 148*, 163*
LAVENDULA s. 37
LEPRA s. 62*
LEPROSUS a. 113*, 146*
LEVISTICUM s. 49*, 61*
LEXIVIUM s. 56*, 141*
LILIUM s. 105*
LINGUA AVIS s. 1, 135*, 137*
LINGUA CERVINA s. 34*, 41*, 111*
LINUM s. SEMEN LINI 39, 63, 90, 70* SUCCUS LINI 70
LIPPITUDO (oculorum) s. 21, 79*
LIQUIRICIA s. 30, 14*, 34*, 39*, 48*, 114*, 151* LIQUIRICA 31 LICORICA 33, 77 LIQUIRI-
    CIUM 0 LIQUORICIUM 80
LOLIUM s. 90
LUTUM s. 55*
MACEDONICUM s. 111*
MACIS[22] s. 49*
MACTA (?) s. 111*
MALVA s. M. MINOR 82* M. AGRESTIS 153*
MARATRUM s. 39*, 80*
MARCIATON[23] s. 5*, 164* MACIATON 148*, 153*
MARUBIUM s. 45, 52, 91
MATER HERBARUM s. 48*
MATRIX s. 48*, 120*, 121*, 157*
MEDULLA s. 37, 94
MEL s. 34, 38, 41, 64, 66, 67, 83, 84, 87, 97, 101, 103, 15*, 53*, 58*, 96*, 97*, 103*, 111*,
    128*, 136*, 138*, 143*, 156*
MENTA s. 37, 41*, 71*, 113*, 146*, 152*
MENTASTRUM s. 48*, 151*
MICA s. 61*
MILLEFOLIUM s. 1, 38
MIRRA s. 97
MORBUS CADUCUS s. 7, 46*, 162*
MORELLA MINOR s. 3*
MORFEA s. 62*
MORTIFERUS a. 26*
MORULA s. 52*
MUSCUS s. 137*
NASTURCIUM s. N. ORTENSE 37 AQUATICUM 37 RUBEUM AQUATICUM 70
NATES s. 12*, 152*
NEPTA s. 48*, 151*
NIDUM s. 34
NIMPHEA s. 75*, 76*
NUX INDIE s. 49* N. INDICE 137*
OLIVA s. OLEUM OLIVE 67*, 141*, 142*, 145*, 153*
OLUS s. O. RUBEUS 1
ORDEUM s. 33*, 41*, 72*, 77*, 82*, 96*, 107*
ORIGANUM s. 37
PARALISIS s. 37, 89*
PASTINATA s. 131*

---

[22] See *ibid.* para.s 770–74.
[23] See Dorveaux, *Antid. Nic.* 75.

PELUSETA s. 128*
PENIDEON [24] s. 129*, 136*
PENNA s. 67*, 141*
PENTAFILON [25] s. 1
PERETRUM s. 37
PERGAMENUM s. 50*
PES LEONIS s. 82*
PETROSILLINUM s. 39*, 48*
PETROSILLUM s. 30, 37, 69*, 106*, 111* P. MACEDONICUM 43
PILA s. 1, 33, 122*, 123*
PILOCELLA s. 46*
PILULA s. 37, 77, 57*
PINGUEDO s. 28, 74, 80 (apri) 6 (auce/ galline/ porci masculi) 19 (caponis) 21, 79* (lactis) 138*
PINNEA s. 137*
PINUS s. 42*
PIPER s. 50, 42*, 68*, 96* P. LONGUS 49*
PIRETA s. 54*
PISA s. 60, 55*
PISCIS s. 84, 111*, 133*
PISTACEA s. 137*
PISTACIUM s. 49*
PISTULA s. 82*, 142*
PIX s. 86
PLANTAGO s. 1, 5, 3*, 41*, 104*
PLASTRUM s. 56*
POPULEON s. 3*
POPULUS (bot.) s. 3*
PORRUM s. 23, 56, 71, 98, 55*
POTAGIUM s. 50*, 117*, 121*, 140*, 161*
PRIMULA VERIS s. 37
PUGILLUM s. 96*
PULEGIUM s. 45 P. MONTANUM 101*
PUTRESCO v.n. 15
PUTRUO v.n. 15
QUERCUS s. 40, 168*
RAFANUS s. 37
RAMNUS s. 1*
RANCLESCO v.n. 15
RANCLO v.n. 15
RAUCEDO s. 68*
RAUCITAS s. 115*
RESALGAR s. 141*
ROSA s. 79 R. RUBEA 14*
ROSACEUS a. AQUA ROSACEA 84*, 137*
RUBEDO s. (oculorum) 5, 21 (palpebrarum) 5, 8
RUBEUS TINCTORIS s. 48*
RUTA s. 22, 55, 65, 79, 92, 15*, 36*, 58*, 147*
SACCULUS s. 12*, 29*, 33*, 56*, 96*, 152*, 153*
SAL s. 52, 84, 78*, 104*, 109*, 144*, 150*
SALGIA s. 42*, 48*, 49*, 89*, 113*, 119*, 128*, 145*, 146*, 151*

---

[24] See *ibid.* 83 and Dorveaux, *Livre* . . . paras. 898–900.
[25] See Dorveaux, *Antid. Nic.* 84.

SALIX s. 59*
SALVIA s. 37, 27*
SAMBUCUS s. 30
SANATIVUS a. 56*, 57*, 113*, 141*
SANDALUS s. 40*
SATURIACIS s. 137*
SATURIO s. 130*, 136*, 137*
SAVINA s. 37, 42*
SAXIFRAGIUM s. 49*, 112*
SCABIES s. 56*, 57*, 63*, 98*
SCARIOLUS s. 48*
SCERUM s. 54*, 152*
SCOLOPENDRIA s. 48*
SENECIUM s. 45*
SEPUM s. 70 (ovinum) 18*, 63*, 64*, 124*, 163*, 164*, 165* (cervinum) 56*, 63* (porcinum) 110*, 116*, 153*, 165*, 166*
SERPILLUM s. 52
SETACUL s. 137*
SETACUM s. 137*
SILER MONTANUM s. 43
SILIGO s. 53*, 161*
SINAPIUM s. 37, 76
SIRPUS s. 65* S. MARINUS 65*
SOLSEQUIUM s. 34*, 57*, 76*
SORBUNCULUS s. 140*
SPINACI s. 137*
STERCUS s. 60, 90, 124*
STERQUILINIUM s. 170*
STINCCUS s. 129*, 133*
SUBFUMIGARE v.a. 144*, 151*
SUBFUMIGATIO s. 152*
SULPHUR s. 90, 56*, 62*
TERCIANUS a. FEBRIS TERCIANA 61*, 104*
TESTICULUS s. 137*
TESTUDO s. T. RUBEA 74, 37*
TIMPUS s. 54, 3*, 16*, 17*, 108*
TORMENTILLA s. 161* TURMENTILLA 147*
TORSIA s. 147*
TORTA s. 90*
TREMULUS s. 47
TRIFOLIUM s. 52*
TRITICEUS a. PASTA TRITICEA 71*
TURBITH s. 40*, 53*
TUSSIS s. 68*
UMBILICUS s. 73*, 148*, 153*
UMBILICUS VENERIS s. 3*
UNCTUM s. 90 (porcinum) 28, 37, 88* (cati, apri, anseris, altilium) 37
UNGUENTUM s. 37, 89, 5*, 56*, 57*, 63*, 88*, 148*, 153*
URINA s. 34, 42, 75, 102, 53*, 78*, 105*, 112*, 156*, 157*
URINALE s. 81*
URTICA s. 48, 49*, 111*, 113*, 146*, 150*
URTICA RUBEA s. 37
UVA s. 109
VEPRIS RUBEA s. 1

VERMIS s. 15, 40, 83, 96, 51*, 53*, 102*, 156*
VERVENA s. 79
VESICA s. 20*
VESPERTILIO s. 141*
VIOLA s. 80*
VIOLARIA s. 3*, 34*
VIRGA s. 58*, 112*, 130*, 137*
VITELLUM (ovorum) s. 67, 84*, 113*, 144*
VITREOLUM VIRIDE s. 84*
WARANCIA s. 1
YDROPISIS s. 0, 143*
YSOPUM s. 85, 49*, 147*, 151*, 160*
ZINZIBER s. 37, 49*, 149*
ZUC(C)URA s. 0, 54*, 101*, 114* SUCURA 149*

GLOSSARY (including notes)

to Chapter 6, pp.264–96

ACCÉS s. 173 attack (of illness)
ACHE s. 2, 6, 7, 62, 93, 95, 98, 100, 117, 127, 168, 182, 235 MENUE A. 99, 137, 215, 219,
    241 wild celery, smallage (Apium graveolens) [FEW 1,105a]
AFFODILLUS s. 180 ramsons (Allium ursinum) [FEW 1,157b]
AFUNDRER v.a. 118 to melt
AGRIMOINE s. 2 AGRIMONE 151 EGREMOINE 103, 108, 111 EGREMOYNE 7, 25 agrimony
    (Agrimonia eupatoria) [FEW 24,270a]
AGUE s. 205 ague
AGUSER v.a. 7 AGUCER 218 to render more active (of medicament)
AIL s. 118 AUS 37 AUZ 134 garlic (Allium sativum) [FEW 24,333a]
AIMANT s. 207 magnet
AISYLLE s. 12 vinegar see also EYSIL(LE
ALISA(U)NDRE s. 93, 168, 170, 201, 218 alexanders, horse parsley (Smyrnium olusatrum)
    [FEW 24,313b]
ALMONIAC s. 7 gum ammoniac [FEW 24,459a]
ALOE EPATIC s. 1 aloes [FEW 24,345b & 4,403b]
ALOEN s. 146 ALOES 158 aloes [FEW 24,345b]
ALOIGNE s. 8, 61, 122, 124, 137, 138, 141, 164, 165, 169, 177 ALOYNE 6, 9, 247 ALOYGNE
    31 ALOINE 235 wormwood (Artemisia absinthium [FEW 24,346a]
ALUN s. 225 common or potash alum [FEW 24,376b]
AMBROSIE s. 7, 108, 111, 219 'ambrosia', applied to a variety of plants esp. hindheal (Teu-
    crium scorodonia) [FEW 24,412b]
AMBROYSE s. 20 AMBROISE 121 see above
AME s. PAR AME 9 approximately
AMEROKE s. 57 AMAROKE 75 AMAROSCHE 237 AMERUSKE 101 LA BRUNE A. stinking
    camomile, mayweed (Anthemis cotula) [FEW 24,383a]
AMEURIR v.a. 5, 144 to ripen
AMIABLE a. 235 gentle, moderate (of heat)
ANDRA s. 95 probably betony (Betonica officinalis)

ANETE s. 85, 164 dill (Anethum graveolens) [FEW 24,559a]

ANGELTWACH(E (ME) s. 86 earthworm, lumbricus

AMIS s. 47 ANISE 168, 169, 180, 227 aniseed (Pimpinella anisum) [FEW 24,599a]

APOSTEME s. 4, 5, 57, 143, 144, 145 impostume, abscess

APOSTOLICON s. 6 Apostles' ointment

ARESTEBEOF s. 67 RESTEBEOF n. 65 restharrow, cammok (Ononis repens) [FEW 1,146b]

ARGENTILLE s. 101 applied to a variety of plants; perhaps silver weed (Potentilla anserina) [FEW 1,136b]

ARGUIL s. 147 argol, tartar of wine, crude potassium bitartrite

ARMOYSE s. 212 mugwort (Artemisia vulgaris) [FEW 1,149a]

ARREMENT s. 61, 118, 199, 202 oak gall

ARUNDE s. 78, 234 swallow

ARSUN s. 148 burn, burning

ARTEMESE s. 231 mugwort (Artemisia vulgaris) [FEW 1,149a] see also ARMOYSE

ARUBRE s. 7 ? error for *marubre* (Marrubium vulgare) [FEW 6,i,377b]

ATTERLOÞEBERIE (ME) s. 102 berry of plant used as antidote, esp. betony and black nightshade (Solanum nigrum)

AUBE ESPINE s. 7, 89 hawthorn (Crataegus monogyana)

AUBE PRUNERE s. 141, 142 plum tree (Prunus domestica)

AUBON s. 35, 202 AUBUN 99, 128, 141, 151, 188, 215 white of an egg

AVENCE s. 2, 7, 8, 9, 97, 108, 109, 110, 111, 112, 113, 121, 129, 218, 219 wood avens (Geum urbanum)

AVEROYGNE s. 23 AVEROIGNE 167, 179 AVERONIE 240 AVEROYNE 47, 160 southernwood (Artemisia abrotanum) [FEW 24,48a]

AYREN (ME) s. pl. 102 eggs

BAGE s. 147 bag, pouch [FEW 1,204a inadequate]

BAIE DE LORER s. 9, 21 BAEES DE L. 59 berry of the bay (Laurus nobilis)

BARDANE s. 205 common burdock (Arctium lappa) [FEW 1,264b]

BATERIE s. 5 battery, beating

BATURE s. 123 viscous mixture of ingredients, a paste or plaster

BERZIZE s. 169 barley malt, wort

BETOYNE s. 18, 27, 73, 129 BETOINE 245 wood betony (Betonica officinalis) [FEW 1,345b]

BISE s. 194 hind

BOCE s. 6 boil, sore

BOILLUN s. 8, 9 (time taken for) boiling

BOLACE s. 105 bullace (Prunus insititia) [FEW 1,624a]

BOLETER v.a. 66, 94 to bolt, sift

BOTUN s. 195 hip

BRAN s. B. DE FORMENT 139, 249 wheat bran

BRER (ME) s. RED B. 102 dog rose (Rosa canina)

BRIONIE s. 137 bryony (Bryonia dioica) [FEW 1,580a inadequate]

BRUÉ s. 227 broth

BRUSURE s. 3, 5, 138 fracture

BRUSWORT (ME) s. 102 daisy (Bellis perennis) or comfrey (Symphytum officinale)

BUGLE s. 2, 7, 109, 121, 129, 219 bugle (Ajuga reptans) sometimes confused with bugloss [FEW 1,600a]

BURE s. 19, 20, 26, 49, 61, 83, 127, 150, 221 butter B. DE MAY 2, 4, 5, 8, 9, 10, 83, 205, 212, 217, 218, 219, 235 may butter

BURJUN s. 205, 217 (poplar) bud

BURNETTE s. 93, 185 n. 30 burnet, great burnet (Sanguisorba officinalis), garden burnet (Poterium sanguisorba), or common pimpernel (Anagallis arvensis) [FEW 15,i,308b]

BUTTRE OF MAY (ME) s. 102 may butter

CALAMENTE s. 8, 47 common calamint (Calamintha officinalis) [FEW 2,i,53a]

CALKETRAPPE s. 18 caltrops (Centaurea melitensis) or star thistle (Centaurea calcitrapa)
     [FEW 2,i,65a]
CAMAMILLE s. 20, 27 common camomile (Anthemis nobilis) [FEW 2,i,148a]
CANCRE s. 114, 115, 116, 120 malignant tumour
CANEVAZ s. 217 linen, canvas
CAPILLUS VENERIS s. 169 maidenhair fern (Adiantum capillus-veneris) [cf. FEW 2,i,250a]
CASTOR s. (7) 19 beaver
CASTORIE s. (7) 9, 218 medicament derived from the scent glands of the beaver, castoreum
     [FEW 2,i,474b]
CAUL s. RED C. 102 red cabbage
CEDEWAL (ME) s. 34 setwall, zedoary
CELIDOINE s. 7, 26, 95, 117, 197 SELIDOYNE 26 greater celandine (Chelidonium majus)
     [FEW 2,i,634a]
CENGLE s. 204 herpes, impetigo or shingles
CENTONICLE s. 47 sea-wormwood (Artemisia maritima) [FEW 11,187a]
CENTORIE s. 73, 97, 166, 193, 223 CENTORYE 6, 43 CENTOYRE 16, 64 common centaury
     (Centaurium erythraea) or yellow centaury (Blackstonia perfoliata) [FEW 2,i,583b]
CEPHALEA s. 245 a variety of the helleborines (Cephalanthera)?
CERFOIL s. 2, 19, 41, 131 CERVOILLE 93 chervil (Anthriscus cerefolium) [FEW 2,i,37b]
CERISE s. 79 cherry
CERISER s. 170 cherry tree
CERLA(U)NGE s. 46, 112, 169, 185, 190, 221, 237 hart's tongue fern (Phyllitis scolopen-
     drium) [FEW 2,i,614b]
CERVOISE s. 18, 42, 43, 44, 57, 61, 95, 109, 111, 121, 129, 164, 166, 169, 185 SERVEISE
     223 SERVEYSE 222 barley beer
CHANVETTE s. 58, 113 and n. 78 hemp (Cannabis) [FEW 2,i,210a]
CHANVRE s. 108, 121 KANVRE 219 hemp (Cannabis) [FEW 2,i,210a]
CHAPUN s. 36 capon
CHENLANGE s. 84 hound's tongue (Cynoglossum officinale) [FEW 5,362a]
CHENULÉ s. 87, 161, 162, 163, 171, 205 henbane (Hyoscyamus niger, 'jusquiamus') [FEW
     2,i,86a]
CHEVREFOIL(LE s. 7, 20, 85 CHEVEREFUR 241 honeysuckle (Lonicera periclymenum / ca-
     prifolium) or red clover (Trifolium pratense) [FEW 2,i,308b]
CHEYURE s. 5 fall [FEW 2,i,26a]
CHIKENEMETE (ME) s. 138 chickweed (Stellaria media)
CHOLET s. ROUGE C. 7, 108, 219 red cabbage (Rubeus olus) C. VERMAIL 121 [FEW
     2,i,535a]
CINCE s. 156 CINSE 103 strip of material, bandage
CIRE s. 1, 19, 235 wax C. VIRGINE 2, 3, 4, 5, 6, 8, 9, 20, 213, 219 virgin wax
CLAREE s. 59 clary, clear-eye (Salvia sclarea) cf. ESCLARÉ
CLOTE (ME) s. 205, 217 common burdock (Arctium lappa)
CLOU s. 143 boil, furoncle, carbuncle [FEW 2,i,771a]
CODE (ME) s. 4 KODE 7 KODE DE NORTWEIE 7 'code', cobbler's wax, mastic
COK s. 152 cock
COLIZ s. 103, 147 cullis, clear strained broth [FEW 2,ii,878b]
COLUMBINE s. 143, 219 columbine (Aquilegia vulgaris) [FEW 2,ii,930a 'Cotgr. 1611' inade-
     quate]
COMIN s. 1, 4, 5, 80, 186, 191 COMYN 227 cumin (Cuminum cyminum) [FEW 2,ii,1526a]
CONFIRE v.a. 235 to prepare, concoct
CONFIRIE s. 2, 102, 128, 129 comfrey (Symphytum officinale) [FEW 2,ii,1030a]
CONSOUDE s. 2, 128, 129, 172 consound, comfrey (Symphytum officinale) LA MENUE C. 7
     'consolida minor', daisy (Bellis perennis) [FEW 2,ii,1076b] C. LA GRANDE 20 'consolida
     maior', comfrey (Symphytum officinale) [FEW 2,ii,1076a]
COPERUN s. 2, 7, 205 top, tip (of plant)

CORIANDRE s. 168 coriander (Coriandrum sativum) [FEW 2,ii,1184a]

CORN DE CERF s. 6, 118 hart's horn; also possibly herb ivy, buck's horn plantain [Plantago coronopus] [FEW 2,ii,1196a]

CORN DE TOR s. 117 horn of a bull

COSTE s. 246 costmary (Chrysanthemum balsamita), sometimes also costus root (root of Saussurea lappa) [FEW 2,ii,1254a]

COSTIVÉ a./ s. 62 costive, constipated (person)

COSTIVEURE s. 61 constipation, costiveness

COUPERE s. 46, 190 COPERE 205 rendered by 'liverwort' in many glossaries, probably Anemone hepatica, see Hunt, *Plant Names*, p.108

COUSLOPPE (ME) s. 201 cowslip (Primula veris)

COYPEL s. 217 cutting, tip (of plant)

CRASE GELINE s. 205 fat hen (Chenopodium bonus Henricus) [FEW 4,39b gives late examples applied to a variety of plants]

CREPPE MALVE (ME) s. 7 CRESPE MALVE 20 curled marrow (Malva crispa)

CRESSUN s. C. DE FONTAYNE 7 water cress (Rorippa nasturtium-aquaticum) [FEW 16,384b]

CROISSIR v.n. 157 to make a crackling sound

CROPPE (ME) s. 102 any part of the plant except the root

CROSTE s. 18 crust

CROULEURE s. 201 unsteadiness, shaking (of the legs)

CROUP s. 121 any part of the plant except the root

CROWESOPE (ME) s. 111, n. 70 soapwort (Saponaria officinalis)

CURSUN s. 66 diarrhoea

CYCOREE s. 46, 190 chicory (Cichorium intybus) [FEW 2,i,665a]

CYREMONTAYNE s. 34 sermountain, hartwort (Seseli montanum) [FEW 11,611a]

CYRUN s. 157 itch mite (Acarus scabiei) [FEW 17,67b]

DATE s. 83, 105, 121, 243 urine

DELIÉ a. 66 fine

DERTE s. 146, 147, DERTRE n. 88 tetter, eczema, herpes [FEW 3,46a]

DESESTOPER v.a. 170 to unblock

DIETER v.a. 179 to diet

DITAINE s. 130 DITAYNE 91 dittany (Origanum dictamnus or Dictamnus albus) [FEW 3,70b]

DRACHE s. 110, 111 solid waste of herbs after removal of juice [FEW 3,156b]

DRAGANT s. 1, 2 tragacanth, gum-dragon

DRAGANTE s. 152 DRAGAUNCE 251 dragonwort (Dracunculus vulgaris)

É s. 41 bee

EBLE s. 12, 16, 61, 63, 137, 149, 182, 201, 218, 252 EBLEE 18, IEBLE 55 dwarf elder, danewort (Sambucus ebulus) [FEW 3,202a]

EGLENTER s. 20 eglantine (Rosa rubiginosa)

EMERAUDES s. pl. 74 haemorrhoids, piles

EMFLURE s. 5 swelling

EMPLASTRE s. 13, 24, 25, 27, 35, 49, 75, 85, 100, 104, 107, 108, 127, 128, 132, 139, 141, 171, 191, 201, 202, 235 ENPLASTRE 64, 127, 235 plaster, salve

EMPLASTRER v.a. 133, 149, 163, 186, 204 to apply plaster to

ENBEU p.p. 205 steeped, soaked

ENCENS s. 6 incense BLAUNC ENCENZ 250

ENCYRER v.a. 9 to wax

ENDIV(I)E s. 46, 190 endive, chicory, wild lettuce (Cichorium intybus and endivia) [FEW 4,784b]

ENPLENTER v.a. 127 to splint

ENREVRE a 174 inflamed, angry

ENTRERUS s. 185 middle bark ('cortex mediana'), alburnum, sapwood

ENTRET s. 2, 3, 4, 5, 6 ENTRETE 124 salve, plaster

ERE s. 29 IERE 14 ivy (Hedera) BAYE DE E. 218 ivy berry GUMME DE IERE 189 ivy gum
   (Y)ERE TERESTRE 7, 21, 23, 28, 35, 177 ground ivy (Nepeta glechoma) [FEW 13,i,262a]

ERMOYSE s. 47, 169 mugwort (Artemisia vulgaris) [FEW 1,149a]

ESCHAUDEURE s. 149 scald

ESCLARÉ s. 43, 193 clary, clear-eye (Salvia sclarea) cf. CLAREE

ESCUMER v.a. 20, 61, 104, 123 to skim

ESPERVIER s. 210 sparrowhawk

ESPIGORNEL s. 184 SPIGURNELE n. 47 ? spignel, baldmoney (Meum athamanticum)

ESPINE s. NEIR E. 6 blackthorn (Prunus spinosa)

ESPOI s. 213 spit

ESQUASSER v.a. 130, 145, 153, 189 to crush

ESQUINANCIE s. 57 quinsy

ESTAL s. 82 urine

ESTAL a. 42, 95, 223 stale

ESTALER v.n. 76, 80 to urinate v.a. 81 to discharge with the urine

ESTANCHER v.a. 65 to staunch, stop the flow of v.n. 156 to cease flowing

ESTOPER v.a. 109, 243 to stop, plug, block

ESTUPES s. pl. 13, 220 ESTOUPES DES LINZ 114 fibres of tow [FEW 12,314b]

ESTUER v.a. 9 to store, reserve

EUFRASYE s. 20 eufrasy (Euphrasia officinalis) [FEW 3,249b]

EURUQUE s. 89 rocket (Eruca sativa) [FEW 3.242b]

EWE BENEITE s. 79, 86, 209 holy water

EWE ROSE s. 20, 162, 170, 198 rose water

EY (ME) s. 102 egg

EYSIL / EISIL s. 6, 15, 24, 28, 29, 31, 33, 37, 38, 70, 135, 160, 186, 189, 205 vinegar

FARCINE s. 214 farcy

FAVEE s. 171 FAVEE DE L'EWE 80 an aquatic plant, perhaps water plantain (Alisma plantago-aquatica); often used to gloss ME *lemke* (brooklime) and Lat. *favida / fabaria*, thus possibly indicating Veronica beccabunga or Sium angustifolium / latifolium, 'water parsnip'.
   [FEW 3,340b suggests Berula angustifolia and Sium angustifolium]

FELUN s. 4, 97, 99, 100, 101, 102, 135, 184, 236 suppurating sore, ulcer, carbuncle

FENEGREC s. 1 FENUGRECH 5 FENIUGREZ 180 fenugreek (Trigonella foenum-graecum)
   [FEW 3,461b]

FENOIL s. 7, 45, 46, 47, 51, 53, 62, 76, 89, 93, 169, 182, 190, 197 FENIL 20, 168, 181, 203
   FENOYL 224, 227 FENUIL 30, 31 fennel (Foeniculum vulgare) [FEW 3,454a]

FENS s. F. DE COLUMB 218, 245 dove droppings

FEOR s. A FEOR DE 142 in the manner of

FESTRE s. 107, 108, 109, 111 fistula, ulcer F. CHANCRÉ 106 cancerous ulcer

FEUGERE DE CHESNE s. 44 polipody of oak, oak fern (Thelypteris dryopteris (L.) Slosson)
   [FEW 3,515a]

FEUGEROLE s. 6 royal fern, osmunda (Osmunda regalis) [FEW 3,515a]

FEU GREGEYS s. 211 Greek fire [FEW 4,210b]

FEUTRE s. 127 (piece of) felt

FEVE s. 136, 198 bean NEIRE FEVES 118, 242 FARINE DE F. 14 bean meal FLUR DE F. 16
   bean flour

FEVRE s. 175, 206, 214 fever F. AGUE 170, 172 ague F. COTIDIANE 174 quotidian fever F.
   TERCEINE 173 tertian fever F. QUARTAYNE 231 quartan fever

FIBRA LINI s. 246 fibres of flax

FIEL s. gall FEIL DE CHEVRE 115 FEIL DE LIEVRE 22 FEL DE TOR 37

FIENTE s. dung, droppings F. DE CHIEVRE 126 F. DE OWE 83 F. DE VACHE 154

FISIKE s. 82 the science of medicine

FLUR (ME) s. WHETENE F. 102 wheat flour

FONDRER v.n. 5 to melt

FORMAGE s, 70 cheese

FORMI s. 189 ant

FRANC ENCENS s. 1, 2, 3, 4, 5, 7, 8, 9, 20, 103, 108, 177 frankincense

FRASERE s. 2, 46, 190 FRASER 230 strawberry plant

FREIDELE s. 116 'spignel' [cf. FEW 1,157], see Rothwell, ZFSL 86 (1976), 241

FRENE s. FREYNE 247 ash ESCORCE DE F. 51, 247 ENTRERUS DE FRESNE 185

FUMETERE s. 45 FUMITERE 172 fumitory (Fumaria officinalis) [FEW 3,857b]

FUNDIZ s. 8 FUNDRIZ 9, 20 residue, dregs

FURMENT s. FLUR DE FL. 65, 99, 100, 123, 180, 215, 229 corn flour FARINE DE F. 94, 127, 140, 142

FUSSELET s. 3 sprig

GALBANUM s. 7 galbanum, a gum resin derived from plants of the genus Ferula [FEW 4,23b]

GARGARISME s. 196 gargle

GARLEC (ME) s. 120 garlic (Allium sativum)

GARZ s. 212 gander

GAZERE s. 8, 9 [f.47r commedatur fructus gazar']? cf. Alphita 84, 9 'gasir .i. seminis junci'; often indicates 'vitis sylvestris'

3EKESSURE (ME) n. 88 cuckoopint (Arum maculatum)

GELINE s. 152, 210 hen

GENEITE s. 8 broom (Sarothamnus scoparius)

GINGIVRE s. 8, 55, 168 GINGEVRE 9 ginger (Zingiber officinale) [FEW 14,663b]

GLANDRE s. 178 glander, swelling of the lymphatics [FEW 4,146b]

GLEDENE (ME) s. 48 and n. 48 sword iris

GLEIRE s. 140, 250 yolk of an egg

GLETONERE s. 217, 238 common burdock (Arctium lappa) [FEW 16,330b]

GLETTE s. 53, 224 mucus, phlegm [FEW 4,157a]

GOMME ARABICH s. 1 GUMME A. 2, 4 gum arabic

G(O)UTE s. 14, 16, 18, 109, 201 gout G. AUGERE 188 dropsy FREIDE G. 7, 8, 212 'gutta frigida' G. EMFLE 10 G. ENOSSÉ 12 gout in the bones G. FESTRE 110, 214 fistular swelling G. CHAIVE 206 'gutta caduca', epilepsy G. PODAGRE 248 podagra, gout in the feet

GRAVELE s. 242 wine lees, tartar [FEW 4,225b]

GROMIL s. 76, 168 GRUMIL 93 common gromwell (Lithospermum officinale) [FEW 2,87a]

GRUNDESWILIE (ME) s. 62 groundsel (Senecio vulgaris)

GRUND YVI (ME) s. 120 ground ivy (Glechoma hederacea)

GWYMALVE s. 20 marshmallow (Althaea officinalis) [FEW 4,422b]

HATEREL s. 159 hattrel, nape of the neck

HERBA MUNDA s. 219 'malva'; in MS Sloane 146 f. 70r it is glossed 'gallice sparge'

HERBE JOHAN s. 7, 8, 20, 169 H. JON 218 St John's wort (Hypericum perforatum) [FEW 5,48a]

HERBE ROBERT s. 100, 108, 110, 111, 113 H. ROBERD 218 Herb Robert (Geranium robertianum) [FEW 10,426a]

HERBE WATER s. 7, 108, 109 ERBE WALTER 219 sweet woodruff (Asperula odorata)

HERBE YVE s. 10, 217 buck's horn plantain (Plantago coronopus)

HERMODACLE s. 104 a dried root of an Asiatic plant Colchicum luteum, also used of meadow saffron / autumn crocus (Colchicum autumnale) [FEW 4,416a]

HONDESTONGE (ME) s. n.129 hound's tongue (Cynoglossum officinale)

HONISOCCLE (ME) s. 85 common honeysuckle (Lonicera periclymenum), also common red clover (Trifolium pratense)

HORSSELLE (ME) s. 183 horseheal, elecampane (Inula helenium)

HORWORT (ME) s. n. 78 cudweed (Filago germanica)

HUAN s. 210 owl

HUNI (ME) s. 102, 120 honey

IBARNT (ME) p.p. 120 burned

JARCER v.a. 16 to scarify

JAUNIZ s. 95, 96 n. 70 jaundice

JUBARBE s. 10, 44, 137, 171, 191, 205, 217 houseleek (Sempervivum tectorum) [FEW 5,78b]
KACIE s. 202 rheum
KANEVAZ s. 9, 20, 205, 218 KANEVAS 11 canvas
KARDUN s. VEIR K. 208 thistle
KAREWY s. 62 KAREWI 168 caraway (Carum carvi) [FEW 2,i,377b]
KERSON s. 36, 64 cress K. EWAGE 19 K. DE EAWE 169 water cress (Rorippa nasturtium-
    aquaticum) K. DE CORTIL 72 K. KE CREST EN KURTIL 232 garden cress (Lepidium
    sativum) [FEW 16,384b] LE RUGE K. 139, 249
KNEPISTEL (ME) s. 51 butcher's broom (Ruscus aculeatus)
LAIT s. 76, 174 LEET 89 DUZ L. 64 LET DUCE 142 L. DE CHEVRE 58, 65, 136 L. DE FEMME
    191
LANCELÉ s. 2, 99 LAUNCELEE 7, 216 ribwort plantain (Plantago lanceolata) [FEW 5,158a]
LANGE DE CERF s. hart's tongue fern (Phyllitis scolopendrium) [FEW 5,361b 'seit 1530']
LARD s. 61, 233 LART 150 fat
LARDUN s. 61 strip of (bacon) fat
LASHANTONWORT (ME) s. 199 groundsel (Senecio vulgaris). In MS Harley 2258 f.184v
    'lastunwort' glosses 'grundeswilie'
LAUREOLE s. 59 bay, laurel (Laurus nobilis)
LAVENDRE s. 7, 8, 9, 20, 129, 218 lavender (Lavandula officinalis)
LEMEKE (ME) s. 138 brooklime (Veronica beccabunga)
LESCHE s. L. DE PAIN 12 slice
LESSIVE s. 192 LESCIVE 208 lye
LETUE s. 45, 89, 163, 205 lettuce
LEVÉ a. 180 well risen, leavened (of bread)
LIE s. 139 LIES 249 lees (of wine)
LIEVRE s. 22, 76 hare
LIMASUN s. 242 snail
LIN s. 203 flax SEMENCE DE L. 135, 141, 142 linseed
LINOIS s. 122, 136, 137, 138 linseed [FEW 5,368b]
LIQUORIZ s. 46, 51, 168, 190 LICORIZ 47, 199, 200 liquorice (Glycyrrhiza glabra) [FEW
    14,173b]
LIVREWORT (ME) s. 190 liverwort, probably Anemone hepatica, see COUPERE
LIZ s. 137 lily
LORER s. 7, 8, 9, 21 FOILLE DE L. 212, 218 BAEES DE L. 59 bay (Laurus nobilis) [FEW
    5,208b]
LOVA(S)CHE s. 7, 8, 30, 218 LOVESCHE 2 LUVESCHE 44, 93, 95 LIVESCHE 164, 168
    lovage (Levisticum officinale) [FEW 5,334b]
LUZ s. 71 pike (ict.)
LYMACHUN s. NEIR L. 11 snail
MALVE s. 20, 141, 154, 201 MAUVE 85 LA GRANT M. 148 LA PETITE M. 148 mallow
    (Malva sylvestris) or marshmallow (Althaea officinalis) [FEW 6,i,129a]
MAMELE s. 86, 87, 88 breast
MANDRAGE s. 161, 205, 217 mandragora, mandrake (Mandragora officinalis) [FEW 6,i,159a]
MANGUE s. 30 scabies, mange
MAROIL s. 54, 182, 193, 240, n.100 MAROYL 42, 43 MAROILE 221 black horehound (Mar-
    rubium nigrum) or common horehound (Marrubium vulgare) [FEW 6,i,377a]
MASELIN s. 18 drinking cup or goblet of veined maple wood
MASTICH s. 4 MASTIK 6, 109, 180 MATIK 7 mastic
MATHEFELUN s. 10, 98, 102 MATHEFELON 191 MATEFELUN 219, 237 MATEFOLON s.
    152 knapweed; greater knapweed (Centaurea scabiosa), lesser knapweed (Centaurea
    iacea/nigra) [FEW 6,i,519b]
ME(I)DENEHER (ME) s. 46, 85, 190 maidenhair fern (Adiantum capillus-veneris or Asple-
    nium trichomanes)
MEDEWRT (ME) s. 7 a herb, probably common balm (Melissa officinalis)

MEK s. 63, whey [FEW 6,ii,43b]

MEL s. 12, 19, 24, 25, 30, 38, 41, 45, 53, 61, 99, 100, 105, 109, 115, 117, 132, 158, 166, 202, 219, 224, 244, 248 MIEL 14, 106 honey

MELLER s. 160 medlar (Mespilus germanica) [FEW 6,ii,44b]

MENESUN s. 65, 66, 72, 74, 228, 230, 232 diarrhoea

MENTE s. 8, 80, 163, 168, 169, 228, 251 mint

MERCH (ME) s. 102 wild celery, smallage (Apium graveolens)

MERCURIAL s. 205 mercurial, mercury; the pot herb allgood (Chenopodium bonus Henricus) or 'annual mercury' (Mercurialis annua) [FEW 6,ii,18a]

MERER v.a. 3, 9 to stir, mix, knead

MEULE s. 194 marrow

MIE s. 74, 140 crumbs, soft part (of bread, pastry)

MILFOIL s. 7, 64, 74, 219, 229, 230 MILFOILLE 84, 186 milfoil, yarrow (Achillea millefolium) [FEW 6,ii,92b]

MOEL s. 74, 100, 127, 188 MOL 248 yolk of an egg

MOL s. M DE SUY 236 pith of the elder [FEW 6,i,635a]

MOLEYNE s. 7, n. 58 MOLEINE 111 mullein (Verbascum thapsus) [FEW 6,iii,52a]

MORELE s. 10, 97, 150, 152, 171, 199, 205, 217, 237, n. 84 M. LA PETITE 137 petty morel, belladonna, deadly nightshade (Solanum nigrum) [FEW 6,i,544a]

MOSCHE s. 153 MUSCHE 209 fly

MOSSEAUS s. pl. 228 small pieces

MUSERE (ME) s. 205 mouse-ear hawkweed (Hieracium pilosella)

NAVELD-ROTE (ME) s. 8, 9 root of the navelwort (Umbilicus rupestris)?

NEP (ME) s. WILDE N. 178 bryony (Bryonia dioica)

NI s. 78, 234 nest

NOGAGE s. 208 walnut, fruit of Juglans regia [FEW 4,36b]

NOIZ s. 41, 121 (wal)nut

NOWEUS DE POME DE PIN s. pl. 212 pine kernels

NUMBIL s. 186 navel

OIGNUN s. 213 onion

OIL(L)E s. 188 oil O. DE LORER 9 O. DE NOIZ 8 O. DE OLIVE 5, 8, 50, 138, 219 O. DE POPI 163 O. ROSIN 245

OINT s. 187 animal fat O. DE CHAPUN 144 O. DE CHAT SAUVAGE 213 O. DE PORC 124, 205, 235 O. DE TESSUN OU DE BUTOR U DE LEUN 18 O. DE VEER 19 O. DE VEIR 17, 144

OPPOPONAC s. 7 opoponax, medicinal gum obtained from the juice or the herb of the genus Opoponax, like Ferula [FEW 7,374b]

OREVALE s. 116 ORVALE 219 orpine (Sedum telephium) and applied to a variety of plants incl. clary (Salvia sclarea) cf. TL 6, 1318 'muskateller Salbei, Scharlei'.

ORGANIE s. 169, 200 one of several plants of the genus Origanum esp. wild marjoram (Origanum vulgare), sometimes also wild thyme or pennyroyal [FEW 7,414b]

ORGE s. 38, 100, 107, 135, 191 barley

ORIGANUM s. 95 a plant of the genus Origanum, see ORGANIE

ORPI(E)MENT s. 117, 146, 189, 241, 244 orpiment, yellow arsenic [FEW 1,182a]

ORTIE s. 16, 36 nettle RUGE O. 8, 9, 19, 76, 150 O. VERMAIL 121 red nettle

OS s. 125, 130 bone O. DE HUME 117

OSMUNDE s. 2, 7, 128, 129 royal osmund, flowering fern (Osmunda regalis)

OWE s. 36, 83, 148, 213 goose

PAPELOTES s. 65 porridge

PARELE s. 84, 94, 133 (que crest en ewe), 146, 172, 183, 235 sorrel, dock (Rumex acetosa) [FEW 7,639a]

PARITARIE s. 109, 110 pellitory of the wall (Parietaria diffusa)[FEW 7,654a]

PARLESYE s. 9 paralysis, palsy

PARLETIK a. 206 paralytic

PASTEL s. 130 poultice

PEIS s. P. RE(I)SINE 1, 5, 6, 7 pitch-resin

PEIVRE s. 30, 54, 55, 76 pepper

PEIZ s. 2, 4 pitch P. NEIR 6

PELOTE s. 94, 121, 205, 220 ball, pellet

PELUEITE s. 7 PELUETTE 113, n. 83 PELUSETTE 109 PYLUETTE 219 mouse-ear hawkweed
(Hieracium pilosella) [FEW 8,504a]

PELUSELE s. 68 PILOSELLE 205 see above

PENIL s. 76 penis

PENIWORT (ME) s. 205 pennywort, 'umblil as dames' (Umbilicus rupestris (Salisb.) Dandy)

PENNE s. 83, 110, 148 (goose) quill

PERCHE DE CERF s. 66 stag's antlers [FEW 8,279b]

PERER s. 170 pear tree

PERSIL s. 20, 45, 47, 51, 76, 93, 98 PERCIL 46, 168, 182, 190 PERCILE 169 common parsley
(Petroselinum crispum / sativum) [FEW 8,325b]

PERVENKE s. 2 periwinkle (Vinca maior and minor) [FEW 14,461b]

PESCHER s. 170 peach tree

PHILAGO s. 109 varieties of cudweed, genus Filago

PIGLE s. 2, 7 greater stitchwort or great starwort (Stellaria holostea)

PIMPERNOLE s. 2 PIMPERNELE 219 'pimpernel', variously applied, esp. the burnets (Sanguisorba officinalis and Paxterium sanguisorba) and pimpernel (Anagallis arvensis) [FEW
8,517a]

PIOYNE s. 95, 158, 206 PYONE 34 peony (Paeonia officinalis) [FEW 7,464b]

PLANTAINE s. 2, 74, 108, 109, 116, 151, 205, 241 PLANTAYNE 10 PLANTAIN 173 PLAN-
TEIN 171 PLAUNTAIGNE 217, 238 PLAUNGTAYNE 230 plantain, waybread (Plantago
maior) [FEW 9,19b]

PLANTE s. 205 PLAUNTE DES PEZ 233, 239 sole (of the foot)

POINTURE s. 154 sting

PO(U)KE s. 9, 11 20 pouch

POLIPODIE s. 19, 169, 227 (crest sur la cheine) polipody (Polipodium vulgare) or oak fern
(Thelypteris dryopteris) [FEW 9,139b]

POMER s. 170 apple tree P. DE BOIS 6 crab-apple tree

POPI (ME) s. 161, 162, 205 poppy (Papaver)

POP(I)LER s. 205, 217 POPELER 241 poplar tree (Populus)

POPILION s. 205 populeon, ointment made with poplar leaves or buds [FEW 9,182a/b]

PORET s. 2 leek (Allium porrum)

POUZ s. 205 pulse

PREENDRE v.a. 2, 5, 7, 10, 110, 196, 205 PREIENDRE 212 to press

PRIMEROLE s. 7, 8, 9, 34, 39, 187, 201, 218 primrose, cowslip (genus Primula) [FEW 9,379a]

PRIMEROSE (ME) s. n.153 primrose (Primula veris)

PRUNELE DÉ BOYS s. 222 sloe (Prunus spinosa) [FEW 9,494b]

PULIOL s. 33, 44, 165, 169 wild thyme (Thymus serpyllum) or pennyroyal (Mentha pulegium) P. REAL 20, 43, 54, 193 pennyroyal P. MONTAIN(E) 43, 193 either of the above
[FEW 9,521a]

PURCEL s. 204 piglet

PURREAL s. 196 leek (Allium porrum)

QUAREL s. 130 bolt (of crossbow)

QUARTERUN s. 1, 137 one fourth of an ounce in apothecaries' weight; also one fourth of a
pound

QUINT(E)FOIL s. 2, 7, 219, 225 cinquefoil (Potentilla reptans) [FEW 2,ii,1481a]

QUITURE s. 109, 202 pus, suppuration

RAIZ s. 77 RAYS 153 radish [FEW 10,27a]

RA(U)NCLE s. 2, 3, 135, 137, 138, 140, 214, 235 impostume, abscess, malignant tumour

RASCURE DE YVOYRE s. 94 scrapings of ivory

RAVRE s. 242 'grappe de raisin depouillee de ses grains' [FEW 16,653b 'seit 1549']

RECETTE s. 5 (medical) receipt

RECHELES (ME) s. 102 incense

RECOUPÉ s. 96 'morsus diaboli', devil's-bit scabious (Succisa pratensis)

RELÉS s. 18 relief (from symptoms of illness)

RESINE s. R. BLANCHE 235 crude resin

RESTEBEOF s. see ARESTEBEOF

RETOR s. 170, 172 recurrence

REUME s. 177 rheum, catarrh [FEW 10,376a]

REVRE a. 76 obstinate, recalcitrant (aphetic form of enrievre, FEW 4,815b)

REYNETTE s. 20 meadow sweet (Filipendula ulmaria) [FEW 10,212a]

RIBBEWORT (ME) s. 102 RIBWORT 120 narrow-leaved plantain (Plantago lanceolata)

ROELE s. 77 round slice, segment

ROIGNE s. 183 scabies

ROSE s. 20, 46, 85, 92, 177, 190, 197 rose

ROULE s. 211 parchment roll

ROVENTELE s. 40 a type of natural rouge

RUBARBE s. 246 rheubarb (Rheum barbarum) [FEW 10,348a]

RUE s. 8, 15, 21, 24, 30, 35, 47, 89, 95, 132, 164, 197, 218 RUWE 240 rue (Ruta graveolens) [FEW 10,597a]

RUNCE s. 2, 7, 164, 195 bramble R. VERMAIL 121 COPERUN DE R. 205 TENDRUN DE R. 108, 219, 241

SAFRAN s. 94, 168, 144 saffron (Crocus sativus) [FEW 19,202a]

SAIM s. 7, 55, 61 (animal) fat S. DE PORK 5, 88, 217, 218, 252 S. DE OES 148

SALPETER s. 211 saltpetre, potassium nitrate [FEW 11,81b]

SALT (ME) s. 120 salt

SANICLE s. 7, 121, 129, 217, 219, 221 wood sanicle (Sanicula europaea) often applied to plants of various genera [FEW 11,183b]

SARCOCOLLE s. 1 sarcocol, gum sarcocolla, produced probably from species of Astragalus

SARRE-PIZ s. 240 angina ?

SARREE s. 19 savory (Satureia hortensis) [FEW 11,252a]

SAUCEFLEUME s. 198 saucefleme, swelling of the face accompanied by inflammation [FEW 11,108b]

SAUGE s. 2, 7, 8, 9, 23, 95, 179, 206, 218, 226, 247 sage (Salvia officinalis) [FEW 11,132a]

SAUSE DE MER s. 151 brine [FEW 11,108b]

SAVINE s. 8, 17, 32, 95, 212, 218 savin, savine (Juniperus sabina) [FEW 11,5b]

SAVON s. 36 SAVUN 40, 124, 146 soap

SAXIFRAGE s. 62, 168 SAXEFRAGE 113 plant of the genus Saxifraga [FEW 11,258a]

SCABIOUSE s. 169 field scabious (Knautia arvensis) [FEW 11,263a]

SCHELLE (ME) s. 120 (egg) shell

SCHEPES SMERE (ME) s. 102 sheep's grease

SEGLE s. 12, 18, 106, 117, 128, 191 rye

SEIGNÉ s. 142 bleeding

SEIGNER v. refl. 52, 206 to have oneself bled

SEL s. 19, 37, 38, 66, 100, 116, 151, 220, salt SEL ARS 117

SENEÇHUN s. 171 SENEISUN 144 SENESUN 138 SENESÇUN 199 groundsel (Senecio vulgaris) [FEW 11,446a]

SEU / SIU s. 134 S. DE BOF 235 S. DE BUK 19 S. DE MOTUN 3, 4, 84, 135, 136, 139, 178, 235, 249 S. DE TOR 37 animal fat

SEU s. 7, 56 SAUZ 211 elder (Sambucus) [FEW 11,6a]

SILOTRE 189 depilatory [FEW 9,501a]

SMEREWORT (ME) s. 2, 205 allgood (Chenopodium bonus Henricus)

SOFT (ME) s. n.129 mullein (Verbascum thapsus)

SOLSECLE s. 179 SOLSICLE 241 marigold (Calendula officinalis) [FEW 12,73a]

SOLUBLE a. 63 free from constipation or costiveness
SORVENUE s. 215 accidental injury, mishap
SOURDOKE (ME) s. SCHORDOCKE n.129 SCORDOCKE n.129 sorrel (Rumex acetosa)
SPARGE s. 7, 109, 110, 113 asparagus (Asparagus officinalis) [FEW 1,156a]
SPIRGRAS (ME) s. 102 applied to various plants incl. 'spearwort' (varieties of Ranunculus) and 'couchgrass' (Triticum repens)
STONCROP (ME) s. 217 n. 97 STANCROP n.101 stonecrop (Sedum acre)
SUCRE s. 45 sugar
SUFFRE s. 211 sulphur
SURSANÉ p.p. 124 scarred, cicatrized
SWINESCRASSE s. n.100 hog's fennel (Peucedanum officinale)
SWINES SMERE (ME) s. 102 swine's grease
SWOM (ME) s. n.100 ? rose-gall
TAN s. 119, 220 tan, crushed bark esp. of oak TAN DUST (ME) 120 [FEW 13,i,82a]
TANESEIE s. 129 TANESY 129 TANESEYE 121 THANESEIE 7 tansy (Chrysanthemum vulgare) [FEW 13,i,79b]
TECCHELURE s. 192 rash
TEIGNUS a. 37 suffering from tinea
TENTE s. 124 tent (med.), pledget
TESTE DE SORIZ s. 205, n. 97 stonecrop (Sedum acre) [FEW 13,i,275b 15th C.]
TESSUN s. 18, 213 THESSUN 218 badger
TETER (ME) s. n. 88 tetter
THIME s. 8, 20 thyme (Thymus serpyllum) [FEW 13,i,317b]
TORMENTINE s. 7 tormentil (Potentilla tormentilla) [FEW 13,ii,44b]
TRIFOIL(LE s. 7, 20, 219 clover, plant of the genus Trifolium [FEW 13,ii,295b]
TRESSE s. TRACE DE AIL 118 TRACE DE AUS 37 bulb of garlic
TRIACLE s. 58 theriac, treacle, antidote[FEW 13,i,308a]
TUILE s. 65 tile
TUNFILLE (ME) s. 131 chervil (Anthriscus cerefolium)
TURTEL s. 18, 106, 229 cake
UMBLIL s. 64, 90, 205 navel
UMBLIL AS DAMES s. 205 pennywort (Umbilicus rupestris (Salisb.) Dandy / Cotyledon umbilicus-veneris L.)
UNGLE DE PORC s. 82 pig's trotter
VALERIANE s. 97 valerian (Valeriana officinalis) [FEW 14,135a]
VANE (ME) s. n. 53 fane, 'saponaria minor'
VEIRE s. 192 VERE 220 glass
VENESUN s. 69 venison
VENTOSER v.n. 16 to cup, bleed
VENTUOSITÉ s. 227 wind, flatulence
VERFLEZ a. 157 ?
VERM s. 64, 86, 186, 195 worm V. DE TERRE 125, 130, 145 earthworm
VERMINE s. 214 parasitic, infestive insects [FEW 14,292b]
VERTE GRECE s. 124 verdigris
VERVEINE s. 2, 43, 193, 197, 209 VERVEYNE 17 vervain (Verbena officinalis) [FEW 14,277a]
VETOINE s. 238, 239 betony, bishopwort (Betonica officinalis) [FEW 14,360a]
VINEGRE s. 50, 103, 105, 108 etc. vinegar
VIOLE s. 130, 205 violet [genus Viola]
VIOLETTE s. 10, 44, 46, 85, 141, 190, 217 violet [genus Viola]
VIVE CHAUZ s. 117, 124, 128 V. KAUZ 220 quicklime
VOMITE s. 53, 224 vomit [FEW 14,631a]
VOMITE s. 55 vomitory [FEW 14,631a]
VOUTHÞISTEL (ME) s. 34 VOUUEÞISTEL 102 card thistle or teasel (Dipsacus sylvestris)
WARENCE s. 108, 113, 121 WARAUNCE 219 madder (Rubia tinctorum) [FEW 17,622b]

WEIBRODE (ME) s. 102 waybread, plantain (Plantago maior)
WIFLEF (ME) s. 102 cinquefoil (Potentilla reptans)
WILDE TESEL (ME) s. 85 WILDE TESLE 107 teasel (Dipsacus sylvestris)
WISPELON s. 209 holy water sprinkler [FEW 17,599b]
WODEROVE (ME) s. 81 woodruff (Asperula odorata)
WYMALVE s. 48, 88, 141, 148, 201, 218, 235 WIMALVE 133, 137 marshmallow (Althaea officinalis) [FEW 4,422b]
YDROPESIE s. 168 dropsy
YSOPE s. 20, 42, 43, 46, 91, 95, 190, 193, 238 hyssop (Hyssopus officinalis) [FEW 4,528a]

SELECT GLOSSARY

to Chapter 7, pp.297–310

Included are all medical and botanical terms. Common words of standard Old French are not recorded. Verbs are listed under the form of the infinitive.

ACHE s. 2, 9, 46 HACHE 26, 64 wild celery, smallage (Apium graveolens) [FEW 1,105a]
AIL s. 72 garlic (Allium sativum) [FEW 24,333a]
ALIS a. PAN A. 9 unleavened bread
ALOINE s. 13, 28, 39, 67 wormwood (Artemisia absinthium) [FEW 24,346a]
ALUM s. 80 ALUN 79 common or potash alum [FEW 24,376b]
AMBROYSE s. 13 ambrosia; various herbs esp. *eupatorium* (hindheal or wild sage), sometimes wood germander (Teucrium scorodonia) [FEW 24,412b]
ANISE s. 52 anise, aniseed (Pimpinella anisum) [FEW 24,599a]   .
APOSTOLICON s. 42 an ointment, apostolicon
ARAGÉ p.p. 53, 54 mad, rabid
ARGENT s. VIF A. 16 quicksilver
ARNEMENT s. 35, 59 ARREMENT 47 oak-gall, or vitriol
AROUÉ p.p. 72 hoarse
ASSEZ s. 57 for *accés*, attack (of illness)
ASTANCHER v.a. 19, 22 to staunch
ASTOPER v.a. 50 to block up, obstruct
ASTRE s. 44 hearth
ASUAGER v.a. 61, 67 to relieve, alleviate
ATRETE s. 13, 42, 67 poultice
AUBE ESPINE s. 55 hawthorn
AUBUN s. 54, 64, 67 white of egg
AUNE s. 83 alder (Alnus glutinosa) [FEW 15,14b]
AVENCE s. 13, 61 wood avens (Geum urbanum)
AVEROIN s. 5 southernwood (Artemisia abrotanum) [FEW 24,48a]
AYSIL s. 60 vinegar
BENEITE a. HERBE B. herb bennet, variously applied e.g. common hemlock (Conium maculatum) and wood avens (Geum urbanum) [FEW 1,323b]
BETOINE s. 84 wood betony (Betonica officinalis) [FEW 1,345b]
BRASIL(L)E s. 79, 80 brazil-wood, red-wood (Sequoia sempervirens [FEW 15,258a]
BRIOYNE s. 21 bryony (Bryonia dioica) [FEW 1,580a]
BUGLE s. 13, 68 BUGLE 61 bugle (Ajuga reptans) [FEW 1,600a]

BURBELETTE s. 49 pustule, boil

BURE s. 18, 53 butter B. DE MAY 14, 15, 78 DE MAY B. 4 May butter

CALEMENTE s. 16, 20 common calamint (Calamintha officinalis) [FEW 2,i,53a]

CANCRE s. 23 carcinoma, tumour

CANELE s. 52 cinnamon [FEW 2,i,202a]

CANEVAS s. 13, 14, 70 canvas

CASTRIZ s. 69 wether

CERFOYLE s. 75 chervil (Anthriscus cerefolium) [FEW 2,i,37b]

CERLANGE s. 4 hart's-tongue fern (Phyllitis scolopendrium) [FEW 2,i,614b]

CHOLET s. ROCHE C. 11 ROUCHE C. 13 red cabbage (rubeus olus) [FEW 2,i,535a]

CINSE s. 31 strip of material, bandage

CIRE s. 11, 13, 14, 17, 31, 42, 66 SIRE 49, 70 wax VIRGINE C. 77 virgin wax

CIROYNE s. 13 wax plaster [FEW 2,i,597a]

CLOU s. C. DE GILOFRE clove [FEW 2,i,771b]

CODE s. 11, 13, 31, 49 'code', cobbler's wax, mastic (ME *cude, code* etc.)

COLER v.a. 4, 79 to strain

CONFIR(E) s. 44, 45, 61 comfrey (Symphytum officinale) [FEW 2,ii,1030a]

CONSAUDE s. 61 consound, comfrey MENU(E) C. 9 daisy (Bellis perennis) [FEW 2,ii,1076b]

COPERUN s. 1 top, tip (of plant)

DEBRUSER v.a. 44 to break, fracture

DECHASSER v.a. 65 to expel

DEMINCER v.a. 60 to chop up

DEPESSER v.a. 13 to fracture

DESTEMPRER v.a. 1, 16; 24, 32, 35, 50, 54, 74 to dissolve in, combine with water or other liquid, to distemper

DESTRESSE s. 74 painful constriction (of the chest)

DIETE s. 69 diet

DITAINE s. 36, 62 dittany (Origanum dictamnus or Dictamnus albus) [FEW 3,70b]

DOCKE, DOCHE s. D. ROCHE 18 RUGE D. 78 red-dock (Rumex sanguineus) [FEW 15,63b]

EBLE s. 15, 26, 73 dwarf elder, danewort (Sambucus ebulus) [FEW 3,202a]

EGREMOYNE s. 54, 65, 68 agrimony (Agrimonia eupatoria) [FEW 1,55a]

EISIL s. 16, 32 vinegar

EMPLATRE s. 7, 8, 17, 26, 45, 76 plaster

ENCENS s. 42, 59 incense

ENDUCIR v.a. 65 to sweeten

ENFLURE s. 24, 29 swelling

ENREVRE a. 65 refractory (to treatment)

ENTEMPRER v.a. 80 to mix, blend

ENTRETE s. 31, 42, 43, 49, 64, 67, 70 ANTRETE 49 salve, plaster

ENT(E)RUS s. 73 middle bark, cortex mediana [FEW 4,763a]

ENVOLUPER v.a. 70 to wrap

ERE s. E. TERESTRE 8, 68 ground ivy (Nepeta hederacea) [FEW 13,i,262a]

ERUKE s. 55 rocket (Eruca sativa) [FEW 3,242a]

ESCALE s. 70 shell

ESCORCE s. 83 SCORCE 41 bark

ESPLENTER v.a. 44, 45, 70 to splint

ESPURGE s. 74 spurge (Euphorbia) [FEW 3,314b]

ESPURGER v.a. 20, 65 to purge

ESTAMPER v.a. 1 to grind, crush

ESTANCHER v.a. 52 STANCHER 60 to staunch v.n. 51 to stop (flowing)

FANC s. 65 marshland

FELUN s. 7, 8, 9, 10, 13 suppurating sore, carbuncle, abscess, ulcer [FEW 3,523a]

FEMETERIE s. 18 fumitory (Fumaria officinalis) [FEW 3,857b]

FENOIL s. 55 fennel (Foeniculum vulgare) [FEW 3,454a]

FERINE s. F. DE ORGE 8 barley-flour F. DE SEGLE 24, 43, 45, 64, 67 rye-flour
FESAUNT s. 69 pheasant
FEVE s. 72 broad bean
FEVERUS a. 58 feverish
FRANC ENCENS s. 14, 18, 26 frankincense
FUR s. 5 oven
GALLIGAL s. 52 galingale (Alpinia officinarum) or English galingale (Cyperus longus) [FEW
    19,61b]
GELINE s. 69 hen
GILOFRE s. CLOU DE G. 52 clove
GLAIOL s. 50 gladden (Iris pseudacorus) [FEW 4,143a]
GLEIRE s. 27 white of egg [FEW 2,i,738a]
GLETINERE s. 9 burdock (Arctium lappa) [FEW 16,330b]
GRESSE s. fat G. DE PORC 14 G. DES OYSEUS 14
GUMME s. 70 gum, resin
HOLIOC (ME) s. 18 marsh mallow (Althaea officinalis)
JAUNE s. 82 applied to a variety of plants [see FEW 4, 25b/26a]
JUBARBE s. 33 houseleek (Sempervivum tectorum) [FEW 5,78b]
KAR s. 69 flesh, meat
KERSUN s. 56 cress
LANCELÉ(E) s. 13, 24, 65 ribwort plantain (Plantago lanceolata) [FEW 5,158a]
LART s. 30, 45, 53 lard, animal fat
LAVENDRE s. 61 lavender (Lavandula officinalis)
LESSIVE s. 76, 80, 81 lye
LET s. 58, 69 milk L. DE CHEVRE 30 goat's milk
LETER v.a. 22 to suckle
LETUE s. 54 lettuce [FEW 5,124b]
LIC(O)UR s. 24, 79 liquid
LIMACEUN s. 78 snail
LUMBRIS s. 32, 33, 34 lumbricus, intestinal worm (Ascaris lumbricoides)
MAROIL s. 4, 13 MARIOL 6 MAROINE 5 horehound (Marrubium vulgare) [FEW 6,i,377a]
MASTIX s. 14 mastic, resin
MATEFELUN s. MATAFELUN 13 METAFELUN 9 one of the varieties of knapweed; matfel-
    lon (Centaurea nigra), greater knapweed (Centaurea scabiosa), lesser knapweed (Centau-
    rea iacea) [FEW 6,i,519b]
MAUVE s. M. DE CORTIL 11, 13, 49 marsh mallow (Althaea officinalis)
MECHE s. 50 whey [FEW 6,ii,43b]
MENE(I)SUN s. 48, 51 diarrhoea
MENTE s. 34, 38, 52 spearmint (Mentha viridis)
MILLEFOILE s. 24 MILFOYLE 37 MILFOILE 51 MILFOYL 54 milfoil, yarrow (Achillea millefo-
    lium) [FEW 6,ii,92b]
MIRE s. 65 doctor
MOEL s. MOUIUEL 9 MOUEL 10 MOUUEL 67 yolk of egg
MOILLER v.a. 60, 70, 79, 83 to steep, wet
MOLUR s. 83 filings [FEW 6,iii,33a]
MORELE s. 7, 8, 26, 41, 53 petty morel, belladonna, deadly nightshade (Solanum nigrum)
    [FEW 6,i,544a]
NAIER v.a. 42, 65, 77 to clean, cleanse
NIER v.a. 65 to clean, cleanse
NIUUELE s. 50 wafer, light cake [FEW 7,70a]
NORISER v.a. 58 to act as wet-nurse to
NORUSE, NURUSE s. 55 wet-nurse
OINT s. 16, 26, 42 WNT 54 UNT 67 animal fat, grease, lard
OLIVE s. 67 olive

OSMUNDE s. HOMUNDE s. 61 royal osmund, flowering fern (Osmunda regalis)

ORTIE s. ROUGE O. 1, 53, 60 red nettle (Lamium purpureum) O. MORTE 37 dead nettle (lamium album?) [FEW 14,68a]

PALESIM s. 5, 65 paralysis [FEW 7,639a]

PARELE s. 15, 16, 65 sorrel, dock (Rumex ssp.) [FEW 7,639a]

PASTEL s. 62 plaster

PÉ DE COLUN s. 9 dovesfoot, wild geranium (Geranium columbinum) [FEW 8,299b]

PÉ DE LEUN s. 74, 76 pes leonis, lion's leaf (Leontice leontopetalum?) or lady's mantle (Alchemilla vulgaris) [cf. FEW 8,299b and 5,256a]

PEIS s. 14, 17 pitch

PEIVRE s. 39 pepper

PERCHE s. P. DE CERF 32 stag's antlers [FEW 8,279b]

PERSIL s. 41 common parsley (Petroselinum crispum / sativum) [FEW 8,325b]

PERTERIS s. 69 partridge

PERTUS s. 13, 31 PERTUSE 31 opening

PILOSE(I)T(T)E s. 65, 66, 71 mouse-ear hawkweed (Hieracium pilosella) [FEW 8,504a]

PIMPERNELE s. 75 applied to a variety of plants, especially the burnets (Sanguisorba officinalis and Paxterium sanguisorba) and pimpernel (Anagallis arvensis) [FEW 8,517a]

PLANTAINE s. 4, 7, 13, 15, 22, 51, 54, 56, 57, 63, 65, 68 broad-leaved plantain, waybread [FEW 9,19b]

POLIPODIE s. 23 common polipody (Polipodium vulgare) or oak-fern (Thelypteris dryopteris) [FEW 9,139b]

POMIZ s. 77 pumice

PRIMEROLE s. 25 variety of the genus Primula [FEW 9,379a]

QUAREL s. 62 crossbow bolt, shaft of an arrow

QUINQUENERVE s. 63 ribwort plantain (Plantago lanceolata)

QUINTEFOYLE s. 51 cinquefoil (Potentilla reptans) [FEW 2,ii,1481a]

QUITURE s. 13 suppuration

RAER v.a. 8, 17, 76 to shave

RANCLE s. 1, 26, 27 impostume, abscess, malignant tumour

RANCLER v.n. 69 to fester, suppurate

RAPHANE s. ROPHANE 4 radish [FEW 10,63b]

REBOYLER v.a. 4 to reboil

RECOPEYE s. 40 devil's-bit scabious (Scabiosa pratensis)

ROINE s. 15, 16, 18, 78 herpes, scabies, eruption of the skin

RUE s. 5, 29, 39 RUWE 38, 55 rue (Ruta graveolens) [FEW 10,597a]

SANER v.a. 42, 43, 59, 69 to heal

SANGUINERE s. 19, 51 applied to a variety of plants with styptic properties, including the genus polygonum, especially knot-grass (Polygonum aviculare), but also used of shepherd's purse (Capsella bursa-pastoris) [FEW 11,164a]

SANICLE s. 15, 61 wood sanicle, often applied to plants of various genera [FEW 11,183b]

SAUGE s. 13, 54, 65 sage (Salvia officinalis) [FEW 11,132a]

SAVINE s. 13, 35, 72 savin, creeping juniper (Juniperus sabina) [FEW 11,5b]

SAVUN s. 80 soap

SEIM s. 11, 45 animal fat, grease SEIM DE CERF 8

SERVEISE s. 4, 29, 39, 61, 65 SERVESE 41 ale

SPARGE s. 15 asparagus [FEW 1,156a]

SU s. 14, 49, 70 SEU DE MOTUN 13, 31, 49, 66 animal fat

SU s. 41 elder (Sambucus) [FEW 11,6a]

SUAGER v.a. 11 ASUAGER 61, 67 ESSUAGER 65 to relieve, alleviate

SUFRE, SOUFRE s. 16, 18 sulphur

SUPPRIUR s. 49 sub-prior

SURVENUE s. 11 accidental injury

TAN s. T. DE CHENE 79, 83 tan, crushed bark of the oak [FEW 13,i,82a]

TANESIE s. 28, 61, 67 tansy (Chrysanthemum vulgare) [FEW 13,i,79b]

TENTE s. 31 lint dressing, tent, pledget

TERTEYNE a. FEVRE T. 40, 57 tertian fever

TEYNNE s. 17 TEINE 76 TEYNE 76 TEIGNE 77 ringworm, tinea, disease of the scalp

TIM s. 65 thyme (Thymus serpyllum) [FEW 13,i,317b]

TISANE s. 9 infusion

TORTRE v.a. 78 to wring out

TOUSE s. 4, 5, 6 TOSE 5 TOUCE 74 cough

TREMBLE s. 73 aspen, asp (Populus tremula) [FEW 13,ii,245a]

TRENCHEISUNS s. pl. 30 stomach pains, tormina, colic [FEW 13,ii,280b]

TRIBLER v.a. 5, 15, 25, 28, 29, 33, 39, 54, 65, 76 TRIMBLÉT 8 TRINBLÉT 67 TRINBLE 70 to triturate, pulverize

VENIM s. 65 venom, poison

VERDEGRIS s. 80 VIDEGRÉS 49 verdigris

VERGE s. 24, 25 penis

VETOINE s. 30, 61, 65, 67 betony, bishopwort (Betonica officinalis) [FEW 14,360a]

VIOLE s. 15, 62, 67 violet

VIRGINEMENT adv. 22 in the manner of a virgin

WADE s. 82 woad [FEW 17,471b]

WILDEWOLDE (ME) s. 81 the plant weld (Reseda luteola) [see OED *weld sb.*[1]1]

WOXINGE (ME) s. 52 hiccuping [see OED *yexing*]

YSOPE s. 4 hyssop (Hyssopus officinalis) [FEW 4,528a]

GLOSSARY

to Chapter 8, pp.311–24

ACHE s. 5, 7, 42, 82, 84, 89, 90 MENU A. 24 PETITE A. 24 wild celery, smallage (Apium graveolens) [FEW 1,105a]

AGRIMONIA s. 56 agrimony (Agrimonia eupatoria) [FEW 24,270a]

AGUE s. 9, 10, 28 ague

AIL s. 20, 45 garlic (Allium sativum) [FEW 24,333a]

AISIL s. 4 vinegar

ALESKE s. 20 strip, slice

ALOCHÉ p.p. 6, 88 dislocated, out of joint

ALOCHURE s. 12 dislocation

ALOEN s. 63 aloes [FEW 24,345b]

ALOEN EPATIK s. 36 A. EPATIC 100 aloes [FEW 24,345b & 4,403b]

ALOINE s. 24, 26, 86 wormwood (Artemisia absinthium) [FEW 24,346a]

AMBROSIE s. 24 wood sage, sage-leaved germander (Teucrium scorodonia) [FEW 24,412b]

AMORROIDES s. pl. 25 haemorrhoids, piles

ANGELICA s. 56 angelica (Angelica archangelica) [FEW 24,560b]

ANGOILLE s. 8 eel

APOPLEXIE s. 10 apoplexy, stroke

APOSTUME s. 23, 72 impostume, abscess

ARGENT s. VIF A. 97 quicksilver

ARKANGELICA s. 26 dead nettle (Lamium album)

AVEINE s. 29, 72 oats

AVENCE s. 15, 20, 22, 34, 37, 51, 54, 56, 58, 66, 79 wood avens (Geum urbanum)

BACUNCELE s. 18, 19 an unidentified plant (read *batuncele?*). MS Exeter Cath. 3519 has 'endivia: baccusella, anglice sowethistyle' and a receipt in MS B. L. Arundel 295 (s.xiv in) f.102r has 'cum suco buglosse et bacuncelle' with a marginal note 'nota viticelle' [= bryony]

BERBELE s. 26 pustule

BETONIE s. 23 wood betony (Betonica officinalis) [FEW 1,345b]

BEVEE s. 3 draught, drink

BILRE (ME) s. 25 an aquatic plant, prob. brooklime (Veronica beccabunga), but also applied to the water parsnip (Sium latifolium) and watercress, Lat. berula

BLANC s. B. DE L'OEF 5, 59, 65, 82, 89, 90 white of an egg

BOEL s. 48 bowel, intestine

BOL s. 100 earth, 'bolus Armenicus' (containing iron oxide)? [FEW 1,428b]

BRIONIE s. 4, 25 BRIANIE 12, 29 bryony (Bryonia dioica) [FEW 1,580a]

BROKE-LEMEKE (ME) s. 96 brooklime (Veronica beccabunga)

BUGLE s. 79 bugle (Ajuga reptans) [FEW 1,600a]

BURE DE MAY s. 3, 16, 36 may butter (unsalted)

BURJUN s. 16 (poplar-)bud

BUSARD s. 107 buzzard

CALAMINE s. 36, 49 calamine, zinc ore

CALKETRAPPE s. 20 KALKETRAP 54 caltrops (Centaurea melitensis) or star thistle (Centaurea calcitrapa) [FEW 2,i,65a]

CANCRE s. 15, 19, 23, 60, 98 malignant tumour

CANEVAZ s. 32, 34 canvas

CANVE s. 5, 12, 77 hemp

CELIDOINE s. 17 CELIDONIE 34, 106 greater celandine (Chelidonium majus) [FEW 2,i,634a]

CENTOIRE s. 24 common centaury (Centaurium erythraea) or yellow centaury (Blackstonia perfoliata) [FEW 2,i,583b]

CERFOIL s. 21, 35, 103 chervil (Anthriscus cerefolium) [FEW 2,i,37b]

CERVEISE s. 9, 15, 20, 37, 53, 90 barley beer

CHANELEE s. 17 CHANLEE 25 henbane (Hyoscyamus niger) [FEW 2,i,86a]

CHARDUN s. VERT C. 21 SALVAGE 21 CHAUDUN 53 a thistle

CHAUZ s. 60, 98 lime

CHEEL s. 78 whelp

CHEENE s. 14 oak

CHIKEMETE (ME) s. 24 69, 96, 102 chickweed (Stellaria media)

CHOLET s. 56 cabbage

CINCE s. 65 strip of material, bandage

CINQUEFOLE s. 56 cinquefoil (Potentilla reptans) [FEW 2,ii,1481a]

CIRANTE s. 81 for *ciroine* (ceroneum), wax plaster?

CIRE s. 100 wax C. VIRGINE 41, 52, 66, 81 virgin wax

CLOFYUNKE (ME) s. 15 crowfoot (Ranunculus) or hellebore (Veratrum)

CLUTE s. 89 patch (of cloth)

COLLIRIE s. 36 collyrium, eye salve

COMFIRIE s. 43, 67 CONFIRIE 90 comfrey (Symphytum officinale) [FEW 2,ii,1030a]

CONFECTIUN s. 100 preparation

CONSEUDE MENDRE s. 20, 90 common daisy (Bellis perennis) PETITE C. 22, 43

CONSOLIDE MENDRE s. 15 'consolida minor', common daisy (Bellis perennis) [FEW 2,ii,1076b]

COPEROSE s. 30 C. BLANC 36 copperas

COPERUN s. 21, 66 top, tip (of plant)

COSTIF a. 85 costive, constipated

CREIE s. 59, 67 chalk

CREMEL s. 28 white or yellow pond lily (Nymphaea alba or Nuphar lutea) cf. crumel p.398

CROP s. 46 any part of the plant except the root

CRUDDEN (ME) s. pl. 15 C. DE LEIT 15 curds

CUIZ s. 49 quoit

CUMIN s. 4, 32, 88, 100 cumin (Cumin cyminum) [FEW 2,ii,1526a]

DELIÉ a. 7, 12 fine (of texture)

DENT DE LEON s. 17, 105 dandelion (Taraxacum officinale) [FEW 5,256a]

DESTEMPERURE s. 5 mixture (in solution)

DISSINTERIE s. 67 dysentery

DRASCHE s. 57 solid waste of herbs after removal of juice [FEW 3,156b]

DRAGAGANT s. 100 tragacanth, gum dragon (Astragalus gummifer) [FEW 13,ii,158a]

EDOCKE (ME) s. 28 see *cremel* above

EGRIMOINE s. 85 agrimony (Agrimonia eupatoria) [FEW 24,270a]

EICUTE (ME) s. 107 buzzard

ELENA CAMPANE s. 62 elecampane (Inula helenium)

ELFKECHEL (ME) s. 87 'elf cake', enlargement of the spleen

ELREN (ME) s. 37, 38, 106 elder (Sambucus)

EMPLASTRE s. 26, 32, 37, 59, 69, 72, 88 ENPLASTRE 51 plaster, salve

EMPLASTRER v.a. 26 to apply plaster to

ENCENS s. 34, 36, 59, 81, 100 incense E. FRONC 46 frankincense

ENFESTRÉ p.p. 26 caused to fester

ENTAMER v.a. 48 to damage, injure

ENTRET s. 93 ENTRETE 43 salve, plaster

ERWIGGE (ME) s. 92 earwig

ESCHALE s. 99 nutshell 106 eggshell

ESCHAMEL s. 25, 68, 102 stool

ESCLICE s. 106 spatula

ESCUME s. E. DE BLAUNC MIEL 4 skim

ESPLENTER v.a. 90 to splint

ESPURGE s. 52 spurge (Euphorbia)

ESQUINANCIE s. 23 quinsy

ESTANCHER v.a. 11, 33, 59, 105 to staunch, stop the flow of

ESTIKE s. 5 stick, stalk, stem

ESTRAMER v.a. 12 to scatter

ESTUPER v.a. to stop, plug, block

ESTUPES s. pl. 7 fibres of tow [FEW 12,314b]

ESTUVER v.n. 23, 102 to cook/bathe in steam v. refl. 25 to take a steam bath

EUFRASIE s. 33 eufrasy (Euphrasia officinalis) [FEW 3,249b]

EWE BENEITE s. 94 holy water

EWE ROSE s. 28, 79 rose water

FARINE s. F. DE ORGE 3 barley flour

FAVEROLE s. 25, 29 brooklime (Veronica beccabunga) or water parsnip (Sium angustifolium)

FEBRIFUGIE s. 86 feverfew (Chrysanthemum parthenium)

FEINGRÉ s. 100 fenugreek (Trigonella foenum-graecum) [FEW 3,461b]

FELTRE s. 90 felt

FELUN s. 82, 99, 104 FELON 104 suppurating sore, ulcer, carbuncle

FENOIL s. 23, 24 FENIIL 102 fennel (Foeniculum vulgare) [FEW 3,454a]

FENS s. F. DE OWE 35 goose droppings

FESTRE s. 15, 57 fistula, ulcer

FEVE s. 43 (as a measure), 75, 86 bean

FEVRE s. F. AGUE 28, 106 ague

FI s. F. SENGLANT 3 FICH SENGLANT 77 ulcerated tumour

FICH s. 75 fig-worm

FIEL s. gall F. DE PORC 24 F. DE TOR 93

FIENS s. dung, droppings F. DE COLUMB BLANS U NEIRS 64 F. DE COLUMB 103 F. DE OWE 103

FILIPENDULA s. 13, 39, 40, 56 dropwort (Spiraea filipendula)

FLUR s. 59 flour F. DE SEGLE 5, 86 rye flour

FORMENT s. 4 wheat

FRESE s. 36 strawberry

FUMITERIE s. 85 fumitory (Fumaria officinalis) [FEW 3,857b]

FUND DE PORK s. 51 see note 46

FUNDEMENT s. 25 anus

FUNTAINE s. 28 fontanel

FURMENT s. FLUR DE F. 67, 69, 82, 89, 90 corn flour FARINE DE F. 42

GALINGAL s. 63 galingale, sweet cyperus (Cyperus longus)

GARGARISME s. 63 gargle

GARSER v.a. 84 to scarify

GELINE s. 33 hen

GILOFRE s. 63 cloves (Eugenia caryophyllata) [FEW 2,i,446b]

GLEIRE s. 42 yolk of an egg

GRATE s. 6 grater

GRATER v.a. 6 to grate, crumb

GRESSE s. 4, 83 fat, grease G. DE CHAPUN OU DE GELINE 41 G. DE PORC 16, 21, 24, 25, 71, 73 G. DE OWE 16 G. DE MUTUN 71 G. DE GELINE 52

GRUE s. 61 crane

GUME s. 100 gum G. ARABIC 100 gum arabic

GUPILLERE s. 24 foxglove (Digitalis purpurea)

GUTE s. 20, 53, 54 gout G. ARTATIK(E 58, 96 arthritis G. EIUERE 21 dropsy G. CHAIVE 55 'gutta caduca', epilepsy G. CHAUDE 16

G. CRAMPE 34 stomach cramp G. ENOSSE 20 gout in the bones G. FESTRE 56, 57 fistular swelling G. MAELE 94 leucoma GUTES RUNGESUNS 29

HEDERE TERRESTRE s. 17 ground ivy (Nepeta glechoma) [FEW 13,i,262a]

HEIHOVE (ME) s. 58 HEYHOVE 96 ground ivy (Nepeta glechoma)

HENNEBANE (ME) s. 87, 90, 102 henbane (Hyoscyamus niger)

HERBE BENEITE s. 37, 96, 102 avens (Geum urbanum) or hemlock (Conium maculatum)

HERBE CORRUBLE DORRÉ s. 99 ?

HERBE CRUISEE s. 56 crosswort (Galium cruciata)

HERBE ORIBLE s. 31 'papwort', identity uncertain, possibly Mercurialis annua

HERBE ROBERT s. 56 Herb Robert (Geranium robertianum) [FEW 10,426a]

HERBE SEINTE FIACRE s. 75 cuckoopint (Arum maculatum)

HERBE SEINT JOHAN s. 24 St. John's wort (Hypericum perforatum) [FEW 5,48a]

HERBIVE s. 20, 54, 96 buck's horn plantain (Plantago coronopus)

HILGARS (ME) s. 3 a plant fatal to sheep

HORSSELLE (ME) s. 21 horseheal, elecampane (Inula helenium)

HUNDESTUNGE (ME) s. 8, 17 hound's tongue (Cynoglossum officinale)

JUBARBE s. 26 houseleek (Sempervivum tectorum) [FEW 5,78b]

JUSQUIAMUS s. 17, 23 JUSQUIAMUM 25, 102 henbane (Hyoscyamus niger)

KAK(E)NELE s. 79, 80- membrane (of the brain)

KERSUN s. 90 KERSUNS DE EWE 17, 22 CHERSUNS DE EWE 29 KERSUNS DE FUNTAINE 25 watercress (Rorippa nasturtium-aquaticum)

KIVIL s. 14 peg, piece of wood

KUKUSPITTE (ME) s. 62, 75 cuckoopint (Arum maculatum)

LAIT s. milk L. DE CHIEVRE 3 L. DE VACHE 3, 44, 67, 70, 72

LARD s. 36 fat

LEMEKE (ME) s. 102 brooklime (Veronica beccabunga) or water parsnip (Sium angustifolium)

LEPRE s. 102 leper

LEU s. 78 wolf (med.), skin disease 'lupus'
LEVEINE s. 37 leaven
LEVRER s. 78 greyhound
LIEVRE s. 43 hare
LIMAÇUN s. snail NEIR L. 76 RUGE L. 83
LIN s. 5 flax
LINOIS s. 69, 70, 72 linseed [FEW 5,368b]
LISE s. 78 hound bitch L. MASTIVE 78 mastiff bitch
LUVESCHE s. 24, 32 lovage (Levisticum officinale) [FEW 5,334b]
MADOC (ME) s. 40, 46 maddock, earthworm
MAELE s. 94 leucoma
MALVE s. mallow (Malva sylvestris) or marshmallow (Althaea officinalis) MALVAS 41
    MAWE 52 MALVES DE CURTIL 24
MAMELE s. 22, 71 breast
MANJUE s. 25 scabies, mange
MARIZ s. 1 womb
MAROIL s. 24, 37, 102 MARRUIL 17 black horehound (Marrubium nigrum) or common
    horehound (Marrubium vulgare) [FEW 6,i,377b]
MASTIC s. 4, 34, 36, 46, 59, 79, 100 mastic
MATEFELUN s. 34, 54 knapweed (Centaurea nigra / Centaurea scabiosa / Centaurea iacea)
    [FEW 6,i,519b]
MENTE s. 74 mint
METTELEVE (ME) s. 53 'blanc chardun' (?) [MS chaudun]
MIEL s. 4, 5, 15, 16, 20, 32, 43, 60, 70, 82, 84, 87, 89, 90, MEL 42 honey
MUEL s. 4 MOEL 82 MOEUS 26 yolk of an egg
MOLEINE s. 17, 24, 45, 96 mullein (Verbascum thapsus) [FEW 6,iii,52a]
MORT MAL s. 93 gangrene
MORUN s. 24, 71 chickweed (Stellaria media) or scarlet pimpernel (Anagallis arvensis)
    [FEW 16,570b]
MUSGE s. 100 musk
NEF SALVAGE s. 50 white bryony (Bryonia dioica)
NEPTE s. 24 catmint (Nepeta cataria)
NOLI ME TANGERE s. 21 skin disease of the face
NUGAGE s. 77 walnut, fruit of Juglans regia [FEW 4,36b]
NUTEHECH (ME) s. 14 NUTEHEHT 12 nuthatch (Sitta caesia)
OBLEE s. 75 holy wafer
OILE s. 35, 103 oil O. DE GRANZ NOIZ 92 O. DE OLIVE 34 O. DE OES 66, 98, 99 cosmetic
    paste, see note 51
OINT s. 47, 62, 69, 97 animal fat
OISTRE s. 104 oyster
OK-NISTLE (ME) s. 55 mistletoe (Viscum album)
ORGE s. 3, 70, 87 barley
ORIBLE s. 32 see *herbe orible* above
ORTIE s. nettle O. DE ULTREMER 5 ROGE O. 62 purple deadnettle (Lamium purpureum) O.
    GRIACHE 17, 24, 58 Greek nettle (Urtica pilulifera?) [FEW 4,211a]
OSMUNDE s. 90 royal osmund, flowering fern (Osmunda regalis)
OWE s. 16 35 goose
(PA)PELOTES s. pl. 3 balls, pellets
PAPWRT (ME) s. 31 name applied to a variety of plants, esp. Mercurialis annua
PARELE s. RUGE P. 62 red-veined dock (Rumex sanguineus)
PARLESIE s. 10, 24 paralysis, palsy
PEIVRE s. 21 pepper
PEIZ s. NEIR P. 100 pitch
PELOTE s. 43 77 ball, pellet

PELUSEE s. 24 mouse-ear hawkweed (Hieracium pilosella) [FEW 8,504a]
PENDANTS s. pl. 44, 70 testicles
PENIL s. 1 penis
PERRE s. P. SANGUIN 36 hematite
PERSIL s. 102 P. SAUVAGE 4 common parsley (Petroselinum sativum) [FEW 8,325b]
PIÇ s. 63 pitch
PIERE s. 64 stone (med.)
PIÉ DE PULEIN s. 17, 23, 24 coltsfoot (Tussilago farfara)
PIGLE s. 79 stitchwort or great starwort (Stellaria holostea)
PLANTEINE s. 24, 47, 69, 89 plantain, waybread (Plantago maior) [FEW 9,19b]
PLANTE s. P. DEL PIÉ 80, 104 sole of the foot
POI s. POI REISIN 81 PORESIN 100 pitch resin
POPUILLER s. 16 poplar tree (Populus)
POR s. 89 pig
PORETTE s. 73 P. DE CURTIL 25 leek (Allium porrum)
POTEL s. 16 small pot (measure)
PRIMEROLE s. P. DE HERBER 24 P. DE PRÉ 17, 24 primrose, cowslip (Primula) [FEW 9,379a]
PRUNER s. 24 BLANC P. 17 plum tree (Prunus domestica)
PULEIN s. 14 foal
PULEINÉ p.p. that has recently foaled [FEW 9,542b]
PULMENT s. 67 pottage
QUAREL s. 5 bolt (of crossbow)
QUARTFOILLE s. 14 a four-leaved plant
QUARTER s. 32, 100 one fourth of an ounce in apothecaries' weight; also one fourth of a pound
QUIVRE s. 49 brass
RANCLE s. 12, 71 impostume, abscess, malignant tumour
RECOPEE s. 24 devil's bit scabious (Succisa pratensis)
REGAL s. 62 cuckoopint (Arum maculatum) cf. MS Wellcome Hist. Med. Libr. 544 (s.xiv) p. 272a 'Pernez le regal cru id est cucukesmete'
REI s. LA MALADIE LE R. 51 ?
RESTA BOVIS s. 17 restharrow, cammok (Ononis repens)
ROINE s. 62 RUINE 82, 102 scabies
RUE s. 24, 26 rue (Ruta graveolens) [FEW 10,597a]
RUMPURE s. 43, 44 rupture
RUNCE s. 21, 46, 56, 66 bramble
SAFRAN s. 9, 10 saffron (Crocus sativus) [FEW 19,202a]
SANATIF a. 5 healing, curative
SARCOCOL s. 100 sarcocol, gum sarcocolla produced by plants of genus Astragalus
SAUGE s. 40, 46, 89 sage (Salvia officinalis) S. SALVAGE 56 wood sage (Teucrium scorodonia)
SAUZ s. 17, 24 elder (Sambucus) [FEW 11,6a]
SAVUN s. 98 soap
SAXIFRAGIE s. 24 plant of the genus Saxifraga [FEW 11,259a]
SEGLE s. 5, 86 rye
SEIGNEE s. 11 bleeding
SEIM s. 98, 99 animal fat S. DE PORC 4, 34
SENEÇUN s. 24, 58, 66 groundsel (Senecio vulgaris) [FEW 11,446a]
SENICLE s. 43, 48, 79 wood sanicle (Sanicula europaea), often applied to plants of various genera [FEW 11,183b]
SEU / SIU s. animal fat S. DE BUK 77 S. DE MUTUN 29, 34, 70, 72, 73, 96
SEU s. 106 elder (Sambucus) [FEW 11,6a]
SIEL s. 12, 60, 65, 74 salt
SOLSEQUIE s. 9, 22, 41, 81 marigold (Calendula officinalis) [FEW 12,73a]

SPALET s. 42 for *spelta* 'spelt'
SPARGE s. 66 asparagus (Asparagus officinalis) [FEW 1,156a]
STANCHE s. 90 shepherd's purse (Capsella bursa-pastoris)
SUFRE s. VIF S. 21 sulphur
SUI s. 37, 38 elder (Sambucus)
SUSTANCE s. 38, 91 solid remains of herbs after extraction of juice
TAN s. 70, 89 crushed bark, esp. of oak
TANESIE s. 24 tansy (Chrysanthemum vulgare) [FEW 13,i,79b]
TEINE s. 97 tinea
TENTE s. 5, 7 tent (med.), pledget
TESTE s. 22 nipple, teat
TORTEL s. 60 TURTEL 60 cake
TRET s. 39 salve, plaster
TUELE s. 77, 102 tile
UMBIL s. 1 UMBLIL 76 navel
VALERIENE s. 95 valerian (Valeriana officinalis) [FEW 14,135a]
VERM s. 15, 40, 46, 75, 92 worm
VERVEINE s. 65 vervain (Verbena officinalis) [FEW 14,277a]
VINEGRE s. 16, 20, 25, 88 vinegar
VIOLETTE s. 80 violet (Viola)
WARANCE s. 56, 81 WARONCE 24 madder (Rubia tinctorum) [FEW 17,622b]
WASTEL s. 6 cake
WATERBIL (ME) s. 25 WATERBILRE 25 see *bilre* above
WDEROVE (ME) s. 21 woodruff (Asperula odorata)
WI DE CHEINE s. 55 mistletoe (Viscum album) [FEW 14,523a]
WILDE TASEL (ME) s. 15 teasel (Dipsacus sylvestris)
WIMALVE s. 24 marshmallow (Althaea officinalis) [FEW 4,422b]
WISMINTE (ME) s. 86 error for *wit minte?*
YSACLE s. 44 error for *sanycle?*

GLOSSARY
to Chapter 9, List A, pp.325–30[1]

ACHE s. 2, 3, 6, 12, 15, 24 wild celery, smallage (Apium graveolens) [FEW 1,105a]
AGAPIS* s. 24 agate stone with medicinal properties
AGARIC* s. 15 larch agaric, tree fungus (Polyporus officinalis) [FEW 24,256a] [LSM 28–32]
AISIL s. 1, 5, 9 vinegar
ALAUSTELOGIE LA REONDE / LA LONGE* s. 12 AROSTROLOGIE REONDE 24 EROSTRO-
   LOGIE LONGE 24 birthwort (Aristolochia rotunda and longa) [FEW 1,139b] [LSM 83–86]
ALMONIAC s. 17 gum ammoniac [FEW 24,459a] [LSM 47–52]
ALOINE s. 2, 9 ALUINE 18, 19 wormwood (Artemisia absinthium) [FEW 24,346a]
ALUM s. 10, 21 alum [FEW 24,376b]

---

[1] A = R. Arveiller, 'Textes médicaux français d'environ 1350', *Romania* 94 (1973), 157–77; LSM = *Livre des simples medecines* ed. P. Dorveaux (Paris 1913); R = W. Rothwell, 'Medical and Botanical Terminology from Anglo-Norman Sources', *ZFSL* 86 (1976), 221–60. An asterisk denotes an earlier dating than is offered in the standard dictionaries of Old French and in etymological works.

AMBRE* s. 24 ambergris [FEW 19,7a] [LSM 87–89] [A 164]

AMEOS* s. 12, 24 ammi, bishopsweed (genus Ammi) [FEW 24,457b]

AMOME* s. 24 amomum, spice, various aromatic plants from the Orient (Amomum carda-momum) [FEW 24,463b]

AMONIACON* s. 1 gum ammoniac obtained from desert plant Ferula or Dorema [FEW 24,459a] [R 226]

ANES s. 15 anise (Pimpinella anisum) [FEW 24,599a]

ANET s. 24 ANETE 12 dill (Anethum graveolens) [FEW 24,559a]

ANGUILLE s. 26 eel [FEW 24,567a]

ANIS s. 12, 14 anise, aniseed (Pimpinella anisum) [FEW 24,599a]

APOPONAC* s. 1 opoponax, medicinal gum obtained from the juice of a herb of the genus Opoponax, like Ferula [FEW 7,374b] [LSM 821–28]

APOSTOLICOM CIRURGICOM s. 1 antiseptic ointment originally comprising twelve in-gredients, Apostles' ointment, see note 3 BASTART 2

ARESCES s. 24 garden orache (genus Atriplex) [FEW 1,166b]

ARGENTINE* s. 4 a variety of plants incl. silverweed (Potentilla anserina) [FEW 1,136b 'seit Ende des 16.Jh.']

AROSTROLOGIE REONDE s. 24 see above, Alaustelogie

ARNEMENT s. 21 ARREMENT 10 oak gall [FEW 1,166a inadequate]

ARTETIKE s. 22, 23 gout, arthritis [FEW 1,149b inadequate] [R 244]

ASARA* s. 12 asarabacca, hazelwort (Asarum europaeum) [FEW 1,151b]

AURA s. 15 gold-coloured plant, centaury ? [cf. FEW 1,178b]

AUS s. pl. 10 garlic (Allium sativum) [FEW 24,333a]

AVANCE s. 3, 7 wood avens (Geum urbanum)

AVERONE* s. 19 southernwood (Artemisia abrotanum) [FEW 24,48a]

BALSAMI* s. 24 aromatic oleoresin, balm yielded by shrubs of genus Commiphora [FEW 1,226a]

BASILICON s. 14, 24 basil (Ocimum basilicum) [FEW 1,271a] [A 165]

BASME s. balm (genus Commiphora) FRUIT DE B. 12, 24 FUST DE B. 24 [FEW 1,226a]

BOL* s. 17 (Armenian) bole, a red astringent earth used as a styptic and antidote [LSM 142–46] [A 165]

BOUC s. 24 goat

BOUELS s. pl. 17 bowels

BRAN s. 19 BREN DE F. 18 bran, wheat bran [FEW 1,513b]

BRIOINE s. 24 bryony (Bryonia dioica) [FEW 1,580a inadequate] [R 229]

BRUSC s. 15 butcher's broom, knee holly (Ruscus aculeatus) [FEW 1,575b]

BUGLE s. 2, 3, 7 bugle (Ajuga reptans), sometimes confused with bugloss [FEW 1,600a]

BURE s. B. DE MAI 3 may butter (unsalted and preserved in May for medicinal use) [FEW 1,663a inadequate]

BURNETE s. 14 burnet, variety of medicinal plants (Sanguisorba officinalis / Poterium san-guisorba / Anagallis arvensis) [FEW 15,i,308b]

BUTOR s. 24 bittern

CALAMENT s. 12, 19 the common calamint (Calamintha officinalis) [FEW 2,i,53a]

CAMEDREOS* s. 12 the common or wall germander (Teucrium chamaedrys) [FEW 2,i,620b 14th C.] [LSM 302–10]

CANCRE s. 10, 21 carcinoma, tumour [FEW 2,i,174b] [R 229]

CANELE s. 13, 24, 25 cinnamon (-bark) [FEW 2,i,202a]

CANELLIE s. 5 henbane (Hyoscyamus niger) [FEW 2,i,86a]

CAPARIS* s. 12, 15 caper (Capparis spinosa) [FEW 2,i,284b c.1390] [A 166] [LSM 234–41]

CARDAMOME s. 24, 25 cardamom (Elettaria cardamomum), various species of Amomum and Elettaria [FEW 2,i,364a] [LSM 225–30] [A 166]

CARVI* s. 14, 24 caraway (Carum carvi) [FEW 2,i,377b 1539!] [LSM 311–13]

CASSIALIGNE* s. 12, 13 cassia bark [not in FEW 2,i,462b] [LSM 263–73]

CENTOIRE s. 9, 24 common centaury (Centaurium erythraea) or yellow centaury (Blackstonia perfoliata) [FEW 2,i,583b]

CERISE s. NOIELS DE C. 14 NOIAUS DE C. 15 cherry stones

CHAUS VIVE s. 10 quicklime

CHEVEUS* s. pl. 10 small roots (of garlic) [FEW 2,i,249a Furetière 1690]

CHIERFOIL s. 7 chervil (Anthriscus cerefolium) [FEW 2,i,37b]

CIPERON* s. 12, 14, 24 CEPERON 13 cyperus, galingale (Cyperus longus) [FEW 2,ii,1613b cyperi, hapax 13th C.] [LSM 333–41] [A 168]

CIRE s. 2, 7, 9, 17 CHIRE 1 wax C. VIRGE 2 VIRGE C. 3, 4 virgin wax

CITRE* s. 24 CITRULE 12 pumpkin [FEW 2,i,720a] [R 232] [A 167] see note 15

CLISTERE s. 18, 19, 20 clyster, enema [FEW 2,i,801b]

COE DE PORCEL s. 12 hog's fennel (Peucedanum officinale) [FEW 2,ii,531b 1559 'queue de pourceau']

COLEURE s. 18, 19, 20 strained material [FEW 2,ii,878a] [A167] [R 234]

COLOFONIE* s. 17 colophony, Greek pitch [FEW 2,ii,921b 14th/15th C.] [R 232]

CONCUNGRE* s. 12 cucumber (Cucumis sativus) [FEW 2,ii,1457b]

CONFIRE s. 7 comfrey (Symphytum officinale) [FEW 2,ii,1030a]

CONSOUDE s. 7 consound C. LE PETITE 3 daisy, 'consolida minor' (Bellis perennis) C. MENUE ET GRANT 17 comfrey, 'consolida maior' (Symphytum officinale) [FEW 2,ii,1076b]

CORIANDRE s. 14 coriander (Coriandrum sativum) [FEW 2,ii,1184b]

CORNE s. horn C. DE CHIEVRE 9 C. DE CERF 10, 23

COST s. 12, 24 costmary (Chrysanthemum balsamita) [FEW 2,ii,1254a] sometimes also costus root (root of Saussurea lappa) [LSM 365–70]

CRESSON s. D. D'EWE 6 watercress (Rorippa nasturtium-aquaticum) [FEW 16,384b]

CROC* s. 24 saffron (Crocus sativus) [FEW 2,ii,1357b]

CRUPE s. 15 any part of the medicinal plant except the root; sprig, sprout etc.

CUBEBE s. 24 cubeb, berry of Cubeba officinalis [FEW 2,i,1b] [LSM 284–87]

CUCUBBITE* s. 12 gourd, esp. fruit of Lagenaria vulgaris [FEW 2,ii,1458a, records this form only with a different sense 1460a]

DAUQUE s. 12, 24 carrot (Daucus carota) [FEW -] [LSM 415–22]

DECOCTION s. 1 coction, thorough cooking; 15, 17 decoction, liquid [FEW 3,26a inadequate]

DELLION s. 24 bdellium, sweet gum from trees of the genus Commiphora [LSM 181] [A 165]

DIAUTÉ s. 3 a salve, ointment made from marsh mallow [A 169]

DRAGAGANT* s. 17 D. BLANC 24 the gum tragacanth [FEW 13,ii,158a] [LSM 404–14] [A 168]

EBLE s. 2 dwarf elder, danewort (Sambucus ebulus) [FEW 3,202a]

EGREMOINE s. agrimony (Agrimonia eupatoria) [FEW 24,270a]

EMPLASTRE s. 17 plaster (med.)

ENCENS s. 1, 4, 7, 10, 16, 17 incense BLANC E. 3 [FEW 4,620b] [A 169]

ENTRESUC* s. 2 sap (hapax)

ERE s. 9 ivy (Hedera) [FEW 13,i,262a]

ERINGES* s. 25 sea holly (genus Eryngium)

ERUC s. E. BLANC 12 rocket (Eruca sativa) or white rocket (Hesperis matronalis) [FEW 3,242a] [LSM 493–94]

ESCREVICHE s. 10 crayfish

ESPARDRE v.a. 7 disperse

ESPARGE s. 7, 12 SPARGE 24 SPARARGE 15 asparagus (Asparagus officinalis) [FEW 1,156a]

ESPERMENT s. 10 experiment [FEW 3,309b]

ESPIC s. 12, 14 SPIC 24 spick, spike, aspic (Lavandula spica) giving aromatic oil [FEW 12,174a]

ESPINE s. NEIRE E. 2 blackthorn (Prunus spinosa)

ESQUINANT s. 14 SQUINANT 12, 24 squinant, schoenanth, camel's hay (Andropogon schoenanthus) [FEW 11,299b]

ESTEIM s. 1 ESTAIM 1 pewter

ESTERNUE* s. 24 applied to various plants, probably sneezewort (Achillea ptarmica), sometimes neezewort, white hellebore (Veratrum album) [FEW 12,262b]

ESTUER v.a. 15 to store, reserve

EUFORBE s. 24 euphorbia, spurge, yielding the gum resin euphorbium [FEW 3,249b] [LSM 456–65]

EWE s. E. ROSE 9 rose water

FENOIL s. 9, 12, 14, 15 FENOILE 24 fennel (Foeniculum vulgare) [FEW 3,454a]

FESTRE s. 10 fistula, ulcer [FEW 3,582b]

FIEL s. F. DE BOEF 22 ox gall

FIENTE s. 10 dung, droppings

FISALIDOS* s. 24 dropwort (Spiraea filipendula)

FLOR s. F. D'ARAIM 10 flowers of brass

FRANC ENCENS s. 2, 9 frankincense

FRAZIERE s. 3 FRAZIER 5 strawberry plant (Fragaria vesca) [FEW 3,748b]

FREGON's. 12 butcher's broom (Ruscus aculeatus) [FEW 3,806a]

FREINE s. 27 ash (Fraxinus excelsior) [FEW 3,771b]

FROISSEURE s. 1 fracture

GAIDE s. 8 woad (Isatis tinctoria) [FEW 17,471b]

GALBANON s. 1, 17 galbanum. a gum resin obtained from plants of the genus Ferula [FEW 4,23b]

GALLITRICOM* s. 10 wild clary (Salvia sclarea) [LSM 525–28]

GALINGAL s. 25 GARENGAL 12 GARINGAL 15 galingale (Cyperus longus) [FEW 19,61b] sometimes the rhizome of Alpinia officinarum

GARIOFILAT s. 15 common avens (Geum urbanum) [cf. FEW 2,i,447a–448b] [LSM 515–18] [A 171]

GELINE s. 2, 4 hen

GENOIVRE s. 12, 14 juniper (Juniperus communis) [FEW 5,74b]

GERMENDREE s. 24 common or wall germander (Teucrium chamaedrys) [FEW 2,i,620a]

GILOFRE s. 2, 24, 25 cloves (Eugenia caryophyllata) or clove-scented plant esp. common avens (Geum urbanum) [A 171]

GINGEBRE s. 12, 24 GINGEMBRE 25 ginger [Zingiber officinale] [FEW 14,663b] [A 171]

GLAIOL s. 13, 24 GLAIOS 12 gladden (Iris pseudacorus); or Acorus calamus [FEW 4,143a]

GLAN s. GLANS DE CHENE 16 acorn [FEW 4,147a]

GOUTE s. 22 gout

GRAVELE* s. 24 gravel (med.) [FEW 4,255b]; 24 G. DE VIN BLANC dried wine lees, tartar [FEW 4,255b 1398] [LSM 1116]

GROMIL s. 24 GRUMIL 12, 14, 15 gromwell (Lithospermum officinale) [FEW 2,87a]

HERBE s. H. FOLLE 7 'herba fullonis' (Dipsacus fullonum) ? H. LINAIRE 7 linary, toadflax, (Linaria vulgaris) [FEW 5,369a] H. ROBERT 7 herb Robert (Geranium robertianum) H. WAUTIER 7 sweet woodruff (Asperula odorata) H. YVE 7 yellow bugle ? buck's horn plantain (Plantago coronopus)

IREOS s. 12, 24 (rhizome of) Florentine iris (Iris florentina) [LSM 561–3]

JUBARBE s. 5 houseleek (Sempervivum tectorum) [FEW 5,78b]

LAITUE s. 13 LETTUE 5 lettuce

LANCELEE s. 3 LAUNCELEE 7 ribwort plantain (Plantago lanceolata) [FEW 5,158a]

LANGE s. L. DE OISEL 14 ash key (winged two-celled seed or samara of the ash tree) [FEW 5,362b langue oisel 'semence de frêne'] [LSM 607–9]

LAPIS LAZULI s. 24 lapis lazuli powdered in medicines and used as a colouring agent [LSM 587–94]

LAPIS LINCIS s. 14, 24 stone formed from the urine of the lynx (belemnite) [LSM 309,914]

LECTUAIRE s. 25 electuary

Notes on pp.384–88

LEUSAVON s. 7 see note 9
LICORIZ s. 24 liquorice (Glycyrrhiza glabra) [FEW 14,173b]
LIEVRE s. 17 LEVRE 17 (LIVRE 10) hare
LIMAILLE s. 24 filings [FEW 5,338b]
LION s. 24 lion
LORIER s. FOILLE DE L. 14, 24 bay leaf (Laurus nobilis) [FEW 5,208b]
LOVACHE s. 9, 12 LOVASCHE 24 (Levisticum officinale) [FEW 5,334b]
LUVERCOST s. 12 an error for *lorier, cost* (see note 16)?
MASTIC s. 1, 9, 10, 17, 24 mastic, resin
MAUVE s. 18, 19, 20, 24 mallow (Malva sylvestris), sometimes marshmallow (Althaea offici-
nalis) [FEW 6,i,129a]
MELON s. 12 melon (Cucumis melo) [FEW 6,i,683b]
MENE s. M. DE PORC 4 a flitch or side of bacon [FEW 6,i,579a]
MENTE s. 24 mint
MERCURIALE s. 18, 19, 20 mercurial, mercury; the pot herb allgood (Chenopodium bonus
Henricus) or dog's mercury (Mercurialis perennis) [FEW 6,ii,18a]
MEU* s. 12 meu, meum, spignel (Meum athamanticum) [FEW 6,ii,64b hapax 14th C.] [LSM
710–13]
MIE s. 8 soft part of bread
MIRE s. 13 MIRRE 16 myrrh, gum resin derived from species of Commiphora esp. Commi-
phora myrrha
MIRFOIL s. 7 milfoil, yarrow (Achillea millefolium) [FEW 6,ii,92b]
MORELE s. 5 petty morel, (Solanum nigrum) belladonna, deadly nightshade (Atropa bella-
donna) [FEW 6,i,544a] [LSM 1040–44]
MOUMIE s. 17 mummy, ointment [FEW 19,130b] [LSM 700–04]
MUGUE s. 2, 24 musk [FEW 19,134a]
NITRE s. 10 sodium carbonate, natron, used in medicaments [FEW 7,152b]
NOIS MUSCADE s. 15, 25 nutmeg (Myristica fragrans) [FEW 19,133b] [A 172]
OIGNION s. OIGNONS ROUGES 22 red onions (Allium cepa) O. DE MER* 12 'cepa marina',
squill or sea-onion (Scilla maritima) [FEW 14,44a 1611]
OILE s. O. COMMUNE 19 O. DE FORMENT 26 O. DEL FREINE 27 O. DE MOEUS DES OES 26
O. LAURINE 9 oil of bays O. D'OLIVE 1 O. MUSCELINE 24 oil of musk O. NARDUS 24 oil
of nard A173 O. SANGUINE 24 O. VIOLAT 23
OINT s. 11 fat grease O. DE PORC 5 O. DE CAPON 4 O. DE GELINE 4
OINZEROLE s. 5 'consolida minor' ? orpin ?[2]
ORIGANE s. 14, 19 marjoram (genus Origanum) [FEW 7,414b]
OROBE* s. 12 a variety of leguminous plants of the genus Vicia or Lathryus, esp. mouse pea
(Lathyrus macrorrhizus) or meadow vetchling (Lathyrus pratensis) [FEW 7,419b 1545]
ORMIEL s. 4 elm (Ulmus) [FEW 14,6b]
ORPIMENT s. 10, 21 orpiment, yellow arsenic [FEW 1,182a]
ORTIE s. 2 nettle O. GRIESSE 14 O. GRIESCE 15 'Greek nettle' (Urtica pilulifera? or Lamium
purpureum?) O. DE OUTRE MER 24
OSMONDE s. 3 royal osmund (Osmunda regalis)
PANNAIE s. 13 parsnip (Pastinaca sativa) [FEW 7,752a]

---

[2]   The identity of the plant so designated is difficult to derive from the examples I have found. J.
Camus, 'Un manuscrit namurois du XVe siècle', *Revue des langues romanes* 38 (1895), 196 has 'Oingteruelle – nom de plante, peut-être l'orpin' and quotes a text 'R. une herbe que on apelle oingteruelle, et si
est d'aukun apelee orpine'. In MS London, B. L. Sloane 5 (s.xiv) f.9vb we read 'ointerrele, anglice
selfhele' and in Sloane 420 (s.xiv) f.109rb 'unctuosa gallice uncturol'. See also *Alphita* ed. Mowat, p.193
'unctuosa gallice u . . . relle, anglice selhele vel smerwort'. Selfheal is Prunella vulgaris and the identification is confirmed by Cotgrave. Smearwort is usually used of Chenopodium bonus Henricus. In MS
London, B. L. Royal 12 B III f.9r 'ointerole' appears in a receipt forming part of the *Lettre d'Hippocrate*.
Mondeville, *Chirurgeria* ed. Pagel, p.476 has 'Consolida minor quae vocatur in Francia oniterola'. P.
Meyer, *Romania* 37 (1908), 365 discards *oientereule* as 'mot corrompu'.

PAVAUT s. 13 poppy (Papaver somniferum) [FEW 7,573b]

PERSIL s. 12 PERESIL 14, 24 PERESIN 15 parsley (Petroselinum crispum) [FEW 8,825b]

PERESIL MACEDOINE s. 14 PERESILE MACEDOINE 24 alexanders (Smyrnium olusatrum, 'Petroselinum macedonicum') [FEW 6,i,3a & 8,325b]

PERVENKE s. 3 periwinkle (Vinca maior or minor) [FEW 14,461b]

PETRE s. 24 pellitory (Pyrethrum orientale) [FEW 9,648b] or the English cowslip, Herb Peter (Primula veris) ?

PIÇ s. 13 pitch [FEW 8,620a]

PIERE s. 12, 14, 15, 24 PERE 13 stone (med.), 'calculus', lithiasis [FEW 8,313b inadequate] P. D'ERMENIE 24 Armenian stone, a blue carbonate of copper

PIGLE* s. 3, 7 stitchwort or great starwort (Stellaria holostea) [R 250]

PIGNON* s. 25 pine kernel [FEW 8,521a 1397] [A 174] [LSM 894–95 (pignole)]

PIMPERNELE s. 14 applied to a variety of plants esp. the burnets (Sanguisorba officinalis and Paxterium sanguisorba) and pimpernel (Anagallis arvensis) [FEW 8,517a]

PINCENART s. 15 spikenard (Nardostachys jatamansi) [FEW 12,174b] [A 170]

PIOINE s. 24 peony (Paeonia officinalis) [FEW 7,465a]

PLANTAIN s. 3, 5, 7 plantain, waybread (Plantago maior) [FEW 9,19b]

PLATIN s. 17 plate

POIS s. 9, 17 pitch P. DONT ON ENGLUE NEFS 1 ship pitch, 'pix navalis' P. GREGOIS(E)* 1 colophony, 'pix greca' [FEW 8,620b 1611] NEIR P. 2 black pitch, 'pix nigra', cedar gum [FEW 8,620b 16th C.] P. BLANCHE 4 crude resin, 'pix alba' [FEW 8,620a]

POIVRE s. P. BLANC 14, 24 white pepper P. LONG 24 powder from fruit spikes of Piper longum [FEW 8,553b] P. NEIR 24 black pepper

POLIPODE* s. 11, 12 common polipody (Polypodium vulgare) or oak fern (Thelypteris dryopteris) [FEW 9,139b 15th C.]

POME s. P. DÉ BOS 9 crab apple, wood apple

POPELION s. 5 populeon, ointment made with poplar leaves or buds [FEW 9,182a/b] [R 252]

POPLIER s. 5 poplar (Populus)

PORET s. FOILES DE P. 3 leek (Allium porrum)

PRINCIPAL a. 24 the most important

PULIOL s. 24 pennyroyal (Mentha pulegium) [FEW 9,521a]

QUINTEFOILLE s. 3, 12, 14 cinquefoil (Potentilla reptans) [FEW 2,ii,1481a]

RAMESE (ME) s. 6 ramsons, wild garlic (Allium ursinum)

RANCLE s. 2, 3 impostume, abscess, malignant tumour [FEW 3,151b]

REE DE MIEL s. 11 honeycomb

REISINE s. BLANCHE R. 9 crude resin

RELIEMENT s. 1 binding, bandaging

REUBARBE s. 15, 24 rheubarb (Rheum barbarum) [FEW 10,348a]

REUPONT* s. 24 a type of centaury (Centaurea rhapontica) or, more probably, species of rheubarb (Rheum rhaponticum) [FEW 10,348b] [LSM 988 (reupontic)]

RONCE s. 5 bramble

ROSEL s. 11 reed

RUE s. 19 rue (Ruta graveolens) [FEW 10,597a]

RUMPURE s. 17 fracture

SAFFRAN s. 15 saffron (Crocus sativus) [FEW 19,202a]

SAIM s. 2, 4 animal fat, grease, lard S. D'ANGUILLE 25 S. DE CAPON 9 S. DE CHEVRE 9 S. DE GELINE 2 S. DE MENE DE PORC 4 S. DE PORC 2, 7

SANATIF* a. 7 healing [FEW 11,146a 1354]

SANC DE DRAGON* s. 10, 17 dragon's blood, juice or resin of the dragon tree (Dracaena draco) [FEW 11,171a hapax 13th C.] [LSM 1070] [R 254]

SANEMONDE* s. 16 avens (Geum urbanum) [FEW 11,145b]

SANICLE s. 2, 3 SENICLE 7 wood sanicle (Sanicula europaea), often applied to plants of various genera [FEW 11,183b]

SAUGEME s. 10 SAUGEMME 19 salgem, rock salt [FEW 4,94a]

SAUSEFRAGE s. 12 saxifrage, a variety of plants of the genus Saxifraga, esp. Saxifraga granulata [FEW 11,257b 1270, Picard] see *Saxifrage* below

SAVINE s. 24 savin, savine (Juniperus sabina) [FEW 11,5b]

SAVON s. S. D'OUTRE MER 21 soap

SAXIFRAGE s. 14, 15, 24 member of the genus Saxifraga, esp. Saxifraga granulata [FEW 11,258a]

SCOLOPANDRE* s. 13 scolopendrium, hart's tongue fern (Scolopendrium vulgare) [FEW 11,317a]

SEMELE s. 10 sole (of shoe)

SENÉ s. 15 senna (Cassia officinalis) [FEW 19,153b]

SERAPIRON* s. 1 gum, resin from Ferula persica [FEW 11,669a] [LSM 1051–56 (*sagapin*)]

SEU s. animal fat S. DE CERF 4, 9 SIU DE MOTON 7, 9 [FEW 11,358b]

SILMONIAC s. 17, sal ammoniac (Ammonium chloride) [FEW 11,77a]

SIMARIN VERT s. 3 ? error for 'romarin'?

SINOCASSIA s. 24 for 'xilocassia', cassis bark, see *cassialigne* above

SIRMONTEIN s. 12 SIRMONTAIN 24 sermountain, hartwort (Seseli montanum) [FEW 11,611a]

SOULIER s. 10 shoe

SPARARGE s. 15 ESPARGE 7, 12 SPARGE 24 asparagus (Asparagus officinalis) [FEW 1,156a]

SPATELE* s. 1 spatula [FEW 12,151b 1377]

SPONGE s. PIERE DE S. 13 sponge [FEW 12,207a] [R 238]

SQUINANT s. 12, 24 ESQUINANT 14 squinant, schoenanth, camel's hay (Andropogon schoenanthus) [FEW 11,299b]

SUFFRE s. 21 sulphur

SUIE s. 21 soot [FEW 12,395b]

TAMARIN s. 12 tamarind (Tamarindus indica) [FEW 19,180a] [A 176]

TARTARON s. 10 tartar, acid potassium tartrate, argol [FEW 13,i,126a *tartharum* hapax 13th C.] [LSM 1116–20 (*tartarum*)]

TERBENTINE s. 1 resin extracted from the terebinth (Pistacia terebinthus), turpentine [FEW 13,i,236a]

TITOLOSE s. 12, 24 crow garlic (Colchicum autumnale) [3]

TORMENTINE s. 7 tormentil (Potentilla tormentilla) [FEW 13,ii,44b]

TORTEL s. 1, 8 cake

TREIFOIL* s. 3 any plant of the genus Trifolium [FEW 13,ii,295b 14th C.]

VALERIENE s. 13, 14 WALERIEN 12 valerian (Valeriana officinalis) [FEW 14,135a]

VERDEGRECE s. 10 VERT DE GRECE 21 verdigris [FEW 14,514a]

VETOINE s. 2 VETOGNE 14 betony (Betonica officinalis) [FEW 14,360a]

VIOLET s. 5 VIOLETE 18 violet

WARANCE s. 9 madder (Rubia tinctorum) [FEW 17,622b]

WIMAUVE s. 9 marshmallow (Althaea officinalis) [FEW 4,422b]

ZUCRE s. 6, 15 Z. DE ALISANDRE 24 [FEW 19,161b]

---

[3] See B. von Lindheim, *Das Durhamer Pflanzenglossar lateinisch und altenglisch*, Beiträge zur englischen Philologie 35 (1941; repr. 1967), p.18, no.322 and p.73; P. Bierbaumer, *Der botanische Wortschatz des Altenglischen* 3 (Frankfurt am Main etc. 1979), pp.61f and p.229, MS London. B. L. Sloane 402 f.117r has 'ermodactula vel titulosa, anglice croulek'.

GLOSSARY

to Chapter 9, List B, pp.330–36

ACCEPTOUS a. SIROP S. 2 syrup of vinegar, see note 25

ACHE s. 7, 8, 9, 11, 17, 25 wild celery, smallage (Apium graveolens) [FEW 1,105a]

AGRIPPE s. 13 'unguentum Agrippa', see note 40

AGUSEMEN s. 5 sharpening, fortifying agent

AGUSER v.a. 1, 3 to render tart, pungent, piquant (and hence more active)

ALASCIER v.a./n. 1 LASSIER 1 ALASCHIER 13 to (cause to) evacuate the bowels

ALEMANDE s. 6 almond

ALEMANDELE s. 1 almond [FEW 24,502b]

ALOINE s. 8 wormwood (Artemisia absinthium) [FEW 24,346a]

ALUM s. 27 common or potash alum [FEW 24,376b]

AMEOS s. 17 ammi (Ammi majus L or Ammi visnaga (L.) Lam.) [FEW 24,457b]; also applied to various umbelliferae

AMIDON s. 18 starch [FEW 24,510a]

ANBLIQUE s. 8 emblic myrobalan, fruit of Phyllanthus emblica, see note 34

ANIS s. 7, 20 anise, aniseed (Pimpinella anisum) [FEW 24,599a]

AREIME s. 25 brass

ARGENT s. VIF. A 10, 25, 27 quicksilver

ARGUEL s. 24 argol, tartar of wine, crude potassium bitartrite

ARRAGUN s. 15 'unguentum Arragon', see note 42

ARTETIKE s. 15 gout

ASEIER v.a. 14 to reduce the swelling of, cause to subside

AUNÉ s. 9, 10, 25 elecampane (Inula helenium) [FEW 4,784b]

AVEROYNE s. 11 southernwood (Artemisia abrotanum) [FEW 24,48a]

BELCRIQUE s. 8 belleric myrobalan, fruit of Terminalia bellerica used medicinally

BEN(E)OITE s. 1, 4, 5 'confectio benedicta', see note 21

BLANC s. B. DE PUILLE 27 whiting

BORAGE s. 8 borage (Borago officinalis) [FEW 1,442a]

BOURACE s. 8 borage (Borago officinalis) [FEW 1,442a]

BRU s. 7 butcher's broom (Ruscus aculeatus) [FEW 1,557b]

BRUET s. 1 broth, soup

BURE s. 22 butter

CALAMENT s. 11, 17 common calamint (Calamintha officinalis) [FEW 2,i,53a]

CANELE s. 17, 22 cinnamon (bark) [FEW 2,i,202a]

CAPON s. 26 capon

CARTATIQUE s. C. EMPERIAL 3, 4, 5 'katharticum imperiale', see note 29

CARDAMOME s. 22 cardamom (Elettaria cardamomum), various species of Amomum and Elettaria [FEW 2,i,364a]

CASSIAFISTULA s. 8 purging cassia, seeds embedded in a laxative pulp used in electuary of senna [FEW 2,i,462b]

CAUDEL s. 6 caudle

CHAMBRE s. ALER A C. v.n. 1, 2 to relieve oneself by evacuating the bowels

CHASTAIGNE s. 18 chestnut (Castanea vesca) [FEW 2,i,463a]

CHAUCHE s. 22 hose, stocking (as strainer)

CHAUVER v.a. 1 to heat

CIPERON s. 11, 22 sweet cyperus, English galingale (Cyperus longus), also Indian species (Cyperus rotundus) [FEW 2,ii,1613b]

CIRE s. 21, 25 wax

CITRIN s. 18 citrul, pumpkin gourd (Cucurbita pepo), perhaps also colocynth (Citrullus colocynthis), see note 15 and FEW 2,i,721a

CLARÉ s. 22 spiced wine sweetened with honey

COLER v.a. 22, 25 to strain, filter

COL(E)RE s. 2, 5 choler, bile

COLOFOINE s. 21 colophony, Greek pitch [FEW 2,ii,921b]

COMIN s. 1 cumin (Cuminum cyminum) [FEW 2,ii,1526a]

COMINEE s. 6 cumin-flavoured stew

CONCONGRE s. 18 cucumber (Cucumis sativus) [FEW 2,ii,1457b]

CONDUIZ s. pl. 6 passages (med.)

CONFIRE v.a. 17, 18, 23 to prepare, concoct

CONSOUDE s. LA PETITE C. 25 'consolida minor', daisy (Bellis perennis) [FEW 2,ii,1076b]

COORDE s. 18 dry fruit or gourd of Cucurbita maxima; also Lagenaria vulgaris – bottle gourd, calabash [FEW 2,ii,1458a]

COUPERON s. 9 top, tip, cutting (of plant)

COVREFEU s. 1 curfew

CRESSON s. 11 (water)cress (Nasturtium officinale) [FEW 16,384b]

CRUPE s. 1, 3 sprig, any part of the plant except the root

DECOCTION s. 6 liquid, decoction

DEGASTER v.a. 10, 21 to use up, consume

DERTRE s. 9, 24 tetter, eczema, herpes [FEW 3,46a]

DIACALAMENT s. 17 drug using calamint, see note 44

DIADRAGANT s. 18 drug using gum tragacanth, see note 45

DIAMORON s. 23 drug using mulberries or similar, see note 50

DIAPENDIDION s. 19 drug using barley sugar, see note 47

DIAUTÉ s. 16, 21 drug using marshmallow, see note 43

DIETE s. 6 diet

DIETER v.a. 1, 6 to put on a diet

DIURETIC a. 7 diuretic, promoting urination

DRAGANT s. D. BLANC 18 gum tragacanth, gum-dragon

DRAGIE s. D. DE PARIS 20 a sweetmeat, a sweet medicinal preparation (often a powder) for the stomach [FEW 13,ii,158b]

EMFLEURE s. 14 ENFLEURE 13 swelling

EMPLASTRE s. 16 plaster (med.)

ENCORPORER v.a. 8 to incorporate

ENTECHIER v.a. 8 to afflict, taint

EPITIMES s. 8 common dodder (Cuscuta epithymum)

ESCAILLE s. 15 (egg)shell

ESCAMONIE s. 1, 3, 5 gum derived from scammony (Convolvulus scammonia), [FEW 11,276a]

ESCARDE s. 1 scale (of fish)

ESCHINE s. 15 backbone

ESCORCE s. E. DE LA POUME 1 apple peel

ESPECETÉ s. 1 thick consistency

ESPIC s. 22 spick, spike, aspic (Lavandula spica) giving aromatic oil, sometimes standing for 'spica nardi', spikenard (Nardostachys Jatamansi) [FEW 12,174b]

ESPLEN s. 14 spleen

ESQUIELE s. 24 bowl, dish

ESQUINANT s. 22 squinant, schoenanth, camel's hay (Andropogon schoenanthus) giving lemongrass oil [FEW 11,299b]

ESREIEMENT s. 19 hoarseness

ESTEIM s. 24 tin, pewter

ESTUER v.a. 7, 8, 23 to store, reserve, set aside

ESTUVE s. 9, 11 herbal or steam bath

ESULE s. 1, 3 ESULA 1 ESLE 5 applied to almost any plant of the genus spurge, not especially leafy spurge (Euphorbia esula)

FENOIL s. 7, 8, 9, 11, 20 fennel (Foeniculum vulgare) [FEW 3,454a]
FEVRE s. 15 F. AGUE 6, 12 acute fever
FEVERUS a. 3 feverish
FIMETERRE s. 8 fumitory (Fumaria officinalis) [FEW 3,857b]
FINEGREC s. 21 fenugreek (Trigonella foenum-graecum) [FEW 3,461b]
FLAUNS s. pl. 15 flanks, thighs
FLEUME s. 1, 5 phlegm
FOLION s. 22 aromatic leaf resembling cinnamon or nard, the 'malabathrum' of Dioscorides
FRANC ENCENS s. 27 frankincense
FREIDEURE s. 14, 15, 17 chill, cold
FREINE s. 24 ash (Fraxinus excelsior)
GALBANUM s. 21 galbanum, gum resin derived from various species of Ferula, esp. Ferula
     galbaniflua [FEW 4,23b]
GALINGAL s. 22 china root, galangal, the rhizome of Alpinia officinarum
GELINE s. 1, 6 hen
GENOIVRE s. 11 juniper (Juniperus communis) [FEW 5,74b]
GERAPIGRE s. 1, 4 the purgative 'hiera pigra' containing aloes, see note 22
GILOFRE s. 20, 22 cloves (Eugenia caryophyllata) [FEW 2,i,446b]
GINGEMBRE s. 17, 20, 22 GINGEBRE 8 ginger (Zingiber officinale) [FEW 14,663b]
GLUTEMENT adv. 1 greedily
GOME s. G. ARABIC BLANC 18 gum arabic G. DE ERE 21 gum ivy
GOUTE s. 14, 15, gout G. ROSE 27 gutta rosacea (pustules)
GOUTE s. 23 drop
GROIN DE PORC s. 6 pig's snout
GRUEL s. 6 broth
HIEVELE s. 9 dward elder, danewort (Sambucus ebulus) [FEW 3,202a]
IRRE DES ARBRES s. 9 common ivy (Hedera helix) [FEW 13,i,262a]
JEUNER v.n. 1 to fast, go without food
JUBARBE s. 6 houseleek (Sempervivum tectorum) [FEW 5,78b]
KENILLIE s. 6 henbane (Hyoscyamus niger) [FEW 2,i,86a]
LAITUAIRE s. 1, 4 LECTUAIRE 17, 18, 19 electuary
LAITUE s. 6 lettuce
LAUNCELÉ s. 25 ribwort plantain (Plantago lanceolata) [FEW 5,158a]
LICUR s. 24 liquid
LIN s. 21 flax
LOINES s. pl. 14 LOIGNES 15 loins
LORIER s. 11 bay (Laurus nobilis) [FEW 5,208b]
LOVASCHE s. 25 lovage (Levisticum officinale) [FEW 5,334b]
LUVETTE s. 23 uvula
LUZ s. 1 pike
MACIS s. 20 mace, outer covering of nutmeg (Myristica fragrans) [FEW 6,12a]
MAIMUINE s. 22 ? an error for mumie 'mummy', a medicinal gum
MANJUE s. 24 mange, scabies
MARCIATON s. 14 a green ointment, see note 41
MASCHER v.a. 1 to chew
MAUVE s. 1, (marsh)mallow (Althaea officinalis) [FEW 6,i,129a]
MANNE s. 8 manna
MEL s. 6 MIEL 17, 22, 23 honey
MELONE s. 18 melon (Cucumis melo) [FEW 6,i,683b]
MENUISE s. 1 sprat, small fish, sometimes applied to plaice and gudgeon [FEW 6,ii,130a]
MERCURIALE s. 1 applied as 'English Mercury' to Chenopodium bonus Henricus and as
     'Dog's Mercury' to Mercurialis perennis and as 'Annual Mercury' to Mercurialis annua
     [FEW 6,ii,18a]

Notes on pp.384–88

MESELERIE s. 8 leprosy

MIE s. 1 loaf of bread, the soft part of a loaf

MIRABOLAN s. the fruit of various species of Terminalia [FEW 6,iii,315b] M. CITRIN 8 Terminalia citrina M. QIEBLE 8 Terminalia chebula M. INDE 8 fruit of Terminalia gathered before completely ripe, see note 34

MOELE s. 7 pith, medulla (of plant)

MOINE s. M. MEDICINE 2, 3 medium (-strength) medicine

MORELE s. petty morel, belladonna (Solanum nigrum, Atropa belladonna) [FEW 6,i,544a]

MORT MAL s. 9 mormal, gangrene ? disease of the skin ? see note 37

MOURE s. 23 mulberry (Morus nigra) [FEW 6,iii,152b]

NERS s. pl. 13, 16 nerves

NETTIER v.a. 8 to cleanse, clean

NIFLE s. 7 medlar [FEW 6,ii,45b]

NIULE s. 1, 6 light cake, wafer [FEW 7,70a]

OIGNE[ME]NS s. pl. 12 ointments

OIGNION DE MER s. 21 squill (Urginea scilla) [FEW 14,44a]

OINT s. 27 animal fat O. DE PORC 10, 25 lard

OLIVE s. 27 olive

ORGE s. PAIN D'ORGE 1 barley bread

ORIGANE s. 11 sweet marjoram (Origanum vulgare) or wild thyme (Thymus serpyllum) [FEW 7,414b]

ORTIE s. ROUGE O. 25 purple dead-nettle (Lamium purpureum) [FEW 14,68a]

OXIMEL s. 1, 7 preparation of herbs, vinegar and honey; oxymel

PALAIS s. 23 palate

PARALISIE s. 14 paralysis

PARELE s. ROUGE P. 25 red-veined dock (Rumex sanguineus) PARELLE D'EWE 25 red- or water-dock (Rumex aquatica)

PAULIN s. 1 'paulinum', see note 20

PESCHER v.n. 5 to conflict, be opposed

PEIVRE s. P. NEIR 17, 22 black pepper P. LONG 17, 22 powder from fruit spikes of Piper longum [FEW 8,553b]

PENIDES s. 18, 19 barley sugar [FEW 8,188b]

PERCHE s. 1, 6 perch [FEW 8,216a]

PERESIL s. 7, 9, 11, 17 persil (Petroselinum crispum) [FEW 8,325b]

PESANTUME s. 12 heaviness

PIECETE s. 10, 20 small piece

PILE s. 1 pill

PIRETRON s. 22 pellitory (Anacyclus pyrethrum) [FEW 9,648b]

PISSER v.n. 13 to urinate

PLANTAINE s. 6 plantain, waybread (Plantago major) [FEW 9,19b]

PLUM s. 27 lead

POIRE s. 6 pear

POIZ RESINE s. 21 pitch resin

POLIPODE s. 1, 7, 8 common polypody (Polypodium vulgare) [FEW 9,139b]

PO(U)ME s. 1, 6 apple

POPULEON s. 6 POPELION 12 ointment made with the leaves or buds of the poplar

POREE s. 1 thick soup

PORGIER v.a. 4 to purge

POSCENET s. 25 cooking pot, vessel

POUS s. 6 pulse

PRESSONS DEL VENTRE s. pl. 1 tormina

PRIENDRE v.a. 21 to press out (juice)

PRUNE s. 6, 8 plum

PURCELEINE s. 6 golden purslane (Portulaca sativa) or garden purslane (Portulaca oleracea)
[FEW 9,226b]
PUSCETTE s. 24 vessel, container [FEW 9,628a]
QUARTAINE s. 15 quartan fever
QUILLIERÉ s. 6 spoonful
RAER v.a. 7 to shave
RELENTIR v.n. 24 to become viscous [FEW 5,253b]
RENCHAIR v.n. 6 to relapse
REQUIRE v.a. 7 to cook again
RESUER v.n. to sweat again
RETRAIT a. 13 strained (of nerves)
RICOLICE s. 8, 20 liquorice (Glycyrrhiza glabra) [FEW 4,173b]
ROCHE s. 1 roach
ROINE s. 8, 9 ROIGNE 24 scabies
ROISIN s. 8 grape
ROSAT a. SIROP R. 2, 6 syrup of roses OILLE R. 12 oil of roses
ROSE s. 6, 8 rose
RUE s. rue (Ruta graveolens) [FEW 10,597a]
RUNCE s. 26 bramble
SAC s. 21 bag, sachet
SANS s. 1 blood
SAUF s. METRE EN S. 8 to reserve, store, set aside
SAUGE SAVAGE s. 8, 11 sage-leaved germander (Teucrium scorodonia) [FEW 11,132b]
SAUGEME s. 6 rock salt; sodium chloride [FEW 11,77a]
SAUSEFLEUME s. 5, 24 saucefleme, 'salt phlegm' [FEW 11,108b]
SAVINE s. 11 savine (Juniperus sabina) [FEW 11,5b]
SCABIE s. 24 scabies
SEL s. 6 salt
SENESCHON s. 25 groundsel (Senecio vulgaris) [FEW 11,446a]
SEUS s. 9 elder (Sambucus)
SER(R)É a. 1, 6 constipated
SIRMONTAIN s. 17 sermountain (Laserpitium siler / Seseli montanum) [FEW 11,612b]
SIROP(E) s. 2, 8 syrup CIROP 18
SOLUBLE a. 1 laxative 2, 6 free from constipation
SOU s. 18 solidus
SOUFRE s. 25 sulphur
SPARAGE s. 7 asparagus (Asparagus officinalis) [FEW 1,156a]
SUER v.n. 12 to sweat
SUPPOSITURE s. 6 suppository
TENDRON s. 26 shoot (of plant)
TEMPRER v.a. 7 v.n. 10 to steep, soak
TERBENTINE s. 21 turpentine, resin extracted from the terebinth (Pistacia terebinthus)
[FEW 13,i,236a]
TESCH s. 24 macula (in the skin)
THAMARINDE s. 8 tamarind (Tamarindus indica) [FEW 19,180a]
TIEGNE DE LIN s. 8 for tim de lin? flax dodder (Cuscuta epilinum)
TIEULE s. 1 tile
TIM s. 17 thyme (Thymus vulgaris / serpyllum) [FEW 13,i,317b]
TISANE s. 6 infusion
TOUSSE s. 18, 19 TOUZ 17 cough
TRIFE ZARAZINE s. 2, 4 'Tryphera sarracenica', see note 27
VEIR s. 24 glass
VERMINE s. 25 parasitic, infestive insects [FEW 14,292b]
VIN EGRE s. 1, 6, 7 vinegar

Notes on pp.384–88

VIOLAT a. SIROP V. 2, 6 syrup of violets OILLE V. 12 oil of violets
VIOLE s. 24 phial
VIOLETTE s. 6, 8 violet
WIMAUVE s. 21, 25 marshmallow (Althaea officinalis) [FEW 4,422b]
YDROPISIE s. 11, 13 dropsy
ZUCRE s. 18 sugar

Index